Clinical Pharmacology for Anaesthetists

Commissioning Editor: Maria Khan
Project Manager: Emily Pillars
Typeset by J&L Composition Ltd, Filey, North Yorkshire
Printed in Hong Kong

Clinical Pharmacology for Anaesthetists

James G Bovill MD, PhD, FFARCSI
Professor of Anaesthesiology, University Hospital Leiden
Leiden, The Netherlands

Michael B Howie MD, MA, FFARCSI
Professor and Vice Chairperson, Ohio State University Medical Center
Columbus, Ohio, USA

W. B. SAUNDERS

London • Edinburgh • New York • Philadelphia • Sydney • Toronto

WB Saunders
An imprint of Harcourt Publishers

First published 1999

ISBN 0–7020–2167–9

British Library Cataloguing in Publication Data
A catalogue record for this book is available from the British Library

Library of Congress Cataloging in Publication Data
A catalog record for this book is available from the Library of Congress

Note
Medical knowledge is constantly changing. As new information becomes available, changes in treatment, procedures, equipment and the use of drugs become necessary. The editors/authors/ contributors and the publishers have, as far as it is possible, taken care to ensure that the information given in this text is accurate and up-to-date. However, readers are strongly advised to confirm that the information, especially with regard to drug usage, complies with the latest legislation and standards of practice

The
Publisher's
policy is to use
**paper manufactured
from sustainable forests**

CONTENTS

CONTENTS

FOREWORD

The spectrum of anaesthesiology is rapidly expanding. In fact, in many areas of the world anaesthesiology is becoming recognised as the specialty of perioperative medicine. Increasingly complex surgical procedures are becoming more commonly performed on an ambulatory basis. In the US, more than 60% of surgery is now performed on an outpatient basis, with predictions that 20% of surgery will soon be performed in the isolated environment of the surgeon's office. Intravenous and inhalational anaesthetic agents are becoming shorter acting and more controllable. The capability to determine real-time plasma concentrations of intravenous agents is just around the corner and the ability to determine CNS effects of many anaesthetic drugs has arrived.

While the landscape of anaesthesiology has changed dramatically, other fields of medicine have not sat idly by. Indeed, advances in other specialties of medicine have been staggering. It is a daunting challenge for anaesthesiologists to remain current with the burgeoning developments in fields such as immunology, oncology, gastroenterology, haematology and infectious disease and the accompanying evolution in pharmacotherapy. Nevertheless, the new drugs taken by surgical patients and the increasingly remote environment where anaesthesia is delivered make such an understanding critical.

In *Clinical Pharmacology for Anaesthetists*, Professors Bovill and Howie offer the anaesthesia community a solution to this challenge. In one comprehensive volume, the editors have assembled an all-star cast of contributors from around the world. Although a substantial portion of contributors maintain anaesthesiology as their specialty, many others emanate from the fields of internal medicine, rheumatology, infectious disease, neurology, immunology and nephrology.

The text begins logically with a review of the principles of drug action at the cellular level and then expands to universal issues of pharmacokinetics and pharmacodynamics. Not surprisingly, the volume focuses on drugs that anaesthesiologists use on a daily basis, including inhalational and intravenous anaesthetics, muscle relaxants and local anaesthetic agents. However, what separates this work from others is the substantial emphasis placed on new developments in clinical pharmacology in related areas of medicine. A wide variety of rapidly advancing fields ranging from immunosuppression to dyspepsia are addressed. Drugs as divergent as antihypertensives, anticoagulants, antihistamines, and antineoplastic agents are discussed in detail with relevant applications to the practice of anaesthesiology. Even modifications in drug therapy for special patient populations, such as the elderly or pregnant patient, have not been forgotten.

This text is intended for the anaesthesiology practitioner the world over. In fact, a clever, concise table early in the text compares nomenclature for drugs in the UK vs. the US. Whether preparing for Board or other postgraduate examinations or simply attempting to maintain a state-of-the-art practice of anaesthesiology in the medical world of the new millennium, this broad-reaching, comprehensive text will prove to be of valuable assistance.

Charles H McLeskey, MD
Professor and Chair, Department of Anesthesiology
Medical Director, Perioperative Services
Scott & White Memorial Hospital & Clinic
Texas A&M University Health Science Centre
Temple, Texas

PREFACE

> There once was a Doctor,
> (No foe to the Proctor,)
> A physic concoctor,
> Whose dose was so pat,
> However it acted,
> One speech it extracted,-
> "Yes, yes", said the Doctor,
> "I meant it for that"!
>
> From *The Doctor*, by Thomas Hood (1799–1845)

The above poem epitomises, albeit in a humorous and tongue-in cheek manner, the shortcomings of pharmacology as practised by physicians in the early 19th century. In those days, and indeed until the first half of the present century, the pharmacological approach to therapy was to a large extent empirical, with little knowledge of how drugs produced their effects. This has changed dramatically in the past decades. Today we have available a wide spectrum of drugs, and knowledge about how they work at cellular and sub-cellular levels has increased by leaps and bounds. Anaesthetists have made a considerable contribution to these advances, and this is not surprising.

In anaesthesia, more than perhaps in any other speciality, drugs that are often extremely potent and potentially very toxic are administered acutely. Some drugs, e.g. some opioids such as sufentanil, are active at plasma concentrations below 1 ng ml^{-1}. It is therefore appropriate that anaesthetists are required to have an in-depth knowledge of pharmacology. And this knowledge needs to extend beyond those drugs used specifically, and often exclusively, during anaesthesia. Other drugs not directly related to anaesthesia, e.g. antibiotics, may also be given during surgery. In addition, many patients will be taking drugs related to their surgical or medical condition before surgery. In some cases these can have important consequences for the conduct of anaesthesia. Anaesthetists are also increasingly involved clinically outside the operating theatre, e.g. in intensive care units, pain clinics or as perioperative physicians. In these situations they also are concerned with non-anaesthetic drugs. Thus while the emphasis in this book is on the pharmacology of those drugs directly related to anaesthetic practise others, such as antibiotics, drugs used in psychiatric disorders and epilepsy, and those used in the treatment of cancer and immune disorders are also included. Many of these agents can have significant toxic effects on vital organ systems, which limit their clinical benefits but also have consequences for patients being treated with these drugs who present for anaesthesia and surgery. Some, such as immunosuppressive agents and anticancer agents, which are not usually covered in conventional anaesthetic pharmacology textbooks, can have significant interactions with anaesthetic drugs and muscle relaxants. Bleomycin, an antibiotic used as an antineoplastic agent, will have a direct impact on the conduct of anaesthesia because of the need to restrict the concentration of inspired oxygen in patients taking this durg. Accordingly it is important that anaesthetists have a good understanding of their actions, interactions and toxic effects.

This book was planned as a comprehensive, clinically orientated textbook intermediate in scope between an undergraduate text and an authoritative pharmacological reference work. The aim was to produce a book that would be valuable both to students preparing for a postgraduate examination in anaesthesia and to existing specialists who want to keep abreast of developments in pharmacology related to anaesthesia. We have tried to produce a text that will allow our readers to easily grasp the key points and issues in pharmacology. Summaries of the salient points of each chapter are reproduced in summary boxes; we hope that this feature will prove useful especially for those revising for examinations.

Pharmacology is a rapidly changing discipline, with new drugs continually becoming available and additional uses being found for existing drugs. Enormous advances also have been made in unravelling of the mechanisms involved in drug actions. The first chapter covers the current concepts of the mechanisms of action of anaesthetic drugs, and descriptions of relevant cellular mechanisms have also been incorporated in the text of other chapters. Although this is a pharmacology textbook, an appreciation of physiology and pathology are important for a full understanding of modern pharmacological concepts. Emphasis has therefore been placed on how changes in physiology and pathology impact on drug actions.

As editors we are indebted to the authors of individual chapters and we express our appreciation of their valuable contributions to this textbook. We also gratefully acknowledge the editorial support and encouragement of the publishers, W.B. Saunders, and in particular Maria Khan, Linda Clark, Louise Cook and Emily Pillars.

James G Bovill
Michael B Howie

DEDICATION

In memory of my father, whose foresight helped me on to the first rung of an academic career.

James G Bovill

To my wife Olga who, like my Mother, Anne Britchford Howie, and my Uncle Edward, showed me that human beings can be gracious, generous and honourable.

Michael B Howie

CONTRIBUTORS LIST

Dr PCM van den Berg
Department of Anaesthesiology
Leiden University Medical Centre
PO Box 9600
2300 RC Leiden
The Netherlands

Professor RJM ten Berge
Renal Trans Unit & Clin and Lab
Immunology Unit
Department of Internal Medicine
Academical Medical Centre
University of Amsterdam
Meibergdreef 9
Amsterdam 1105 AZ
The Netherlands

Dr NC Bhaskaran
Department of Anaesthetics
Royal Hallamshire Hospital
C Floor OPD
Glossop Road
Sheffield S10 2JF

Dr WP Blunnie
Department of Anaesthesia & Intensive Care
Mater Misericordiae Hospital
Eccles Street
Dublin Ireland 7

Professor JG Bovill
Department of Anaesthesiology
Leiden University Medical Centre
PO Box 9600
2300 RC Leiden
The Netherlands

Dr P Bowen
Assistant Professor of Anaesthesiology
Emory University School of Medicine
Department of Anesthesiology

Grady Memorial Hospital
Box 26074, 80 Butler Street
Atlanta GA 30335 USA

Dr PJ van den Broek
Department of Infectious Diseases
Leiden University Medical Centre
Building 1, C5-P
Rijnsburgerweg 10
Postbus 9600
Leiden 2300 RC
The Netherlands

Professor AGL Burm
Department of Anaesthesiology
Leiden University Medical Centre
PO Box 9600
Leiden 2300 RC
The Netherlands

Dr FL Christofi
Department of Anesthesiology
Ohio State University Medical Center
N416 Doan Hall
410 W 10th Avenue
Columbus OH 43210 USA

Dr DP Desiderio
Department of Anesthesiology
Memorial Sloan-Kettering Cancer Center
1275 York Avenue
New York NY 10021
USA

Dr P Dorinsky
Department of Anesthesiology
The Ohio State University Medical Center
Columbus, Ohio 43210-1228
USA

Dr FHM Engbers
Department of Anaesthesiology
Leiden University Medical Centre
PO Box 9600
23 RC Leiden
The Netherlands

Dr med C Frenkel
Klinik & Poloklinik für Anäesthesiologie
Rheinische Friedrich-Wilhelms Universität Bonn
& Spezielle Intensivmedizin
Sigmund Freud Strasse 25
Bonn D-53105 Germany

Dr MA Gerhardt
Department of Anesthesiology
The Ohio State University Medical Center
Columbus
Ohio 43210–1228
USA

Dr RL Harter
Department of Anesthesiology
Ohio State University Medical Center
N416 Doan Hall
Columbus OH 43210
USA

Professor A Hoeft
Klinik und Poliklinik fur Anasth und
spezielle
Institut für Anäesthesiologie der
Universität
Sigmund-Freud Strasse 25
Bonn D-2300 Germany

Professor MB Howie
Professor and Vice Chairperson
Department of Anesthesiology
Ohio State University Medical Center
410 West 10th Avenue
Columbus OH 43210–1228
USA

Professor MFM James
Head: Department of Anaesthesia
Faculty of Health Sciences
Observatory
Cape Town
South Africa 7925

Professor RM Jones
Professor of Anaesthetics
St Mary's Hospital
Academic Department of Anaesthetics
London W2 1NY
United Kingdom

Dr ZP Khan
St Mary's Hospital
Imperial College of Science and Technology
Medical School
Norfolk Place
London W2 1PG
United Kingdom

Professor Dr JW van Kleef
Chairman
Department of Anaesthesiology
Leiden University Medical Centre
PO Box 9600
Leiden 2300 RC
The Netherlands

Dr RD Latimer
Department of Cardiothoracic Anaesthesia
Papworth Hospital NHS Trust
Papworth Everard
Cambridge CB3 8RE
United Kingdom

Professor J Marty
Hôpital Beaujon
Service d'anesthèsie-réanimation
100 bd du Gal-Leclerc
Clichy 92118 CEDEX
France

Dr H Mattie
Department of Infectious Diseases
Leiden University Medical Centre
Building 1, C5-P
Rijnsburgerweg 10
Postbus 9600
Leiden 2300 RC
The Netherlands

Professor C Meistelman
Department d'Anesthesie-Reanimation
Hôpital de Brabois
rue du Morvan
Vandoeuvre France 54511 CEDEX

Dr QJW Milner
Department of Cardiothoracic Anaesthesia
Papworth Hospital NHS Trust
Papworth Everard
Cambridge CB3 8RE
United Kingdom

Professor LH Opie
Department of Medicine
University of Cape Town
Medical School
Observatory
Cape Town
South Africa 7925

Dr PS Pagel
Department of Anesthesiology
Medical College of Wisconsin
MEB-462C
8701 Watertown Plank Road
Milwaukee WI 53226
USA

Dr JE Peacock
Department of Anaesthetics
Royal Hallamshire Hospital
C Floor OPD
Glossop Road
Sheffield S10 2JF

Dr M Pfaffendorf
Department of Pharmacotherapy
Academical Medical Cente, University of Amsterdam
Meibergdreef 15
Amsterdam 1105 AZ
The Netherlands

Dr B Plaud
Department d'Anesthesie-Reanim
Hôpital de Brabois
chez Professor Meistelman
rue du Morvan
Vandoeuvre
54511 CEDEX France

Dr A Reeves
Department of Neurology
The Ohio State University
University Medical Center
410 West 10th Avenue
Columbus OH 43210–1228
USA

Dr D Royston
Consultant in Cardiothoracic Anaesthesia
Harefield Hospital
Harefield Middlesex UB9 6JH
United Kingdom

Professor E Samain
Service d'anesthèsie-réanimation

Hôpital Beaujon
100 bd du Gal-Leclerc
Clichy 92118 CEDEX
France

Dr PThA Schellekens
Department of Internal Medicine
Academical Medical Centre, University of Amsterdam
Clinical and Laboratory Immunology Unit
Meibergdreef 9
Amsterdam 1105 AZ The Netherlands

Dr AW Schuster
Clinical Assistant Professor of Medicine
The Ohio State University
N-416 Doan Hall 410 West 10th Avenue
Columbus Ohio 43210
USA

Dr AJ Scurr
Department of Anaesthetics
Newham General Hospital
Glen Road
Plaistow
London E13 8SL
United Kingdom

Professor PS Sebel
Department of Anesthesiology
Grady Health System
80 Butler Street, SE
Atlanta, GA 30335–3801 USA

Professor RN Sladen
Professor & Vice Chair
Department of Anesthesiology; PH. 527
Cardiothoracic Surgical ICU
Columbia-Presyterian Medical Center
630 West 168th St
New York NY 10032
USA

Dr AJ Souter
Department of Anaesthesia
Royal United Hospital
Bath BA1 3PQ
United Kingdom

Dr JG van der Stroom
Department of Anaesthesia
Academical Medical Centre, University of Amsterdam
Meibergdreef 9
Amsterdam 1105 AZ
The Netherlands

S Surachno
Dept of Internal Medicine
Clinical and Laboratory Immunology Unit
Academical Medical Centre, University of Amsterdam
Meibergdreef 9
Amsterdam 1105 AZ
The Netherlands

Dr BJ Swanton
Senior Registrar in Anaesthesia
Rotunda Hospital
Dublin
Ireland

Dr MB Vroom
Department of Anaesthesia
Academical Medical Centre, University of Amsterdam
Meibergdreef 9
Amsterdam 1105 AZ
The Netherlands

Dr J Vuyk
Staff Anaesthesiologist
Department of Anaesthesiology
Leiden University Medical Centre
PO Box 9600
2300 RC Leiden
The Netherlands

Professor DC Warltier
Department of Anesthesiology
Medical College of Wisconsin
MEB-462C
8701 Watertown Plank Road
Milwaukee WI 53226
USA

Dr HB van Wezel
Department of Anaesthesia
Academical Medical Centre
University of Amsterdam
Meibergdreef 9

Amsterdam 1105 AZ
The Netherlands

Dr M White
Department of Anaesthesiology
Leiden University Medical Centre
PO Box 9600
2300 RC Leiden
The Netherlands

Professor PF White
Professor and Chairman
Department of Anesthesia & Pain Management
Southwestern Medical Center at Dallas
5323 Harry Hines Blvd
Dallas, TX 75235–9068
USA

Professor JM Wilmink
Department of Internal Med F4–215
Academical Medical Centre, University of Amsterdam
Renal Transplant Unit
Meibergdreef 9
Amsterdam 1105 AZ
The Netherlands

Dr A Windsor
Nuffield Department of Anaesthetics
John Radcliffe Hospital
Headington
Oxford
United Kingdom

Dr RP Woda
Assistant Professor
Department of Anesthesiology
Ohio State University Medical Center
N416 Doan Hall
410 W 10th Avenue
Columbus OH 43210
USA

ABBREVIATIONS

a_2-PI	a_2-plasmin inhibitor	DA	dopamine (peripheral receptor)
A	adenosine (receptor)	DAD	delayed afterdepolarization
AAG	a_1-acid glycoprotein	DAG	diacylglycerol
AC	adenylyl cyclase	DBI	diazepam binding inhibitor
ACE	angiotensin-converting enzyme	DBS	double-burst stimulation
ACh	acetylcholine	DI	diabetes insipidus
AChE	acetylcholinesterase	DKA	diabetic ketoacidosis
ACT	activated clotting time	DM	diabetes mellitus
ACTH	adrenocorticotrophic hormone	DNA	deoxyribonucleic acid
ADH	antidiuretic hormone	DTH	delayed-type hypersensitivity
ALA	aminolaevulinic acid	E_{max}	maximum effect
AMPA	a-amino-3-hydroxy-5-methyl-4-isoxazole propionate	EAD	early afterdepolarization
		ECG	electrocardiogram
ANP	atrial natriuretic peptide	ED_{50}	dose producing 50% of maximum effect
ANS	autonomic nervous system	EEG	electroencephalogram
APC	antigen-presenting cell	ELISA	enzyme-linked immunosorbent assay
APTT	activated partial thromboplastin time	EPP	endplate potential
ARDS	adult respiratory distress syndrome	ER	endoplasmic reticulum
AT	antithrombin	ERP	effective refractory period
ATG	antithymocyte globulin	ET	endothelin
ATP	adenosine triphosphate	5-FC	5-fluorocytosine
ATPase	adenosine triphosphatase	FENa	fractional excretion of sodium
AUC	area under the curve	G protein	guanine nucleotide-binding protein
AV	atrioventricular	GABA	γ-aminobutyric acid
BCDFE	2-bromo-2-chloro-1, 1-difluoroethylene	G-CSF	granulocyte colony-stimulating factor
BUN	blood urea nitrogen	GDP	guanosine diphosphate
cAMP	cyclic adenosine monophosphate	GFR	glomerular filtration rate
CBF	cerebral blood flow	GI	gastrointestinal
CD	cluster of differentiation	GM-CSF	granulocyte–macrophage colony-stimulating factor
cGMP	cyclic guanosine monophosphate		
Cl	total plasma clearance	GORD	gastrooesophageal reflux disease
$CMRO_2$	cerebral metabolic oxygen utilization	GR	glucocorticoid receptor
CNS	central nervous system	GTN	glyceryl trinitrate
CO	cardiac output	GTP	guanosine triphosphate
COMT	catechol-O-methyltransferase	GTPase	guanosine triphosphatase
COX	cyclooxygenase	GX	glycine xylidide
CPB	cardiopulmonary bypass	H	histamine (receptor)
CSF	cerebrospinal fluid	HG	haemoglobin
CT	computed tomography	HIT	heparin-induced thrombocytopenia
CTZ	chemoreceptor trigger zone	HIV	human immunodeficiency virus
CVP	central venous pressure	5-HT	5-hydroxytryptamine
CVS	cardiovascular system	I	imidazoline (receptor)
D	dopamine (central receptor)	ICP	intracranial pressure

ICU	intensive care unit	PK–PD	pharmacokinetic–pharmacodynamic
IL	interleukin	PLC	phospholipase C
IP_3	inositol 1,4,5-triphosphate	PPHN	persistent pulmonary hypertension of the newborn
IPSP	inhibitory postsynaptic potential		
IR	insulin receptor	p.p.m.	parts per million
ISDN	isosorbide dinitrate	PPX	pipecoloxylidide
ISMN	isosorbide mononitrate	PSVT	paroxysmal supraventricular tachycardia
KIU	kallikrein inactivator unit	PTC	posttetanic count
LMWH	low molecular weight heparin	PTU	propylthiouracil
M	muscarinic receptor	PVC	polyvinyl chloride
M3G	morphine-3-glucuronide	PVR	peripheral vascular resistance
M6G	morphine-6-glucuronide	PZI	protamine zinc insulin
MAC	minimum alveolar concentration	RAS	renin–angiotensin system
MAM	monoacetylmorphine	RAST	radioallergosorbent test
MAP	mean arterial pressure	RBF	renal blood flow
MBC	minimum bactericidal concentration	REM	rapid eye movement
MEGX	monoethylglycine xylidide	RIMA	reversible inhibitor of monoamine oxidase A
MEN	multiple endocrine neoplasia		
MEPP	miniature endplate potential	rPF4	recombinant platelet factor 4
MHC	major histocompatibility complex	RyR	ryanodine-sensitive calcium-release (channels)
MI	myocardial infarction		
MIC	minimum inhibitory concentration	SA	sinoatrial
MMR	masseter muscle rigidity	SE	spectral edge
6-MP	6-mercaptopurine	SIADH	syndrome of inappropriate antidiuretic hormone secretion
MRI	magnetic resonance imaging		
MRT	mean residence time	SLE	systemic lupus erythematosus
mTAL	medullary thick ascending loop of Henle	SND	sinus node dysfunction
nAChR	nicotinic acetylcholine receptor	SNP	sodium nitroprusside
NANC	nonadrenergic noncholinergic	SR	sarcoplasmic reticulum
NDMR	nondepolarizing muscle relaxant	SSKI	saturated solution of potassium iodide
NHP	neutral protamine Hagedorn	SSRI	selective serotonin-reuptake inhibitor
NK	natural killer	T_3	triidothyronine
NMDA	N-methyl-D-aspartate	TCR	T-cell receptor
NOS	nitric oxide synthetase	TEE	transoesophageal echocardiography
NSAID	nonsteroidal antiinflammatory drug	TFA	trifluoroacetyl halide
NTS	nucleus tractus solitarius	TFPI	tissue factor plasma inhibitor
NYHA	New York Heart Association	TOF	train-of-four
PA	pulmonary artery	tPA	tissue plasminogen activator
Pa_{O_2}	arterial partial pressure of oxygen	TR	thyroid receptor
PAF	platelet-activating factor	TSH	thyroid-stimulating hormone
PBP	penicillin-binding protein	UDP	uridine diphosphate
PG	prostaglandin	UFH	unfractionated heparin
PIP_2	phosphatidylinositol 4,5-biphosphate	V_d	volume of distribution
PKA	protein kinase A	VES	ventricular extrasystole
PKC	protein kinase C	VOC	voltage-operated channel

COMPARISON OF UK AND US TERMINOLOGY FOR DRUG NAMES

UK	USA
Adrenaline	Epinephrine
Diamorphine	Heroin
Frusemide	Furosemide
Hyoscine	Scopolamine
Isoprenaline	Isoproterenol
Lignocaine	Lidocaine
Methohexitone	Methohexital
Noradrenaline	Norepinephrine
Orciprenaline	Metaproterenol
Paracetamol	Acetaminophen
Pethidine	Meperidine
Pentobarbitone	Pentobarbital
Rifampicin	Rifampin
Salbutamol	Albuterol
Sodium cromoglycate	Cromolyn sodium
Suxamethonium	Succinylcholine
Thiopentone	Thiopental

Section 1
BASIC PRINCIPLES

1

JG Bovill

CELLULAR MECHANISMS OF DRUG ACTION

Summary box 1.1 Receptors

- Large proteins that bind specific molecules (ligands) stereoselectively.

- Ligands may be either agonists, antagonists or inverse agonists.

- Agonist – binding to receptor triggers a pharmacological response:

  - full agonist produces maximum response (intrinsic activity = 1)

  - partial agonist cannot produce maximum response (intrinsic activity < 1).

- Antagonist – binding to receptor does not produce response (intrinsic activity = 0):

  - competitive antagonist – block of receptor can be overcome by increasing concentration of agonist

  - noncompetitive antagonist – block cannot be overcome by increasing concentration of agonist.

- Inverse agonist – ligand binding produces opposite effects to those of an agonist.

An organism depends on a fully operational communication system for its proper functioning. Many drugs produce their pharmacological actions by interacting with regulatory proteins whose function is to convey signals from one cell to another. Other drugs interact with enzymes (e.g. cholinesterase inhibitors). The cell membrane is a highly specialized structure containing ion channels and receptors involved in cell signalling. Receptors are specialized proteins that bind with specific molecules to control cellular behaviour.

PROPERTIES OF RECEPTORS AND LIGANDS

Two essential properties of a receptor are signal recognition and signal transduction. Recognition involves the ability of the receptor to bind specific molecules, known as ligands, with high affinity and specificity. Ligands, compounds that have affinity for a receptor, may be classified as agonists or antagonists. An agonist has affinity for the receptor and produces a response as a result of the ligand–receptor interaction. This ability to produce a response is known as efficacy or intrinsic activity. An antagonist binds to the receptor but lacks intrinsic activity, i.e. has zero efficacy. Antagonists usually have high affinity – indeed this is essential if they are to displace the agonist from the receptor. If the binding of the ligand increases the probability of receptor interaction with a transduction protein, for example a G protein, then the ligand is said to have positive efficacy. If the ligand decreases the probability of receptor–transducer association it has negative efficacy, and is referred to as an inverse agonist. The best known examples of inverse agonists are certain compounds that bind to the γ-aminobutyric acid (GABA)$_A$ benzodiazepine receptor, but inverse agonists acting on β-adrenoceptors have also been described.[1] Inverse agonists produce pharmacological effects opposite to those of the agonists; for example, for benzodiazepines they produce anxiety rather than relieving it. Agonists may be full agonists or partial agonists. A full agonist is able to cause a maximum response which corresponds to an activity of unity, whereas partial agonists cannot produce the maximum response so have intrinsic activities of less than unity (Fig. 1.1). Not all full agonists have equal efficacy: some may produce a maximum response when only 5% of the available receptors are occupied, whereas less efficient agonists may need to occupy 30% or more to obtain a full response.

There are two types of antagonists: competitive and unsurmountable. Competitive antagonism implies that the agonist and the antagonist bind at the same site on the receptor, so that the binding is mutually exclusive. Provided the binding is freely reversible, then the blocked response caused by the presence of the antagonist can be fully overcome by sufficiently increasing the concentration of the agonist, i.e. the antagonism is *surmountable*. When the effect of an antagonist cannot be fully overcome by increasing the concentration of the agonist, the antagonism is said to be *unsurmountable*. This often arises with covalent bonding between antagonist and receptor. Covalent bonds are very strong, requiring considerable energy to break. They result in irreversible binding between ligand and receptor, so that the receptor is rendered nonfunctional. The effects of irreversibly bound drugs will persist until new receptors are synthesized, a process that takes several days. Examples of drugs that bind irreversibly by means of covalent bonding are the α-adrenoreceptor antagonist, phenoxybenzamine, and aspirin.

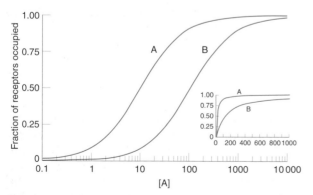

Fig. 1.1 Fractional receptor occupancy (E_A/E_M) as a function of agonist concentration [A], in the absence (A) and presence (B) of a competitive antagonist. The graphs are plotted on a semilogarithmic axis for [A], yielding sigmoid curves. The insert shows the same data plotted on a linear scale for [A], yielding hyperbolic curves.

RECEPTOR KINETICS

The binding of an agonist to a receptor is a chemical process and the interaction between agonist (A) and receptor (R) can be described by the equation:

$$A + R \rightleftharpoons AR \qquad [1]$$

At equilibrium, the law of mass action gives the equilibrium dissociation constant, K_d:

$$K_d = \frac{[A][R]}{[AR]} \qquad [2]$$

K_d reflects the affinity of the agonist for the receptor; high values of K_d denote low affinity, low values high affinity. To determine the fraction of receptors occupied by the agonist [AR], the number of receptors is assumed to be finite, say R_T (= [R] + [AR]). Substitution for [R] in eqn [2] and rearranging gives:

$$\frac{[AR]}{[R_T]} = \frac{[A]}{[A] + K_d} \qquad [3]$$

Eqn [3] shows that when $[AR]/[R_T]$ = 0.5 (50% of receptors occupied), K_d equals [A]. That is, K_d is numerically equal to the free ligand concentration when half the receptors are occupied.

If it is assumed that the magnitude of the pharmacological response is proportional to fractional receptor occupancy, then the response elicited by agonist binding may be expressed as:

$$\frac{E_A}{E_m} = \frac{[AR]}{[R_T]} = \frac{[A]}{[A] + K_d} \qquad [4]$$

where E_A is the observed response to agonist A and E_m is the maximum response obtainable. The graph of E_A/E_m versus [A] is a rectangular hyperbola, but a semi-logarithmic plot of E_A/E_m versus log [A] yields a sigmoid relationship (Fig. 1.1). This simple model can be modified to allow for the concept of receptor reserve, or 'spare', receptors, whereby an agonist with high efficacy need occupy only a fraction of the total available receptors to produce a maximum response.

COMPETITIVE ANTAGONISTS

When a competitive antagonist (I) is present concurrently with an agonist, the antagonist competes with the agonist for binding sites on the receptor. Since an antagonist has no intrinsic efficacy there will be a reduction in the response produced by the agonist. This interaction can be expressed as:

$$I + R \rightleftharpoons IR$$

or, applying the law of mass action:

$$\frac{[I][R]}{[IR]} = K_I$$

In the presence of an antagonist the occupancy Eqn [3] becomes:

$$Y_d = \frac{[A]/K_d}{1 + [A]/K_d + [I]/K_I}$$

where $Y_d = [AR]/R_T$. When negligible antagonist is present, this equation reduces to eqn [3]. As the concentration of the antagonist increases, the concentration of the agonist required to maintain the same occupancy increases (i.e. its value of K_d appears to increase). This can be seen as a displacement of the agonist occupancy curve to the right (Fig. 1.1).

STEREOISOMERISM

Most hormones and neurotransmitters, and many drugs, exhibit the phenomenon of stereoselectivity, with actions markedly dependent on their spatial configuration. Substances with the same elementary chemical composition but with the elements occupying different positions in space are called isomers. Structural isomers are compounds with the same numbers of chemical elements which differ in their position and arrangement. As such they are different chemical and biological substances. Examples are enflurane and isoflurane and the β-adrenoceptor antagonists, practolol and atenolol. More important in pharmacology are the two classes of stereoisomers: optical and geometrical isomers.

Optical isomers

Optical isomers are compounds differing only in their ability to rotate the plane of polarized light. The (+), or dextrorotatory (d), isomer rotates light to the right (clockwise) and the (–), or laevorotatory (l), isomer rotates light to the left (anticlockwise). Optical isomers or *enantiomers* (Greek *enantios morphe*, meaning opposite shape) arise when molecules contain atoms or groups forming an asymmetrical chiral centre (Greek χειρ, meaning hand), arranged so that the molecules differ only as does the right hand from the left, i.e. they are nonsuperimposable mirror images (Fig. 1.2). A 50 : 50 mixture of (+) and (–) enantiomers is a racemic mixture, which has no effect on polarized light. The commonest asymmetrical centre is a carbon atom with four different groups attached. Enantiomers have identical chemical and physical properties but may have different physiological or pharmacological activities. If more than one asymmetrical centre is present in the molecule (*diasteromer*) then physical properties will differ. Labetalol has two chiral centres and is a mixture of two racemates, i.e. labetalol is a mixture of four stereoisomers. When giving labetalol, four drugs are being administered, not one.

In addition to the prefixes (+) and (–), or d- and l-, other terminologies refer to the spatial configuration of the atoms or groups around the chiral centre. The D (dextro) and L (laevo) nomenclature, not to be confused with the lower-case d and l, was chosen arbitrarily to coincide with the (+) and (–) isomers of glyceraldehyde, with the D configuration assigned to the (+) glyceraldehyde. However, except for the simplest molecules, this system is ambiguous. Modern nomenclature uses the R, S system based on the Cahn, Ingold and Prelog convention. For a chiral atom, the four substituents are assigned relative priorities according to atomic weights, the group with the highest sum of weights being given the highest priority. The molecule is then rotated so that it is viewed from the side opposite the group with the lowest priority and the symbol R, for *rectus* (right), is assigned if the remaining groups follow descending priorities in a clockwise order about the centre. If the order from highest to lowest is anticlockwise then the symbol S, for *sinister* or left, is assigned (Fig. 1.2). Note that the chirality (right- or left-handedness) of a configuration is no guide to the optical rotation of polarized light. Thus the R-configuration may rotate light clockwise (+) or anticlockwise (–), for example R(–)-ketamine and S(+)-ketamine but R(+)-bupivacaine and S(–)-bupivacaine.

Differences in the pharmacological activities

Summary box 1.2 Isomers

- Substances with the same chemical composition but different spatial arrangements of molecular elements.

- Structural isomers – compounds with the same numbers of chemical elements which differ in their position and arrangement; they are different chemical and biological substances.

- Stereoisomers:

  - optical – molecules with a chiral centre; differ only in ability to rotate polarized light. Have same chemical but different pharmacological properties. A 50:50 mixture of (+) and (–) enantiomers is a racemic mixture.

  - geometric – molecules with a site of restricted rotation (e.g. double bond or rigid ring system). Unlike optical isomers, are not mirror images.

- Conformational isomers are atoms with a nonidentical spatial arrangement of their atoms resulting from rotation about single bonds, and allowing folding of the molecule.

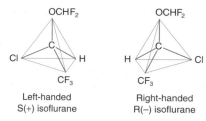

Fig. 1.2 The enantiomers of isoflurane. The molecular weights of the relevant groups are H = 1, Cl = 35, $OCHF_2$ = 67, CF_3 = 69. See text for derivation of R and S configurations.

between enantiomers can be considerable. Thus (+)-lofentanil is a μ-opioid agonist while (–)-lofentanil is a μ antagonist. In some barbiturates the (–) isomer is a depressant whereas the (+) form is a convulsant. Dobutamine is a racemic mixture in which both enantiomers contribute to the inotropic effect of the drug. R(+)-dobutamine is an agonist at β_1 and β_2 receptors while S(–)-dobutamine is a potent α_1-adrenoceptor agonist.

Naturally occurring compounds are usually single enantiomers (e.g. *l*-morphine, *l*-hyoscine). Atropine is an exception. Although synthesized in the belladonna plant as *l*-atropine, it is partly converted in the extraction process to the *d*-isomer (chiral inversion), and is administered as a racemic mixture. During this process its anticholinergic activity is approximately halved since the *d*-isomer has little activity. In contrast to biological synthesis, organic synthesis usually results in racemic mixtures. Up to 90% of β-adrenergic agents, antiepileptics and oral anticoagulants, and about 50% of antihistamines and antidepressants, are racemic mixtures. More than half of the drugs used in anaesthesia are chiral. Of the five inhalation anaesthetics in use today, only sevoflurane does not possess a chiral centre. The anaesthetic potency of S(+)-isoflurane is about 53% greater than that of the R(–)-enantiomer.[2]

Among the intravenous anaesthetics, stereoselectivity was first observed with the barbiturates. In general, for the barbiturates, the S isomer is about twice as potent as the R isomer. Etomidate is also chiral but is marketed as R(+)-etomidate. S(–)-etomidate has minimal hypnotic activity. In the case of ketamine, S(+)-ketamine is about three times more potent than R(–)-ketamine. The R(–) isomer is also responsible for the psychotimimetic effects.[3] Many amide local anaesthetics are chiral and, with the exception of ropivacaine, are used clinically as the racemic mixtures. The cardiotoxicity of bupivacaine is predominantly due to the R(+)-isomer, which also has greater central nervous system (CNS) toxicity.[4]

Geometric isomers

Geometric isomers form a second type of stereoisomerism (but not necessarily optical isomerism). Geometric isomers arise when there is restricted rotation in a molecule, either around a double bond or a rigid ring system. Stereoisomerism arising from the presence of a double bond is indicated by using Z (German *zusammen*, meaning together) or E (German *entgegen*, meaning opposite). These correspond in general (but not always) to the older *cis* and *trans* configurational designations. The two forms arise when the substituents are on the same side (Z or *cis*) or on the opposite sides (E or *trans*) of the double bond.

Z/E conformations are not mirror images and have different physicochemical and pharmacological properties. Mivacurium is a mixture of three geometrical isomers, *cis–cis*, *trans–trans* and *cis–trans*. The *cis–cis* isomer has only about 10% of the potency of the other two isomers. The recently introduced *cis*-atracurium is one of the 10 stereoisomers of atracurium.

Conformational isomers

Conformational isomerism is the nonidentical spatial arrangement of atoms in a molecule resulting from rotation about one or more single bonds, and allowing folding of the molecule. Acetylcholine, for example, has three centres of rotation allowing several spatial configurations. Binding to the muscarinic and nicotinic receptors involves different conformational isomers of the acetylcholine molecule.

ION CHANNELS AND RECEPTORS

Many receptors have been cloned and their amino acid sequences determined. This has led to the recognition of four superfamilies of receptors:

1. Ligand-gated ion channels that contain a transmitter binding site as part of the ion channel.
2. G protein-coupled receptors linked to a second messenger system by a guanine nucleotide protein.
3. Ligand-activated receptors with intrinsic enzyme activity.
4. Nuclear receptors that alter DNA transcription.

With the exception of the nuclear receptors, receptors span the cell membrane, allowing transmission of information from the external milieu to the inside of the cell. Transmembrane receptors contain distinct domains with polar hydrophilic surfaces exposed to the aqueous environment on either side of the membrane, separated by a transmembrane nonpolar hydrophobic region.

ION CHANNELS

Ion channels are membrane-spanning proteins containing a central water-filled pore through which ions can traverse the cell membrane. When activated, there is a change in the ionic conductance, resulting in either membrane depolarization or hyperpolarization. Opening of the channel allows selected ions (Ca^{2+}, Na^+, K^+ or Cl^-) to flow down their electrical or chemical gradients. The rate of ion flow is very fast, so that response times are very short – a few milliseconds. Ion channels are found when speed is essential to the signalling process, as in nerve cells and pacemaker cells in the heart.

There are two types of ion channels: voltage gated and ligand gated. Voltage-gated ion channels open and close in response to changes in membrane potential. The channels are named according to the ion they selectively control. Ligand-gated ion channels are generally complex protein structures, often with several ligand binding sites, for example the $GABA_A$ and N-methyl-D-aspartate (NMDA) receptor complexes. Some (e.g. $GABA_A$) are selective for a single ion (Cl^-); others can modulate the passage of several ions. The ion currents generated by ligand-gated channels often provide the stimulus for the subsequent opening of voltage-gated ion channels.

VOLTAGE-GATED ION CHANNELS

The voltage-gated ion channels have important structural features in common and may be derived from a common ancestral ion channel. This primitive ancestor was probably a protein similar to the single domain of the K^+ channel, which is believed to be the most primitive of the voltage-gated ion channels.[5] Voltage-gated ion channels consist of motifs with six membrane-spanning α helices formed by predominantly hydrophobic amino acids. These motifs are repeated four times in the Ca^{2+} and Na^+ channels, whereas K^+ channels contain only one motif. However, four such motifs are required to make a single functioning K^+ channel. The fourth transmembrane helix contains arginine and lysine, the most positively charged of the amino acids, arranged in every third position among otherwise neutral amino acids. These charged amino acids are thought to act as the voltage sensor controlling gating of the channel. Rotational and longitudinal movement of this segment in response to a change in transmembrane potential causes the ion pore to open. The intracellular sequence connecting the third and fourth repeats of the motif swings into the mouth of the channel after the membrane has been depolarized, preventing further ion flow so that the channel becomes inactive. This is known as the 'ball and chain model' of channel inactivation (Fig. 1.3).

SODIUM ION CHANNELS

Sodium channels exist in one of three states: closed (or resting), open and inactivated. The trigger for opening is an increase in the intracellular potential to approximately –55 mV. This causes a voltage-dependent change in the conformation of the channel. The opening of the sodium channel is very transient: within less than 1 ms it closes spontaneously and enters the inactivated state. It can return to its resting state only

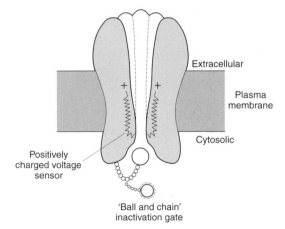

Fig. 1.3 Proposed structure of a voltage-gated ion channel consisting of four subunits. The inactivation gate at the cytosolic opening of the channel pore, the 'ball and chain', is thought to be formed by the intracellular loop connecting the third and fourth transmembrane subunits.

Summary box 1.3 Ion channels

- Membrane-spanning proteins with a central pore through which ions can traverse the cell membrane. Very fast response times (ms).

- Two types:

  - voltage-gated channels open and close in response to changes in membrane potential. Examples are Ca^{2+}, Na^+ and K^+ channels; there are several subtypes of each of these.

  - ligand-gated channels open in response to binding of specific ligand. Often have several ligand-binding sites. Examples are nicotinic ACh, $GABA_A$ and NMDA channels.

when the membrane potential returns to near the resting potential. The same potential changes that lead to the opening of sodium channels also open potassium channels. These, however, open more slowly than the sodium channels and become fully open when the sodium channel has almost returned to the inactivated state. The outward flow of potassium ions is responsible for the repolarization of the neuron. Although an action potential is associated with large changes in membrane potential, the number of sodium ions entering and potassium ions leaving the cell is very small and ionic equilibrium is rapidly restored by the $Na^+–K^+$ pump. When a squid axon has been poisoned with cyanide so that ion pumping is abolished, the axon can fire nearly 100 000 action potentials before failing.

Local anaesthetics act on Na^+ channels, and there is extensive evidence that inhalational and intravenous anaesthetics also act on these channels. Local anaesthetics bind tightly to the inactivated state, stabilizing this form of the channel. The closed or resting state has the least affinity for local anaesthetics. This differential affinity explains the phasic or frequency-dependent neuronal block produced by local anaesthetics.[6] An important mechanism of the class I antiarrhythmic drugs, including lignocaine, is inhibition of the fast inward depolarizing currents carried by sodium ions.

POTASSIUM ION CHANNELS

K^+ channels are a very diverse family of membrane proteins, with numerous subtypes both in the CNS and peripheral tissues, in particular in the heart. Although of fundamental physiological importance, they have had limited pharmacological significance since, until recently, no drugs were available for human use with specific actions on them. This situation is, however, changing with the introduction of the potassium channel openers.

A particularly important potassium channel in terms of pharmacology is the adenosine triphosphate (ATP)-sensitive K^+ channel, K_{ATP}, whose opening is inhibited by intracellular ATP. First discovered in cardiac muscle,[7] it has since been found in endocrine cells, smooth and skeletal muscle cells, and the central and peripheral nervous systems. These channels regulate the secretion of hormones such as insulin, prolactin and growth hormone, and influence the excitability of cardiac, skeletal and vascular smooth muscle. K_{ATP} channels are opened by negative regulators of insulin secretion such as somatostatin and galanin, and are inhibited by sulphonylurea antidiabetics such as glibenclamide and tolbutamide. They are of particular importance during ischaemia in both the heart and the brain, where they reduce or delay cell death.[8]

K_{ATP} channels are activated by a chemically diverse group of agents named potassium channel opening drugs. To this group belong cromakalin and its active enantiomer levcromakalin, bimakalin and celikalin, nicorandil, pinacidil, aprikalim, minoxidil and diazoxide. These drugs produce smooth muscle relaxation and vasodilatation. They are used in treating various cardiovascular conditions as well as asthma, urinary incontinence and certain skeletal muscle myopathies. In cardiac myocytes, K_{ATP} channels remain permanently closed owing to the tonic block produced by high levels of intracellular ATP. When the cells become ischaemic, or are treated with metabolic inhibitors such as cyanide, K_{ATP} channels open and the flow of K^+ shortens the action potential, preventing Ca^{2+} entry during the plateau phase to conserve ATP and to prevent Ca^{2+} accumulation that would lead to cell death. Potassium channel opening drugs have been shown to improve recovery of contractile function on reperfusion and reduce infarct size. The hypoxic vasodilatation of the coronary arteries is mediated by K_{ATP} channels. In the renal tubule cells, K_{ATP} channels contribute to potassium balance and K_{ATP} blocking drugs may have potential as potassium sparing diuretics. Glibenclamide, a sulphonylurea which inhibits K_{ATP} channels, induces significant sodium diuresis without urinary potassium loss.

CALCIUM ION CHANNELS

To date six distinct Ca^{2+} channel types have been defined both electrophysiologically and pharmacologically,[9] designated T, L, N, P, Q and R. They have different voltage thresholds for activation and different kinetics for opening and closing, and also exhibit distinct selectivities for blocking compounds (Table 1.1). Although under certain circumstances these channels permit the passage of Na^+ and K^+, they are highly selective for Ca^{2+}, by a factor greater than 1000. This is due to selective binding of calcium ions to two sites within the channel, which leads to the exclusion of Na^+ and K^+.[10]

T-type calcium channels.

These are found on both central and peripheral neurons as well as in nonneuronal tissues such as muscle and secretory cells. T-type channels are activated by low voltages and have short open times, hence the designation T – for transient. Recently a new class of calcium entry blocker has been introduced, mibefradil. Mibefradil blocks both L- and T-type calcium channels, but is 10 times more potent at blocking T channels than L channels.[11] The first drug known to block T channels, mibefradil is selective for the coronary circulation but has no negative inotropic properties.[12] T-type channels are also inhibited by volatile anaesthetics, although it is

Table 1.1 Characteristics of voltage-gated Ca^{2+} channels				
	Ca^{2+} channel			
	L	T	N	P
Activation range	+ve to −10 mV	+ve to −70 mV	+ve to −20 mV	+ve to −40 mV
Rate of inactivation	Slow	Very fast	Fast	Slow
Conductance (pS)	25	8	15	12
Specific inhibitor	DHP	NA	ω-CTX	FTX
Anaesthetics	Sensitive	Sensitive	Sensitive	? Sensitive

NA, none available; DHP, dihydropyridines; ω-CTX, ω-conotoxin; FTX, funnel web spider toxin.

uncertain whether this contributes to the mechanism of general anaesthesia.[13]

L-type calcium ion channels

L-type channels are activated by high voltages (more positive than −10 mV) and exhibit little inactivation. When activated they have long open times – L for 'long lasting'. Although the open times of L channels are relatively long lasting, there is a very wide variability between channels in different tissues. L-type currents in cardiac muscle are considerably faster than those in smooth muscle and in many neurons.[10] In the CNS, they are located predominantly on neuronal cell bodies. L channels in the cardiovascular system are important in cardiovascular pharmacology. The group of drugs known as calcium entry blockers, or calcium antagonists, selectively inhibit L-type channels. These include dihydropyridines (e.g. nifedipine), phenyl-alkylamines (e.g. verapamil) and benzothiazepines (e.g. diltiazem). Distinct, but allostererically interacting, receptors exist for each of these structurally different classes on the same $α$ subunit of the L channel. L channels are particularly sensitive to the dihydropyridine class, such as nifedipine. Although evidence for an action by anaesthetic drugs on neuronal L channels is conflicting,[14] both volatile and intravenous anaesthetics depress L current in skeletal and cardiac muscle.

N-type calcium ion channels.

N-type channels are distributed widely in the nervous system, where they are localized mainly on the presynaptic terminals of peripheral neurons. They are also present in endocrine cells. They were initially given the designation 'N' because they were neither T nor L type. Nowadays the N is often taken to refer to 'neuronal' in view of their particular importance in neurons. N-type channels are sensitive to the toxin, ω-conotoxin, from the marine mollusk *Conus geographus*. This toxin has little effect on other Ca^{2+} channel types. N-type channels play an important role in the control of neurotransmitter release.

P-type calcium ion channels

These channels are designated P since they were first described in cerebellar Purkinje cells. They are the most common (approximately 80%) voltage-sensitive Ca^{2+} channel in mammalian nerve terminals. P channels are selectively blocked by the FTX toxin from the funnel-web spider. Like N and L high voltage-activated channels, they are not affected by dihydropyridines. They appear not to be influenced by general anaesthetics.

Intracellular Ca^{2+} channels

The internal membranes of cells also contain calcium channels. These are important for releasing Ca^{2+} into the cytosol, for the regulation of cell function.[10] Two types of internal Ca^{2+} channels have been identified: one releases calcium in response to inositol 1,4,5-triphosphate (IP_3) and another is very sensitive to a plant alkaloid, ryanodine. Ryanodine-sensitive calcium-release (RyR) channels are located on the sarcoplasmic reticulum (SR) and mediate the rapid release of Ca^{2+} from intracellular stores, a fundamental part of the excitation–contraction coupling in cardiac, skeletal and smooth muscle. In skeletal muscle RyR channels are coupled to L-type Ca^{2+} channels on the plasma membrane. Depolarization causes the L channel to undergo a conformational change, which generates a signal to the RyR channel to open. How this information is passed between the two channels is unknown. Actions of halothane on the RyR channels in skeletal muscle are thought to underlie malignant hyperthermia.[15] Patients who develop malignant hyperthermia may have a defect in this channel.[16]

LIGAND-GATED ION CHANNELS

The physiological stimulus for activation of ligand-gated ion channels is the binding of a neurotransmitter (ligand) to a receptor on the channel protein, causing the channel to change its conformation, opening the channel and allowing ions to cross the cell membrane. This allows the membrane potential to change very rapidly (0.1–0.2 ms), and postsynaptic ligand-gated ion channels are responsible for the rapid dialogue between neurons of the peripheral and central nervous systems. They transfer the chemically transmitted signal of a neurotransmitter of one cell into an electrical signal, which is then rapidly conducted along the nerve fibre of a second cell. Ligand-gated ion channels may be either excitatory or inhibitory. Excitatory receptors (e.g. nicotinic acetylcholine receptors, NMDA glutamate receptors and 5-hydroxytryptamine ($5-HT)_3$ receptors, when activated open channels that allow the passage of Na^+, K^+ or Ca^{2+} ions. This causes depolarization of the postsynaptic membrane. GABA and glycine bind to ligand-gated chloride channels, causing hyperpolarization of the postsynaptic membrane and inhibition. Members of the ligand-gated ion channel family are composed of five subunits, each subunit consisting of four membrane-spanning a helices (Fig. 1.4).

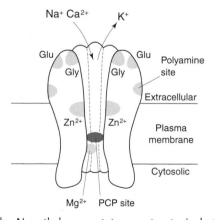

Fig. 1.4 The N-methyl-D-aspartate receptor, typical of ligand-gated ion channels, consists of five membrane-spanning domains. This model of the receptor shows the proposed sites of interaction for glutamate (Glu), glucine (Gly), polyamine, Zn^{2+} and Mg^{2+}. Glutamate requires the presence of glycine to open the receptor channel. Polyamine positively modulates, and Zn^{2+} and Mg^{2+} negatively modulate, the opening of the channel. Ketamine and phencyclidine bind to the site labelled PCP.

NICOTINIC ACETYLCHOLINE RECEPTORS

Acetylcholine (ACh) is an example of an endogenous neurotransmitter that binds to more than one receptor type: the nicotinic acetylcholine receptor (nAChR), which preferentially binds nicotine, and the muscarinic receptor, which binds muscarine, a mushroom alkaloid. The latter is a G protein-coupled receptor whereas the nAChR is an excitatory ligand-gated ion channel which transports Na^+ ions. Nicotinic cholinergic receptors are found in autonomic ganglia and at the neuromuscular junction of skeletal muscles.

Activation of the channel occurs in two steps. First, two molecules of ACh bind sequentially to specific sites on the $α$ subunit of the channel protein. This is followed by a conformational change in the channel from a resting, nonconducting (closed) state to an open, conducting state. The channel can exist in two other states, desensitized and blocked. In the desensitized state the receptor is closed and must revert to the resting state before it can be activated. ACh binds with high affinity to the desensitized state but the channel in this state does not open, and has to revert to the resting state before it will do so. The resting state is more stable than the open state in the absence of ACh, but once ACh has bound to the receptor the open state becomes the most stable. Continued presence of ACh converts the receptor to the most stable state of all, the desensitized state. Anaesthetics have complex actions on the nAChR, involving allosteric changes to the channel and/or changes induced by perturbation of the lipid membrane bilayer.[17] High concentrations of anaesthetics are able to stabilize the desensitized receptor, by a mechanism independent of agonist binding sites.

GABA_A RECEPTORS

The overall activity of the brain is basically governed by two superior functions, excitation and inhibition. The major excitatory neurotransmitter in the mammalian nervous system is the amino acid, L-glutamate. GABA is the major inhibitory transmitter in the CNS.[18] Several GABA receptor subtypes have been identified: $GABA_A$, $GABA_B$ and receptors that have been termed $GABA_C$ or 'non-$GABA_A$, non-$GABA_B$ receptors'. $GABA_A$ and $GABA_B$ receptors are found presynaptically and postsynaptically on GABA and non-GABA terminals, including those also containing NMDA receptors. The $GABA_B$ receptor is a G protein-linked receptor coupled to calcium or potassium ion channels. It has been suggested that at least two GABA molecules must bind to the receptor for full activation.[19]

Binding of GABA to the $GABA_A$ receptor increases membrane conductance for Cl^-, resulting in a Cl^- current into the cell, membrane hyperpolarization and a reduction in neuronal excitability. GABA regulation of the chloride channel is not a simple gating between an open and closed state: there are three open states, 10 closed states and one desensitized state. The average open duration increases with increasing GABA concentration due to a shift in the type of opening. At low GABA concentration the majority of openings are 0.5 ms in duration, whereas at higher concentration openings of longer duration are more frequent. Bursts composed of repeated openings into the same open state are interrupted by brief closures. Drugs may enhance $GABA_A$ current by increasing channel conductance, increasing channel open and burst frequencies, and/or increasing channel open and burst duration. Several anaesthetic drugs, including barbiturates, benzodiazepines, steroids, propofol and volatile anaesthetics, bind to $GABA_A$ receptors and augment $GABA_A$-mediated inhibition via allosteric modulation of receptor function.

Barbiturates bind to distinct sites on the $GABA_A$ receptor. They facilitate the response to GABA and mimic GABA by opening the receptor chloride channel in the absence of GABA. The enhancement of GABA action is manifest by an increase in GABAergic inhibitory postsynaptic potentials (IPSPs). This is brought about by prolonging bursts of channel openings, increasing the mean channel open. Etomidate is even more potent than barbiturates in activating $GABA_A$ receptor channels, with a potency comparable to that of GABA.[20] A similar potentiation of $GABA_A$ action is produced by steroid anaesthetics. Steroids bind to different domains of the $GABA_A$ complex from those of the barbiturates. At least some of the anaesthetic properties of propofol are mediated via the $GABA_A$ receptor complex.[21] Propofol binding to the $GABA_A$ receptor is at a site distinct from those for barbiturates, benzodiazepines or steroids.

Benzodiazepines bind to a distinct site on the $GABA_A$ receptor complex, often referred to as the benzodiazepine receptor. Benzodiazepines alone do not have any effect on chloride currents in the absence of GABA or GABA agonists. When GABA is present, they increase chloride ion flux. In contrast to the barbiturates, benzodiazepines increase channel current by increasing receptor open and burst frequency, but average open and burst durations are not altered. Benzodiazepines also enhance the probability of the $GABA_A$ channel opening in bursts of long duration. Inverse agonists reduce the chloride channel open and burst frequencies.[19]

NMDA RECEPTORS

The amino acid L-glutamate, the most important excitatory neurotransmitter in the mammalian CNS, activates three broad subtypes of excitatory amino acid receptors: a-amino-3-hydroxy-5-methyl-4-isoxazole pro-

pionate (AMPA) receptors, NMDA receptors and a non-NMDA receptor activated by kainite. A fourth family of glutamate receptors are the metabotrophic receptors. Metabotrophic glutamate receptors do not contain an ion channel but stimulate a G protein when activated. NMDA receptors are widely distributed throughout the brain and spinal cord, with the highest densities in the cerebral cortex and hippocampus, and have very widespread physiological functions.[22] N-methyl-D-aspartate (NMDA) receptors control ion channels that permit entry of monovalent (mainly Na^+) and divalent (mainly Ca^{2+}) ions into the cell. Calcium flux is by far the most important. In addition to a binding site for L-glutamate, the NMDA receptor has binding sites for glycine, Mg^{2+} and Zn^{2+}. A recognition site for phenylcyclidine and ketamine lies in the opening of the ion channel (Fig. 1.4), and these drugs are noncompetitive antagonists of the NMDA receptor.

The NMDA receptor is unique in that it is the only ligand-gated ion channel whose probability of opening depends strongly on the voltage across the membrane. The receptor is inoperative when the neuron is in the resting state, with a negative intracellular membrane potential. This puts an important restriction on Ca^{2+} flux through the ion channel by imposing a voltage-dependent Mg^{2+} block on the channel. Presynaptically released glutamate cannot activate any significant ion flow through the channel unless the postsynaptic membrane is sufficiently depolarized to remove this Mg^{2+} block.

The NMDA receptor is involved in a number of functions relevant to anaesthesia, including sensory information processing, memory and learning, locomotion, and regulation of vasomotor tone and blood pressure, and is also involved in the pathophysiology of cellular damage or death associated with ischaemia, traumatic head injury or stroke. NMDA receptors also have an important role in nociception, in particular neuronal plasticity associated with chronic pain, tissue injury and inflammatory states. Chronic pain, with high-frequency or sustained afferent input to the dorsal horn, produces a prolonged depolarization so that the Mg^{2+} block on spinal NMDA receptors is removed, allowing NMDA activation and an influx of Ca^{2+}. In animals subjected to repeated peripheral nerve stimulation of sufficient intensity to activate C fibres, the responses of a proportion of neurons in the spinal dorsal horn increase with each subsequent stimulus. This phenomenon, referred to as 'wind-up' is associated with facilitation of spinal nociceptive reflexes or hyperalgesia. It is closely related to the NMDA receptor. Wind-up of dorsal horn nociceptive neurons is selectively reduced by NMDA antagonists, including ketamine.

THE 5-HT₃ RECEPTOR

The 5-HT$_3$ receptor is the only monoamine neurotransmitter receptor that functions as a ligand-gated ion channel, controlling the flux of Na^+ and K^+ ions. 5-HT$_3$ receptors are located on parasympathetic nerve terminals in the gastrointestinal tract, and high densities are found in areas of the brain associated with the emetic response, such as the area postrema. The antiemetic effects of 5-HT$_3$ antagonists, such as ondansetron, result from actions at these sites. Indeed, the only clearly established therapeutic role for 5-HT$_3$ receptor antagonists is that of antiemesis, and they appear to be selective in their action. 5-HT$_3$ receptors in the dorsal horn of the spinal cord have been implicated in nociception, and development of new 5-HT$_3$ receptor-related compounds may have potential as nonopioid, nonaddictive analgesics. Various studies also indicate the potential for the anxiolytic antipsychotic and antidepressant effects of 5-HT$_3$ receptor antagonists.[23]

G PROTEIN-COUPLED RECEPTORS

INTRACELLULAR SIGNALLING MECHANISMS

The binding of ligands to many receptors leads to an increase or decrease in the concentration of intracellular molecules called *second messengers*, which trigger changes in the activity of other intracellular enzymes or proteins producing the final cellular response. Five second messengers are currently known; cyclic adenosine monophosphate (cAMP), cyclic guanosine monophosphate (cGMP), IP$_3$, diacylglycerol (DAG) and calcium. Many second messengers are generated through an intermediate signal transducing G protein (guanine nucleotide proteins, hence the 'G' terminology).

More than 20 G proteins have been identified, the most important being G$_s$, G$_i$, G$_o$ and G$_q$. G proteins consist of three subunits, α, β and γ, associated with the cystolic face of the cell membrane, and contact both the receptor and an effector molecule such as adenylyl cyclase. They exist in two states: an inactive state in which guanosine diphosphate (GDP) is bound to the α subunit, and an active form when the GDP is replaced by guanosine triphosphate (GTP). When the receptor is activated by binding of an agonist, it interacts with the G protein, triggering the release of GDP and binding of GTP. The activated α-GTP subunit then dissociates from the β/γ subunit and interacts with the effector molecule. The activation of the effector molecule is brief (a few seconds) because G proteins have intrinsic guanosine phosphatase (GTPase) activity and GTP on the α subunit is rapidly hydrolysed to GDP, with inactivation of the G protein.

Bacterial toxins that specifically catalyse the Gα subunits are used to identify G$_s$ or G$_i$ proteins. Pertussis toxin (from *Bordetella pertussis*, the bacterium causing whooping cough) uncouples G$_i$ proteins from their receptors (hence these G proteins are referred to as pertussis sensitive) whereas cholera toxin activates G$_s$ protein by inactivation of its intrinsic GTPase activity.

G protein-coupled receptors are characterized by seven hydrophobic membrane-spanning domains connected by three extracellular and three intracellular loops (Fig. 1.5). The transmembrane domains are folded with a pocket formed by the third, sixth and seventh domains where ligand binding occurs. The intracellular loop between domains five and seven and the C-terminus are binding sites for the G protein (Fig. 1.5). The receptors coupled to G proteins are summarized in Table 1.2 and discussed below. Opioid receptors are covered in Chapter 7 and the histamine receptors in Chapter 19.

The adenylyl cyclase pathway

Activation of G$_s$ or G$_i$ proteins results in stimulation or inhibition, respectively, of the membrane enzyme adenylyl cyclase (AC), by GTP-α_s or GTP-α_i (Fig. 1.6). Activated AC catalyses the formation of cAMP from ATP. cAMP diffuses into the cytoplasm where it binds to the regulatory subunits of cAMP-dependent protein kinases, otherwise known as protein kinase A (PKA). PKA mediates the diverse cellular effects of cAMP by phosphorylating the terminal phosphate group in ATP

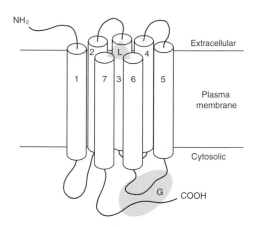

Fig. 1.5 Model of a G protein-coupled receptor with seven membrane-spanning domains. These domains are folded in the membrane so that a pocket is formed for ligand binding on the extracellular surface of the receptor by the third, sixth and seventh domains (L). The intracellular loop connecting domains five and seven, together with the C-terminus, is the likely site (G) for binding to the G protein.

to the hydroxyl group in serine, threonine and tyrosine residues of substrate enzymes, markedly increasing their activity.

$$ATP + protein\text{-}OH \xrightarrow{PKA} ADP + protein\text{-}O\text{-}PO_3$$

Among the responses mediated by cAMP are increases in contraction of cardiac and skeletal muscle and glycogenolysis in the liver by adrenaline. PKAs consist of two regulatory (R) and two catalytic (C) subunits, and binding of cAMP to the R subunits causes the C subunits to dissociate and initiate phosphorylation. Each R subunit binds two cAMP molecules, but binding of the first molecule increases the binding affinity for the second subunit so that small changes in the cytostolic concentration of cAMP can produce large changes in the number of C subunits and hence in PKA activity. This, together with the ability of a single activated receptor to effect the conversion of up to 100 inactive G_s proteins to the active form (and each of these results in the synthesis of several hundred cAMP molecules), results in considerable signal amplification. For example, adrenaline concentrations as low as 10^{-10} mol l^{-1} can stimulate the release of glucose sufficient to increase blood glucose by 50%.

Activation of G_i protein-coupled receptors results in inhibition of AC and a fall in the intracellular concentration of cAMP. For example, noradrenaline acting on β-adrenoceptors (G_s coupled) increases cAMP levels, but when it acts on a_2 adrenoceptors (G_i coupled) it decreases cellular cAMP concentration. In addition to stimulating or inhibiting AC, G_s can directly stimulate voltage-gated Ca^{2+} channels in the atria in response to muscarinic M_2 receptor stimulation. Further, ion channel activity can be modified by increased or decreased channel phosphorylation subsequent to changes in intracellular levels of cAMP.

The phospholipase C pathway

This pathway is activated by binding of ligands to receptors coupled to either G_o or G_q proteins (Fig. 1.6). Among neurotransmitters using this pathway are acetylcholine (muscarinic M_1, M_3 or M_5 receptors), noradrenaline (a_{1A-C} adrenoceptors), histamine (H_1 receptor) and serotonin (5-HT_{1C} and 5-HT_2 receptors).

Table 1.2 G protein-coupled receptors, their effector systems and intracellular second messengers

G protein	Effector	Second messenger	Receptor
G_s	Adenylyl cyclase (+) Ca^{2+} channels (+)	↑ cAMP ↑ $[Ca^{2+}]_i$	Adrenergic (β_{1-3}) Dopamine (D_1, D_3, DA_1) Histamine (H_2) Adenosine (A_2) Serotonin (5-$HT_{4, 6, 7}$)
G_i	Adenylyl cyclase (−) K^+ channels (+)	↓ cAMP Hyperpolarization	Acetylcholine (M_2, M_4) Adrenergic (a_2) Dopamine (D_{2A}, D_3, D_4, DA_2) Adenosine (A_1) Histamine (H_3) Opioids (μ, δ, κ) Serotonin (5-$HT_{1A, 1C}$) $GABA_B$
G_q/G_o	Phospholipase C (+)	↑ IP_3, DAG	Acetylcholine (M_1, M_3, M_5) Adrenergic (a_1) Histamine (H_1) Adenosine (A_3) Dopamine (D_{2A}) Serotonin (5-HT_2)
$G_?$	Phospholipase A_2	↑ Arachidonic acid	Adrenergic (a_1) Adenosine (A_2) Serotonin (5-HT_{2A})

IP_3, inositol triphosphate; DAG, diacylglycerol; $[Ca^{2+}]_i$, intracellular Ca^{2+} concentration; cAMP, cyclic adenosine monophosphate; 5-HT, 5-hydroxytryptamine; GABA, γ-aminobutyric acid.

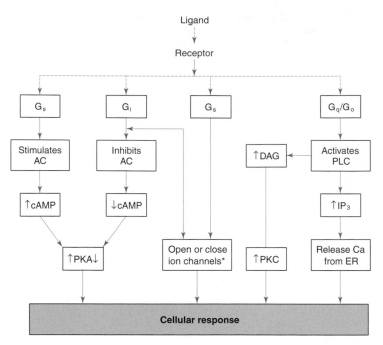

Fig. 1.6 Pathways involved in cellular signalling initiated by agonist binding to G protein-coupled receptors.* G_s-coupled receptors open Ca^{2+} and close K^+ channels, depolarizing the cell, while G_i-coupled receptors close Ca^{2+} and open K^+ channels, hyperpolarizing the cell. PKA, protein kinase A or cyclic adenosine monophosphate (cAMP)-dependent protein kinases; PKC, protein kinase C; ER, endoplasmic reticulum; AC, adenylyl cyclase; PLC, phospholipase C; IP_3, inositol triphosphate; DAG, diacylglycerol.

G_o and G_q proteins activate phospholipase C (PLC), which hydrolyses phosphotidylinositol 4,5-bisphosphate (PIP_2), one of several inositol phospholipids found in the cytosolic leaflet of the plasma membrane. Hydrolysis of PIP_2 yields two second messengers: IP_3 and DAG. IP_3, which is water soluble, diffuses through the cytoplasm and interacts with IP_3-sensitive Ca^{2+} channels in the membrane of the endoplasmic reticulum (ER), stimulating the release of stored calcium. The calcium binds to cytostolic calmodulin, which then activates other enzymes (e.g. myosin in muscle). Each calmodulin molecule binds four calcium ions in a cooperative fashion (i.e. binding of one Ca^{2+} facilitates binding of additional ions), so that a small change in cytosolic Ca^{2+} concentration leads to a large change in the level of active calmodulin, another example of signal amplification. The PLC–IP_3 pathway is also stimulated by receptor tyrosine kinases. IP_3 is rapidly degraded, within 1 s of its formation, to inactive inositol diphosphate and then to inositol.

In muscle cells and neurons a second mechanism exists for the release of intracellular Ca^{2+}, involving ryanodine receptors in the ER membrane. This pathway is activated by an action potential opening a plasma membrane voltage-gated Ca^{2+} channel, allowing a small influx of extracellular Ca^{2+}. Binding of Ca^{2+} to the ryanodine receptor triggers a massive release of Ca^{2+} from the ER stores.

The DAG produced by the hydrolysis of PIP_2 by PLC remains in the plasma membrane where it activates a family of membrane-associated protein kinases collectively termed protein kinase C (PKC). Activation of PKC requires a rise in the intracellular levels of both Ca^{2+} and DAG. Activated PKC produces a variety of cellular responses, including the regulation of protein synthesis and key metabolic pathways.

ACETYLCHOLINE MUSCARINIC RECEPTOR

Acetylcholine is the physiological agonist for two receptors, the nicotinic receptor and the muscarinic receptor. These receptors are completely different entities: the nicotinic receptor is a ligand-gated ion channel whereas the muscarinic receptor is a G protein-coupled receptor. Therapeutically, drugs acting at this receptor include muscarinic antagonists such as atropine and anticholinesterases (e.g. neostigmine and edrophonium) which stimulate the receptor indirectly by preventing the breakdown of acetylcholine.

To date, five muscarinic acetylcholine receptor sub-types have been identified, M_1 to M_5. Muscarinic receptors are widely distributed throughout the CNS, in cardiac and smooth muscle, and in exocrine, endocrine and paracrine glands. The M_1, M_3 and M_5 receptors are coupled to G_o and G_q proteins, and activate IP_3 and DAG to mediate hydrolysis of membrane phospholipids and release of Ca^{2+} from intercellular stores. This opens a calcium-gated K^+ channel and hyperpolarizes the cell.

The M_2 and M_4 muscarinic receptors activate G_i proteins to decrease cAMP concentration. In the heart M_2 receptor activation also opens inwardly, rectifying K^+ channels via a direct action of G_i proteins on the channel, and this is responsible for the cardiac side-effects of anticholinergic drugs.[24] Anticholinergic drugs such as atropine are nonselective antagonists at all five muscarinic receptors, although the increase in heart rate caused by atropine may be mediated selectively through M_2 receptor-mediated action on K^+ channels. The tachycardia produced by pancuronium and gallamine may also be due to a similar mechanism. Brain muscarinic signalling is important in the modulation of consciousness, and in learning and memory, and actions of anaesthetic agents at these sites probably contribute to the mechanisms of general anaesthesia.[24] Muscarinic receptors in the spinal cord are involved in nociception, and intrathecal administration of cholinergic agonists or anticholinesterases produces a potent antinociceptive effect.[25]

ADRENERGIC RECEPTORS

Since Ahlquist first proposed the existence of two adrenoceptor subtypes, α and β, in 1948 this class of receptors has been investigated extensively and a large number of valuable drugs have been introduced that are either agonists or antagonists at one or other of these receptors. The number of known receptors has also expanded considerably, and at present nine distinct adrenoceptor subtypes have been identified. There are two subtypes of the α receptor (α_1 and α_2, with subfamilies of each of these) and three subtypes of the β receptor (β_1, β_2 and β_3). The adrenoceptors are G protein-coupled receptors, but second messenger and G-protein linkage differ between the subtypes. α_1-Adrenoceptor activation increases the level of PLC via a G_q protein, resulting in an increase in intracellular calcium.

Another mechanism of α_1-adrenoceptor-mediated responses involves the influx of extracellular calcium through voltage-gated Ca^{2+} channels. This mechanism is possibly more important for α_1 agonists with lower intrinsic efficacy. It has been postulated that α_1 receptors in vascular smooth muscle are linked to two G proteins, one mediating PLC activation, the other linked to a Ca^{2+} channel. Full agonists can activate both G proteins, while partial agonists can activate only the latter. α_2-Adrenoceptors are coupled to a G_i protein and inhibit AC. The three β adrenoceptors mediate G_s protein-linked stimulation of AC, although in cardiac muscle there may also be a direct link between the G_s protein

and a voltage-gated calcium channel. While many drugs act directly on adrenergic receptors, others act indirectly by influencing the synthesis, uptake or metabolism of endogenous cathecholamines such as monoamine oxidase inhibitors, tricyclic antidepressants and ephedrine.

The α_1 and β adrenoceptors are located on the postsynaptic junction of sympathetic nerve terminals innervating smooth muscles and endocrine glands or cardiac cells (β_1). Most vasoconstrictor responses to sympathetic stimulation are mediated by α_1 adrenoceptors. In general α_2 and β_2 receptors are prejunctional adrenergic neuronal membranes, and inhibit and facilitate, respectively, the release of noradrenaline. Prejunctional α_2 adrenoceptors also exist on cholinergic neurons and inhibit the release of acetylcholine. The three β-adrenoceptor subtypes have markedly different tissue distribution. The β_1 adrenoceptor is present mainly in the heart, where it is the target for β-adrenoceptor antagonists and agonist inotropic drugs. The β_2 adrenoceptor is found in skeletal muscle, the uterus and in bronchial smooth muscle, where β_2 agonists act as bronchodilators. The main location for the β_3 adrenoceptor is adipose tissue, where it seems to regulate noradrenaline-induced changes in energy metabolism and thermogenesis.[26] The physiological role of this receptor in other tissues is unclear.

DOPAMINE RECEPTORS

Dopamine is a major neurotransmitter which acts on multiple receptors. It can activate both α and β adrenoceptors in addition to acting on specific dopamine receptors. These are widely distributed throughout the CNS and are also present in the renal tubules and in renal and mesenteric blood vessels, and many dopaminergic drugs are used in the treatment of Parkinson's disease, in psychiatric disorders, as antiemetics and for renal protection. Neuroleptic drugs such as haloperidol and droperidol are dopamine receptor antagonists.

Six CNS and two peripheral dopamine receptors have been identified by pharmacological means. CNS receptors are designated 'D' and those in the periphery as 'DA'. Those in the CNS are postsynaptic receptors, belonging to two major classes, D_1 and D_2, but recent cloning experiments have expanded this number to D_3, D_4 and D_5. The new receptors appear to have restricted localization to the limbic and frontal cortical areas of the brain. They all bind neuroleptic drugs, and the D_4 receptor has a notably high affinity for clozapine. They may thus be involved in the aetiology of schizophrenia. Presynaptic dopamine receptors appear to be exclusively D_2. Central D_1 and D_3 receptors and peripheral DA_1 receptors increase, whereas D_{2A}, D_3, D_4 and DA_2

receptors decrease, the level of cAMP. D_{2A} receptor activation also increases intracellular IP_3 and DAG levels. The antiemetic agent, metoclopramide, is a dopamine antagonist whose central effects are mediated via D_2 receptors in the chemotherapeutic trigger zone (CTZ) in the area postrema.

The effect of low concentrations of dopamine in enhancing urine output is due to its action on DA_1 receptors in the renal vasculature. Dopexamine, which is especially useful in preserving the mesenteric circulation in shock states, is a DA_1 agonist with β_2-adrenoceptor agonist properties. Fenoldopam, a recently developed selective dopaminergic DA_1 receptor agonist, is a rapidly acting vasodilating agent effective in the management of severe, including postoperative, hypertension, and may be a useful alternative to currently available standard therapies such as nitroprusside.[27] Unlike dopamine, it provides maximum dopaminergic effects without adrenergic stimulation.

ADENOSINE RECEPTORS

Adenosine belongs to a biologically important group of substances known as autacoids, which act on their cell of origin or on neighbouring cells. The term autocoid is derived from the Greek *autos* ('self') and *akos* ('medicine' or 'remedy'). Adenosine is a purine nucleotide found throughout the body, but with highest concentrations in the CNS. It is a potent peripheral vasodilator in all vascular beds except the kidney and placenta, where it produces vasoconstriction through A_2 receptor activation. In the heart adenosine has anti-arrhythmic properties, possibly due to a shortening of the atrial action potential duration and membrane hyperpolarization resulting from increased K^+ conductance.

Adenosine interacts with at least four different G protein-coupled receptors, A_1, A_{2A}, A_{2B} and A_3. The A_1 receptor is coupled to the inhibitory G_i protein and the A_2 receptor to the stimulatory G_s protein, and respectively inhibit or activate AC, whereas the A_3 receptor mediates G protein-dependent activation of PLC. There is antagonistic interaction between adenosine A_{2A} and dopamine D_2 receptors, whereby stimulation of A_{2A} receptors decreases the affinity of agonists for the D_2 receptor. There may also be an interaction at the second messenger level, since A_{2A} receptor activation stimulates while D_2 receptor activation inhibits AC.[28] This mechanism may play a role in the behavioural response to xanthines such as caffeine and theophylline. These are adenosine A_{2A} receptor antagonists and they mimic the motor stimulation produced by dopamine secondary to block of adenosine actions. A few cups of coffee contains sufficient caffeine to occupy 50% of adenosine receptors, antagonizing adenosine-induced neuronal inhibition.

The physiological role of the A_3 receptor is unclear, but one function is to facilitate degranulation of mast cells, and a role for mast cells and A_3 receptors in mediating myocardial preconditioning has been proposed. Selective A_3 antagonists might, therefore, have potential for the treatment of allergic, inflammatory and possibly ischaemic disorders. Adenosine is normally present in the extracellular fluid of the brain, as in most body tissues, and its concentration increases rapidly following ischaemia. There is evidence that in cerebral ischaemia adenosine may have protective effects, since it inhibits the release of many excitatory neurotransmitters such as glutamate, and it also stabilizes the membrane potential. In addition, adenosine may improve cerebral blood flow and depress the formation of free oxygen radicals. Both A_1 and A_2, and possibly A_3, receptors may be involved in this neuroprotective effect. Unfortunately, adenosine has an extremely short half-life, but recently nucleoside (adenosine) transport inhibitors (e.g. nitrobenzyl-thioinosine, draflazine) have been developed which prevent the endothelial uptake and breakdown of adenosine and prolong its beneficial effects. Nucleoside transport inhibitors also have myocardial protective properties and may have an important role in organ preservation before transplantation.[29] Adenosine also has an antinociceptive function and various adenosine analogues have antinociceptive activity, which correlates with their affinity for the A_1 receptors, although a delayed analgesic effect associated with A_2 receptors has been described.[30] This antinociceptive action probably involves interactions between NMDA, adenosine and nitric oxide in the spinal cord.

5-HT (SEROTONIN) RECEPTORS

Serotonin (5-hydroxytryptamine, 5-HT) is another neurotransmitter that binds to multiple types of receptors. At least 14 subtypes of 5-HT receptors have been described, belonging to seven families, 5-HT_1 to 5-HT_7, widely distributed throughout the CNS and the cardiovascular and gastrointestinal systems. Apart from 5-HT_3 (a ligand-gated ion channel), 5-HT receptors are G protein-coupled receptors (Table 1.3).

5-HT_{1A} and 5-HT_{1D} receptors function as 'autoreceptors' that control the release of 5-HT and other neurotransmitters. A class of second-generation anxiolytics, the azapirones (buspirone, ipsapirone, gepirone), are selective agonists or partial agonists at the 5-HT_{1A} receptor. These drugs have a weak affinity for dopamine receptors but no activity at $GABA_A$ receptors. They cause minimal sedation and do not appear to have potential for drug abuse or dependence. Ketanserin is the prototype 5-HT_2 antagonist. It blocks 5-HT_{2A} receptors potently and has no significant effect on other 5-HT receptors. However, ketanserin also has high

Table 1.3 Summary of interactions between 5-HT and G proteins

Receptor subtype	G protein	Action on effector protein	Second messenger
5-HT$_{1A}$ 5-HT$_{1B}$	G$_i$	Inhibits AC	↓ cAMP
5-HT$_{1A}$	G$_k$	Opens K$^+$ channel	↑ K$^+$ current
5-HT$_{1C}$ 5-HT$_2$	G$_q$/G$_o$	Activates PLC	↑ IP$_3$, ↑ DAG
5-HT$_{2A}$	G$_?$	Activates PLA$_2$	↑ Arachidonic acid
5-HT$_4$ 5-HT$_6$ 5-HT$_7$	G$_s$	Stimulates AC	↑ cAMP

AC, adenylyl cyclase; cAMP, cyclic adenosine monophosphate; PLC, phospholipase C; PLA$_2$, phospholipase A$_2$; IP$_3$, inositol triphosphate; DAG, diacylglycerol; 5-HT, 5-hydroxytryptamine.

affinity for α adrenoceptors and histamine H$_1$ receptors. The physiological function of the 5-HT$_4$ receptor is as yet unknown but may be involved in the regulation of gastrointestinal function. The only currently available 5-HT$_4$ agonist is cisapride, which activates excitatory presynaptic 5-HT$_4$ receptors of cholinergic neurons in the gastrointestinal tract, increasing the release of acetylcholine from the nerve terminals. Cisapride is thus a prokinetic drug and is used to increase gastro-intestinal contractions and propulsion. A number of other selective 5-HT$_4$ agonists are in various stages of development for the treatment of gastrointestinal disorders.

Alterations in 5-HT neurotransmission may be involved in a variety of neuropsychiatric disorders, including depression and generalized anxiety disorders. Although the precise role of 5-HT in the aetiology of these diseases is still unclear, many of the drugs used in their treatment in some way alter the serotonergic system. Tricyclic antidepressants and electroconvulsive therapy sensitize postsynaptic neurons to 5-HT, monoamine oxidase inhibitors increase the availability of 5-HT, while the newer selective serotonin reuptake inhibitors (e.g. fluoxetine, sertraline) increase the efficacy of 5-HT neurons by desensitizing 5-HT auto-receptors located on 5-HT nerve terminals.[31] Some of the newer drugs used in the treatment of schizophre-nia, such as clozapine and risperidone, are combined 5-HT$_{2A/2C}$ and dopamine D$_2$ receptor antagonists. Clozapine also has a high affinity for 5-HT$_6$ and 5-HT$_7$ receptors, but it is unclear whether this contributes to its clinical actions. The appetite-suppressant drugs, fluoxetine and D-fenfluramine, alter feeding behaviour by increasing extracellular brain 5-HT levels and also by acting directly at 5-HT$_{2C}$ receptors and possibly at other 5-HT receptors.

Methysergide, used for the prophylactic treatment of migraine and other vascular headaches, is a 5-HT$_{2A/2C}$ antagonist, although it is not selective and also blocks 5-HT$_1$ receptors. It inhibits the vasoconstrictor and pressor effects of 5-HT. The newest and most effective drug for the treatment of acute migraine attacks is sumatriptan, a selective 5-HT$_{1D}$ receptor agonist. Its antimigraine effect is thought to be due to constriction of intracranial blood vessels, restoring vascular tone and/or blockade of neural transmission and neurogenic inflammation.[32] An additional benefit is that, unlike most other antimigraine drugs, it inhibits rather than enhances the emetic symptoms normally associated with a migraine attack.

GABA$_B$ RECEPTORS

GABA$_B$ receptors are located on the presynaptic nerve terminals of neurons that secrete neurotransmitters such as GABA, glutamate, 5-HT or noradrenaline, and operate as neuromodulators. They are coupled via G proteins to K$^+$ and Ca^{2+} ion channels and mediate late IPSPs, inhibiting neurotransmitter and neuropeptide release. GABA$_A$ and GABA$_B$ receptors are both present in the spinal cord where they are involved in nociception and maintenance of muscle tone. Baclofen, the only currently available selective GABA$_B$ receptor agonist, is used to treat muscle spasticity. GABA$_B$ recep-tor antagonists may have therapeutic potential as anti-depressants, anticonvulsants and for the improvement of memory and cognitive function.[33]

RECEPTORS WITH INTRINSIC ENZYME ACTIVITY

This is a large group of ligand-activated receptors that pass through the plasma membrane of the cell only once. Ligand binding on the extracellular domain effects activation of the cytosolic domain, which possesses the intrinsic enzyme activity. These receptors fall into two main classes: protein kinases that phosphorylase either tyrosine or serine residues in their target proteins and whose endogenous ligands include insulin and a variety of other growth-related factors, and guanylyl cyclase. Ligand binding to kinase receptors initiates multiple intracellular events with both immediate (e.g. activation of PLC) and long-term (e.g. cell growth) consequences. In addition, receptor activation can stimulate the generation of IP_3 and DAG second messengers by a mechanism that is distinct from that of G protein-coupled receptors.

The other family of receptors with intrinsic enzyme activity is the membrane-bound guanylyl cyclase. This family includes cell membrane receptors activated by atrial, cardiac or brain natriuretic factors, and cytosolic receptors associated with nitric oxide. These receptors catalyse the formation of cGMP from cGTP. cGMP acts as a second messenger and can either act directly on target molecules (e.g. ion channels) or activate cGMP-dependent phosphorylation of many proteins, resulting in a wide variety of metabolic changes. For example, a cGMP phosphodiesterase can be activated that lowers the intracellular concentrations of cAMP. Activation of soluble guanylyl cyclase to produce cGMP is one of the primary ways in which nitric oxide, now recognized as an important cellular messenger, mediates cellular and intracellular communication.[34]

INTRACELLULAR RECEPTORS

In addition to plasma membrane receptors, some cells also have receptors on the membrane of the nucleus or soluble receptors in the cytosol. Examples are steroids, thyroid hormones, and vitamins A and D, which exert their effects by binding to intracellular receptors that control specific gene transcription and expression. The steroid receptor in its inactive form is present in the cytoplasm associated with other proteins. Binding of a steroid molecule results in dissociation of the receptor, exposing a specific recognition site for binding to DNA. The activated hormone – receptor complex then enters the nucleus where it binds to specific regions of DNA called the hormone response elements. This initiates the transcription of genetic material resulting in new protein production. When the receptor is not occupied by a steroid it has a negative regulatory function to prevent the gene from being transcribed, so no proteins are produced. One of the characteristics of hormone and drug effects mediated by intracellular receptors is a comparatively slow response time (minutes to hours) because of this requirement of new protein synthesis. Conversely, the effects persist after withdrawal of the agonist.

REFERENCES

1. Chidiac P, Hebert TE, Valiquette M, Dennis M, Bouvier M. Inverse agonist activity of β-adrenergic antagonists. *Mol Pharmacol* 1994; **45**: 490–499.
2. Lysko GS, Robinson JL, Casto R, Ferrone RA. The stereospecific effects of isoflurane isomers in vivo. *Eur J Pharmacol* 1994; **263**: 25–29.
3. White PF, Schuttler J, Shafer A, Stanski DR, Horai Y, Trevor AJ. Comparative pharmacology of the ketamine isomers. Studies in volunteers. *Br J Anaesth* 1985; **57**: 197–203.
4. Denson DD, Behbehani MM, Gregg RV. Enantiomer-specific effects of an intravenously administered arrhythmogenic dose of bupivacaine on neurons of the nucleus tractus solitarius and the cardiovascular system in the anesthetized rat. *Reg Anesth* 1992; **17**: 311–316.
5. Katz AM. Cardiac ion channels. *N Engl J Med* 1993; **328**: 1244–1251.
6. Catterall WA. Structure and function of voltage-sensitive ion channels. *Science* 1988; **242**: 50–61.
7. Noma A. ATP-regulated K$^+$ channels in cardiac muscle. *Nature* 1983; **305**: 147–148.
8. Lazdunski M. ATP-sensitive potassium channels: an overview. *J Cardiovasc Pharmacol* 1994; **24** (Suppl. 4): S1–S5.
9. Godfraind T, Govoni S. Recent advances in the pharmacology of Ca^{2+} and K$^+$ channels. *Trends Pharmacol Sci* 1995; **16**: 1–4.
10. Terrar DA. Structure and function of calcium channels and the actions of anaesthetics. *Br J Anaesth* 1993; **71**: 39–46.
11. Mishra SK, Hermsmeyer K. Selective inhibition of T-type Ca^{2+} channels by RO 40–5967. *Circ Res* 1994; **75**: 144–148.
12. Clozet J-P, Pordy R, Pitt B. Miberfradil: the first L- and T-calcium antagonist. In: Messerli FH (ed.) *Cardiovascular Drug Therapy*, 2nd edn. Philadelphia: WB Saunders, 1996: Ch. 108, pp. 1009–1015.
13. McDowell TS, Pancrazio JJ, Lynch C. Volatile anesthetics reduce low-voltage-activated calcium currents in a thyroid C-cell line. *Anesthesiology* 1996; **85**: 1167–1175.
14. Hirota K, Lambert DG. Voltage-sensitive Ca^{2+} channels and anaesthesia. *Br J Anaesth* 1996; **76**: 344–346.
15. Louis CF, Zualkernan K, Roghair T, Mickelson JR. The effects of volatile anesthetics on calcium regulation by malignant hyperthermia-susceptible sarcoplasmic reticulum. *Anesthesiology* 1992; **77**: 114–125.
16. Nelson TE. Halothane effects on human malignant hyperthermia skeletal muscle single calcium-release channels in planar lipid bilayers. *Anesthesiology* 1992; **76**: 588–595.
17. Tonner PH, Miller KW. Molecular sites of general anaesthetic action on acetylcholine receptors. *Eur J Anaesthesiol* 1995; **12**: 21–30.
18. Krogsgaard-Larsen P, Frølund B, Jørgensen FS, Schousboe A. GABA$_A$ receptor agonists, partial agonists and antagonists. Design and therapeutic prospects. *J Med Chem* 1994; **37**: 2489–2505.
19. MacDonald RL, Olsen RW. GABA$_A$ receptor channels. *Annu Rev Neurosci* 1994; **17**: 569–602.
20. Robertson B. Actions of anaesthetics and avermectin on GABA$_A$ chloride channels in mammalian dorsal root ganglion neurons. *Br J Pharmacol* 1989; **98**: 167–176.
21. Hales TG, Lambert JJ. The actions of propofol on inhibitory amino acid receptors of bovine adrenomedullary chromaffin cells and rodent central neurones. *Br J Pharmacol* 1991; **104**: 619–628.

22. Daw NW, Stein PSG, Fox K. The role of the NMDA receptors in information processing. *Ann Rev Neurosci* 1993; **16**: 207–222.

23. Greenshaw AJ. Behavioural pharmacology of 5-HT$_3$ receptor antagonists: a critical update on therapeutic potential. *Trends Pharmacol Sci* 1993; **14**: 265–270.

24. Durieux ME. Muscarinic signalling in the central nervous system. *Anesthesiology* 1996; **84**: 173–189.

25. Collins JG. Spinally administered neostigmine – something to celebrate. *Anesthesiology* 1995; **82**: 327–328.

26. Strosberg AD, Pietri-Rouxel F. Function and regulation of the β_3-adrenoceptor. *Trends Pharmacol Sci* 1996; **17**: 373–381.

27. Hill AJ, Feneck RO, Walesby RK. A comparison of fenoldopam and nitroprusside in the control of hypertension following coronary artery surgery. *J Cardiothorac Vasc Anesth* 1993; **7**: 279–284.

28. Ongini E, Fredholm BB. Pharmacology of adenosine A$_{2A}$ receptors. *Trends Pharmacol Sci* 1996; **17**: 364–371.

29. Masuda M, Sukehiro S, Mollhoff T, Van Belle H, Flameng W. Effect of nucleoside transport inhibition on adenosine and hypoxanthine accumulation in the ischemic human myocardium. *Arch Int Pharmacodyn Ther* 1993; **322**: 45–54.

30. Lipkowski AW, Maszcz-Yuska I. Peptide, *N*-methyl-D-aspartate and adenosine receptors as analgesic targets. *Curr Opin Anaesth* 1996; **9**: 443–448.

31. Blier P, de Montigny C, Chaput Y. A role for the serotonin system in the mechanism of action of antidepressant treatments: preclinical evidence. *J Clin Psychiatry* 1990; **51** (Suppl 4): 14–21.

32. Ferrari MD, Saxena PR. Clinical and experimental effects of sumatriptan in humans. *Trends Pharmacol Sci* 1993; **14**: 129–133.

33. Bittiger H, Froestl W, Mickel S, Olpe HR. GABA$_B$ receptor antagonists: from synthesis to therapeutic applications. *Trends Pharmacol Sci* 1993; **14**: 391–394.

34. Schmidt HHHW, Lokmann SM, Walter U. The nitric oxide and cGMP signal transduction system: regulation and mechanism of action. *Biochim Biophys Acta* 1993; **1178**: 153–175.

PRINCIPLES OF PHARMACOKINETICS

Anaesthetists, more than any other medical professionals, are responsible for the acute administration of potent drugs with profound consequences for the vital functions of their patients. It is crucial that such drugs are administered in a manner that avoids systemic toxicity resulting from overdosing but, at the same time, achieves adequate anaesthesia. To meet these requirements, drug concentrations must be kept within a narrow therapeutic range. During operation, drug concentrations need to be increased or decreased depending on surgical or anaesthetic circumstances. At the end of the operation the concentrations must be reduced to levels that permit fast return of consciousness. Pharmacokinetics is the study of drug disposition and deals with the processes of absorption, distribution, metabolism and elimination. The purpose of this chapter is to discuss these processes and to develop some of the principles that describe their kinetics.

DRUG ABSORPTION

To reach their site of action, most drugs must first enter the systemic circulation (unless injected intravenously), from where they must be transported to a target organ and subsequently act at a cellular or subcellular level. This requires that the drug successfully traverses one or more cellular membranes.

THE CELL MEMBRANE

The typical cell membrane is 10 nm thick and is composed of a bimolecular layer of phospholipids. Phospholipid molecules consist of a polar or hydrophilic (water attracting) region connected to a nonpolar or hydrophobic (water repelling) region. The molecules are arranged in parallel, oriented such that the polar regions face either to the outside or the inside of the cell, whereas the inner part of the membrane consists of a lipid hydrophobic core. The membranes contain proteins, some of which serve as ion channels or receptors for endogenous substances or drugs. The membrane is a dynamic structure whose primary function is to maintain a constant environment within the cell by selectively transporting substances into and out of the cell. Drugs cross cell membranes by a process of either *simple diffusion* or *carrier transport*.

Simple diffusion

This is a passive process whereby a drug moves under the influence of a concentration gradient. The rate of diffusion is directly proportional to the magnitude of the concentration gradient, the cross-sectional area over which the process occurs, and inversely proportional to the thickness of the membrane. The rate of diffusion is also related to the nature of the membrane, and some membranes pose more of an obstacle than others. The basement membrane upon which the endothelial cells of the brain capillaries are attached and through which drugs must pass to reach the brain (the *blood–brain barrier*) is tightly applied to the underlying astrocyte cells. The endothelial cells themselves are tightly bound to one another by so-called 'tight junctions'. This membrane is a more formidable obstacle than the membrane of endothelial cells at other sites in the body.

Carrier transport

The drug combines with a carrier protein and the drug–protein complex is transported across the membrane, whereafter the drug is released and the carrier protein returns to the exterior of the membrane. Carrier-mediated transport is characterized by the net movement of a substance against a concentration gradient, which may be large. Carrier transport mechanisms are more important in elimination or secretory processes than for absorption. They tend to be energy dependent, specific and unidirectional.

DRUG PENETRATION OF THE CELL MEMBRANE

The ability of a drug to penetrate cell membranes is determined by its chemical structure and physico-chemical properties. Three properties are of particular importance: degree of ionization, protein binding and lipid affinity. The ability of a drug to cross the cell membrane is determined by its overall profile with respect to each of these properties and not necessarily by any one of them taken in isolation.

Degree of ionization

Most drugs are either weak acids or weak bases (Table 2.1) and exist in physiological fluids in both ionized and un-ionized states. The un-ionized drug is 1000 to 10 000 times more lipid soluble than the ionized state and thus is able to penetrate the cell membrane more easily. An acid is a substance that donates protons more readily than it accepts them, whereas a base accepts protons more readily than it donates them. Weak acids or bases are those that do not completely dissociate in solution. For an acid, dissociation in solution is represented by:

$$\text{HA} \quad \rightleftharpoons \quad \text{H}^+ + \text{A}^-$$
$$\text{un-ionized} \qquad\quad \text{ionized}$$

The dissociation constant, K_a, defined by the equation

$$K_a = \frac{[\text{H}^+][\text{A}^-]}{[\text{HA}]}$$

is a measure of the strength of an acid. Most acidic drugs are weak acids with pK_a ($= \log_{10}[K_a]^{-1}$) values greater than 7 (Table 2.1). Rearranging the above equation and converting to logarithmic form gives the *Henderson–Hasselbach equation*:

$$pK_a = \log_{10}\frac{[\text{HA}]}{[\text{A}^-]} + pH$$

or

$$\log_{10}\frac{[\text{HA}]}{[\text{A}^-]} = pK_a - pH$$

This equation describes the relationship between the proportion of un-ionized and ionized forms of drug and pH (Fig. 2.1a). For example, thiopentone is a weak acid with pK_a of 7.6. In solutions with a pH lower than 7.6, the ratio [HA]/[A$^-$] is greater than 1 and thus the drug exists predominantly as the un-ionized [HA] form. When pH = pK_a, the term $\log_{10}$ [HA]/[A$^-$] = 0 so that [HA]/[A$^-$] = 1 and the ionized and un-ionized fractions are equal. This gives an alternative definition of pK_a as the pH of a solution in which a substance is 50% ionized and 50% un-ionized. When pH is greater than

Bases	pK_a	Acids	pK_a
Table 2.1 pK_a of some drugs used in anaesthesia			
Weak		Strong	
Diazepam	3.7	Salicylic acid	3
Etomidate	4.1	Frusemide	3.9
Midazolam	6.15		
Alfentanil	6.5		
Ketamine	7.5	Thiopentone	7.6
Lignocaine	7.8	Methohexitone	7.9
Bupivacaine	8.2	Atropine	8.9
Fentanyl	8.4	Paracetamol	9.5
Morphine	8.6		
		Propofol	11
Strong		Weak	

pK_a the ionized [A$^-$] form predominates. At pH 7.4 thiopentone is 61.3% un-ionized, and it is this form that is able to penetrate the blood–brain barrier to reach the site of action.

For a base:

$$\text{BH}^+ \quad \rightleftharpoons \quad \text{H}^+ + \text{B}^-$$
$$\text{ionized} \qquad\quad \text{un-ionized}$$

with the dissociation constant K_a defined by the relationship:

$$K_a = \frac{[\text{B}][\text{H}^+]}{[\text{BH}^+]}$$

The Henderson–Hasselbach equation for a base is:

$$\log_{10}\frac{[\text{B}]}{[\text{BH}^+]} = pH - pK_a$$

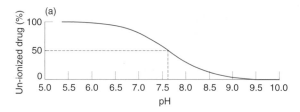

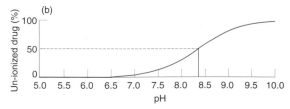

Fig. 2.1 Relationship between pH and the percentage of drug in the un-ionized form, for (a) a weak acid (thiopentone; pK_a 7.6) and (b) a weak base (fentanyl; pK_a 8.4).

The relative proportion of the base that is un-ionized can thus be calculated for a given pH. A base exists predominantly as the ionized form at pH less than pK_a, and when pH is greater than pK_a the un-ionized form predominates. This is illustrated in Fig. 2.1b for the basic drug fentanyl (pK_a 8.4).

Protein binding

Most drugs are bound to plasma proteins. Acidic drugs tend to have a high affinity for albumin whereas basic drugs have a high affinity for a_1-acid glycoprotein (AAG). AAG is present in only small amounts in the plasma and can easily be saturated by high concentrations of drug. Only the nonprotein-bound fraction or 'free' concentration of a drug is pharmacologically active since the large size of the binding protein precludes its penetration of the cell membrane.[1] Protein binding is the mechanism whereby lipid-soluble drugs are carried to their site of action. The binding reaction is usually reversible:

Drug–protein complex ⇌ Free drug + Protein

In the tissues, where the concentration of free drug is low, the drug–protein complex dissociates. Certain physiological or pathological situations can significantly alter the concentration of plasma proteins and thereby alter the concentration of 'free' drug available for pharmacological action. These can be classified as follows.

Decreased Plasma Proteins

| Age: | Serum albumin concentration tends to decrease with age. AAG concentration is low in the neonate. |

Malnutrition:	May result from poor diet or as a consequence of hyper-catabolic states (e.g. after major surgery, trauma or burns), hepatic disease or cachexia due to malignancy.
Dilutional states:	Excessive fluid therapy, pregnancy.
Protein-losing diseases:	Enteropathies, nephropathies.

Increased Plasma Protein

Disease states. AAG is an acute-phase reactant whose concentration is raised as a response to numerous acute and chronic conditions (e.g. trauma, burns, myocardial infarction, malignancy) and inflammatory diseases such as ulcerative colitis and rheumatoid arthritis.

Displacement reactions. Drugs may compete for the same binding sites on carrier proteins and thus one drug can displace a less tightly bound one and thereby increase the 'free' concentration of the second drug. Thus warfarin can displace salicylates, tolbutamide and sulphonamides from albumin. The consequences of these disturbances will usually be significant only for drugs that are highly protein bound. For example, for a drug that is only 40% bound, a 20% decrease in binding capacity will increase the unbound fraction from 60% to 68%, an increase of 13%. For a drug that is 95% bound the concentration of free drug will increase from 5% to 24%, an increase of 480%. However, the extra 'free' drug will be 'diluted' in the body water so that the increase in free drug concentration will be less than expected. The extra free drug will also be available for elimination or binding to alternative tissue sites. The net result is to mitigate the consequences of the initial displacement reaction (Fig. 2.2).

The *diffusible fraction* is the product of the nonbound fraction and the un-ionized fraction. As an example, the diffusible fractions of four opioids are shown in Table 2.2. It is apparent that the diffusible fraction alone does

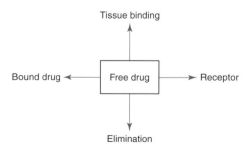

Fig. 2.2 Diagram showing possible interactions for the 'free' form of a drug, i.e. drug not bound to protein.

not determine overall membrane-penetrating potential since the diffusible fraction of morphine is only half that of alfentanil and twice that of sufentanil or fentanyl, while these drugs have very different clinical profiles in terms of potency and onset of action. The reason for this difference lies partly in the differing fat solubilities of these drugs.

Lipid solubility

Since cell membranes are lipid structures, it is not surprising that lipid solubility plays an important role in drug transport across the membrane. Small, un-ionized, lipid-soluble drugs can penetrate cell membranes with ease. Ionized forms of all drugs are poorly lipid soluble and therefore play little part in membrane transport. Lipid solubility is characterized by the partition coefficient between oil and water or between an alcohol such as octanol and water (λ_{ow}).

DRUG ADMINISTRATION AND ABSORPTION

When a drug is given intravenously, all of the drug immediately enters the systemic circulation (the drug is 100% *bioavailable*). However, for administration by other routes, the process whereby the drug eventually reaches the bloodstream must be considered. The purpose of this section is to discuss these alternative routes of administration, which, in contrast to the intravenous route, have potentially slower, less complete and less predictable bioavailability to the systemic circulation.

ENTERAL ADMINISTRATION

The oral route has the advantages of convenience and patient acceptability. However, many drugs are susceptible to degradation or modification at the low pH in the stomach. Absorption from the stomach is notoriously variable and is highly dependent on the way in which a drug is formulated. The gastrointestinal transit time is a further source of variability. Absorption of drug through the gastric mucosa is highly dependent on the un-ionized fraction at gastric pH (approximately 2). Acidic drugs tend to be completely un-ionized at this pH and diffuse readily, whereas basic drugs are predominantly ionized and are therefore poorly absorbed from the stomach. In the small intestine, where the pH is 6–7, basic drugs will be better absorbed than acidic drugs.

After absorption through the gastric or intestinal mucosa, drugs pass via the portal vein to the liver. For drugs that undergo extensive hepatic metabolism, only a proportion of the drug presented to the liver will enter the systemic circulation. This is known as *first-pass* or *presystemic metabolism*. Drugs that undergo extensive presystemic metabolism usually demonstrate significant interindividual variability in drug absorption. Food intake increases liver blood flow and can increase the bioavailability of drugs such as propranolol by increasing the amount of drug presented to the liver above its capacity to metabolize it. Alternative routes of drug delivery such as rectal, sublingual or transdermal administration avoid presystemic metabolism.

SUBLINGUAL ADMINISTRATION

The sublingual surface area is relatively small but has a rich blood supply. The major advantage of this route is avoidance of intestinal destruction and hepatic first-pass metabolism. However, absorption can be highly variable; critical factors are the residence time of the drug in the mouth and saliva flow. Premature swallowing or excessive saliva production preclude efficient absorption. Nitroglycerin, nifedipine, propranolol and buprenorphine are all available as sublingual preparations.

RECTAL ROUTE

The venous drainage of the upper part of the rectum drains to the portal system, whereas the lower part

Table 2.2 **Diffusible fraction of opiate analgesics at pH 7.4**			
	Nonprotein bound (%)	Un-ionized (%)	Diffusible fraction (%)[*]
Alfentanil	10	89	8.9
Sufentanil	10	20	2
Fentanyl	20	9	1.8
Morphine	80	5	4

[*] Product of the nonbound and un-ionized fractions.

drains directly into the systemic venous system. Drugs given rectally can thus partly avoid hepatic first-pass metabolism. The rectal route is valuable for drugs that cause gastric irritation or erosions (e.g. nonsteroidal antiinflammatory analgesics), or in patients with nausea and vomiting. To facilitate rectal absorption drugs must be formulated either as a suppository, a gelatine capsule or an enema. Patient acceptability of this route is variable between countries and cultures.

TRANSDERMAL DELIVERY

Transdermal delivery is suitable for small, potent, generally lipophilic molecules that require low input rates to achieve effective plasma concentrations (Table 2.3). This route avoids stomach or intestinal modification or degradation and also first-pass metabolism by the liver. It is usually advisable regularly to change the site of drug delivery to reduce the risk of local adverse reactions. There may be a slow rate of increase of concentration if the drug forms a depot in the skin. Depot formation will also result in a slow decrease in concentration when the system is removed from the skin. In addition, to drug transport across the skin by simple diffusion, techniques have been developed that use iontophoresis, i.e. the molecules are actively carried across the skin by a small electrical current.[2] This provides a faster and more controllable transfer of drug.

INTRAMUSCULAR OR SUBCUTANEOUS ADMINISTRATION

In contrast to the epithelial lining of the intestines, the capillary walls in subcutaneous tissues and muscle offer little impedence to drug absorption, even for drugs that are polar and ionized. For example, gentamicin, which is water soluble and ionized, is poorly absorbed from the gastrointestinal tract but is rapidly and completely absorbed following intramuscular injection. The rate of absorption of drug from muscular or subcutaneous tissues is, however, heavily dependent on regional blood flow. A patient who is peripherally vasoconstricted due to hypovolaemia or hypothermia will absorb drug poorly when it is administered intramuscularly or subcutaneously; for example, care needs to be taken when

administering morphine by this route to a patient in shock. Absorption can be deliberately slowed by dissolving the drug in an emulsion or converting water-soluble drugs into water-insoluble complexes (e.g. insulin–zinc complexes). These sustained-release forms have a smoother onset and longer duration of action, avoiding the necessity and discomfort of repeated injections. Certain drugs (e.g. thiopentone and digoxin) can cause local tissue damage when inadvertently injected via these routes.

INHALATION

The alveolar capillary membrane is normally very thin, has a huge surface area and a large blood supply. Drugs given by this route, such as bronchodilators and pulmonary steroids, are rapidly absorbed into the bloodstream. This is also the route for administering the inhalational anaesthetics. The uptake of anaesthetic vapours by the lungs is described in Chapter 4.

DRUG DISTRIBUTION

After absorption, a drug enters the systemic circulation and subsequently undergoes the simultaneous processes of dilution by the blood and distribution to the tissues. A few compounds, such as indocyanine green, a dye used in indicator–dilution measurements of organ blood flow, cannot penetrate the endothelial membrane and are confined to the circulating blood. Drugs that do pass the endothelial membrane diffuse into the peripheral tissues. The extent to which this process occurs is very variable. Highly polar drugs are largely confined to the extracellular water (approximately 12 litres for a 70-kg individual) and the drug will be diluted by this volume (Table 2.4). However, if the volume in which a nonpolar drug is evenly dispersed is simply considered as the amount of drug in the body divided by the concentration, then after full distribution has occurred a volume is calculated that, for many drugs, is considerably in excess of total body volume. For example, the apparent volume of distribution of propofol in a healthy adult is about 700–1000 litres. The reason for this is that drugs bind to proteins not only in the blood but even more extensively, and by the same processes, in the tissues. This bound drug is effectively 'lost' when volume is measured, and for this reason the calculated volume is referred to as an *apparent volume* of distribution, defined as a hypothetical volume into which a drug would have to be dispersed to produce the observed blood or plasma concentration. Apparent volumes of distribution are calculated with respect to the concentration in blood or plasma, and indicate the volume in which the drug would be dispersed were it to have the same concentration as in blood or plasma. The value of the

Table 2.3 Transdermal delivery systems
Glyceryl trinitrate
Oestradiol
Clonidine
Fentanyl
Nicotine
Scopolamine
Oestradiol/norethisterone

Table 2.4 Distribution volume (V_d)		
	V_d (litres per 70 kg)	Examples
Confined to plasma	3	Indocyanine green: 3 litres
Confined to ECF	12	Tubocurarine: 10 litres
Less than TBW	40–60	Phenytoin: 40 litres
Greater than TBW	> 60	Thiopentone: 84 litres Nortriptyline: 1540 litres

ECF, extracellular fluid; TBW, total body water.

apparent distribution is that it provides a method of estimating the amount of drug in the body at some time after administration based on the concentration, since amount = concentration $\times$ volume. Thus, if the plasma concentration of a drug with a V_d of 500 litres is 10 ng ml^{-1}, then the amount in the body will be 500 000 ml $\times$ 10 ng, or 5 mg. The determination of volume of distribution will be discussed in more detail below.

MECHANISMS OF DRUG METABOLISM AND EXCRETION

The principal objective of drug metabolism is to make a drug available for excretion by urine or bile. The renal and biliary systems can excrete polar (water soluble) forms of a drug without the absolute necessity for the drug first to be metabolized, whereas nonpolar (water insoluble) drugs must first be converted to a polar form before they can be excreted efficiently. Drug metabolism, therefore, is principally, but not exclusively, of importance for drugs that are nonpolar. Metabolism usually results in inactivation of the drug but there are exceptions; for example, diazepam is metabolized to an active metabolite, desmethyldiazepam, which has a much longer duration of action than the parent compound.

DRUG METABOLISM

The liver is the principal site of drug metabolism. Hepatic drug metabolism is usually classified into two distinct phases. *Phase I* consists of metabolic modification of the drug by either oxidation, reduction or hydrolysis. One of the most important systems that catalyse oxidation are the family of haem-containing cytochrome P450 enzymes. The name is derived from the absorbance spectrum of a solution of P450 enzymes equilibrated with carbon monoxide, which has a peak absorbance at 450 nm. Cytochrome P450 catalyses a reaction whereby one oxygen atom is incorporated into the drug substrate to form a hydroxyl group (Fig. 2.3).

Phase II reactions consist of a synthetic conjugation reaction involving the product of phase I metabolism and a second carrier molecule such as glucuronic acid, glycine, glutamine, sulphate or acetate. Conjugates are more polar than the parent compound and can be removed more readily by renal or biliary excretion. For some drugs (e.g. morphine) phase II conjugation reactions are the primary means of biotransformation.

ENZYME INDUCTION

Many of the cytochrome P450 enzymes are inducible, i.e. their activity can be enhanced by certain substances. This increased activity represents *de novo* enzyme synthesis and involves deoxyribonucleic acid (DNA) transcription since it is blocked by actinomycin D (a polypeptide antibiotic that binds to DNA, preventing it from acting as a template for ribonucleic acid (RNA) synthesis; DNA replication is unaffected). More than 200 substances, including barbiturates, polycyclic hydrocarbons, steroids, polychlorinated insecticides, nicotine, ethanol, food dyes and preservatives, and inhalational anaesthetics, have been found to enhance the metabolism of drugs by the cytochrome P450 systems. Common inducing drugs in humans are the antiepileptics phenobarbitone, carbamazepine and phenytoin, and the antibiotic rifampicin. A practical consequence of enzyme induction is that the inducing agent will accelerate the metabolism of a second drug. An example of such a phenomenon is the decreased effectiveness of oral contraceptive drugs when rifampicin is concurrently taken as part of antituberculous therapy, resulting in unwanted pregnancy. Other substances inhibit P450 activity. The clinical implications of enzyme induction and inhibition are discussed in Chapter 28.

PHARMACOGENETICS

Pharmacogenetics is the study of unusual or idiosyncratic drug responses which have a hereditary

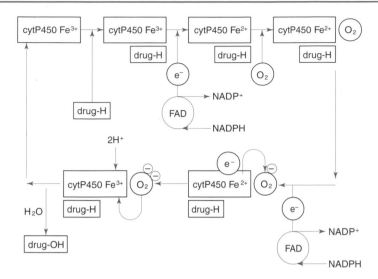

Fig. 2.3 Phase I oxidation by the cytochrome P450 enzyme system. The drug combines with the oxidized (Fe^{3+}) form of P450 to form a complex which is reduced to the (Fe^{2+}) form by transfer of an electron. The Fe^{2+} form of the complex is capable of binding molecular oxygen. Once bound, the molecular oxygen becomes activated by addition of electrons from nicotinamide adenine dinucleotide (NAD) and Fe^{2+}, eventually regenerating the oxidized (Fe^{3+}) form of P450 together with the release of the hydroxylated form of the drug. FAD, flavine adenine dinucleotide.

basis. Some of the enzymes responsible for drug metabolism are susceptible to genetically determined variation (Table 2.5). This may be inherited in the same way as metabolic disorders but with the principal distinction that the disorder becomes manifest (it is hitherto said to be 'silent') only when a particular drug is encountered (which may never happen).

Chromosomes, other than the sex chromosomes, are called *autosomes*. The *phenotype* refers to the outward manifestation of a genetic trait (e.g. eye colour) whereas *genotype* refers to the characterization of the gene pair. An individual is said to be *homozygous* if the two complementary genes are identical (*A/A* or *a/a*) and *heterozygous* when not (thus *A/a*). If a normal autosomal gene is dominant over an abnormal (mutant) gene, the disorder is inherited in an *autosomal recessive* manner, whereas if the mutant gene predominates over the normal one the disorder is inherited in an *autosomal*

dominant manner. For autosomal recessive disorders a problem arises only when both parents are *heterozygous* with respect to the mutant allele, whereas an autosomal dominant disorder can be inherited if either of the parents possesses the abnormal gene. If one allele is not dominant over the other, the mechanism of inheritance is termed *additive*, and this mechanism is the one most commonly encountered in genetically determined enzyme disorders.

Polymorphism

This is a stably inherited trait associated with variable characteristics of an enzyme system within a population. Affected individuals appear to be completely healthy but have sharply distinctive characteristics with respect to drug metabolism. The metabolic abnormality is diagnosed only after drug administration (the abnormality may either be a laboratory finding without associated symptoms or be manifested by symptoms or abnormality precipitated by drug treatment). It is not possible within the context of this chapter to review this subject comprehensively, but some examples will be discussed to illustrate the general principles.

Butyrylcholinesterase (Plasma Cholinesterase or Pseudocholinesterase) Deficiency

This enzyme is responsible for the metabolic breakdown of the muscle relaxant succinylcholine (suxamethonium) to the pharmacologically inert succinyl monocholine. The mechanism of inheritance is

Table 2.5 **Some genetically variable enzymes of drug metabolism**
Butyryl cholinesterase (pseudocholinesterase)
Debrisoquine/sparteine oxidase (CYP2D6)
Alcohol dehydrogenase
Glucuronyl transferase
N-acetyl transferase
Catechol-*O*-methyl transferase
Glucose 6-phosphate dehydrogenase

additive. Individuals who are genotypically homozygous with respect to a mutant gene for the enzyme have serious deficiencies of the active form of this enzyme.[3] The enzyme is often present in normal amounts, but its affinity for succinylcholine is greatly reduced compared with the normal form of the enzyme.

There are several variants of atypical plasma cholinesterase (Table 2.6) and they all appear to arise from a single locus on chromosome 3.[3] The *atypical* gene mutation can be diagnosed in the laboratory on the basis of inhibition of cholinesterase by a 10^{-5} mol l^{-1} concentration of the local anaesthetic cinchocaine (dibucaine) using benzoylcholine as substrate. Cinchocaine is an inhibitor of the normal form of plasma cholinesterase, whereas the abnormal form is approximately 20 times less sensitive to such inhibition. The degree of inhibition, expressed as a percentage, is called the 'dibucaine number'. Based on the cinchocaine number, individuals can be classified into three groups: normal individuals (dibucaine number between 71 and 85), intermediate (dibucaine number approximately 60) and atypical (dibucaine number approximately 20). Those in the intermediate group are heterozygous (A/U) with a frequency of about 1 in 25, and do not normally show significant sensitivity to succinylcholine or ester drugs. The frequency of the atypical homozygotes (A/A) is 1 in 3000 to 1 in 10 000, and they are sensitive to succinylcholine. These are the patients who develop 'scoline apnoea'.

Another variant of plasma cholinesterase deficiency gene is characterized by resistance to inhibition by fluoride ion. Fluoride resistance is determined by a different *allele* of the same gene (i.e. a mutation occurs at a different location within the same gene). Patients who are homozygote F/F are moderately sensitive to succinylcholine. Homozygotes for the 'silent gene' have little or no cholinesterase activity and are extremely sensitive to succinylcholine.

Acetylation Polymorphism

Acetylation is responsible for the metabolism of a wide range of drugs and other environmental chemicals in humans and animals. The reaction is catalysed by *N*-acetyltransferase and involves the transfer of an acetyl group to an acceptor amine with the production of an amide. Acetylation polymorphism was first recognized in tuberculous patients treated with isoniazid, which is metabolized principally to acetyl isoniazid. If the plasma concentration of isoniazid is determined at a fixed time after a standardized dose, a bimodal distribution of drug concentration is obtained (Fig. 2.4). Each individual can accordingly be classified as either a fast or slow acetylator. The proportion of fast and slow acetylators varies widely between ethnic groups. About 50–60% of endogenous Europeans, but only 5% of Japanese, are slow acetylators. There is a strong correlation between various side-effects of isoniazid therapy (e.g. peripheral neuropathy, skin reactions) and slow acetylator status, although the precise nature of the relationship is unclear. Acetylation polymorphism also occurs for

Table 2.6 Summary of the more common inherited variants of the plasma cholinesterase gene (modified from Davis et al.[3] with permission)

Variant	Gene label	Allele frequency	Plasma activity	Sensitivity to succinylcholine
Usual	U	0.98	Normal	Normal
Atypical	A	0.02	Activity decreased by 70%	Homozygotes very sensitive; 2 h paralysis
Silent	S	0.0003	No activity	Homozygotes extremely sensitive; 3–4 h paralysis
Fluoride	F	0.003	Activity decreased by 60%	Homozygotes only moderately sensitive; 1–2 h paralysis
H type	H	ND	Activity decreased by 90%	Homozygotes very sensitive; 2–3 h paralysis
K type	K	0.13	Activity decreased by 30%	Homozygotes only mildly sensitive; < 1 h paralysis
J type	J	ND	Activity decreased by 66%	Homozygotes only moderately sensitive; 1 h paralysis

ND, frequency not determined.

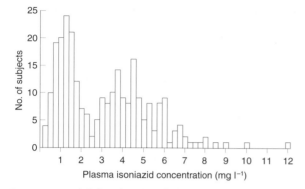

Fig. 2.4 Bimodal distribution of plasma isoniazid concentrations in 483 subjects given oral isoniazid 9.8–10 mg kg^{-1}. From Evans *et al.*[8]

several other drugs, including hydralazine, nitrazepam, phenelzine and procainamide.

Cytochrome P450 polymorphism

Multiple hepatic cytochrome P450 enzymes play an important role in the oxidative biotransformation of a vast number of structurally diverse drugs. The synthesis of these enzymes is controlled by a family of genes called *CYP*, and genetic variability with respect to these proteins has been demonstrated. The enzyme CYP2D6 (debrisoquine 4-hydroxylase) is one of the best known examples of cytochrome P450 polymorphism and is of particular importance with respect to drugs metabolized by this enzyme, such as antipsychotic drugs, anti-arrhythmics, antihypertensives, β-adrenoceptor antagonists and some morphine derivatives. CYP2D6 polymorphism is responsible for highly variable pharmacokinetics following administration of these drugs. New molecular biological techniques such as gene expression assays now make it theoretically possible to genotype individuals, allowing identification of those potentially at risk because of CYP2D6 deficiency.

DRUG EXCRETION

When a drug or its metabolite is rendered suitably polar, it is usually excreted in either the urine or the bile.

RENAL EXCRETION

Renal excretion occurs either by filtration at the glomerulus, by secretion into the proximal tubule or by diffusion into the distal tubule. Glomerular filtration is a passive process which permits free passage of non-protein-bound drugs or drug metabolites into the tubular lumen. Drugs that are nonpolar at the pH of the urine tend to be reabsorbed into the proximal tubule, whereas polar compounds are 'trapped' within the

tubule and excreted in the urine. Proximal tubular secretion, on the other hand, is an active process requiring expenditure of energy and involves two principal carrier systems, one of which is specific for acidic drugs while the other is responsible for secretion of basic drugs. Competition between drugs may exist for the carrier transport mechanisms and this may be employed to pharmacological advantage; for example, probenecid prolongs the duration of action of penicillin by competing for a common secretory mechanism in the proximal tubule.

In the distal tubule, diffusion is the principal mechanism whereby nonpolar drugs are either secreted into or reabsorbed from the tubular lumen. The pH of the urine can significantly influence the reabsorption of drugs (Fig. 2.5) as this determines the degree of ionization. Excretion of acidic drugs is promoted by alkalinization of urine, whereas excretion of basic drugs is promoted by acidification (in both cases the drugs are less ionized). Therapeutic alkalinization of the urine is occasionally used to promote salicylate excretion after overdosing whereas acidification is less commonly used, for example following overdosage of a weak acid such as amphetamine.

BILIARY EXCRETION

Secretion of drugs or their metabolites by hepatocytes into the biliary canaliculi is an energy-dependent and carrier-specific process. Biliary excretion is of major importance for the excretion of drugs and metabolites that are predominantly ionized (e.g. muscle relaxants or antibiotics) since this route of excretion is not dependent on solubility in the lipid membrane of the hepatocyte. Some drugs that are excreted in the bile as conjugates may subsequently be reabsorbed from the bowel following hydrolysis by bacterial flora in the

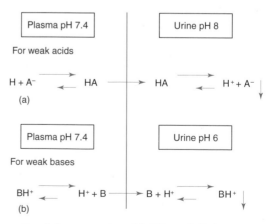

Fig. 2.5 Renal drug excretion. (a) Effect of alkalinization of urine to promote excretion of acidic drug and (b) acidification of urine to promote excretion of alkaline drug.

bowel lumen. This process is referred to as *enterohepatic recirculation*. Biliary excretion is a relatively minor excretory route for substances with a molecular weight of less than 500 Da.

KINETICS OF DRUG DISPOSITION AND ELIMINATION

Pharmacokinetics is the study of the uptake, distribution and elimination of drugs expressed as a function of time and expressed in the language of mathematics. The principal objective is to describe the relationship between dose and the time course of drug concentration in the blood and tissues. *Pharmacokinetics* describes the dose–concentration relationship, whereas *pharmacodynamics* refers to the dose–effect relationship, and is discussed in Chapter 3.

Knowledge about what doses or infusion rates of drug are appropriate and safe, how long it will take for the drug to produce an effect, and the possible duration of that effect can be learnt from practical experience, without any conception of the actual drug concentrations achieved in a particular patient. However, such an empirical approach has severe limitations. It is usually not possible empirically to predict what happens when a familiar dosing schedule is altered or an unfamiliar drug is given. The science of pharmacokinetics, on the other hand, develops a conceptual approach or mathematical 'model' of drug handling which is applicable to *all* drugs and for *all* drug input regimens regardless of their complexity. The nature of the drug and the method of administration may be varied but the basic principles that govern the operation of the selected model do not.

It is a feature of many processes in nature that, over a fixed time interval, termed the *half-life* ($t_{1/2}$), the amount of a given entity decreases to 50% of its original value (Fig. 2.6). Such a process is termed *exponential decay* and its principal feature is that a constant fraction of the original quantity decreases per unit time. It is said to be of *first order*. Put another way, the rate of decrease at any time is directly proportional to the amount present at that time. First-order exponential processes are very common in pharmacokinetics. They can be expressed mathematically using calculus notation. If the concentration of a drug at time t is $C(t)$, then the rate of change of C with time is given by the expression:

$$\frac{dC(t)}{dt} = -k \cdot C \text{ where } k \text{ is a constant} \qquad [1]$$

This can be solved for $C(t)$ using standard techniques of integration to give

$$C(t) = C_o e^{-kt} \qquad [2]$$

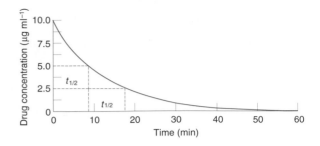

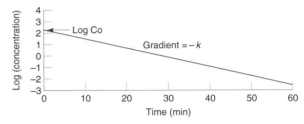

Fig. 2.6 (a) Exponential decay of a drug following bolus intravenous injection showing the concept of half life; (b) semilogarithmic plot of drug decay.

where C_o is the concentration at time $t = 0$, and e is the irrational number 2.71828 ... An irrational number is one that cannot be defined to a finite number of decimal places. In the above equations it is assumed that the body is modelled as a single compartment in which the drug is uniformly distributed. Compartmental models are commonly used in pharmacokinetics. The compartmental approach implies that the body comprises of one or more interconnected compartments and that the drug diffuses backwards and forwards between these compartments along concentration gradients.

ONE-COMPARTMENT MODEL
Although drugs that have one-compartment pharmacokinetics are uncommon, this model is discussed in some detail because it has the advantage of relative simplicity and thus the principles are easier to understand than for the more complicated two- and three-compartment models.

Bolus administration
In this model the body is regarded as a single, evenly mixed, compartment with a volume of distribution V_d (Fig. 2.7). This model describes the behaviour of only a very few drugs (e.g. indocyanine green) which are almost totally confined to the circulation and are unable to diffuse into the tissues. It is assumed that removal of an amount of drug, X, from the system is a first-order process governed by the equation:

$$\frac{dX}{dt} = -k_{10} \cdot X \qquad [3]$$

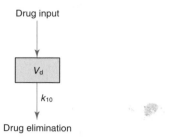

Drug input

V_d

k_{10}

Drug elimination

Fig. 2.7 One-compartment pharmacokinetic model.

where k_{10} is the *rate constant* and the subscript ascribes the direction in which the constant operates (i.e. from compartment 1 to the outside of the system). The rate constant has dimensions of reciprocal time (t^{-1}) and expresses the fractional change in concentration per unit time. Thus if $k_{10} = 0.1\ \text{min}^{-1}$, the concentration in the compartment will decrease by 10% every minute. Solving eqn [3] yields:

$$X(t) = X_o \cdot e^{-k_{10}t} \qquad [4]$$

where X_o is the initial amount of drug. If a dose of drug X_o is administered and mixed instantaneously, the initial concentration of drug will be $C_o = X_o/V_d$. The equation can be rewritten in terms of concentration by dividing both sides by V_d to give an equation describing the concentration–time relationship for the drug:

$$C(t) = C_o \cdot e^{-k_{10}t} \qquad [5]$$

Eqn [5] can be converted to one that is analytically more useful by taking logarithms:

$$\log_e \frac{C(t)}{C_o} = -k_{10}t \qquad [6]$$

A plot of $C(t)$ against t using semilogarithmic axes is a straight line with gradient $-k_{10}$ and y intercept C_o (which allows calculation of V_d) (Fig. 2.6b). Thus, all the model parameters that are specific to the drug can be determined experimentally and all further values of interest are merely functions of these parameters. In the particular situation where C is half C_o, $t = t_{1/2}$ and

$$\log_e \left(\frac{1}{2}\right) = \log_e(1) - \log_e(2) = -k_{10}t_{\frac{1}{2}} \qquad [7]$$

and since $\log_e (1) = 0$ and $\log_e (2) = 0.693$, this gives:

$$t_{\frac{1}{2}} = \frac{0.693}{k_{10}} \qquad [8]$$

The *clearance* (*Cl*) of a drug is defined as the rate of drug elimination per unit drug concentration. In eqn [3], k_{10} defines the rate of decline of drug amount but does not provide information on how much drug is eliminated. The equation can be rewritten:

$$\frac{dX}{dt} = -k_{10} \cdot C \cdot V_d \qquad [9]$$

By definition:

$$Cl = \frac{dX/dt}{C} = k_{10}V_d \qquad [10]$$

Here the negative sign has been neglected since clearance is always positive. Thus, clearance equals the product of the elimination constant and the volume of the compartment, and therefore has the dimensions of volume per unit time. Clearance can also be regarded as the volume of the compartment that is completely cleared of drug per unit time. Clearance can also be calculated from the area under the concentration curve (AUC) following bolus administration:

$$Cl = \frac{\text{Dose}}{C_o} \cdot k_{10}, \quad \text{since} \quad C_o = \frac{\text{Dose}}{V_d} \qquad [11]$$

and

$$\text{AUC} = \int_{t=0}^{\infty} C \cdot dt = \int_{t=0}^{\infty} C_o \cdot e^{-k_{10}t} \cdot dt$$
$$= \left[\frac{C_o}{-k_{10}} \cdot e^{-k_{10}t} \right]_{t=0}^{\infty} = \frac{C_o}{k_{10}} \qquad [12]$$

and substitution gives:

$$Cl = \text{Dose} \cdot \frac{k_{10}}{C_o} = \frac{\text{Dose}}{\text{AUC}} \qquad [13]$$

We now know how to calculate the two parameters, k_{10} and V_d, which describe the behaviour of the drug within the one-compartment model. It therefore becomes possible to describe the concentration–time relationship for any administration scheme.

Infusion

The concentration–time profile following a fixed rate infusion Q can be calculated. According to the model, drug is now also being added while simultaneously being removed by elimination:

$$\frac{dX}{dt} = \text{Rate}_{into} - \text{Rate}_{out} = Q - k_{10}X \qquad [14]$$

When the drug concentration at the start of the infusion is zero, this differential equation can be solved to give (after dividing by V_d to convert to concentrations):

$$C(t) = \frac{Q}{k_{10}V_d}(1 - e^{-k_{10}t}) \qquad [15]$$

When, instead of being zero, the starting concentration is C_o:

$$C(t) = \frac{Q}{k_{10}V_d}(1 - e^{-k_{10}t}) + C_o \cdot e^{-k_{10}t} \qquad [16]$$

These calculations are not easy to perform manually. They are, however, readily managed by computers, and can be conveniently performed within a commercial spreadsheet or graphics program.

The concentration–time curve generated by zero-order infusion into a one-compartment model has the form of an exponential wash-in curve, whereby eventually a steady-state concentration of drug is reached (C_{ss}). When t is large or tends to infinity then the exponential term tends to zero and the steady-state concentration becomes:

$$C_{ss} = \frac{Q}{k_{10} \cdot V_d} = \frac{Q}{Cl} \quad [17]$$

For a fixed rate infusion, 95% of this steady-state concentration will be reached in approximately 4.5 half-lives after starting the infusion.

TWO-COMPARTMENT MODEL

Bolus administration

The disposition of many drugs can be modelled adequately by a two-compartment model (Fig. 2.8). Addition of drug to the system and elimination from the system occurs via the first or central compartment. This compartment comprises the circulating blood and organs with high blood flows. The drug is perceived as instantaneously distributing itself within the first compartment while distribution to the second or peripheral compartment is a much slower process governed by the rate constants k_{12} and k_{21}. For this model the concentration–time relationship following bolus intravenous injection may be fitted to a function that contains two exponential terms and the drug's behaviour is referred to as *biexponential*:

$$C(t) = Ae^{-at} + Be^{-\beta t} \quad [18]$$

The graph of $C(t)$ against time after bolus administration has two distinct phases (Fig. 2.9). During the a phase there is a steep decline in concentration immediately following the bolus owing to rapid distribution of the drug into the second compartment. The β phase, the final portion of the decay curve, is less steep. A, B, a and β in eqn [18]

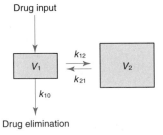

Drug input

V_1 k_{12} ⇄ k_{21} V_2

k_{10}

Drug elimination

Fig. 2.8 Two-compartment pharmacokinetic model.

are constants whose values can be determined experimentally.

As t progressively becomes larger and tends to infinity, each of the exponential terms in eqn [18] approaches zero. However, because by convention $a > \beta$, the contribution of the first term decreases more rapidly than that of the second term, and becomes progressively less significant. We can use this fact to 'strip' the overall concentration–time relationship into two separate components, C_a and C_b (this is termed the *method of residuals*) such that $C(t) = C_a + C_b$, where $C_a = A \cdot e^{-a t}$ and $C_b = B \cdot e^{-\beta t}$. Since, during the β phase, the contribution from C_a can be ignored, we can study the C_b term in isolation. If the data are plotted on semilogarithmic axes, the terminal β phase is a straight line. Extrapolation of this line to the concentration axis gives an intercept equal to B in eqn [18]. From the a phase of the curve, where the contribution of the first exponential term is significant, we can calculate C_a since this equals $C(t) - C_b$. Subtracting the (extrapolated) data points of the β phase from C_t (this is the process of 'stripping') yields another straight line, which when extrapolated to the concentration axis gives the intercept A in eqn [18] (Fig. 2.9). This follows since, on the $C(t)$ axis, $t = 0$ and the value of each exponential term becomes unity. The slopes of the curves are, respectively, $-\beta$ and $-a$. The constants A, B, a and β can be used to determine the other relevant parameters (k_{10}, k_{12}, k_{21}, V_1 and V_2) that govern the two-compartment model:

$$k_{21} = \frac{A \cdot \beta + B \cdot a}{A + B}$$

$$V_2 = V_1 \cdot \frac{k_{12}}{k_{21}}$$

$$k_{12} = a + \beta - (k_{21} + k_{10})$$

$$V_1 = \frac{Dose}{A + B}$$

$$k_{10} = \frac{(a \cdot \beta)}{k_{21}}$$

It is also possible to calculate the concentration of drug in the second compartment. Immediately after administration of a rapid intravenous bolus the concentration of drug in compartment 1 declines as a result of two simultaneous processes: elimination from the first compartment and distribution to the second compartment, which is initially empty (Fig. 2.10). Eventually the concentration in compartment 2 (C_2) becomes greater than that in compartment 1 (C_1) and then the flow of drug reverses, from compartment 2 to 1.

The response of a two-compartment system to an infusion of rate Q is given by:

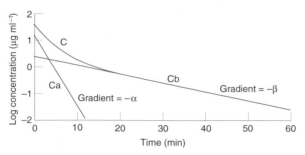

Fig. 2.9 Biexponential decay of drug (semilogarithmic plot) illustrating the two phases and derivation of the pharmacokinetic parameters A, B, α and β.

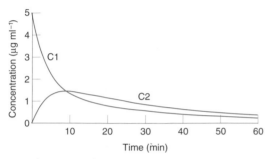

Fig. 2.10 Changes in drug concentration in compartments 1 (C1) and 2 (C2) following bolus intravenous injection: biexponential decay.

$$C_1(t) = \frac{Q}{V_1 \cdot k_{10}}\left(1 + \frac{\beta - k_{10}}{a - \beta}e^{-at} + \frac{k_{10} - a}{a - \beta}e^{-\beta t}\right) \quad [19]$$

The curve generated by this equation is again of an exponential wash-in form, but now with two exponential components. When the infusion is discontinued, the amount of the drug in the second compartment influences the decay of concentration in the first compartment. After stopping the infusion, redistribution of drug from compartment 2 to compartment 1 competes with the elimination from compartment 1. The longer the duration of the infusion, the greater the amount of drug in the second compartment and the slower the decay process after stopping the infusion. Hughes *et al.*[4] introduced the term *context-sensitive half-time*, the time from stopping an infusion until the plasma concentration has decreased by 50%, to describe this phenomenon. The term emphasizes that the behaviour of a drug in the central compartment is always dependent on the current disposition of drug throughout the model and not merely on the concentration of drug in the central compartment (Fig. 2.11).

THREE-COMPARTMENT MODELS

The pharmacokinetics of many drugs used in anaesthesia, such as hypnotics and analgesics, can best

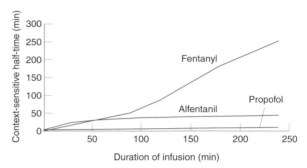

Fig. 2.11 Context-sensitive half-times for fentanyl, alfentanil and propofol. Context-sensitive half-time relates the time required for the plasma concentration to decrease by 50% after stopping an infusion of a drug to the duration of the infusion.

be described by a three-compartment model. For this model the change in plasma drug concentration after a bolus intravenous injection is described by a triexponential equation:

$$C(t) = Ae^{-at} + Be^{-\beta t} + Ce^{-\gamma t}$$

The parameters A, B, C and α, β and γ can be obtained in a similar manner as described for the two-compartment model, but the mathematics are considerably more complex than for the two-compartment model and will not be considered here. Interested readers are referred to standard textbooks on pharmacokinetics, or the review by Hull.[5]

NONCOMPARTMENTAL OR MODEL-INDEPENDENT APPROACHES TO PHARMACOKINETICS

Noncompartmental analysis uses techniques analogous to statistical moment theory to describe the disposition of a drug in the body, which is considered as a homogeneous kinetic space. The area under the $C(t)$ against time curve (AUC) following a single injection is analogous to the *zero* moment, and the area under the $C(t) \cdot t$ against time curve (AUMC) is analogous to the *first* moment. The ratio AUMC/AUC is the mean residence time (MRT), defined as the average time taken by drug molecules injected into the kinetic system to leave the system. The MRT is equivalent to the time constant of a one-compartment model, and indicates the time taken for 62.5% of a dose to be eliminated from the body, i.e. $t_{1/2} = 0.693$ MRT since concentration decreases by 62.5% in two time constants. The apparent volume of distribution at steady state (V_{ss}) is calculated as $V_{ss} = Cl \cdot$ MRT, where $Cl =$ dose/AUC.

PITFALLS OF PHARMACOKINETICS

Pharmacokinetics employs mathematical models as conceptual frameworks to gain insight into the complex process of drug handling. It is, however, impossible to define a model that describes each and every aspect of the overall process. A compromise has to be reached between model sophistication and its overall utility, and it has to be accepted that all of the currently available models have their pitfalls.[6]

ESTIMATION OF COMPARTMENT VOLUME

One of the commonest problems encountered is that each model assumes that the drug is instantaneously mixed with the contents of the central compartment after administration. This is evidently not so since a finite time is required for complete mixing to occur. Failure to recognize this problem leads to gross underestimation of the central compartment volume. Anaesthetic drugs, in particular, tend to have very rapid initial distribution phases and thus extrapolation techniques to estimate the volume of the central compartment after bolus administration are often markedly inaccurate.

SAMPLING POINT

As long as the drug is being added to or removed from the body, concentration gradients will exist between different sampling points. The most extreme example of this is seen when sampling downstream from the point of injection (e.g. from a central vein when the drug is infused peripherally). Such effects are readily demonstrated during drug infusion and tend to become less apparent following cessation of infusion.

NONLINEARITY

Pharmacokinetics are said to be nonlinear when one or more of the parameters vary according to either dose, concentration or with time. This can result from drug-induced changes in haemodynamics, changes in regional blood flow and also temperature and metabolic changes. The other source of nonlinear pharmacokinetics is high drug concentrations that saturate the ability of the liver enzymes to metabolize the drug. Common examples are ethanol and phenytoin, or when high doses of barbiturates are given for cerebral protection. When pharmacokinetics become nonlinear, the amount of drug eliminated per unit time is constant rather than a constant fraction of the amount in the body, as for the linear situation.

PATIENT HETEROGENEITY

There exists wide inter- and intra-patient variability in respect of drug handling and it is unreasonable to expect that a single set of pharmacokinetic parameters will predict accurately the concentration of drug under all conditions in every patient. One way to improve the predictive capability of a model is through the use of population pharmacokinetics, which allows adjustment of model parameters for specific patient attributes such as age or sex.[7]

CONCLUSION

Lord Kelvin (1824–1907), the distinguished Scottish physicist (natural philosopher), often declared: 'If ye cannae make a model, ye dinnae understan' it'. It has been the principal purpose of this chapter to demonstrate the wisdom of these words and the usefulness of modelling concepts in describing both the qualitative and quantitative aspects of drug handling. The science of pharmacokinetics based on such concepts has led to new insight into the way that drugs are handled by patients, to novel drug development and safer drug administration.

REFERENCES

1. du Souich P, Verges J, Erill S. Plasma protein binding and pharmacological response. *Clin Pharmacokinet* 1993; **24**: 435–440.
2. Berner B, John VA. Pharmacokinetic characterisation of transdermal delivery systems. *Clin Pharmacokinet* 1994; **26**: 121–134.
3. Davis L, Britten JJ, Morgan M. Cholinesterase. Its significance in anaesthetic practice. *Anaesthesia* 1997; **52**: 244–260.
4. Hughes MA, Glass PSA, Jacobs RR. Context sensitive half-time in multicompartment pharmacokinetic models for intravenous anesthetic drugs. *Anesthesiology* 1992; **76**: 334–341.
5. Hull CJ. Compartmental models. *Anaesth Pharmacol Rev* 1994; **2**: 188–203.
6. Mather LE, Bjorkman S. Pitfalls in pharmacokinetics. *Anaesth Pharmacol Rev* 1994; **2**: 260–270.
7. Whiting B, Kelman AW, Grevel J. Population kinetics. *Clin Pharmacokinet* 1986; **11**: 387–401.

3

JG Bovill, FHM Engbers

PHARMACODYNAMICS OF DRUG ACTION

Drugs are administered in order to achieve a desired pharmacological effect, which is related to the drug concentration at an effect site, sometimes referred to as the biophase. The process that describes the relationship between the dose of a drug and the resulting concentration–time course in a compartment of the body where drugs can be measured (e.g. plasma or blood) is the subject of pharmacokinetics and is dealt with in Chapter 2. Pharmacodynamics is concerned with the relation between the concentration of a drug and its effect.

Although drug concentrations are readily measured in the blood or plasma, this is the site of action for only very few drugs. To relate plasma concentration to clinical effect a link is needed between the concentration in the plasma and at the effect site. Pharmacokinetic–pharmacodynamic (PK–PD) models have been developed that incorporate this link. These have proven extremely useful in explaining many of the clinical observations about drug actions, such as the time delay between achieving a particular concentration of a drug in the blood and the effect. PK–PD models are increasingly used in the initial development of new drugs, before they are tested in humans. Simulations using PK–PD modelling can help to predict doses that may produce adverse responses even when actual pharmacokinetic or pharmacodynamic data about the drug are limited. This approach has been described by one member of the United States Food and Drug Administration as a tool that 'like a lantern on a dark night, is valuable for the illumination it provides'.[1] The objective of this chapter is to introduce and explain the relevant terminology used in the science of pharmacodynamics, to illustrate how pharmacodynamic principles can be used

in anaesthesia, and to provide the background to read and understand scientific articles about pharmacodynamics.

CONCENTRATION–EFFECT RELATIONSHIPS

The binding of a drug with a receptor is a chemical reaction governed by the law of mass action. If D is the number of free (unbound) drug molecules, R_t the total number of receptors and DR the number of occupied receptors, then the fraction of occupied receptors can be expressed by the equation:

$$\frac{[DR]}{[R_t]} = \frac{[D]}{[D] + K_D} \qquad [1]$$

where $[D]$, $[R]$, and $[DR]$ represent the molar concentrations of D, R and DR, and K_D is the equilibrium dissociation constant for the reaction, i.e. the drug concentration at which 50% of the receptors are occupied (see Chapter 1). Classical occupation theory, accepted until the 1950s, stated that the pharmacological effect of a drug is directly proportional to the number of receptors occupied (DR) and that the maximum effect (E_{max}) is achieved when all receptors

---

Summary box 3.1   Pharmacodynamics

- Pharmacodynamics describes the relationship between the concentration of a drug and its pharmacological effect.

- For many drugs there is a time delay between the time-course of drug effect and plasma drug concentration.

- PK–PD models can be used to quantify this delay. They use a first-order rate constant (k_{eo}) which characterizes the temporal aspect of equilibrium between plasma concentration and drug effect.

- For intravenously administered drugs the parameter k_{eo} is an important determinant of the onset time, time to reach maximum effect and the duration of the clinical effect.

are occupied, i.e. $E = E_{max}$ only when $[DR] = [R_t]$. Eqn [1] refers to the binding of a ligand to a receptor. For drug-induced changes in a tissue or intact animal, the corresponding equation is the E_{max} equation in which the effect (E) of a drug concentration (C), expressed as a fraction of E_{max}, is given by:

$$E = E_{max} \cdot \frac{C}{C + EC_{50}^{y}} \qquad [2]$$

where EC_{50} is the concentration that results in 50% of the maximum response (corresponding to the K_D parameter for ligand–receptor binding in eqn [1].

Eqn [2] is the equation of a rectangular hyperbola, and if it is assumed that the pharmacological response is proportional to the fraction of receptors occupied, then there will be a hyperbolic relationship between drug concentration (or dose) and response. As the drug concentration increases, the fraction of receptors that are occupied will increase progressively and asymptotically approach 1, and the effect E will approach E_{max} asymptotically. If this graph is plotted with log concentration against effect, a sigmoid concentration–response curve is obtained (Fig. 3.1). Potency is characterized by the EC_{50}: the more potent a drug, the lower the EC_{50}. Drug A in Fig. 3.1 is more potent than drug B. Note that potency is defined by the dependency of effect on concentration. Traditionally, in pharmacology, potency has been related to dose rather than concentration, i.e. based on ED_{50} (dose producing 50% of maximum effect). However, the dose–effect relationship involves both pharmacokinetic and pharmacodynamic components, whereas the concentration–effect relationship involves only the pharmacodynamics of a drug.

Drugs with similar potencies for one pharmacological effect may have a very different potency ratio for another effect, and for the same drug potency may differ markedly for different pharmacological endpoints. The plasma concentrations of alfentanil (combined with 66% nitrous oxide) required to prevent

responses in 50% of patients were 475 ± 28 ng ml^{-1} for laryngoscopy and tracheal intubation, 279 ± 20 ng ml^{-1} for skin incision and 150 ± 13 ng ml^{-1} for skin closure.[2] The EC_{50} of alfentanil for suppressing responses to intraoperative stimuli was also higher in patients undergoing upper abdominal surgery (412 ± 135 ng ml^{-1}) than in those having lower abdominal procedures (309 ± 44 ng ml^{-1}) or undergoing breast surgery (270 ± 63 ng ml^{-1}).

The E_{max} parameter in eqn [2] characterizes the agonist properties of a drug. Drugs that are full agonists can cause a maximum response at sufficiently high concentrations (drugs A and B in Fig. 3.1). Pure antagonists produce no response at all. Partial agonists effect responses that are less than those produced by full agonists, even at very high concentrations (drug C, Fig. 3.1). The ability of a drug to produce a biological response after binding to a receptor depends on its affinity for the receptor (determined by simple intermolecular forces), and a subsequent change in the receptor that leads to the response. The degree (fraction of maximum) to which a drug can activate a biological system is characterized by a parameter called *intrinsic activity* or *efficacy*. Full agonists are assigned an intrinsic activity value of 1, pure antagonists 0 and partial agonists a value between 0 and 1. Efficacy is, however, only one of the factors that determine the final response. Other factors of importance are the total number of receptors available for combining with the drug molecules and the nature of the coupling between the activated receptor and the final cellular response (transduction). Agonists combine with a receptor to produce a response, i.e. they have both affinity and intrinsic efficacy. An antagonist, on the other hand, has affinity (usually high) but zero intrinsic efficacy.

According to classical occupation theory, a drug with an intrinsic activity of 1 produces its maximum response when all available receptors are occupied. Since the work of Stephenson[3] and Nickerson[4] in 1956, it has been realized that most (if not all) full agonists produce their maximum response when only a fraction of the available receptors is occupied, i.e. there are 'spare receptors' or receptor reserve. Partial agonists, on the other hand, do not cause a maximum response even with 100% receptor occupancy (Fig. 3.2). Spare receptors are frequently encountered when the receptor activation–signal transduction–response process involves considerable amplification. For example, a single G protein-coupled receptor can activate hundreds of G proteins in some systems.

Partial agonists, because they compete with agonists for available receptors, can produce either agonist or antagonist effects, depending on the circumstances in which they are used. In low concentrations they usually produce agonist effects, and in the presence of low

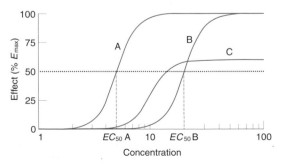

Fig. 3.1 Plasma concentration–response curves for full agonists (A and B) and for a partial agonist (C). Drug A is more potent than drug B (EC_{50} of A is lower than that of B).

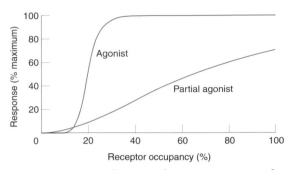

Fig. 3.2 Response as a function of receptor occupancy for a full agonist and a partial agonist. Note that for the full agonist maximum response occurs when only 35% of the receptors are occupied while for the partial agonist maximum response does not occur even when all receptors are occupied.

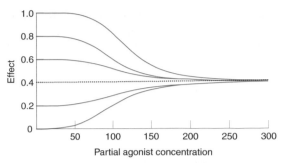

Fig. 3.3 Hypothetical concentration–response curves for the combined effects of a partial agonist, with a maximum effect (intrinsic activity) of 0.4, and a full agonist. The lower curves show the response when increasing concentrations of the partial agonist are added to a low concentration of the full agonist; the combined response increases asymptotically to the E_{max} of the partial agonist. When increasing concentrations of the partial agonist are added to a high concentration of the full agonist, the combined response decreases asymptotically to the E_{max} of the partial agonist.

concentrations of a full agonist the effect will be additive. When, however, the concentration of the full agonist is high, addition of a partial agonist with an affinity for the receptor similar to or greater than that of the full agonist will displace the latter from the receptor. Since the response produced by the partial agonist is less than that of the full agonist, the overall effect will be a reduction of the response, and the partial agonist acts as a competitive reversible antagonist (Fig. 3.3). This mechanism explains why nalorphine, a partial μ-opioid agonist, can be used to reverse the effects of a full opioid agonist such as fentanyl.

PHARMACODYNAMIC MODELS

Several pharmacodynamic models have been used to describe the relationship between drug concentrations and effect. The most widely used is the sigmoid E_{max} model:

$$E = E_{max} \cdot \frac{C^{\gamma}}{C^{\gamma} + EC_{50}^{\gamma}} \qquad [3]$$

where γ is a dimensionless parameter that determines the slope of the concentration response curve (Fig. 3.4). When $\gamma = 1$ the equation is identical to the E_{max} equation (eqn [2]). Drugs with a high value of γ will have steep concentration–response curves, and a small increase in concentration (or a small additional dose) will result in a marked increase in clinical response. This is of benefit during anaesthesia (e.g. a small bolus of an opioid will be sufficient to restore analgesia). In other circumstances it can increase the risk of side-effects. A small additional bolus of an opioid in the postoperative period may result in respiratory depression. While the simple E_{max} equation produces a hyperbolic curve when E is plotted against C on a linear scale, the corresponding curve for eqn [3] is sigmoid shaped. Although the

concentration–effect relationship is hyperbolic for some drugs, for most drugs the relationship is best described by the sigmoid E_{max} model. Eqn [3] was developed by Hill to describe the association between haemoglobin and oxygen, and is often referred to as the Hill equation.

Eqns [2] and [3] describe the situation in which the effect of a drug produces a graded increase in pharmacological effect with increasing concentration. In other situations a drug produces an inhibitory effect, for example a reduction in heart rate by propranolol or the slowing of the electroencephalographic (EEG) frequency by an opioid. The model can easily be adapted to deal with this situation. In the inhibitory E_{max} model the effect of the drug is subtracted from the response when no drug is present (E_0):

$$E = E_0 - E_{max} \cdot \frac{C^{\gamma}}{C^{\gamma} + EC_{50}^{\gamma}} \qquad [4]$$

The models described above relate to pharmacodynamic responses that are continuous. Many types

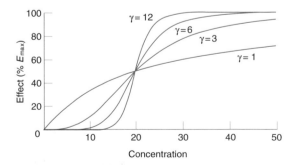

Fig. 3.4 Influence of the slope factor, γ, on the shape of the sigmoid E_{max} concentration–response curve.

of response, however, are quantal (a response is either present or absent), for example movement in response to a noxious stimulus. Quantal data can be modelled in a similar way using techniques such as that described by Waud.[5]

PHARMACOKINETIC–PHARMACODYNAMIC MODELS

These models combine concentration–time and concentration–effect relationships. If the equilibrium between drug in the circulation and at the effect site was instantaneous then plasma drug concentrations could be plugged directly into eqn [3] to link concentration, response and time. This would allow determination of the drug input required for a desired response. Often, however, there is a distinct time lag in the occurrence of the pharmacological effect relative to the plasma concentration. This time delay between the time-course of drug effect and plasma drug concentration gives rise to an anticlockwise hysteresis loop in the effect–concentration plot when effect–plasma concentration data pairs measured, for example during and after a short intravenous infusion, are connected in time order (Fig. 3.5). Hysteresis arises because a drug requires a finite time to pass from the bloodstream to the effect site. This delay is determined mainly by the physico-chemical properties of the drug such as pK_a, lipid solubility, etc. Further delays may arise as a result of signal transduction processes at the cellular level, i.e. between drug activation of the receptor and the biological response (see Chapter 1).

For anaesthetic drugs the equilibrium delay between plasma concentration and corresponding drug effect is clinically relevant and thus important to characterize. This delay explains the differences in the time to maximum effect between, for example, fentanyl and remifentanil. The equilibrium delay can be character-ized by means of PK–PD models, which use mathemat-ical functions to describe the relationship between drug concentration and effect. A link is made between the pharmacokinetic response and the pharmacodynamic (or effect) response by postulating an effect compart-ment linked to a conventional pharmacokinetic com-partmental model. Effect compartment models were originally developed by Hull et al.[6] in 1978 and subse-quently extended by Sheiner et al.[7] Both groups defined their models using muscle relaxants, which have the advantage that the effect can be readily and directly mea-sured. The effect site compartment is considered as another kinetic compartment linked to the central com-partment of a pharmacokinetic model by first-order processes, but with negligible volume (usually taken as 1/1000 or 1/10 000 of V_1) and receiving only a negligi-ble amount of the drug (Fig. 3.6). This also means that

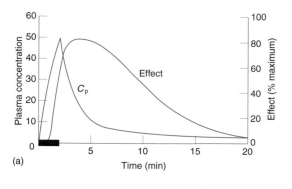

(a)

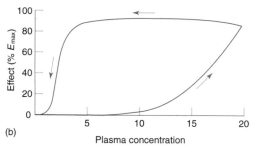

(b)

Fig. 3.5 The concept of hysteresis. (a) Changes in plasma concentration (C_p) and the resulting pharmacological effect during and after stopping a fixed rate intravenous infusion (black bar). There is dissociation between the concentration and effect curves due to delay in the equilibration of drug between plasma and effect site. This results in a hysteresis loop when the effect is plotted against C_p (b). The direction of the hysteresis loop is shown by the arrows.

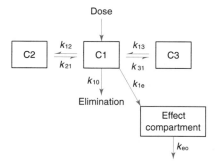

Fig. 3.6 Three-compartment pharmacokinetic model with a linked effect compartment.

negligible drug returns from the effect compartment to the plasma and thus the pharmacokinetic model is not changed significantly by adding the effect compart-ment. The output from this compartment is a first-order rate constant (k_{eo}) which characterizes the temporal aspect of equilibrium between plasma concentration and drug effect. The time-course of effect site concentration is a function of k_{eo} and of the pharmacokinetic parameters that describe the disposition of the plasma or blood concentration. As for other pharmacokinetic rate constants, k_{eo} can be converted to a half-life:

$$t_{1/2}k_{eo} = \frac{\ln 2}{k_{eo}} = \frac{0.693}{k_{eo}}$$

If the plasma concentration of a drug were instantaneously increased to a higher steady-state concentration, it would take 4–5 times the $t_{1/2}k_{eo}$ for the effect site concentration to reach 90–95% of its steady-state concentration.

The rate constant k_{eo} can be determined from simultaneously measured plasma concentrations and drug effect, for example during and after a short intravenous infusion. Two approaches may be used. The parametric method involves a priori defining appropriate pharmacokinetic and pharmacodynamic models (the correct choice of both models is crucial), and nonlinear regression techniques are used to link the effect data directly to plasma concentrations and to provide estimates of both pharmacokinetic and dynamic parameters (e.g. E_0, E_{max} and EC_{50} for the pharmacodynamic model). An alternative approach is semiparametric or nonparametric modelling, which make no a priori assumptions about the pharmacodynamic model. In these methods the value of k_{eo} is iterated until the area within the hysteresis loop between concentration and effect is minimized (Fig. 3.7). The putative concentration in the effect site can then be plotted directly against the effect and the concentration–effect relationship evaluated directly (Fig. 3.7d).

PK–PD models are a powerful tool in pharmacology and their use in the early stages of new drug development has become almost as mandatory as conventional pharmacokinetic analysis. In addition to predicting drug effects in response to a variety of different drug inputs from single-dose data, they can also provide insight into the mechanisms of drug interaction and for designing optimum dosage regimens when two or more drugs are administered, for example the combination of propofol and an opioid (and see Chapter 28).[8] Algorithms have been developed for computer-controlled intravenous infusion systems to allow control of a target effect site concentration instead of the more conventional plasma concentration.[9,10]

FACTORS INFLUENCING PHARMACODYNAMICS

The pharmacodynamics of a drug may be influenced by factors such as age, sex and disease, just as these factors can influence a drug's pharmacokinetics. The pharmacodynamics are also significantly affected by the choice of pharmacodynamic endpoint.

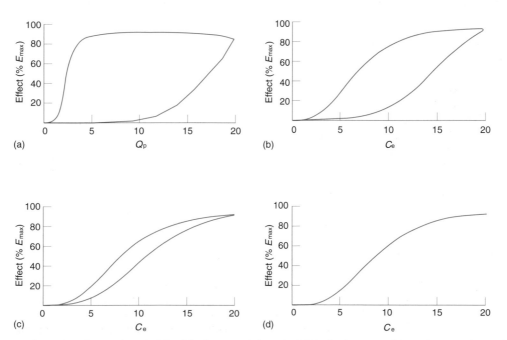

Fig. 3.7 Nonparametric approach to estimating k_{eo}. The hysteresis loop in (a) is the same as that in Fig. 3.5. (b) and (c) show the hysteresis loops for effect site concentration (C_e) calculated using estimates of k_{eo} that are too large. The correct choice of k_{eo} results in the collapse of the hysteresis loop (d).

AGE

It is a common clinical experience that elderly patients require a lower dose of an anaesthetic drug for induction and maintenance of anaesthesia than younger patients. Because of the changes in pharmacokinetics with increasing age, it is often difficult to separate the confounding influence of pharmacokinetics and pharmacodynamics. However, a definite influence of age on the pharmacodynamics of several drugs has been demonstrated, although the mechanisms for these changes are poorly understood. Changes in receptor numbers or sensitivity may account for some of the observed changes in the elderly. Perhaps the best-documented age-related pharmacodynamic change is the decrease in the minimum alveolar concentration (MAC) of inhalational anaesthetic agents (see Chapter 4). For intravenous anaesthetics the picture is less clear. The decreased dose of thiopentone required for induction of anaesthesia in the elderly appears to be due to altered pharmacokinetics rather than pharmacodynamics.[11] Similar findings have been reported for etomidate. The dose of benzodiazepines needed to achieve a given degree of anxiolysis or hypnosis is lower in most elderly subjects than in younger subjects. Also the intravenous dose of midazolam required for induction of anaesthesia is lower in elderly patients. These changes have been attributed more to an age-related increase in pharmacodynamic sensitivity than to alterations in pharmacokinetic distribution or clearance processes. The midazolam EC_{50} for response to verbal command decreased significantly with increasing patient age, from 598 ng ml^{-1} at 40 years to 139 ng ml^{-1} at 80 years (Fig. 3.8), demonstrating that aging increases pharmacodynamic sensitivity to the hypnotic effects of midazolam independently of pharmacokinetic factors.[12]

For the opioids there are conflicting reports on the alterations in pharmacodynamics with age. Scott and Stanski[13] found that the brain sensitivity to the EEG effects increased linearly with age for fentanyl and alfentanil. In contrast, Lemmens et al.[14] could not demonstrate an age dependency for alfentanil plasma concentration–effect relations based on responses to intraoperative surgical stimuli, and attributed changes in dose requirements to age-related changes in pharmacokinetics and/or sex-related differences. The differences between these studies may reflect the differences in the measures used to define drug effect. While EEG-induced changes may be more sensitive markers of pharmacodynamic effects than clinical measures, the endpoints used by Lemmens et al. are likely to be more clinically relevant. Although there are age-related differences in the actions of sufentanil, these cannot be explained by changes in the drug's pharmacokinetic properties and must be assumed to be caused by changes in its pharmacodynamics with age. The k_{eo} and EC_{50} of remifentanil, based on the EEG spectral edge (SE_{95}) as a measure of drug effect, decrease with increasing age.[15]

Neonates often have very different (usually much lower) dose requirements for many centrally acting drugs than infants or older children. This probably reflects differences in both pharmacokinetics and pharmacodynamics. Factors affecting the pharmacodynamics of drug may include the increased permeability of the blood–brain barrier and immaturity of drug receptors in premature infants and neonates.

SEX

It has recently become evident that there are important sex-related differences in the response to anaesthetics and analgesics. Women have a higher incidence of awareness during anaesthesia compared with men and tend to emerge faster than men from general anaesthesia. κ opioids produce significantly more analgesia in women than men[16] while μ opioids produce less analgesia in female than in male animals. Women are more sensitive to respiratory depression induced by morphine.[17] The mechanisms of these differences are probably related to sex-related differences in the sensitivity of the brain to anaesthetics and analgesics. Many studies in humans have demonstrated differences in pain sensitivity between the sexes.[18] These differing sensitivities may be due to direct hormonal differences or to differences in brain neurobiology and structure (sexual dimorphism).

DISEASE

Renal and hepatic disease. In their original paper describing PK–PD modelling, Sheiner et al.[7] suggested that the pharmacodynamic parameters for tubocurarine were different between normal subjects and

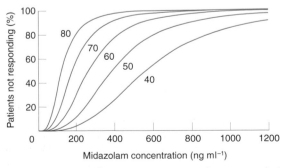

Fig. 3.8 Percentage of patients not responding to a verbal command versus steady-state midazolam plasma concentrations at different ages. Curves were simulated using the model P (response) $= 1/(1 + e^{-23.96 + 3.05 \ln (C_p) + 0.115 \times age})$ described by Jacobs et al.[12]

patients with renal failure. More recently it has been shown that subjects with severe chronic liver disease are more sensitive to the ventilatory depressant effects of remifentanil.[19] The EC_{50} value (the remifentanil concentration that depresses carbon dioxide minute ventilation by 50%) in the control and hepatic disease groups were 2.52 and 1.56 ng ml^{-1} respectively. The pharmacokinetics of remifentanil are unchanged in those with liver disease. Such patients may be more sensitive to the ventilatory depressant effects of remifentanil, a finding of uncertain clinical significance considering the extremely short duration of action of the drug. The EC_{50} values were lower in subjects with hepatic disease, suggesting that they may be more sensitive to the ventilatory depressant effects of remifentanil. The mechanism of the altered EC_{50} in patients with liver disease is unknown. The increased alfentanil requirement in patients with Crohn's disease have been attributed to a change in pharmacodynamics rather than pharmacokinetics.[20]

DRUG INTERACTIONS

Drug combinations are of increasing importance in modern medicine, and particularly in anaesthesia where drugs are given acutely and usually intravenously. An important type of drug interaction with a predominantly pharmacodynamic mechanism commonly arises between drugs that have overtly similar pharmacological actions, such as hypnosis or analgesia. Similar actions mean that each drug produces the same effect even if the common effect is due to different mechanisms. Because pharmacodynamic variability is much greater than pharmacokinetic variability, pharmacodynamic interactions are much more important from the clinical point of view compared with pharmacokinetic interactions (see Chapter 28).

PK–PD modelling has proved a valuable tool for determining the optimum concentrations of combinations of opioids and intravenous anaesthetics to ensure adequate anaesthesia and recovery.[8] Pharmacodynamic interactions occur as a result of several mechanisms, most of which are poorly understood. At the cellular level one drug may enhance the binding of a second drug to its receptor, or conversely inhibit its binding (e.g. agonist–antagonist interaction). A drug may also alter the intracellular signal transduction pathway of another drug, for example the potentiation of the arrhythmogenic effects of catecholamines by halothane as a result of both increasing adenylyl cyclase activity. Probably the most common cause of pharmacodynamic interactions is two drugs acting on separate receptor systems that have a final common cellular pathway.

CLINICAL APPLICATION OF PHARMACODYNAMICS

An understanding of pharmacodynamic principles is of practical value and can improve insight into many clinical observations. For intravenously administered drugs the parameter k_{eo} is an important determinant of the onset time, time to reach maximum effect and the duration of the clinical effect. The changes in the effect site concentrations following two bolus injections of propofol, one double the dose of the other, are shown in Fig. 3.9a. With the higher dose, the peak effect site concentration is twice that of the lower dose, but the time to peak concentration is the same in both cases. Fig. 3.9b shows the effect of different values of k_{eo} on the disposition of the effect concentration following the lower dose of propofol. As the value of k_{eo} is reduced ($t_{1/2}$ k_{eo} increases), the onset time and the duration of action of the drug become progressively longer and the peak effect site concentration (and thus the pharmacological effect) becomes lower. For drugs with an intermediate value of k_{eo}, such as midazolam, the onset time can be

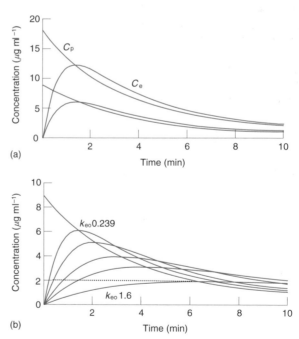

Fig. 3.9 (a) Relationship between plasma and effect site concentrations (C_e) following a single intravenous bolus of a drug. The upper curves are the result of giving twice the dose used to produce the lower set of curves; note that with the higher dose the peak C_e is twice as high but the time at which the peak concentration occurs is the same. Increasing the dose will, however, allow a given threshold C_e (horizontal line) to be reached in a shorter time. (b) Effect of different values of k_{eo}, from 0.293 to 1.6 min^{-1}, following the lower bolus dose in (a).

reduced by increasing the dose but at the price of prolonged action. The values of k_{eo} and $t_{1/2}k_{eo}$ for several anaesthetic drugs are given in Table 3.1.

The rate of administration of an intravenous drug is an important variable determining the total dose administered when the infusion is continued until a given endpoint has been reached. For anaesthetic induction agents, slower infusion rates are associated with lower doses to achieve loss of consciousness but at the cost of longer induction times.[21,22] To understand why this is so, consider a hypothetical drug administered at varying infusion rates with cessation of the infusion when consciousness is lost (Fig. 3.10). It is assumed that consciousness is lost when the effect site concentration reaches a threshold, and that this is also the concentration at which consciousness is regained in the absence of other drugs. The fastest infusion rate results in loss of consciousness after 40 s with return of consciousness at 10 min. As the infusion rate is slowed, the time required for the effect site concentration to reach the threshold level for loss of consciousness becomes longer and the time to awakening shorter. The total dose of the drug needed for induction with the lowest infusion rate is reduced by 50% compared with the highest infusion rate. Note that as the infusion rate is slowed the peak effect site concentration becomes lower, until a rate is reached at which the effect

concentration just attains the threshold level. At this rate the induction time will be prolonged and the period of unconsciousness very short. This is obviously not an ideal situation for induction of anaesthesia. However, administering drugs such as intravenous anaesthetic agents by slow infusion rather than fast bolus injection has advantages in ill patients. The slower rate of administration results in a lower total dose and the lower peak effect site concentration can reduce the risk of adverse central nervous system side-effects. Lower peak plasma concentrations will minimize adverse cardiovascular and other side-effects directly related to the plasma concentration.

Table 3.1 Pharmacodynamic parameters for some drugs used in anaesthesia		
Drug	$k_{eo}(min^{-1})$	$t_{1/2}k_{eo}(min)$
Thiopentone	0.59	1.17
Etomidate	0.43	1.6
Propofol	0.2	3.5
Ketamine	1.03	0.67
Midazolam	0.144	4.8
Diazepam	0.43	1.6
Morphine	0.041	17
Fentanyl	0.105	6.6
Sufentanil	0.112	6.2
Alfentanil	0.77	0.9
Remifentanil	0.595	1.16
Pancuronium	0.21	3.3
Vecuronium	0.187	3.7
Atracurium	0.117	5.9

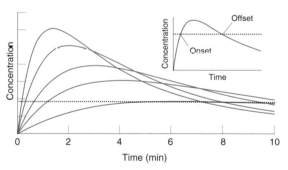

Fig. 3.10 Simulations of the disposition of drug concentration in the theoretical effect site due to administration of a drug by intravenous infusion at increasing infusion rates. The infusion was stopped when the effect concentration reached the threshold for loss of consciousness (horizontal dotted line). Note that for all but the slowest infusion rate the effect concentration continues to rise after the infusion is stopped.

REFERENCES

1. Jacobs JR, Reves JG. Effect site equilibration time is a determinant of induction dose requirement. *Anesth Analg* 1993; **76**: 1–6 (editorial).

2. Ausems ME, Stanski DR, Hug CC, Burm AGL. Plasma concentrations of alfentanil required to supplement nitrous oxide anesthesia for general surgery. *Anesthesiology* 1986; **65**: 362–373.

3. Stephenson RP. A modification of receptor theory. *Br J Pharmacol* 1956; **11**: 379–393.

4. Nickerson M. Receptor occupancy and tissue response. *Nature* 1956; **178**: 697–698.

5. Waud DR. On biological assays involving quantal responses. *J Pharmacol Exp Ther* 1972; **183**: 577–607.

6. Hull CJ, Van Beem B, McLeod K, Sibbald A, Watson MJ. A pharmacodynamic model for pancuronium. *Br J Anaesth* 1978; **50**: 1113–1123.

7. Sheiner LB, Stanski DR, Vozeh S *et al*. Simultaneous modeling of pharmacokinetics and pharmacodynamics: application to *d*-tubocurarine. *Clin Pharmacol Ther* 1979; **25**: 358–371.

8. Vuyk J, Mertens MJ, Olofsen E, Burm AGL, Bovill JG. Propofol anesthesia and rational opioid selection: determination of optimal EC_{50}–EC_{95} propofol–opioid concentrations that assure adequate anesthesia and a rapid return of consciousness. *Anesthesiology* 1997; **87**: 1549–1562.

9. Shafer SL, Gregg KM. Algorithms to rapidly achieve and maintain stable drug concentrations at the site of drug effect with a computer-controlled infusion pump. *J Pharmacokinet Biopharm* 1992; **20**: 147–169.

10. Jacobs JR, Williams EA. Algorithm to control 'effect compartment' drug concentration in pharmacokinetic model-driven drug delivery. *IEEE Trans Biomed Eng* 1990; **40**: 993–999.

11. Stanski DR, Maitre PO. Population pharmacokinetics and pharmacodynamics of thiopental: the effect of age revisited. *Anesthesiology* 1990; **72**: 412–422.

12. Jacobs JR, Reves JG, Marty J, White WD, Bai SA, Smith LR. Aging increases pharmacodynamic sensitivity to the hypnotic effects of midazolam. *Anesth Analg* 1995; **80**: 143–148.

13. Scott JC, Stanski DR. Decreased fentanyl and alfentanil dose requirements with age. A simultaneous pharmacokinetic and pharmacodynamic evaluation. *J Pharmacol Exp Ther* 1987; **240**: 159–166.

14. Lemmens HJM, Bovill JG, Hennis PJ, Burm AGL. Age has no effect on the pharmacodynamics of alfentanil. *Anesth Analg* 1988; **67**: 956–960.

15. Minto CF, Schnider TW, Egan TD *et al*. Influence of age and gender on the pharmacokinetics and pharmacodynamics of remifentanil. I. Model development. *Anesthesiology* 1997; **86**: 10–23.

16. Gear RW, Miaskowski C, Gordon NC, Paul SM, Heller PH, Levine JD. Kappa-opioids produce significantly greater analgesia in women than in men. *Nature Med* 1996; **2**: 1248–1250.

17. Dahan A, Sarton E, Teppema L, Olievier C. Sex-related differences in the influence of morphine on ventilatory control in humans. *Anesthesiology* 1998; **88**: 903–913.

18. Unruh AM. Gender variations in clinical pain experience. *Pain* 1996; **65**: 123–167.

19. Dershwitz M, Hoke JF, Rosow CE *et al*. The pharmacokinetics and pharmacodynamics of remifentanil in volunteer subjects with severe liver disease. *Anesthesiology* 1996; **84**: 812–820.

20. Gesink van der Veer BJ, Burm AGL, Vletter AA, Bovill JG. Influence of Crohn's disease on the pharmacokinetics and pharmacodynamics of alfentanil. *Br J Anaesth* 1993; **71**: 827–834.

21. Peacock JE, Lewis RP, Reilly CS, Nimmo WS. Effect of different rates of infusion of propofol for induction of anaesthesia in elderly patients. *Br J Anaesth* 1990; **65**: 346–362.

22. Gentry WB, Krejcie TC, Henthorn TK *et al*. Effect of infusion rate on thiopental dose–response relationships. *Anesthesiology* 1994; **81**: 316–324

Section 2

DRUGS ACTING ON THE CENTRAL NERVOUS SYSTEM

4

AJ Scurr, ZP Khan, RM Jones

INHALATIONAL ANAESTHETICS

During the 1840s diethyl ether and nitrous oxide were first used for dental and surgical procedures to render patients oblivious to pain. The initial use of both agents was the result of observations of their analgesic properties during recreational use (e.g. 'ether frolics'). In the first decade thereafter, American pioneers such as Crawford Long, Wells and Morton were simply sedating their patients but the concept of general anaesthesia quickly developed, the term 'anaesthesia' being conceived by Oliver Wendell Holmes.[1]

During the nineteenth century the principal agents were nitrous oxide, diethyl ether and chloroform. In the twentieth century others, such as trichloroethylene, ethyl chloride and divinyl ether, and the gas cyclopropane, were introduced. Initially, these were used as sole agents in the provision of the anaesthetic triad of hypnosis, analgesia and muscle relaxation. The modern trend is to provide for each of these requirements with a separate agent, the so-called 'balanced anaesthesia' technique.

The evolution of inhaled anaesthetic agents has been marked by the search for safer and more effective agents. With the introduction of surgical diathermy the search for nonflammable agents was intensified. It was appreciated in the 1930s that fluorination of molecules decreased flammability and toxicity, but it was not until the 1950s that the first fluorinated anaesthetics were introduced. More recently agents entirely halogenated with fluorine have been developed, but the search for the ideal agent continues. None of the currently available anaesthetic agents fulfils all the requirements of the ideal agent.[2]

Summary box 4.1 Properties of the ideal inhaled anaesthetic agent

- Pleasant smell and nonirritant, allowing smooth inhalational induction.

- Adequate potency for effective use in high oxygen concentrations.

- Respiratory and cardiovascular effects should be minimal and predictable.

- No systemic toxicity.

- Central neurological effects should be reversible and there should be no excitatory activity.

- A low blood:gas partition coefficient ensuring rapid induction and recovery characteristics and easy adjustment of depth of anaesthesia.

- Should not be metabolized.

- Stable in light, heat and alkali, not flammable or explosive.

- Stable in soda lime and noncorrosive.

- Should be obtainable at reasonable cost in its pure form and have a good shelf-life.

PHYSICAL PROPERTIES

Inhalation anaesthetic agents are either gases or vapours. In the gaseous phase a compound is considered a vapour when it is below its critical temperature and a gas when it is above its critical temperature. The critical temperature of a compound is the temperature above which it cannot be liquefied by the application of pressure alone. Thus the anaesthetic agents halothane, enflurane, isoflurane, desflurane, sevoflurane and nitrous oxide are properly referred to as vapours.

Vapours in the gaseous phase exert a measurable pressure, referred to as vapour pressure. In common with gases the vapour pressure is the result of the kinetic energy of the molecules. When a vapour overlies a volume of the liquid agent in an enclosed space, the kinetic energy of the molecules will result in the development of a dynamic equilibrium, with some molecules escaping from the liquid surface and entering the gaseous phase and others impinging on the gas–liquid interface and returning to the liquid phase. At equilibrium the vapour achieves maximum pressure and is referred to as saturated. The vapour pressure at saturation is the saturated vapour pressure.

Mixtures of gases and vapours will behave in such a way that the total pressure exerted by the mixture will equal the sum of the partial pressures exerted by each of the components if present alone and occupying the same volume as the mixture (Dalton's law). In other words, the partial pressure of each component of the mixture will be determined by the fractional concentration of that compound, as well as its specific physical characteristics.

A solution of a gas or vapour will also exert a partial pressure within that solution which is equivalent to the partial pressure that the agent in solution would support in a gas–liquid equilibrium, as described above (and is therefore a measure of the kinetic energy of the molecules and their resulting potential to equilibrate between gaseous and liquid phases). The partial pressure thus exerted in solution is referred to as tension.

When a substance is in contact with two different phases (e.g. blood, lipid or gas) it will be proportioned between the two phases depending on its affinity for each phase. The partition coefficient (λ) is the ratio of the proportions at equilibrium and it is constant for different liquids. The Ostwald solubility coefficient is the volume of gas dissolving in a unit volume of liquid at a stated temperature and is numerically identical to the partition coefficient.

The state of anaesthesia is related to the tension (partial pressure) of the anaesthetic in the brain. A rapid increase or decrease in brain tension will lead to rapid induction and recovery. The rate of increase in tension is more rapid for an agent with a low solubility than for one of higher solubility. In Fig. 4.1 a liquid in a enclosed container is in equilibrium with two gases at a pressure of 100 kPa. Gas A is present in 20 volumes % (vol%) and, according to Dalton's law, it exerts a partial pressure of 20 kPa. Gas B is present in 80 vol% and will exert a partial pressure of 80 kPa. *Note:* For the sake of simplicity the partial pressure of the liquid vapour has been ignored. Gas A has partition coefficient of 3.0 and is therefore more soluble than gas B, which has a solubility coefficient of 0.5. Since:

$$\lambda = \frac{\% \text{ in liquid phase}}{\% \text{ in gas phase}}$$

gas A is present in the liquid at a concentration of 20 × 3.0 = 60 vol%, whereas gas B is present in 40 vol%. As

the system is in equilibrium, the tensions that the two gases exert must be identical to that which they exert in the gas phase, i.e. gas A exerts a tension of 20 kPa and gas B 80 kPa. However, even though the tension of gas A is less than that of gas B, the concentration of gas A is greater.

PHARMACOKINETICS

The uptake and elimination of inhalational anaesthetics by the lungs leads to a predictable and controllable kinetic profile, and thus accurate and safe drug administration. Alveolar concentration and thus tension depend on inspired concentration, alveolar ventilation and pulmonary capillary blood flow (i.e. the balance between delivery to the alveolar gas space and its removal in pulmonary capillary blood). Initially the ratio of alveolar to inspired anaesthetic concentration is zero. Over time alveolar concentration increases and approaches the inspired concentration, eventually approaching unity. Pulmonary capillary blood tension forms an equilibrium with alveolar partial pressure, and the rate at which this occurs determines the rate of increase in tension of the agent within the brain, and so the speed of onset of anaesthesia.

Fig. 4.2 shows a comparison of uptake for inhaled anaesthetic agents. The rate of increase in alveolar concentration with respect to inspired concentration, expressed as the ratio F_A/F_I plotted against time, represents the exponential wash-in functions of the anaesthetic agents. The rate of change of an exponential function is expressed in terms of its time constant. This is the theoretical time the process would take to complete if the initial rate of change had been

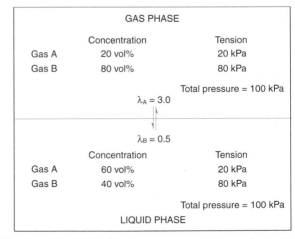

GAS PHASE

	Concentration	Tension
Gas A	20 vol%	20 kPa
Gas B	80 vol%	80 kPa

Total pressure = 100 kPa

$\lambda_A = 3.0$

$\lambda_B = 0.5$

	Concentration	Tension
Gas A	60 vol%	20 kPa
Gas B	40 vol%	80 kPa

Total pressure = 100 kPa

LIQUID PHASE

Fig. 4.1 Relationship between concentration, tension and solubility (λ). A closed container at approximately atmospheric pressure contains a liquid, above which is a mixture of two gases A and B. See text for details.

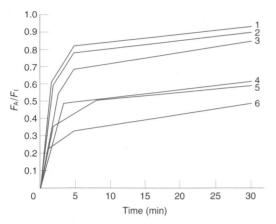

Fig. 4.2 Rate of increase of alveolar fractional concentration (F_A) with respect to inspired F for different inhaled anaesthetics. 1, Nitrous oxide; 2, desflurane; 3, sevoflurane; 4, isoflurane; 5, enflurane; 6, halothane.

maintained. Fig. 4.3 shows the theoretical exponential wash-in curve for an anaesthetic agent of low solubility. A tangent drawn to the curve at time zero allows the time constant to be estimated (in this example 10 min). It can be seen that after one time constant has elapsed the wash-in process is 63% complete, after two time constants the process is 86% complete, and so on. The curve is asymptotic to unity and so, in theory, a true equilibrium is never attained. It is also clear that as wash-in progresses the rate of increase of alveolar tension decreases with the gradient of inspired to alveolar tension. Wash-out progresses at a rate proportional to the difference between the alveolar concentration and the concentration in the inspired gas.

Solubility, blood flow and concentration gradient are the major factors affecting inhalational anaesthetic

uptake. Less soluble agents (low blood : gas solubility coefficient) have a more rapid onset of anaesthesia because brain tension increases faster than with more soluble agents. Increasing the cardiac output increases the amount of anaesthetic taken up but decreases the alveolar concentration. Increasing the alveolar ventilation increases the alveolar concentration and therefore increases the speed of onset. The effect of changes in cardiac output and alveolar ventilation are illustrated in Figs 4.4 and 4.5. In the lung the most important gradient affecting rate of uptake is the alveolar to mixed venous partial pressure difference. During the initial phase the mixed venous partial pressure will be small and uptake will be most rapid. Hypercarbia will increase the rate of uptake of anaesthetic by the brain by causing cerebral vasodilatation and hence increasing cerebral blood flow.

CONCENTRATION EFFECT

It can be demonstrated that the higher the inspired concentration the more rapid the relative increase in

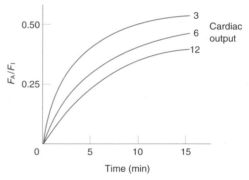

Fig. 4.4 Rate of increase in alveolar concentration to approach inspired concentration (F_A/F_I) plotted against time for halothane. Alveolar ventilation remains constant and cardiac output is altered.

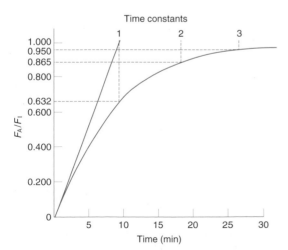

Fig. 4.3 Wash-in exponential function demonstrating time constants for the process.

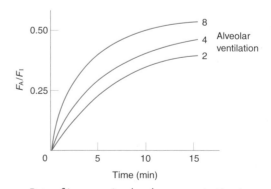

Fig. 4.5 Rate of increase in alveolar concentration to approach inspired concentration (F_A/F_I) plotted against time for halothane. Cardiac output remains constant and alveolar ventilation is altered.

alveolar concentration. The more rapid increase is due to the greater volume of gas absorbed when higher concentrations are administered. If, when breathing 5% nitrous oxide, 10% of the administered nitrous oxide is absorbed and the tidal volume is 500 ml, then 2.5 ml of nitrous oxide is absorbed per breath. In contrast, when breathing 75% nitrous oxide 37.5 ml will be absorbed per breath. If the respiratory rate is $10 \, min^{-1}$ this represents the absorption of $375 \, ml \, min^{-1}$ of nitrous oxide from the alveoli, compared with only 25 ml when breathing 5%. The absorption of this volume of nitrous oxide causes inspired gas to be drawn into the alveoli to replace that absorbed. The net effect is that of a relative increase in alveolar ventilation and thus of alveolar concentration of agent. This is called the concentration effect. It is of significance only with nitrous oxide and possibly desflurane, of which 3 MAC (minimum alveolar concentration) represents about 20% inspired desflurane. Although the more rapid increase observed when breathing higher concentrations of agent is interesting, it is not of particular clinical significance in the majority of situations.

DIFFUSION HYPOXIA

The reverse phenomenon occurs after cessation of high concentrations of nitrous oxide and return to breathing of air. Now large volumes of nitrous oxide enter the alveoli from the blood, to be replaced by nitrogen. But since nitrogen is less soluble in blood than nitrous oxide, more nitrogen will enter the alveoli than nitrous oxide will leave. The net result, according to Dalton's law, will be a dilution effect on alveolar oxygen, i.e. a reduction in the tension of oxygen, known as diffusion hypoxia (Fink effect). The administration of 100% oxygen on cessation of nitrous oxide anaesthesia prevents hypoxia by increasing alveolar oxygen concentration.

SECOND GAS EFFECT

The second gas effect is a phenomenon related to the concentration effect. If F_A/F_I is measured during the uptake of any potent agent, such as isoflurane, in the presence or absence of higher concentrations of nitrous oxide (i.e. 1% isoflurane in 100% oxygen compared with 1% isoflurane in 70% nitrous oxide and 30% oxygen), the increase is more rapid if nitrous oxide is present than if it is absent. Two mechanisms are responsible for this phenomenon. First, there is a relative increase in alveolar ventilation consequent upon the absorption of a significant volume of nitrous oxide, as in the concentration effect. Second, the absorption of nitrous oxide causes the relative concentration of the second vapour to increase.

The measured elimination is not the mirror image of measured uptake (Fig. 4.6). One of the reasons for this is that at the end of administration all compart-

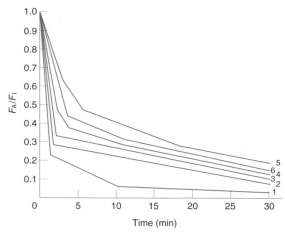

Fig. 4.6 Rate of elimination of inhaled anaesthetics. Rate of decrease in alveolar concentration (F_A) with respect to the last alveolar concentration (F_{AO}) during administration of different inhalational agents. 1, Nitrous oxide; 2, desflurane; 3, sevoflurane; 4, isoflurane; 5, enflurane; 6, halothane.

ments of the body will contain different tensions of anaesthetic depending on the solubility of the agent in those tissues and the length of exposure. Sevoflurane and desflurane both have low blood:gas solubility coefficients, but sevoflurane is significantly more soluble in other body tissues and recovery from sevoflurane anaesthesia is slower than that following desflurane anaesthesia. In addition, all anaesthetics undergo some degree of metabolism and excretion in the urine.

In the case of halothane the considerable degree of metabolism that occurs has a measurable influence on its apparent pulmonary elimination kinetics. As with uptake, increased alveolar ventilation leads to more rapid recovery. However, the effect of cardiac output on elimination is the reverse of its effect during uptake, an increase in cardiac output hastening recovery.

POTENCY AND MOLECULAR MECHANISMS OF GENERAL ANAESTHESIA

The most useful estimate of the potency of an anaesthetic is the minimum alveolar concentration (MAC), defined as the partial pressure of an anaesthetic that produces immobility in 50% of unpremedicated subjects when exposed to a standard noxious stimulus such as skin incision. It is measured at an ambient pressure of 1 atmosphere as a single agent administered in oxygen. Such a measure allows comparison of potencies between agents.

In the clinical situation 1.3 MAC will provide surgical anaesthesia in the majority of patients. MAC is decreased by concomitant use of nitrous oxide (reduces

MAC by about 1% per 1% nitrous oxide, i.e. 60% nitrous oxide decreases the MAC by about 60%), opioids and other sedatives, increasing age, pregnancy and hypothermia. Hyperthermia and alcoholism increase MAC. The duration of anaesthesia, sex and hypocapnia do not affect MAC.

There is good correlation between the potency of anaesthetics and their lipid solubility (oil : gas partition coefficient). This was the basis for the Meyer and Overton postulate, which implied a hydrophobic site for their action. Although general anaesthetics at sufficiently high concentrations can act nonspecifically, current opinion favours the action of inhaled anaesthetics at a relatively small number of selective targets in the central nervous system. At clinical concentrations they appear to have a significant action on ligand-gated ion channels (γ-aminobutyric acid receptors), with potentiation of postsynaptic inhibitory activity, as well as some possible modulation of second messengers such as free calcium.[3]

METABOLISM AND TOXICITY OF INHALATIONAL ANAESTHETIC AGENTS

Toxic reactions are rare and unpredictable complications of inhalational anaesthesia, but when such reactions occur they can cause severe hepatic or renal damage, which can be fatal.[4] The potential of the polyhalogenated compounds to cause toxicity is a consequence of their metabolism by cytochrome P450 enzymes in the liver to form reactive metabolites.[5]

HALOTHANE

Halothane is metabolized by the 2E1 isoform of hepatic cytochrome P450 to the extent of 20–50% in humans. Oxidative metabolism is the major route of biotransformation; reductive metabolism plays a minor role but is favoured at reduced oxygen tensions. Both pathways proceed by formation of reactive metabolites.

There are two distinct forms of liver damage caused by halothane. Mild hepatic impairment is a common but self-limiting consequence of halothane exposure, usually of subclinical severity and evidenced only by a rising serum transaminase level in about 25% of patients. Of much greater concern is the more severe form of halothane hepatoxicity, halothane hepatitis. The incidence of halothane hepatitis lies between 1 in 3000 and 1 in 30 000. Patients who develop halothane hepatitis usually have a history of repeated halothane exposure and suffer with symptoms of delayed onset after 2–5 days. They develop pyrexia, arthralgia, malaise, a rash, eosinophilia, autoantibody formation and immune complex disease, and develop the symptoms and signs of fulminating hepatic failure. The incidence is highest in middle-aged obese women. Because data

relating to the incidence of halothane hepatitis have been collected retrospectively, the omission of just a few cases would have a significant influence on its reported incidence. For this reason children may not, as was once thought, be less prone to halothane hepatitis.

During the oxidative pathway of biotransformation a reactive acyl halide intermediate (CF_3–CO–Cl) is produced which can either be hydrolysed to trifluoroacetic acid or bind covalently to amino groups on hepatic proteins and phospholipids. This latter probably leads to modification of hepatocyte-specific antigens within the endoplasmic reticulum and on the hepatocyte cell membrane. The antibody response elicited by the many hepatocyte-specific halothane-modified antigens is highly complex, and cellular immunity and the action of activated cytotoxic T lymphocytes probably also play a role in the development of the resulting hepatic necrosis.

Halothane is not significantly defluorinated. When halothane is used in a low-flow system in the presence of soda lime it is converted to 2-bromo-2-chloro-1,1-difluoroethylene (BCDFE). BCDFE can, by a complex series of biochemical events known as the β-lyase pathway, form compounds that may cause nephrotoxicity. The final step in the pathway is the conversion of a cysteine conjugate, which is bioactivated in the proximal tubular cells, to an unstable thiol by the enzyme cysteine conjugate β-lyase. Evidence of dose-dependent direct nephrotoxicity has been shown in rats but not in humans, in whom the β-lyase enzyme has 10 times lower activity.

ENFLURANE

Enflurane is a more stable molecule than halothane, and only 2–8% is metabolized in the liver. However, the fluorine atom on the β-ethyl carbon of enflurane is vulnerable to cleavage by liver cytochrome P450 2E1 isoenzymes. This results in peak fluoride levels of 25 μmol l^{-1} or greater, which are 10 times those seen after halothane or isoflurane. The levels are dose dependent and are higher in obese patients or if anaesthesia is prolonged. Even when peak concentrations exceed 100 μmol l^{-1}, renal toxicity appears not to develop because plasma concentrations of inorganic fluoride peak early and decrease rapidly. However, the fluorine element is very reactive because of its electronegativity and it may inhibit the action of antidiuretic hormone on the distal tubule and collecting duct. After prolonged methoxyflurane anaesthesia, high excretion of inorganic fluoride resulted in high output renal failure. It can be argued that, although enflurane-induced renal toxicity is rare, enflurane is best avoided in patients with renal impairment, those on liver cytochrome P450 2E1-inducing drugs such as isoniazid, and those with high intake of alcohol.

The incidence of liver damage is of the order of 1 in 800 000 with exposure to enflurane. When enflurane hepatitis does occur, it is similar to halothane hepatitis; the mechanism of hepatotoxicity may also be due to enflurane metabolite-modified hepatic protein antigens. The lower incidence compared with halothane hepatitis is due to the expression of lower concentrations of metabolite antigens in the enflurane-exposed patients, which is a result of less biotransformation of enflurane.

ISOFLURANE

Isoflurane is a stable molecule and less than 0.2% is metabolized by the liver. Isoflurane, like halothane and enflurane, can form a covalently bound metabolite hapten, but its low extent of metabolism is reflected in its extremely low incidence of hepatotoxicity. However, if anaesthesia with isoflurane is longer than 12 h or when it is used for sedation in intensive care unit, the degree of metabolism increases and plasma fluoride ions may reach $20–25\,\mu$mol l^{-1}. Presumably, with time a greater proportion of isoflurane is metabolized, possibly related to isoflurane-induced hepatic enzyme induction.

DESFLURANE

The extent of metabolism of desflurane in humans is 0.02%. It is remarkably resistant to biotransformation, so its potential for toxicity is negligible. Levels of metabolite-modified proteins expressed in the liver are extremely low, and raised plasma or urinary levels of inorganic fluoride have not been detected in humans.

SEVOFLURANE

About 3–5% of an inhaled dose of sevoflurane is metabolized, but because of its very low tissue solubility it is eliminated from the body very rapidly by pulmonary excretion. Thus, peak metabolic products peak early and decline rapidly. The principal breakdown products are hexafluoroisopropanol and fluoride ions. Animal studies have demonstrated that sevoflurane is neither hepatotoxic nor nephrotoxic. However, one recent study reported a transient increase in plasma glutathione S-transferase in patients receiving sevoflurane anaesthesia, presumably reflecting a minor degree of impaired hepatocellular integrity.[6] Increased levels of inorganic fluoride have been detected in patients anaesthetized with sevoflurane, in some cases exceeding 50 μmol l^{-1}. Sevoflurane appears not to cause nephrotoxicity, presumably because the levels of inorganic fluoride in plasma decrease rapidly after discontinuation of anaesthesia.[7]

In the presence of soda lime or Baralyme, sevoflurane undergoes a nonenzymatic degradation to a group of five products, called compound A to E. Only compound A accumulates in rebreathing systems at anything other than negligible concentrations. Compound A is a vinyl ether that has been detected in anaesthetic gases during low-flow sevoflurane anaesthesia in the presence of the carbon dioxide absorbents soda lime (peak about 30 p.p.m.) or Baralyme (peak about 40 p.p.m.).[8] The lower the fresh gas flow and the more heat is generated, the more compound A is generated. Compound A causes necrosis of the renal tubules in rats and a concentration of 1000 p.p.m. is lethal after 1 h. The mechanism of nephrotoxicity may be via the β-lyase pathway described above. Human studies undertaken to date have not revealed evidence of clinical organ toxicity in patients anaesthetized with low-flow sevoflurane anaesthesia for prolonged periods.

NITROUS OXIDE

Nitrous oxide has the potential to oxidize the cobalt atom in vitamin B_{12}, which prevents B_{12} acting as a methyl-binding intermediary, a function that it performs in a number of biochemical reactions. The enzyme methionine synthase, which requires B_{12} as a cofactor, is essential for the synthesis of the DNA base, thymidine (Fig. 4.7). Nitrous oxide, by inhibiting this process, can inhibit the production of DNA. Clinically this has been observed to cause leucopenia after some 72 h of exposure to nitrous oxide, and after further exposure patients may develop agranulocytosis.

A neuropathic disorder with clinical manifestations of peripheral neuropathy and degenerative change in

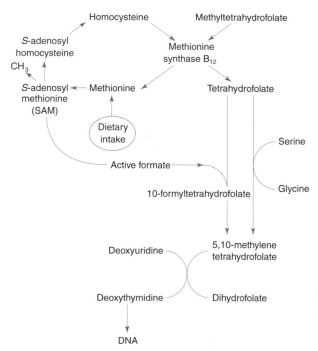

Fig. 4.7 Metabolic pathway of vitamin B_{12}–methionine synthase.

the posterior and lateral columns of the spinal cord has been described in patients after long-term exposure to nitrous oxide, a syndrome indistinguishable from that seen in severe vitamin B_{12} deficiency. This disorder is thought to be caused by the reduction of B_{12} activity as this vitamin is a cofactor necessary for the production of myelin. However, studies carried out in large populations of dental and operating theatre staff have shown the development of this condition to be very rare and it is concluded that such neuropathy or spinal cord degeneration is unlikely to be a complication of nitrous oxide administration in patients.

MALIGNANT HYPERTHERMIA

Malignant hyperthermia is a rare but serious complication of anaesthesia with a mortality rate of around 25%. It is a heritable trait (autosomal dominant) and is triggered by a wide number of agents, probably including all the volatile anaesthetic agents. Susceptible individuals develop a rapid and progressive increase in core temperature because of hypermetabolism and muscle rigidity. Tachycardia, cyanosis, acidosis and hyperkalaemia develop as oxygen supply rapidly becomes insufficient to meet tissue requirement. There is a profound increase in expired carbon dioxide, and plasma levels of creatine kinase are grossly raised. It is believed that the fundamental problem is an increase in myoplasmic calcium concentration: the myocyte becomes depleted of adenosine triphosphate, there is activation of calcium-dependent phosphorylases and loss of integrity of the sarcoplasmic reticulum wall with further entry of calcium. There is thought to be a link with chromosome 19 in humans, which encodes for the ryanodine receptor controlling the calcium release channel in skeletal muscle. There is genetic heterogeneity in this disorder.

Management of this condition includes the identification of affected families and the testing of their members by the in vitro challenge of a muscle biopsy specimen with caffeine and halothane. During an episode of malignant hyperthermia, the triggering agent must be withdrawn and resuscitation with 100% oxygen and fluid replacement instituted. Active cooling measures may be necessary. Dantrolene sodium is administered; this stabilizes cell membranes and damps down hypermetabolism by lowering intracellular calcium ion availability.

AGENT-SPECIFIC DESCRIPTIONS

HALOTHANE

Summary box 4.2 Halothane pharmacology

- Blood : gas solubility 2.3.

- Impairs cerebral vascular autoregulation:

  - contraindicated in patients with raised intracranial pressure.

- Negative inotropic and chronotropic effects.

- Increased blood catecholamine levels can cause reentry arrhythmias.

- Causes respiratory depression:

  - tidal volume reduced

  - respiratory rate unchanged or increased.

- Causes bronchodilatation by an effect on bronchial smooth muscle and inhibition of vagal tone.

- Impairs pulmonary macrophage activity and bronchial ciliary mucous transport.

- Relaxes uterine smooth muscle.

- Trigger for malignant hyperpyrexia.

- Can cause hepatitis:

  - incidence between 1 in 3000 and 1 in 30 000

  - usually associated with repeated exposure

  - symptoms may be delayed for 2–5 days

  - can result in fulminant hepatic failure.

Halothane is a clear nonflammable colourless liquid of moderate stability. Commercially it is supplied with 0.1% thymol as a stabilizing agent. Unlike other agents in current usage, it is a straight-chain halogenated alkane (2-bromo-2-chloro-1,1,1-trifluoroethane). Its lack of pungency renders it nonirritant to the upper airway. The greater blood–gas solubility (Table 4.1) in comparison with the newer agents renders its wash-in and wash-out significantly slower, thus retarding its onset of action and recovery and making rapid changes in depth of anaesthesia more difficult.

Under halothane anaesthesia the electroencephalogram (EEG) shows marked slow-wave activity of high amplitude which progressively replaces the fast low-voltage activity of consciousness with increasing depth of anaesthesia. Cerebral metabolism and oxygen

Agent	Molecular weight (Da)	Boiling point (°C)	SVP at 20°C (kPa)	λ		MAC (%)		Extent metabolized (%)
				Blood:gas	Oil:gas	In O_2	In 70% N_2O	
Halothane	197.4	50.2	32.4	2.3	234	0.75	0.56	20–50
Enflurane	184.5	56.5	22.9	1.9	96	1.58	0.57	2–8
Isoflurane	184.5	48.5	31.9	1.4	91	1.15	0.56	0.2
Sevoflurane	200.5	58.5	21.3	0.6	53	2	0.8	3–5
Desflurane	168	23.5	88.3	0.42	19	6–9	2.5–3.5	0.02
Diethyl ether	74.1	34.6	59.1	12.1	65	1.92	–	6
Nitrous oxide	44	−88.0	5200	0.47	1.4	105	–	–

Table 4.1 Physical properties of the inhalational anaesthetic agents

SVP, saturated vapour pressure; λ, partition coefficient; MAC, minimum alveolar concentration.

requirement are reduced. There is a dose-dependent cerebral vasodilatation and increase in cerebral blood flow, unless systemic blood pressure decreases markedly. There is impairment of autoregulation and a rise in cerebrospinal fluid (CSF) pressure. Halothane is contraindicated in patients with raised intracranial pressure.

Halothane is negatively inotropic in a dose-dependent manner, reducing cardiac output and increasing left atrial pressure. There is little effect on systemic vascular resistance and the net result is a dose-related decrease in arterial blood pressure. Interestingly, there are different effects on regional blood flow in different organs. Thus cerebral blood flow is increased whereas splanchnic and liver blood flow are diminished, and there is probably a slight reduction in renal blood flow. However, halothane has little effect on myocardial blood flow, and coronary autoregulation remains relatively unaltered.

Halothane also has a negative chronotropic effect secondary to a reduction in sympathetic tone and there is also a direct effect on the sinoatrial pacemaker and His–Purkinje conducting system. Under certain circumstances a reduction of automaticity and slowing of conduction may predispose to the development of reentry arrhythmias. An increase in endogenous or exogenous catecholamines will exacerbate the likelihood of significant reentry arrhythmias occurring. Baroreceptor reflexes are obtunded by halothane anaesthesia, which may impair circulatory reflexes such as those normally seen in acute blood loss.

Halothane has a respiratory depressant effect, and patients breathing spontaneously will develop a rise in arterial carbon dioxide tension. Tidal volume is diminished but respiratory rate is somewhat increased. The respiratory depression seen during halothane anaesthesia is less pronounced than with other agents, except sevoflurane. Chemoreceptor reflexes are obtunded, with respiratory responses to hypoxia and hypercapnia diminished. At deep levels of halothane anaesthesia, brainstem function is also depressed.

Halothane causes bronchodilatation by an effect on bronchial smooth muscle and inhibition of vagal tone. It also inhibits histamine-related bronchospasm in an effect that can last as long as 24 h after anaesthesia. However, pulmonary macrophage activity and bronchial ciliary mucous transport are impaired, possibly contributing to respiratory complications after anaesthesia and surgery.

Halothane anaesthesia augments the effects of muscle relaxant drugs as well as reducing muscle tone as a result of central depression. Many of these effects of halothane may be explained on the basis of reduced calcium ion flux which is responsible for excitation–contraction coupling in skeletal, cardiac and smooth muscle. Similarly, uterine muscle is relaxed. The inhibition of calcium ion flux may also contribute to the development of malignant hyperpyrexia in subjects with this inherited trait.

During halothane anaesthesia there is a reduction in renal blood flow and glomerular filtration rate. This is probably secondary to the general circulatory depression rather than being due to a direct action of halothane on the kidney.

ENFLURANE

Cl F F
| | |
H—C—C—O—C—H
| | |
F F F

Summary box 4.3 Enflurane pharmacology

- Blood : gas solubility 1.9.

- Structural isomer of isoflurane.

- Can cause central nervous system excitation and seizure activity:

  - avoid in patients with epilepsy.

- Impairs cerebral vascular autoregulation:

  - contraindicated in patients with raised intracranial pressure.

- Fewer negative inotropic and chronotropic effects than halothane.

- Causes respiratory depression.

Enflurane is a halogen-substituted methyl-ethyl ether (2-chloro-1,1,2-trifluoroethyl difluoromethyl ether), a structural isomer of isoflurane. It is a clear, colourless, nonflammable liquid which is chemically stable, allowing storage without preservative.

The blood : gas partition coefficient is 1.9 (Table 4.1) so that the onset of anaesthesia and recovery is faster than with halothane. Enflurane may encourage seizure activity, and disturbed EEG morphology may be seen for many hours following enflurane administration. This effect is more marked when it is delivered in high concentration in association with hypocarbia. Seizures have been reported in patients receiving enflurane, so it is probably best avoided in subjects known to suffer from epilepsy. In common with halothane, cerebral autoregulation is impaired, with cerebral vasodilatation and an increase in CSF pressure and intracranial pressure. Cerebral metabolic activity and the cerebral metabolic oxygen requirement are reduced.

Enflurane is less negatively inotropic than halothane but depresses peripheral vascular resistance to a greater degree. Systemic blood pressure is thus depressed by a fall in cardiac output together with a decrease in peripheral vascular resistance.[9] In the sinoatrial node and His–Purkinje system enflurane reduces automaticity and conduction to a lesser degree than halothane. Baroreceptor reflexes are obtunded, but a degree of tachycardia is often seen, perhaps reflecting differential effects in the autonomic nervous system.

Enflurane, in common with the other halogen-substituted ethers, does not have the arrhythmogenic activity of the halogen-substituted alkanes (halothane and trichloroethylene) and the cardiac rhythm remains remarkably stable, as it also does during isoflurane anaesthesia. Coronary vascular resistance decreases but there appears to be no evidence that coronary artery ischaemia may occur due to the 'coronary steal' phenomenon.

In common with halothane, enflurane obtunds respiratory chemoreceptor-mediated reflexes. Thus the hypoxic and hypercapnic respiratory drives are diminished, and similarly at high tension there is inhibition of brainstem activity resulting in further respiratory and circulatory depression. It is widely held that the respiratory depressant action of enflurane is more potent than that of other inhalational agents. Bronchodilatation, consequent on smooth muscle relaxation, pulmonary macrophage and mucociliary transport depression, also occurs.

ISOFLURANE

F Cl F
| | |
F—C—C—O—C—H
| | |
F H F

Summary box 4.4 Isoflurane pharmacology

- Blood : gas solubility 1.4.

- Structural isomer of enflurane.

- Stable molecule, less than 0.2% metabolized.

- Extremely low incidence of hepatic or renal toxicity.

- Fewer negative inotropic effects than halothane or enflurane.

- Potent coronary vasodilator; may cause 'coronary steal' in patients with coronary artery disease if used in high concentrations.

- Respiratory depression intermediate between that of halothane and enflurane.

Isoflurane is a halogen-substituted methy-ethyl ether (1-chloro-2,2,2-trifluoroethyl difluoromethyl ether). It is chemically stable and nonflammable, and forms a clear colourless liquid. It is presented free of preservative and does not react with soda lime; it is stable in ultraviolet light and does not react with metals. The industrial preparation of isoflurane is complex and expensive as a number of isomers are created and azeotropic mixtures are formed which are difficult to separate, requiring many distillations. The onset of anaesthesia and recovery is faster than with enflurane as predicted by its blood : gas partition coefficient of 1.4 (Table 4.1).

Isoflurane reduces cerebral metabolism and consequently lowers cerebral metabolic oxygen requirement. Unlike enflurane it has no convulsant properties and produces no epileptiform change in the EEG. Unlike both enflurane and halothane, low concentrations of isoflurane do not increase cerebral blood flow. Above 1.0 MAC there is a dose-dependent rise in cerebral blood flow and intracranial pressure, but this is of much lower degree than that with either halothane or enflurane.[10]

In early laboratory testing during development, rats developed hepatic tumours after exposure to isoflurane. Later it was demonstrated that a contaminant of the feed given to the rats was the true cause of these tumours (these were polybrominated biphenyls which are known teratogens). This unfortunate occurrence delayed the release of isoflurane for several years.

The negative inotropic effects of isoflurane are appreciably lower than those of halothane and enflurane, probably because of a lesser effect of isoflurane on transmembrane calcium flux, so that calcium-mediated excitation–contraction coupling is less impaired. Tachycardia is usually seen during isoflurane anaesthesia and this may be related to a lesser effect on baroreceptor-mediated circulatory reflexes. There is a decrease in peripheral vascular resistance and a decrease in arterial pressure which is slightly offset by the reflex tachycardia. Isoflurane does not exhibit the effect on myocardial sensitivity to catecholamines seen with halothane, and the heart rhythm remains largely unaffected. This is because of a marked lack of effect on automaticity and conduction in the His–Purkinje system, so that arrhythmias do not occur as reentry phenomena or as a result of altered automaticity.

There has been some concern about the use of isoflurane in patients with coronary artery disease as it is a powerful coronary vasodilator and thus has the potential to produce a significant coronary steal effect with the resulting development of myocardial ischaemia.[11] The net coronary blood flow is determined by the coronary perfusion pressure and coronary vascular resistance. During isoflurane anaesthesia, peripheral vascular resistance and systemic blood pressure tend to decrease and thus the coronary perfusion pressure will also decrease, although this is to some extent offset by coronary vasodilatation. It was envisaged that diseased or stenosed coronary vessels could not dilate effectively and that the balance of myocardial perfusion might be altered by decreasing tissue vascular resistance in other areas leading to redistribution of myocardial perfusion away from diseased regions, resulting in myocardial ischaemia. This is the basis of the coronary steal effect. However, provided blood pressure is maintained and excessive concentrations are avoided, isoflurane is considered safe for patients with coronary artery disease. Indeed, it is widely used in cardiac anaesthesia for patients undergoing coronary artery surgery.

Isoflurane is intermediate in terms of ventilatory depression between halothane and enflurane. Similarly, the ventilatory responses to hypoxia and hypercapnia are obtunded. Isoflurane causes bronchodilatation. It is safe to use β_2 agonists and aminophylline in patients with asthma who are receiving isoflurane as the arrhythmic potential for this agent is negligible. Pulmonary vascular resistance is slightly diminished in humans and isoflurane has been used with benefit in subjects with primary pulmonary hypertension.[12]

DESFLURANE

Summary box 4.5 Desflurane Pharmacology

- Exceptionally low blood : gas solubility (0.42) resulting in very fast wash-in and wash-out characteristics.

- Irritating to airways, so not suitable for induction of anaesthesia.

- Low boiling point and high saturated vapour pressure:

  - needs special, electrically heated vaporizer.

- Haemodynamic effects are complex:

  - causes direct myocardial depression

  - sympathetic stimulation helps to maintain heart rate, myocardial contractility and blood pressure

  - rapid increases in inspired concentration can lead to reflex tachycardia and hypertension.

- May be trigger for malignant hyperthermia.

Desflurane is a fluorine-substituted methyl-ethyl ether with a structure similar to that of isoflurane (difluoromethyl-1-fluoro-2,2,2-trifluoroethyl either).[13] Desflurane is stable and does not react with soda lime. It has an exceptionally low blood:gas partition coefficient (Table 4.1) and this results in wash-in and wash-out characteristics with very short time constants, leading to very rapid induction and recovery from anaesthesia. Rapid equilibration in the lung allows the partial pressure of desflurane in the blood, and consequently in the brain, to be altered quickly by manipulation of inspired tension, and this gives good control of depth of anaesthesia.

The low boiling point and resulting high saturated vapour pressure at room temperature (Table 4.1) make desflurane unsuitable for delivery using a conventional vaporizer design. A novel method is used in which the vaporizer is heated electrically to a stable temperature at which the vapour pressure is higher, but held relatively constant, and electronic servo methods are used to control output. Desflurane vaporizers therefore require an electrical supply.

Desflurane decreases cerebrovascular resistance and increases cerebral blood flow comparable with isoflurane. Cerebral oxygen requirement falls in parallel, allowing for adequate cerebral perfusion even during episodes of desflurane-induced hypotension. There may be a dose-dependent suppression of EEG activity. No evidence of epileptiform change in the EEG has been observed.

In physiological preparations desflurane causes depression of myocardial contractility comparable with that of isoflurane. However, in the intact animal the haemodynamic effects of desflurane are complex.[14] Desflurane seems to enhance sympathetic autonomic tone, and this helps to maintain heart rate, myocardial contractility and systemic blood pressure. This effect was initially thought to be a reflex to the noxious and stimulating effect of desflurane on the airway. Later studies have shown that when administered in a cardiopulmonary bypass circuit (thus eliminating airway stimulation) desflurane still enhances sympathetic tone, suggesting reflex autonomic activity initiated in the periphery. Rapid increases in inspired concentrations of desflurane can elicit a reflex tachycardia and hypertension in anaesthetized patients.

Desflurane forms a somewhat acrid vapour which is irritating to the airway and may cause breath-holding, increased airway secretion, coughing, bronchospasm and laryngospasm when administered at high concentration. These properties make it unsuitable for inhalational induction of anaesthesia. In common with the other halogenated anaesthetic agents, desflurane is a respiratory depressant producing a dose-dependent reduction in tidal volume and increasing respiratory rate. The respiratory reflexes associated with falling arterial oxygen tension are obtunded and in spontaneously breathing patients the arterial carbon dioxide tension increases with depth of anaesthesia.

Desflurane significantly depresses neuromuscular function and augments the action of both non-depolarizing and depolarizing muscle relaxants. Initial studies in volunteers suggest that the degree of augmentation of both depolarizing and non-depolarizing relaxants is similar to that during isoflurane anaesthesia. It has been reported to be a trigger of malignant hyperthermia in the animal model of susceptible pigs and it is mandatory to avoid the use of desflurane in patients at risk.

SEVOFLURANE

Summary box 4.6 Sevoflurane pharmacology

- Low blood:gas solubility (0.6) and absence of airway irritation gives rapid induction characteristics.

- Tissue solubility higher than that of desflurane, so recovery somewhat slower.

- Cardiovascular effects broadly comparable to those of isoflurane.

- May cause less respiratory depression than other inhalational agents.

- 3–5% metabolized, but current evidence is that it causes neither hepatic nor renal toxicity.

- Interacts with soda lime and Baralyme to form compound A:

  - compound A is nephrotoxic in animals

  - no evidence of nephrotoxicity in humans anaesthetized with low-flow sevoflurane for prolonged periods.

Sevoflurane (fluoromethyl 2,2,2-trifluoro-1-(trifluoromethyl) ethyl ether) has a blood:gas partition coefficient of 0.6 (Table 4.1) leading to rapid induction characteristics.[15] However, tissue solubility throughout the body is somewhat higher than for desflurane and the load of sevoflurane absorbed is correspondingly greater, rendering the recovery phase somewhat longer than for desflurane.

Early reports indicate that the EEG effects are similar to those of other inhaled anaesthetics. The influence of this agent on cerebral blood flow and intracranial pressure in humans is similar to that of the other halogen-substituted ethers. With regard to effects on the cardiovascular system, in animal and volunteer studies the agent appears similar to isoflurane, but it may be associated with less marked changes in heart rate and may have less potential to cause coronary circulatory changes. In acutely instrumented newborn pigs and chronically instrumented dogs, sevoflurane caused a dose-related decrease in myocardial contractility and mean arterial pressure. The incidence of cardiac arrhythmias during sevoflurane anaesthesia are similar to those seen with isoflurane. Reports of its use in patients with phaeochromocytoma indicate that it does not sensitize the myocardium to catecholamines.

Although all potent inhaled anaesthetics are respiratory depressants, and sevoflurane is no exception to this, it has been suggested that it causes less increase in respiratory rate with a larger tidal volume and longer inspiratory and expiratory times. If this observation is supported by other studies, the cardiorespiratory profile of sevoflurane may prove to be the most benign of all halogenated anaesthetics. The agent does not irritate the upper airway and is similar to halothane in this respect. This absence of airway irritation combined with a very fast onset of action make it very useful as an inhalational induction agent, especially in children.

Sevoflurane potentiates nondepolarizing relaxants to a similar degree as isoflurane and it is likely that it potentiates depolarizing relaxants, but this awaits confirmation. There is one published case report of a 4-year-old child developing malignant hyperthermia during sevoflurane anaesthesia for correction of bilateral ptosis, and the agent should be avoided in all potentially susceptible individuals.

NITROUS OXIDE (N_2O)

Nitrous oxide is a colourless, sweet-smelling agent which is stored under compression in steel cylinders. It is not flammable or explosive but may support the combustion of coadministered flammable compounds. At normal ambient temperature nitrous oxide is below its critical temperature (36.5°C) and is thus a liquid within the cylinder. On release from the cylinder it forms a vapour at ambient atmospheric pressure. The pressure in the cylinder is approximately 51 bar and remains at this level (the saturated vapour pressure of nitrous oxide at room temperature) until all the liquid in the cylinder has evaporated. Thus the gauge pressure on a cylinder of nitrous oxide is not indicative of the amount of nitrous oxide it contains.

Nitrous oxide is produced commercially by heating ammonium nitrate to 270°C, causing the ammonium nitrate to decompose into nitrous oxide and water. Ammonia, nitric oxide and nitrogen dioxide can result as by products. Such compounds have been observed as contaminants in industrially prepared nitrous oxide and may cause significant morbidity and mortality when administered inadvertently. They produce bronchospasm and laryngospasm, accompanied by hypoxia, pulmonary oedema and later a chemical pneumonitis, together with the development of circulatory shock. This results from the reaction between nitric oxide with alveolar water to produce nitric acid.

The low blood : gas solubility (Table 4.1) results in a very fast uptake, with alveolar concentration approaching inspired concentration quickly. Rapid equilibration means that arterial blood saturation rises rapidly and with it effective partial pressure in the brain.

During nitrous oxide anaesthesia, enclosed air spaces, such as those in the middle ear or gut, preexisting pneumothorax or venous air embolus, will fill with nitrous oxide by diffusion from tissue capillaries. Such enclosed air spaces are normally rich in nitrogen, which is 34 times less soluble in blood than nitrous oxide. In distensible air spaces the volume of these spaces will increase, whereas in nondistensible spaces, such as the middle ear, the pressure will rise. These effects may be clinically significant; for instance, if developing pneumothorax or venous air embolism is suspected, nitrous oxide should be withdrawn and appropriate measures instituted. Diffusion of nitrous oxide into the middle ear with resulting pressure increase has been suggested as contributing to postoperative nausea and vomiting.

Nitrous oxide exerts a dose-dependent depressant effect on the central nervous system while increasing cerebral blood flow and intracranial pressure. It is only a weak anaesthetic with a MAC value of 105% and so can produce clinical anaesthesia only when administered in oxygen under hyperbaric conditions. Nitrous oxide is also available as a 50% mixture in oxygen (Entonox) which can be used to provide analgesia during labour or for the transport of trauma victims. Entonox has a minimal effect on the level of consciousness.

Nitrous oxide has a direct negative inotropic effect which can be demonstrated in vitro using isolated papillary muscle. In volunteer studies a weak negative inotropic effect has been shown, with a reduction in ventricular function. Cardiac output and heart rate are reduced, but systemic vascular resistance increases slightly to maintain the blood pressure, suggesting a weak sympathomimetic effect. When given in combination with one of the halogen-substituted ethers, less depression of cardiovascular parameters is seen than when MAC-equivalent mixtures of the halogen-substituted ether alone with oxygen are used.

XENON

Molecular weight	131.3 Da
Boiling point	−108.1°C
Critical temperature	16.6°C
MAC	approx. 70%

Xenon is a nonexplosive, colourless and odourless gas.[16] It has a blood : gas partition coefficient of 0.14, which is low compared with nitrous oxide (0.47); therefore it has a very rapid uptake and elimination. It is an inert gas, which does not undergo any biotransformation and it is devoid of toxic or haemodynamic side-effects. The MAC value is of the order of 70% and it is a potent analgesic. Its use has been limited because xenon is expensive (1 litre costs about £10). With the increased popularity of low-flow systems, there has been a renewed interest in xenon, and it is possible that it will enter routine clinical practice within the next few years.

REFERENCES

1. Vandam LD. Early American anesthetists – the origins of professionalism in anesthesia. *Anesthesiology* 1973; **38**: 264–274.
2. Heijke S, Smith G. Quest for the ideal anaesthetic agent. *Br J Anaesth* 1990; **64**: 3–6.
3. Franks NP, Lieb WR. Molecular and cellular mechanisms of general anaesthesia. *Nature* 1994; **367**: 607–614.
4. Kenna JG, Jones RM. The organ toxicity of inhaled anaesthetics. *Anesth Analg* 1995; **81**: S51–S66.
5. Kharasch ED, Thummel KE. Identification of cytochrome P450 2E1 as the predominant enzyme catalyzing human microsomal defluorination of sevoflurane, isoflurane and methoxyflurane. *Anesthesiology* 1993; **79**: 795–807.
6. Ray DC, Bomont R, Mizushima A *et al*. Effect of sevoflurane anaesthesia on plasma concentrations of glutathione S-transferase. *Br J Anaesth* 1996; **77**: 404–407.
7. Koboyashi Y, Ochiai R, Takeda J *et al*. Serum and urinary inorganic fluoride concentrations after prolonged inhalation of sevoflurane in humans. *Anesth Analg* 1992; **74**: 753–757.
8. Frink EJ, Malan TP, Morgan SE *et al*. Quantification of the degradation products of sevoflurane in two CO_2 absorbants during low flow anaesthesia in surgical patients. *Anesthesiology* 1992; **77**: 1064–1069.
9. Takeshima R, Dohi S. Comparison of arterial baroreflex function in humans anesthetised with enflurane or isoflurane. *Anesth Analg* 1989; **69**: 284–290.
10. Adams RW, Cucchiari RF, Fronet GA *et al*. Isoflurane and cerebrospinal fluid pressure in neurosurgical patients. *Anesthesiology* 1981; **54**: 97–99.
11. Priebe HJ. Coronary circulation and factors affecting coronary 'steal'. *Eur J Anaesthesiol* 1991; **8**: 177–195.
12. Cheng DCH, Edelists G. Isoflurane and primary pulmonary hypertension. *Anaesthesia* 1988; **43**: 22–24.
13. Jones RM, Nay PG. Desflurane. *Anaesth Pharmacol Rev* 1994; **2**: 51–60.
14. Jones RM, Cashman JN, Mant TCK. Clinical impressions and cardiorespiratory effects of a new fluorinated anaesthetic, desflurane (I-653) in volunteers. *Br J Anaesth* 1990; **64**: 11–15.
15. Frink EJ, Brown BR. Sevoflurane. *Anaesth Pharmacol Rev* 1994; **2**: 61–67.
16. Kennedy RR, Stokes JW, Downing P. Anaesthesia and the 'inert' gases with special reference to xenon. *Anaesth Intensive Care* 1992; **20**: 66–70.

5

A Windsor, P Bowen, P Sebel

INTRAVENOUS ANAESTHETICS

In 1665 it was reported to the Royal Society that Sir Christopher Wren, following a discussion with Robert Boyle (of Boyle's law fame), administered opium to dogs using a bladder and quill. This was within 40 years of William Harvey's description of the circulation. News of the intriguing 'stupefying' effect soon spread, and the report tells of a foreign ambassador in London who tried it upon 'a malefactor, that was an inferior servant'. The unfortunate underling survived and we are told that many successful experiments were subsequently performed.

Pirogoff, a Russian surgeon, unsuccessfully infused ether around the time of its inception as an inhalational agent (1846). The manufacture of the hypodermic needle by the Dublin surgeon Francis Rynd in 1845 and the syringe by Scotsman Dr Alexander Wood and Mr Ferguson of London in 1855 provided the necessary technology for successful intravenous administration of drugs. The Frenchman Pierre-Cyprien Oré reported on the use of intravenous chloral hydrate for anaesthesia in 1875. However, large-scale intravenous anaesthetic administration possibly began with Krawkow in St Petersburg (1905), who administered hedonal, a urethrane derivative, resulting in widespread adoption of the technique in Europe. In 1921 the first barbiturate, Somifen (a mixture of the diethlyamines of diethyl and diallyl barbituric acid), was used clinically. A number of other barbituric acid derivatives was developed, amongst which was thiopentone, initially administered in 1934. Intravenous induction of anaesthesia became increasingly common, and the concept of combining drugs to minimize side-effects evolved. This concept was propounded by George Crile as early as 1901, and John Lundy introduced the term 'balanced anaesthesia'

in 1926. In the past 50 years many agents have been introduced, but none yet meets the full specifications for the ideal intravenous anaesthetic.

> **Summary box 5.1 Properties of the Ideal Intravenous Anaesthetic Agent**
>
> - Short context-sensitive half-time.
> - No active metabolites.
> - Elimination unaffected by severe organ failure.
> - Analgesic at subanaesthetic doses.
> - Amnesic at subanaesthetic doses.
> - Sedative at subanaesthetic doses.
> - Produce moderate muscle relaxation.
> - Preserve haemodynamic stability.
> - Preserve coronary and cerebral autoregulation.
> - Be an effective anticonvulsant.
> - No histamine release and low incidence of anaphylactic reactions.
> - Nonirritant and nonthrombogenic.

BARBITURATES

For many years thiopentone has been the most popular anaesthetic induction agent. It was first manufactured in 1903 but not used clinically until 1932. During the 1941 Pearl Harbour attack, inappropriate overdoses of thiopentone in haemodynamically unstable casualties led to a high mortality rate. This initial lack of understanding of the pharmacodynamics of thiopentone was subsequently rectified.[1]

The chemical precursor of thiopentone, barbituric acid, synthesized from malonic acid and urea, has no hypnotic activity, but substitution of organic groups confers the hypnotic effect. Thiobarbitures such as thiopentone are prepared by using thiourea rather than urea in the synthesis process. Thiamylal, secobarbitone and pentobarbitone were also developed from barbituric acid, but methohexitone is the only other barbiturate still commonly used as an induction agent. Thiopentone and methohexitone have the most rapid distribution and elimination half-lives of all the barbiturate-derived induction agents. The induction dose of thiopentone is 3–5 mg kg^{-1} and for methohexitone 0.75–1.5 mg kg^{-1}.

MECHANISMS OF ACTION

Although the mechanism of barbiturate anaesthesia has been studied extensively, the precise details are still unknown. However, it is apparent that the γ-aminobutyric acid GABA$_A$ receptor has an important role in the actions of barbiturates as well as benzodiazepines, propofol and etomidate on the central nervous system (see Chapter 1).[2] It is unclear how much of the anaesthetic action of barbiturates is mediated by the GABA mechanism rather than other pathways. However, this would appear to provide a mechanism for the anticonvulsant properties of thiopentone, the benzodiazepines and propofol.

Summary box 5.2 Key points of barbiturate pharmacology

- Barbiturates bind to a specific site on the GABA$_A$ receptor, depressing neuronal excitability.

- They reduce cerebral blood flow (CBF), cerebral metabolic rate (CMRO$_2$) and intracranial pressure. The reduction in CMRO$_2$ is brought about by decreased electrical activity in neurons. CBF decreases with decreased CMRO$_2$ since flow–metabolism coupling is preserved.

- Cerebral protective effects of barbiturates are controversial.

- Barbiturates cause myocardial depression and vasodilatation leading to hypotension and decreased cardiac output.

- Respiratory effects include transient hyperventilation followed by prolonged hypoventilation, chiefly through reduction in tidal volume. The slope of the ventilatory response to hypercarbia is decreased.

PHYSICAL CHARACTERISTICS

The properties of the various barbiturate compounds depend on the substitution of the 1, 2 and 5 loci on the barbiturate ring (Fig. 5.1). Thiopentone is a thiobarbiturate with a sulphur substitution at C2, whereas methohexitone is an oxybarbiturate with an oxygen molecule at the same site. A branched side-chain at C5 has increased hypnotic action with increasing chain length, until the chain exceeds six carbons, when convulsant properties may result. The speed of onset is increased by methylation of N1 but at the expense of excitatory movement, as observed with methohexitone.

Both methohexitone and thiopentone are weak acids formulated as sodium salts in an alkaline solution with a pH greater than 10. The sodium salts are water soluble whereas the free acid forms are virtually insoluble in water. Sodium carbonate is the buffering agent. The high pH results in marked tissue damage if the solution is injected subcutaneously or intra-arterially. It also necessitates caution as an eye splash is extremely irritant. Admixture with most other drugs, such as suxamethonium, results in precipitation which can cause occlusion of intravenous infusion lines. The pH also makes these solutions a poor culture medium if left to stand. However, a methohexitone solution may deteriorate on exposure to the atmosphere since, unlike thiopentone, it is oxygen sensitive.

PHARMACOKINETICS AND PHARMACODYNAMICS

As with the other intravenous anaesthetics, thiopentone undergoes rapid redistribution after a single bolus injection. The terminal elimination half-life, however, is very long, about 10–12 h, so that there is marked accumulation of the drug following repeated administration or when given by a continuous intravenous infusion (Fig. 5.2). Elimination is exclusively hepatic as high lipid solubility results in extensive renal tubular resorption. Metabolism is largely via oxidation to thiopentone carboxylic acid. A small amount of the active drug, pentobarbitone, is produced. In the first 15 min after a bolus dose, less than 20% of the drug is removed by metabolism. The hepatic extraction ratio of thiopentone is 0.2. Protein binding is 65–85%, principally to albumin. Aspirin, indomethacin and mefenamic acid can decrease thiopentone protein binding. However, this is of little clinical relevance at the concentrations seen during induction of anaesthesia.

The pK_a of thiopentone is 7.6, and 61% is un-ionized at pH 7.4. The pK_a of methohexitone is 7.9 and the un-ionized fraction 75%. The high lipid solubility of these drugs, coupled with the predominantly un-ionized fractions, allows for rapid transfer across the blood–brain barrier and fast onset of action. Systemic acidosis results in an even higher un-ionized fraction, allowing a greater proportion of the lipid-soluble drug to cross into cells, so increasing the volume of distribution and intracerebral concentrations.

Increasing age results in a lower induction dose requirement. This may be a combination of reduced

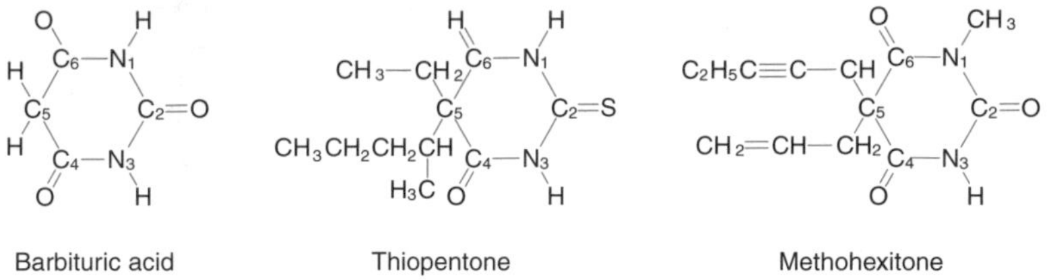

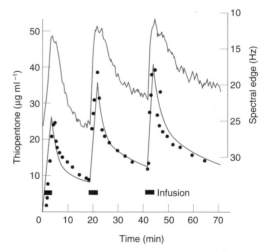

Fig. 5.1 Chemical structures of barbituric acid, thiopentone and methohexitone.

central volume of distribution and slower drug transfer from the central compartment of other compartments. Pregnancy increases the volume of distribution and slows elimination, but does not change protein binding significantly.

Methohexitone is shorter acting and more potent than thiopentone. Until propofol became available, it was commonly used for procedures of short duration. The pharmacokinetic difference from thiopentone is the result of an increased hepatic extraction ratio (from 0.5 to 0.6). Protein binding is similar to that of thiopentone, but the elimination half-life is only 4 h.

CENTRAL NERVOUS SYSTEM

Thiopentone produces a fast onset of anaesthesia when given rapidly. The induction dose can be reduced by giving the drug at a slower rate. Methohexitone produces a less smooth induction with a higher incidence of coughing and hiccoughing. Neither drug is as rapid as propofol for depressing laryngeal reflexes to allow for laryngeal mask insertion.

Thiopentone is popular in neuroanaesthesia for several reasons. Its anticonvulsant activity, probably mediated via the drug's GABA receptor interaction, is useful in any patient with a lowered epileptogenic threshold. It is one of the most effective drugs for treatment of status epilepticus. A dose-dependent decrease in cerebral metabolic oxygen utilization (CMRO$_2$), cerebral blood flow and intracranial pressure occurs following administration of thiopentone. The drug also lowers intraocular pressure. At high doses thiopentone produces electroencephalographic (EEG) burst suppression (periods of EEG quiescence interrupted by short bursts of EEG activity). This reflects depression of synaptic transmission and consequent reduced oxygen consumption. Thiopentone can maximally reduce cerebral oxygen consumption only by about 50%, since the remainder of CMRO$_2$ is for maintenance of the metabolic integrity of cellular structures, on which it has no effect.

It has been suggested that the reduction in CMRO$_2$ can be valuable in reducing anoxic damage in areas of the brain where oxygen delivery has been jeopardized. This hypothesis has been reevaluated in the light of better understanding of the mechanisms of ischaemic injury. A rise in extracellular excitatory neuro-transmitters (particularly glutamate) following ischaemia results in recurrent depolarization of the neurons. This leads to intracellular calcium accumulation, depletion of cellular adenosine triphosphate and phosphocreatinine levels, uncoupling of mitochondrial oxidative metabolism and cerebral blood flow, and irreversible neuronal injury. Animal models of anoxic injury reveal improved preservation of function and reduced extracellular accumulation of the potentially neurotoxic glutamate by thiopentone. Other agents, such as isoflurane, can also induce EEG burst suppression and reduce synaptic transmission, but they do not improve histochemical or neurological outcome. Therefore, it may be that simple reduction in CMRO$_2$ is not

Fig. 5.2 Thiopentone serum concentration (solid dots, measured concentrations; solid line, model-fitted concentrations) and resulting EEG effect (as measured by 95% spectral edge frequency) versus time. Spectral edge frequency plot has been inverted for visual clarity; the frequency decreases as concentration increases (see scale at right). Timing of thiopentone infusion (150 mg min^{-1}) is indicated along lower portion of graph. The EEG effect does not return to baseline after the third dose because of drug accumulation. From Hudson RJ, Stanski DR, Saidman LJ, Meathe E. A model for studying depth of anesthesia and acute tolerance to thiopental. *Anesthesiology* 1983; **59**: 301–308, with permission.

the only way in which thiopentone is cerebroprotective. Indeed, metabolic depression might be thought to be an effect of limited duration, and ineffective in severe global ischaemia. Barbiturates are of no value in severe global ischaemia such as during cardiopulmonary resuscitation. Therefore, decreased excitatory neurotransmitter levels during reperfusion, or diminution of their recurrent depolarizing action, may be an important cerebroprotective mechanism of thiopentone.

At subclinical doses thiopentone is hyperalgesic. In contrast, the action of thiopentone at the spinal level is antinociceptive and mediated by $GABA_A$ receptors. The GABA-like action is not observed at low concentrations and this may explain the lack of analgesic effect of thiopentone at subanaesthetic doses.

CARDIOVASCULAR SYSTEM

Interpreting the effect of any induction agent on a patient's cardiovascular system must take into account any existing cardiovascular pathology and drug therapy. The response of the extremely sick patient to the drug may differ considerably from that in a healthy patient. The effect of barbiturates on the cardiovascular system is similar to that of propofol and the benzodiazepines, although the extent of any effect differs from one drug to another. In healthy patients there is a decrease in cardiac output and a compensatory tachycardia. Methohexitone produces a greater tachycardia than thiopentone. Both drugs decrease cardiac output by a direct negative inotropic action, reduced preload (due to capacitance vessel dilatation), reduced afterload and diminished central nervous system sympathetic outflow. Dilatation of resistance vessels (afterload) is less than that of capacitance vessels (preload) in the healthy patient. Normally, increased myocardial oxygen consumption results from the tachycardia, but this does not result in an increased coronary arteriovenous oxygen content difference since coronary vascular resistance falls and blood flow increases to meet the increased oxygen demand.

The reduction in cardiac output will be greater in a patient who cannot produce a compensatory tachycardia or already has poor cardiac output. High doses of barbiturates are dangerous in the hypovolaemic patient, since the compensatory mechanisms on which the patient depends may be abolished or significantly attenuated. Slow, cautious administration with appropriate dose reduction is necessary. If ensuing hypotension and tachycardia are excessive, coronary artery perfusion is significantly reduced and fatal arrhythmias may result.

RESPIRATORY EFFECTS

Induction doses of thiopentone typically cause transient hyperventilation followed by more prolonged reduction in minute ventilation, chiefly through reduction in tidal volume. There is a reduction in the ventilatory response to hypercapnia (Fig. 5.3). Concurrent opioids and other respiratory depressants increase the likelihood of apnoea after induction doses.

OTHER

Intravenous barbiturates are relatively painless on injection. However, subcutaneous thiopentone can be extremely painful and arterial injection may lead to arterial spasm, thrombosis and distal limb ischaemia. If a patient complains of pain, the injection should be stopped and the injection site examined. Persisting pain or clinical signs suggesting that the peripheral limb circulation is jeopardized requiring treatment. Arterial injection of lignocaine (10 ml of 1%) may provide analgesia and vasodilatation. A brachial plexus block will have the same action for a more prolonged period.

Papaverine, 40–80 mg in 20 ml saline, is an

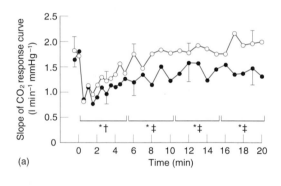

(a)

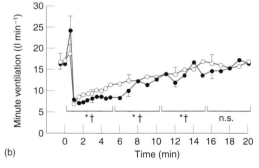

(b)

Fig. 5.3 Ventilatory response to (a) carbon dioxide and (b) minute ventilation over time after thiopentone 4 mg kg^{-1} (○) and propofol 2.5 mg kg^{-1} (●) in eight volunteers. Values are mean ± SEM. Propofol produces longer-lasting depression of ventilatory response to carbon dioxide but similar depression of minute ventilation with these doses. *$P < 0.05$ versus baseline for propofol. †$P < 0.05$ versus baseline for thiopentone. ‡$P < 0.05$ propofol versus thiopentone. n.s., Not significant. From Blouin R, Conard PF, Gross JB. Time course of ventilatory depression following induction doses of propofol and thiopental. *Anesthesiology* 1991; 75: 940–944, with permission.

effective vasodilator. Finally, anticoagulation with heparin should be commenced. Methohexitone does not result in thrombosis, although arterial injection may be painful.

All barbiturates should be avoided in patients with porphyria. The porphyrias are a group of inherited or acquired metabolic disorders involving enzymatic defects in the production of haem (Fig. 5.4). The rate-limiting step in the biosynthesis of haem is the activity of the enzyme aminolaevulinic acid (ALA) synthetase. One of the factors in the manifestation of porphyria is an increased activity of ALA synthetase, which leads to the formation of porphyrins, highly reactive oxidants which are inadequately metabolized and cause toxic neurological sequelae. Barbiturates may trigger an acute attack of porphyria since they induce ALA synthetase activity. The exception is porphyria cutanea tarda which has no neurological complications. Nausea, vomiting, abdominal pain, acute psychoses and lower motor neu-

ron palsies can occur during an acute attack. Management of an acute attack includes administration of glucose, which suppresses ALA synthetase. Diazepam has also been reported as a triggering agent; the other induction agents appear not to induce attacks.[3]

PROPOFOL

Introduced in 1977, propofol rapidly became a significant addition to the clinician's armamentarium, largely due to pharmacokinetic features that result in a short duration of action. This allows its use as both an induction agent and an intravenous maintenance agent. Propofol is also an effective sedative, anxiolytic and amnesic at plasma concentrations lower than those that induce loss of consciousness. The drug also possesses antipruritic and antiemetic actions. Propofol, like thiopentone, acts partly via $GABA_A$ receptors at both supraspinal and spinal sites. Positron emission tomography shows that it produces a global effect on the cerebral cortex and subcortical areas.[4] The binding site of propofol to the $GABA_A$ receptor may differ from that of barbiturates and benzodiazepines.

PHYSICAL CHARACTERISTICS

Propofol is a substituted isopropyl phenol, insoluble in water (Fig. 5.5). It is stable at room temperature and is not light sensitive. The initial formulation of the drug

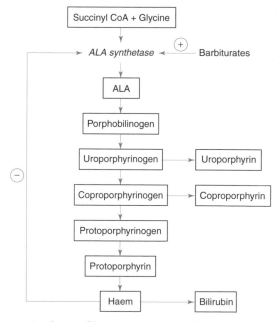

Fig. 5.4 Synthesis of haem. Enzymatic defects in haem biosynthesis result in increased accumulation of uroporphyrin or coproporphyrin in the tissues, depending on which enzyme is affected. CoA, coenzyme A; ALA, aminolaevulinic acid.

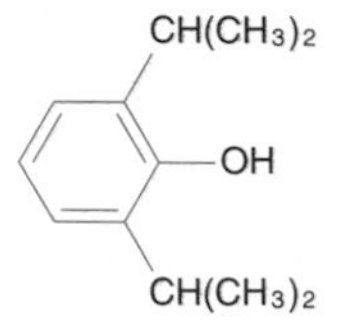

Fig. 5.5 Structure of propofol.

was in cremophor EL, but a high incidence of anaphylactic reactions to the cremophor resulted in a new formulation in 10% soybean oil, egg lecithin, egg phosphatide and glycerol. This is a viscous, milky-white emulsion that requires a sterile technique when being handled, as it is a good culture medium for bacteria. The pK_a of propofol is 11; the emulsion is isotonic and has a pH of 7–8.5. Propofol undergoes oxidative degradation in oxygen, so is packaged with nitrogen to prevent this.

PHARMACOKINETICS AND PHARMACODYNAMICS

As a lipid-soluble drug, propofol is almost entirely metabolized, with less than 1% being excreted unchanged in the urine and 2% in the faeces. It is conjugated to a glucuronide or sulphate before elimination. Plasma protein binding is 98%. Propofol has a large central compartment volume (20–70 litres) and steady-state volume of distribution (150–700 litres). The plasma clearance ($2\,l\,min^{-1}$) exceeds hepatic blood flow, suggesting extrahepatic metabolism. Chronic hepatic and renal disease do not significantly reduce

---

> ### Summary box 5.4 Key points of propofol pharmacology
>
> - The high clearance rate of propofol (approximately $2\,l\,min^{-1}$) permits rapid emergence after continuous infusions of the drug.
>
> - Central nervous system effects include reduction in cerebral blood flow, $CMRO_2$ and intracranial pressure (ICP). Cerebral perfusion pressure may be lowered, despite the reduction in ICP, because of the reduction in mean arterial pressure.
>
> - Propofol decreases blood pressure, cardiac output and systemic vascular resistance to a greater extent than thiopentone at equipotent doses.
>
> - Respiratory effects include an initial brief increase followed by a decrease in minute ventilation, very similar to thiopentone. The reduction in minute ventilation is chiefly through reduction in tidal volume.

plasma clearance. The terminal elimination half-life is long, 4–6 h. In children the volume of the central compartment and plasma clearance is higher than that in adults. As a result children need a higher induction dose and an increased maintenance infusion rate. The rapid recovery from propofol anaesthesia, even after prolonged infusion, is due to its rapid distribution from the blood to the peripheral tissues, and the slow elimination from these tissues has little relevance for the clinical situation. Increased sensitivity in the elderly is probably due to an age-related reduction in the volume of distribution rather than altered pharmacodynamics.

CENTRAL NERVOUS SYSTEM

The onset of action with a bolus injection is rapid, although slightly slower than with thiopentone. The usual dose required to produce loss of consciousness in healthy adults is $1–3\,mg\,kg^{-1}$. The blood propofol concentration at which patients loose consciousness (and thus also the induction dose) is reduced by concomitant administration of opioids[5,6] (Fig. 5.6) and by a slow rate of administration. The reduced dose at slower infusion rates is related to the time required for equilibration between the drug concentration in the blood and the effect site in the brain. At plasma concentrations lower than those that induce loss of consciousness, propofol is an effective anxiolytic and amnesic useful in supplementing regional anaesthetic techniques. It can be administered as an infusion, intermittent bolus or via a patient-controlled device with an efficacy similar to that of midazolam. It can also induce an extroverted, euphoric state at low infusion rates of $1–2\,mg\,kg^{-1}\,h^{-1}$.

Excitatory movements may be observed, particularly in children. These are not associated with cortical excitatory EEG activity and most likely are caused by activation of subcortical sites. They are less frequent at a higher ($5\,mg\,kg^{-1}$) than lower ($3\,mg\,kg^{-1}$) dose, possibly due to an additional inhibitory action of propofol at higher doses or greater sensitivity of the inhibitory pathways to propofol. The incidence of excitatory movements is lower with propofol than with thiopentone and methohexitone.[7] Despite the drug causing excitatory movements, its muscle-relaxant effect has been used successfully in the treatment of tetanus, and techniques have been described utilizing propofol to achieve intubating conditions in combination with alfentanil but no muscle relaxant. The drug causes more depression of laryngeal reflexes than thiopentone and greatly facilitates insertion of a laryngeal mask airway.

Whether propofol can cause epileptic fits remains controversial. Most of the evidence claiming that it causes seizures are case reports, many in circumstances that involved the administration of other drugs that can

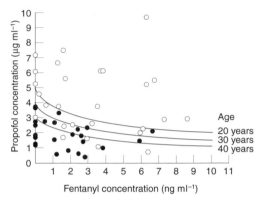

Fig. 5.6 Increasing fentanyl plasma concentration lowers the propofol concentration required to produce loss of consciousness in 50% of patients (Cp50$_{sleep}$). ○, Asleep; ●, awake. The effect reaches a plateau for fentanyl concentrations greater than 4–5 ng ml^{-1} at all ages. From Smith C, McEwan AI, Jhaveri R *et al*. The interaction of fentanyl on the Cp50 of propofol for loss of consciousness and skin incision. *Anesthesiology* 1994; 81: 820–828, with permission.

cause convulsions or in patients with neurological pathology. Fits occurred up to hours or, in one case, 5 days after administration of the drug. Paradoxically propofol has been used successfully in patients with resistant status epilepticus. There is no EEG evidence of propofol-induced cortical epileptiform activity, and significant burst suppression can be achieved in the high clinical dosage range. It also shortens the duration of convulsions after electroconvulsive therapy compared with methohexitone. The investigative data, rather than the clinical case reports, suggest that, in the absence of neurological pathology, propofol has significant anticonvulsant action.

The incidence of emesis is reduced by propofol. The mechanism of this action is unknown, but may be due to a central antiemetic effect. Apart from a residual effect following perioperative use, propofol has also been effective as a subhypnotic infusion in patients receiving chemotherapy and as a 10–15-mg bolus in the recovery area. Propofol has also been used for the treatment of pruritus from both opioids and cholestasis. The mechanism of opioid- and cholestatic-induced pruritus may be similar, as cholestatic pruritus is not related directly to bilirubin levels and both forms are relieved by naloxone, suggesting an opioid-like action of the causative agent in cholestatic pruritus. Propofol suppresses activity in both the anterior and posterior spinal cord and a 10-mg intravenous dose acts for around 1 h in both situations.

Both intracranial pressure and CMRO$_2$ are reduced by propofol; in patients with raised intracranial pressure a drop in cerebral perfusion pressure may result from a concomitant drop in mean arterial blood pressure. Propofol also reduces intraocular pressure.

CARDIOVASCULAR SYSTEM

Propofol decreases blood pressure, cardiac output and systemic vascular resistance to a greater extent than thiopentone at equipotent doses. This is due to a combination of reduced venous and arterial tone and a negative inotropic effect on the myocardium. However, with the usual clinical doses the predominant haemodynamic changes are more likely due to peripheral vasodilatation than myocardial depression.

The decrease in blood pressure and systemic vascular resistance can result in a compensatory tachycardia in healthy patients, although not infrequently a bradycardia occurs. This may be because propofol depresses the baroreceptor reflex more than other intravenous induction agents. Bradycardia is more likely when propofol is given together with an opioid. The hypotensive effect is also increased in the presence of an opioid. With propofol infusions, both myocardial blood flow and oxygen consumption are diminished, preserving the supply : demand ratio.

RESPIRATORY SYSTEM

Apnoea during induction of anaesthesia is more common with propofol than with the other induction agents, and a reduced tidal volume combined with tachypnoea is produced by infusion. As with other induction agents, the addition of opioids increases the period of apnoea and prevents tachypnoea. Propofol alone diminishes sensitivity to arterial partial pressure of carbon dioxide for a greater duration than thiopentone alone (see Fig. 5.3); it causes an initial brief increase followed by a decrease in minute ventilation very similar to that of thiopentone.

OTHER FEATURES

Propofol can cause considerable pain and discomfort on intravenous injection, and mixing the emulsion with lignocaine (2 ml 2%) or priming the vein with a lignocaine injection has been recommended. Although the incidence of hypersensitivity reactions to propofol is low compared with thiopentone and suxamethonium, a number of severe reactions have been described on first and second exposure to the drug. Histamine and adrenocorticotrophic hormone (ACTH) levels are usually unaffected by propofol. Limited experience in patients susceptible to malignant hyperpyrexia suggests it is not a strong triggering agent.

KETAMINE

Ketamine, a phencyclidine derivative, is an induction agent distinctly different from the other intravenous

---

Summary box 5.5 Key points of ketamine pharmacology

- Site of action appears to be primarily in the thalamus and limbic systems, acting via the NMDA receptor as a noncompetitive antagonist.

- Ketamine produces a rise in cerebral perfusion pressure by increased sympathetic outflow causing a rise in mean arterial pressure.

- The drug causes direct depression of the myocardium and vasodilatation on direct exposure to smooth muscle. However, central sympathetic stimulation can counteract these effects.

- Ketamine is a bronchodilator, preserves airway reflexes, and increases tracheobronchial and salivary secretions.

- Emergence phenomena, including vivid dreams, floating sensations and delirium, can occur following ketamine administration. They are more common in adults than children, and are reduced by benzodiazepine or barbiturate administration.

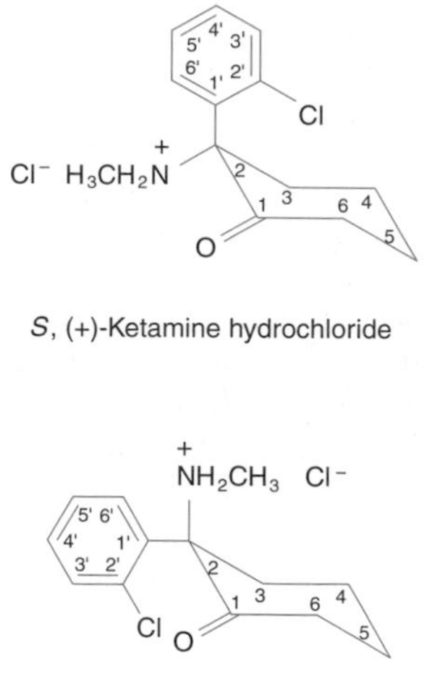

S, (+)-Ketamine hydrochloride

R, (−)-Ketamine hydrochloride

Fig. 5.7 Ketamine isomers. From White PF, Way WL, Trevor AJ. Ketamine – its pharmacology and therapeutic uses. *Anesthesiology* 1982; **56**: 119–136, with permission.

anaesthetics. It has an analgesic action and can preserve airway reflexes even when a patient is fully anaesthetized. It appears to act only on certain regions of the brain, in contrast to the more global effect of drugs such as thiopentone or propofol. The unusual clinical state induced by ketamine has been described as 'dissociative anaesthesia', although this state can also be achieved with phenothiazine–opioid combinations.

PHYSICAL CHARACTERISTICS

Ketamine is soluble in water and is prepared as a sodium salt with benzethonium chloride as a preservative. It is a basic compound and is dissolved in an acidic solution of pH 3.5–5. The ketamine molecule contains an asymmetrical carbon atom with two optical isomers (enantiomers) and is commercially available as the racemate (Fig. 5.7). The $S(+)$ isomer is about three times more potent and longer acting as an anaesthetic than the $R(-)$ isomer; the latter may be responsible for some of the undesirable side-effects, especially psychotomimetic effects. The $S(+)$ isomer is currently undergoing clinical trials.

PHARMACOKINETICS AND PHARMACODYNAMICS

Ketamine can be administered intravenously (1–3 mg kg^{-1}), intramuscularly (3–5 mg kg^{-1} in adults and up to 8 mg kg^{-1} in children), rectally (7–15 mg kg^{-1}) or orally. The bioavailability with intramuscular administration is 93% and peak plasma levels are reached at around

20 min. Intramuscular ketamine, 0.5 mg kg^{-1}, provides 1–2 h of analgesia, although it is less effective than morphine. The oral dose has only 15% bioavailability owing to hepatic first-pass metabolism. Biotransformation is complex, with both hepatic demethylation and hydroxylation as potential routes. Urine excretion of ketamine is minimal. The metabolites are pharmacologically active, but as potentially eight or more metabolites are generated, their relative potencies have not yet been determined. The volume of distribution is 0.5–3 l kg^{-1} with a distribution half-life of around 15 min and elimination half-life of 2–3 h. Ketamine has a low affinity for plasma protein, only 12% being protein bound.

CENTRAL NERVOUS SYSTEM

Ketamine's site of action appears to be primarily in the thalamus and limbic systems, acting via the *N*-methyl-D-aspartate (NMDA) receptor as a noncompetitive antagonist. It does not depress respiratory drive unless high doses are used, and preserves the protective airway reflexes. The patient can sometimes exhibit movement of the limbs or head, apart from movement to skin incision, which can interfere with surgery. The eyes frequently remain open with a slow nystagmic gaze and preservation of the corneal and light reflexes. Glucose utilization in the auditory and somatosensory systems is reduced, suggesting selective deprivation of these senses, and the thalamic and limbic regions show increased utilization. Bizarre, distressing, emergence phenomena can occur following ketamine administration, including vivid dreams (these can occur for several days after anaesthesia), floating sensations and delirium. These emergence phenomena, more common in adults than children, are an undesirable feature of ketamine that detract from its more useful features. They are reduced by concurrent benzodiazepine or barbiturate administration, and by benzodiazepine premedication. Ketamine is not a strong anterograde amnesic in subanaesthetic dosage. The drug produces high-amplitude slowing of the EEG, and case reports of successful treatment of status epilepticus exist.

The effect of ketamine on intracranial pressure is currently being reevaluated. The previously accepted explanation was that the rise in mean arterial pressure resulted in a rise in cerebral perfusion pressure and consequent rise in intracranial pressure, especially in patients with already increased intracranial pressure. For this reason ketamine was contraindicated in patients with potentially raised intracranial pressure. The physiology is more complicated than this and a rise in intracranial pressure does not always occur. The presence of background induction agents may reduce $CMRO_2$ and haemodynamic responsiveness.

The corollary to whether ketamine has an effect on intracranial pressure is also whether it has a specific indication in neurosurgical anaesthesia. Experimental data have shown ketamine to decrease cerebral infarct volume and improve outcome in experimentally head-injured rats. Clinical and experimental exploration of the protective role of NMDA antagonists in head injury and cerebrovascular ischaemia has produced conflicting results. The mechanism of ischaemic injury is polymodal and the contribution of one receptor antagonist may be limited. Antagonism of the effects of extracellular neurotoxic glutamate may be a mechanism of action. An alternative explanation is that the NMDA antagonists simply induce cerebral vasodilatation, so improving perfusion of the watershed areas adjacent to the injury.

CARDIOVASCULAR SYSTEM

Blood pressure and heart rate are frequently raised after administration of ketamine, although a converse hypotensive response can occur following sequential doses. This response is blunted by benzodiazepines and opioids. The drug causes direct depression of the myocardium[8] and vasodilatation on direct exposure to smooth muscle. However, the direct myocardial depression in an animal model is less than that with other commonly used induction agents. The haemodynamic changes in vivo may result from central nervous system stimulation: a rise in noradrenaline levels is detectable in the blood after ketamine administration, and the pressor response is blocked by α- and β-adrenoceptor antagonists and sympathetic ganglion blockade. Ketamine inhibits catecholamine uptake at sympathetic

nerve terminals. Because of its cardiovascular profile, ketamine has been advocated as a drug suitable for haemodynamically unstable patients. Pulmonary vascular resistance also tends to rise and an increase in pulmonary shunting can occur in patients with cardiac septal defects.

RESPIRATORY SYSTEM

Apnoea is unusual unless a large dose is administered rapidly or another respiratory depressant drug (e.g. an opioid) is given. Airway reflexes and skeletal muscle tone are preserved, but salivary and tracheobronchial secretions are increased. Silent aspiration is still a potential hazard despite the retention of protective reflexes. Ketamine has a bronchodilator action that may be mediated either via an increase in blood catecholamines or by its direct smooth muscle relaxant effect. This is a potentially valuable property for induction of anaesthesia in a patient with status asthmaticus.

OTHER

Ketamine is commonly used in developing countries. The combination of analgesia with preservation of respiration that it provides allows for the delivery of an anaesthetic with the economy of drugs and equipment necessitated by sparsely equipped hospitals. The same properties make it useful for providing onsite analgesia in trauma cases.

ETOMIDATE

Etomidate was introduced clinically in 1972. It has a relatively rapid recovery profile and elimination half-life compared with thiopentone, the other commonly used induction agent available at that time. Initially it was popular as both an induction and a maintenance agent owing to its more rapid elimination, combined with concerns about the toxicity of inhalational agents. However, the ability of etomidate to inhibit corticosteroid synthesis has now resulted in restriction of its use to induction of anaesthesia only. It is commonly perceived as offering improved haemodynamic stability during induction in the haemodynamically unstable patient, and as a result still retains a place in clinical practice. This feature will be examined more closely.

PHYSICAL CHARACTERISTICS

Etomidate is an imidazole with two stereoisomers but is marketed as $R(+)$-etomidate. The $S(-)$ enantiomer has minimal hypnotic activity (Fig. 5.8). Although slightly water soluble, it is formulated in 35% propylene glycol with a pH of 8. It is also marketed with lipofundin (medium-chain triglycerides) as the solvent.

Summary box 5.6 Key points of etomidate pharmacology

- Etomidate reduces intracranial pressure, cerebral blood flow and CMRO$_2$.

- The involuntary movements, tremors and dystonia that may occur during induction and recovery are not associated with an epileptiform EEG pattern.

- Etomidate causes less myocardium depression and hypotension than other induction agents.

- It depresses the slope of the ventilatory response to carbon dioxide in a manner similar to that of barbiturates and propofol. However, minute ventilation increases, chiefly through an increase in respiratory rate.

- Etomidate inhibits the hepatic enzyme 11β-hydroxylase, which is essential in the production of both corticosteroids and mineralocorticoids. However, clinically significant reductions in steroid production occur only with prolonged infusions or repeated dosing.

PHARMACOKINETICS AND PHARMACODYNAMICS

Patient recovery occurs 5–7 min after an induction bolus. A typical induction dose is 0.3 mg kg^{-1}. The elimination half-life is around 4 h. Metabolism is by hydrolysis of the ethyl ester by plasma esterases and hepatic microsomal enzymes, the major metabolite being an inactive carboxylic acid ester. About 80% of a bolus dose of the drug is excreted in the urine in the form of the carboxylic acid ester and only a very small proportion of the active drug is excreted unchanged. Some metabolite is excreted in the bile. Protein binding is 75% and hypoproteinaemia increases the volume of distribution. In the elderly the volume of distribution appears to be reduced and a reduction in the induction dose may be required to avoid excessive free (unbound) plasma concentrations.

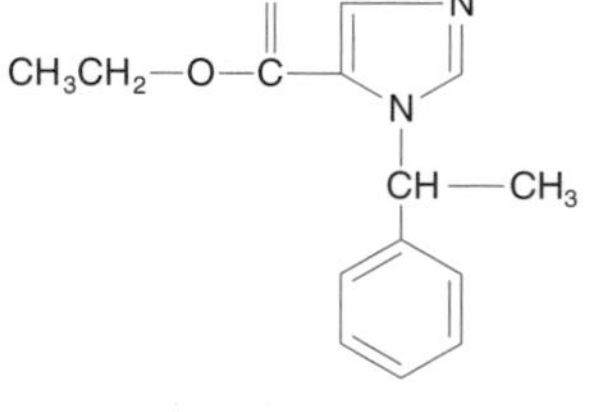

Etomidate

Fig. 5.8 Structure of etomidate.

CENTRAL NERVOUS SYSTEM

Etomidate, like many other induction agents, interacts with the GABA$_A$ receptor, although the precise mode of action is not fully understood. Induction is less smooth than with thiopentone, hiccoughs and involuntary myoclonic movements being more common. The involuntary movements, tremors and dystonia, which may also be seen during recovery, are diminished by opioid premedication and are not associated with epileptiform EEG patterns. In one study excitatory effects, including myoclonus, tremor and dystonic posturing, occurred in 86.6% of patients receiving etomidate.[7] Multiple spikes appeared on the EEG in 22.2%, but were not associated with myoclonic activity. The frequency of excitatory effects was 16.6% after thiopentone, 12.5% after methohexitone and 5.5% after propofol. None of the patients receiving thiopentone, methohexitone or propofol developed myoclonic or seizure activity. The authors concluded that etomidate should be used with caution in patients with epilepsy or cerebral cortical lesions. The drug has been reported both to cause seizures and to treat status epilepticus effectively. However, it produces longer seizure patterns on the EEG than either propofol or methohexitone when given for electroconvulsive therapy. The risk of inducing seizures, although low, may be higher than for other agents but the evidence is equivocal. Etomidate reduces intracranial pressure, cerebral blood flow, CMRO$_2$ and intraocular pressure.[9,10] It may be appropriate to use etomidate in patients with raised intracranial pressure if the desirable feature of cardiovascular stability is an important clinical consideration.

CARDIOVASCULAR SYSTEM

Etomidate's lack of significant cardiovascular depression is often emphasized. Animal studies using isolated heart preparations suggest that etomidate causes minimal effect on myocardial contractility.[8,11] However, the cardiostability of etomidate may not be as complete as previously suggested. Price et al.[12] found a greater decrease in cardiac index (16%) and an increase in systemic vascular resistance (12%) 1 min after induction of anaesthesia with etomidate than with propofol, methohexitone or thiopentone in patients with American Society of Anesthesiologists grade 1. None the less the balance of evidence suggests that etomidate probably does not disturb haemodynamics as much as other induction agents, although this may not be true in every clinical situation where changing haemodynamics will influence the drug effect. The drug is often used in trauma patients with suspected hypovolaemia or unstable haemodynamics because of the presumed cardiovascular stability, but there are few studies to corroborate this purported advantage.

RESPIRATORY SYSTEM

Etomidate does not commonly cause a significant rise in plasma histamine levels in patients with normal or reactive airways. It has little action on pulmonary vascular resistance in clinical doses. The slope of the ventilatory response to carbon dioxide is depressed in a manner similar to that of methohexitone, thiopentone and propofol, indicating depression of medullary respiratory centres responsible for sensitivity to carbon dioxide (Fig. 5.9). However, it causes increased minute ventilation, chiefly through an increase in respiratory rate, presumably by direct stimulation of other respiratory centres responsible for maintenance of ventilation.[13] In the absence of concomitant opioids, etomidate is better suited for induction than barbiturates or propofol where maintenance of spontaneous ventilation is desired. Hiccoughs and laryngospasm can result in

a difficult laryngeal mask insertion unless supplemented by an opioid or adequate alveolar volatile concentrations.

INHIBITION OF CORTISOL SYNTHESIS

In 1983 a letter in the *Lancet* from Ledingham and Watt[14] reported that the mortality rate was almost double in a subgroup of intensive care patients sedated with etomidate by intravenous infusion. This has subsequently been explained by inhibition by etomidate of the adrenocortical enzyme 11β-hydroxylase (Fig. 5.10). This mitochondrial enzyme is essential in the production of both corticosteroids (cortisol) and mineralocorticoids (aldosterone).[15] Following an induction dose, the responsiveness of adrenal production of cortisol to ACTH is depressed for around 6 h owing to inhibition of the enzyme. This effect does not appear to be clinically significant unless etomidate is continuously infused rather than given as a single bolus.

OTHER

The incidence of postoperative nausea and vomiting is higher following etomidate than after thiopentone or methohexitone. The drug is also painful on injection and can cause thrombophlebitis. This is less when lipofundin is used as the solvent rather than propylene glycol.

STEROID ANAESTHETIC AGENTS

At present there are no intravenous steroid anaesthetics in use, although much research has been performed on these compounds over the past 50 years. In 1941 Selye discovered that large doses of intraperitoneal steroids rendered rats unconscious. Since then several hundred steroid derivatives have been tested and a small number have been available to anaesthetists for clinical use.[16]

The initial agent (pregnandione) was esterified to improve aqueous solubility but had an extremely slow onset time. The search for a rapid-onset steroid that was soluble resulted in Althesin, marketed in 1969. This consisted of alphaxalone plus a smaller amount of alphadolone, a less potent steroid that enhanced solubility. They were dissolved in cremophor EL. A high incidence of anaphylactoid reactions, probably to cremophor, led to its withdrawal in 1984. Minaxolone, which was soluble in water at pH 4, was withdrawn before registration because of toxicity following long-term administration in rats. Most recently eltanolone, a natural derivative of progesterone has been developed. Solubility problems were overcome by dissolving the drug in a formulation identical to that for propofol, and clinical trials confirmed it as an effective induction agent. Eltanolone was withdrawn due to reports of urticaria and a possible risk of hypersensitivity reactions.

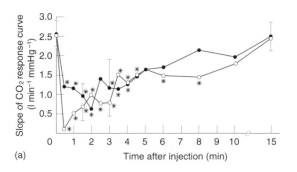

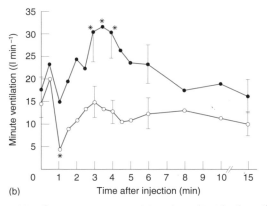

Fig. 5.9 Ventilatory response to (a) carbon dioxide ($l\ min^{-1}\ mmHg^{-1}$) and (b) minute ventilation ($l\ min^{-1}$) versus time after comparable induction doses of etomidate (●) and methohexitone (○) in volunteers. Values are mean ± SEM. Effects on ventilatory response to carbon dioxide are similar, but etomidate increases minute ventilation through an increase in respiratory rate whereas methohexitone decreases it through a decrease in tidal volume. *$P < 0.05$ versus preinjection value. From Choi SD, Spaulding BC, Gross JB, Apfelbaum JL. Comparison of the ventilatory effects of etomidate and methohexital. *Anesthesiology* 1985; **62**: 442–447, with permission.

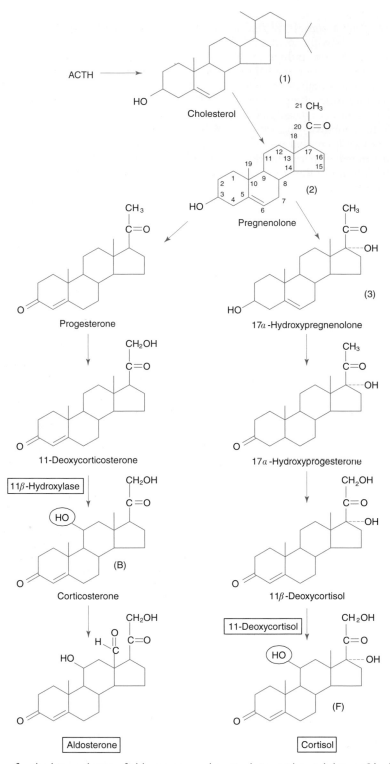

Fig. 5.10 Pathways for the biosynthesis of aldosterone and cortisol. Etomidate inhibits 11β-hydroxylase. ACTH, adrenocorticotrophic hormone. From Ungar F. Biochemistry of hormones. I: Hormone receptors, steroid and thyroid hormones. In: Devlin TM (ed.) *Textbook of Biochemistry: With Clinical Correlations*, 2nd edn. New York, John Wiley, 1986: 570–580, with permission.

Table 5.1 Pharmacokinetic data for intravenous anaesthetic agents					
	Thiopentone	Methohexitone	Propofol	Etomidate	Ketamine
Active metabolites	Yes	No	No	No	Yes (norketamine)
Protein binding (%)	65–85	65–85	98	75	12
Hepatic extraction	0.2	0.5–0.6	> 0.9*	0.9	> 0.9
$V_{d_{steady\ state}}$ (l kg−1)	2.3–3.5	2.3–3.7	3–12	2.5–4.5	3
Elimination half-life (h)	10–12	4	1–6	4	3
Effect of reduced creatinine clearance	Little	Little	Little	Little	Little

* Extrahepatic clearance.

REFERENCES

1. Dundee JW. Fifty years of thiopentone. *Br J Anaesth* 1984; **56**: 211–213.
2. Tanelian DL, Kosek P, Mody I, MacIver MB. The role of the GABA$_A$ receptor/chloride channel complex in anesthesia. *Anesthesiology* 1993; **78**: 757–776.
3. Jensen NF, Fiddler DS, Striepe V. Anesthetic considerations in porphyrias. *Anesth Analg* 1995; **80**: 591–599.
4. Alkire MT, Haier RJ, Barker SJ, Nitin KS, Wu JC, Kao YJ. Cerebral metabolism during propofol anesthesia in humans studied with positron emission tomography. *Anesthesiology* 1995; **82**: 393–403.
5. Vuyk J, Engbers FH, Burm AGL *et al*. Pharmacodynamic interaction between propofol and alfentanil when given for induction of anesthesia. *Anesthesiology* 1996; **84**: 288–299.
6. Smith C, McEwan AI, Jhaveri R *et al*. The interaction of fentanyl on the Cp50 of propofol for loss of consciousness and skin incision. *Anesthesiology* 1994; **81**: 820–828.
7. Reddy RV, Moorthy SS, Dierdorf SF, Deitch RD, Link L. Excitatory effects and electroencephalographic correlation of etomidate, thiopental, methohexital, and propofol. *Anesth Analg* 1993; **77**: 1008–1011.
8. Stowe DF, Bosnjak ZJ, Kampine JP. Comparison of etomidate, ketamine, midazolam, propofol, and thiopental on function and metabolism of isolated hearts. *Anesth Analg* 1992; **74**: 547–558.
9. Artru AA. Intracranial volume–pressure relationship following thiopental or etomidate. *Anesthesiology* 1989; **71**: 763–768.
10. Cold G, Eskesen V, Eriksen H, Amtoft O, Madsen JB. CBF and CMRO$_2$ during continuous etomidate infusion supplemented with N$_2$O and fentanyl in patients with supratentorial cerebral tumour. A dose–response study. *Acta Anaesthesiol Scand* 1985; **29**: 490–494.
11. Kissin I, Motomura S, Aultman DF, Reves JG. Inotropic and anesthetic potencies of etomidate and thiopental in dogs. *Anesth Analg* 1983; **62**: 961–965.
12. Price ML, Millar B, Grounds M, Cashman J. Changes in cardiac index and estimated systemic vascular resistance during induction of anaesthesia with thiopentone, methohexitone, propofol and etomidate. *Br J Anaesth* 1992; **69**: 172–176.
13. Choi SD, Spaulding BC, Gross JB, Apfelbaum JL. Comparison of the ventilatory effects of etomidate and methohexital. *Anesthesiology* 1985; **62**: 442–447.
14. Ledingham IM, Watt I. Influence of sedation on mortality in critically ill multiple trauma patients. *Lancet* 1983; **i**: 270 (letter).
15. Wagner RL, White PF, Kan PB. Inhibition of adrenal steroidogenesis by the anesthetic etomidate. *N Engl J Med* 1984; **310**: 1415–1421.
16. Sear JW. Steroid anesthetic agents: old compounds, new drugs. *J Clin Anesth* 1996; **8** (Suppl.): 91S–98S.

6

PCM van den Berg, JG Bovill

HYPNOTICS AND SEDATIVES

Hypnotic and sedative drugs are widely used in the general population, and in anaesthesia they are used for premedication to produce sedation, anxiolysis and amnesia, and some are used as intravenous induction agents. They are also used to produce sedation and anxiolysis in critically ill patients to augment patient comfort and to increase the acceptance of artificial ventilation and as an adjunct to minor procedures in the intensive care unit. Although both sedatives and hypnotics depress the function of the central nervous system (CNS), there are important distinctions between them. A sedative drug decreases cerebral activity, moderates excitement and calms the recipient, whereas a hypnotic drug produces drowsiness and facilitates the onset and maintenance of a state that resembles natural sleep.

The classical CNS depressants, the barbiturates, have largely been replaced by the benzodiazepines because of their superior margin of safety. Sedation is a side-effect of many agents that are not primarily CNS depressants (e.g. antihistamines), but which may be used to augment the effects of CNS depressants. Some sedative drugs have predominantly anxiolytic activity, such as the benzodiazepines and buspirones. Recently new classes of drugs, zopiclones and azapirones, have been developed with clinical effects similar to those of the benzodiazepines.

Summary box 6.1 Benzodiazepines

- Important pharmacological effects:
  - anxiolysis
  - sedation
  - antiepileptic activity
  - muscle relaxation
  - anterograde amnesia.
- Act by binding to specific binding site (benzodiazepine receptor) on $GABA_A$–chloride channel complex:
  - enhance action of GABA
  - no action themselves in absence of GABA
  - compounds that are ligands at benzodiazepine receptor may be agonists, partial agonists, competitive antagonists or inverse agonists
  - partial agonists and inverse agonists have no therapeutic roles.
- Endogenous benzodiazepines believed to exist:
  - diazepam binding inhibitor (peptide)
  - endozepines (nonpeptide).
- Active orally.
- With exception of midazolam, poorly water soluble.
- Many long-acting benzodiazepines have active metabolites.
- Relatively safe in overdose.
- Tolerance and dependence can develop with chronic use.

BENZODIAZEPINES

The term benzodiazepine refers to the structure composed of a benzene ring fused to a seven-membered diazepine ring (Figs 6.1 and 6.2). Benzodiazepines are moderate sedatives with potent anxiolytic and amnesic effects. They also produce muscle relaxation and have anticonvulsant activity. Although they do not have specific antidepressant effects, the relief of anxiety may be beneficial in depressed patients. Each benzodiazepine possesses a unique profile such that the magnitude of the diverse effects differs between the different compounds. Benzodiazepine compounds are classified as full agonists, partial agonists, antagonists and inverse agonists. Partial agonists and inverse agonists have no therapeutic role.

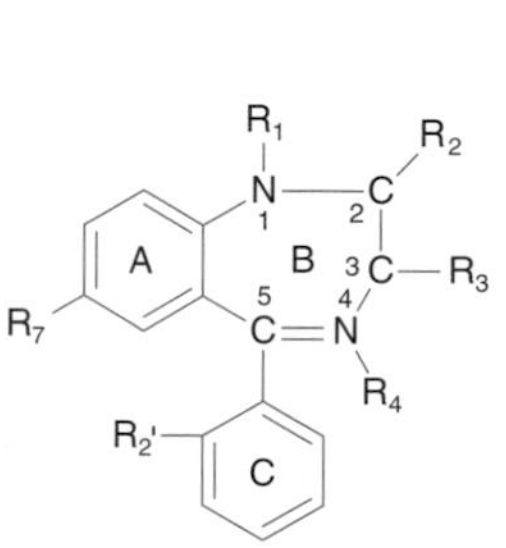

MECHANISMS OF ACTION

The pharmacological actions of benzodiazepines result from activation of specific binding sites, the benzodiazepine receptor, in the γ-aminobutyric acid (GABA)$_A$ receptor complex. GABA$_A$ receptors are located in the cerebral cortex, thalamus, hippocampus, hypothalamus, cerebellar cortex and spinal cord. The GABA$_A$ receptor is a large macromolecule with binding sites for GABA, benzodiazepines and barbiturates. Activation of the GABA$_A$ receptor increases the flux of chloride ions, resulting in hyperpolarization and reduced response to neuronal excitatory stimulation. Three benzodiazepine binding sites have been identified. Two, designated ω_1 and ω_2, are found on the GABA$_A$ complex and may represent variants of the α subunit of the GABA$_A$ receptor. The third subtype, the ω_3 receptor, is not associated with this complex but is found in both the periphery and the brain. Unlike barbiturates, benzodiazepines do not directly gate GABA receptors but enhance the effects of GABA in increasing chloride conductance. Indeed, binding studies have shown that there is a mutual interaction between benzodiazepines and GABA, each increasing the affinity of the other for their respective binding sites. Benzodiazepines alone do not have any effect on

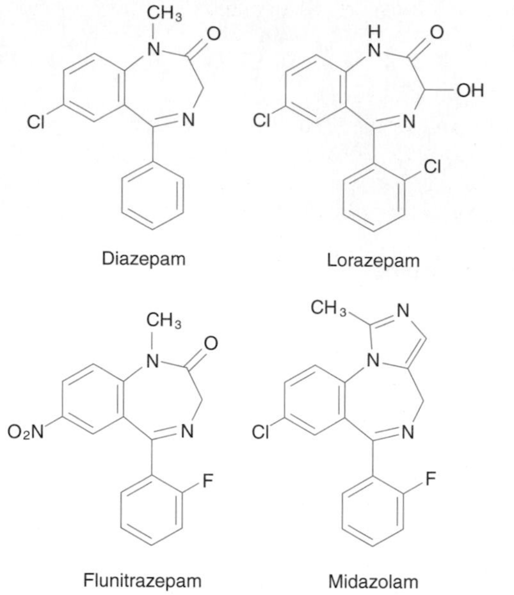

Fig. 6.2 Chemical structures of four benzodiazepines available for intravenous use.

chloride currents in the absence of GABA or GABA agonists.

Inverse agonists produce opposite pharmacological effects to those of the agonists. They are anxiogenic and proconvulsant. Several benzodiazepine inverse agonists have been identified, although as yet no therapeutic role has been found for them. Whereas benzodiazepine agonists increase the GABA response, inverse agonists decrease it.

The presence of a specific binding site for benzodiazepines on the GABA$_A$ receptor, and the fact that benzodiazepines also bind with high affinity to nonGABA sites in the brain and some peripheral tissues, has led to speculation as to the existence of endogenous benzodiazepine ligands. Possible candidates for endogenous benzodiazepine ligands include diazepam binding inhibitor (DBI), a polypeptide[1] and a group of low molecular weight, nonpeptide substances known as endozepines.[2] Hepatic encephalopathy is associated with an increase in the brain content of endozepines[3] and flumazenil ameliorates the neurological signs of this syndrome.

Not all the clinical effects of the benzodiazepines can be explained by their binding to the GABA receptor. Benzodiazepines inhibit neuronal uptake of adenosine, and are associated with the inhibition of Ca^{2+} currents. Benzodiazepine binding sites are present in the myocardium, and are responsible for the coronary vasodilatation produced by high doses of benzodiazepines. However, the clinically relevant effects of

Fig. 6.1 General chemical structure of a benzodiazepine molecule. Ring B is the seven-member diazepine moiety.

benzodiazepines are all explained by activation of the GABA$_A$ receptor.

PHARMACOLOGICAL EFFECTS

All benzodiazepines have a similar action on the CNS, and differences between individual drugs are related largely to potency and pharmacokinetics. They are anxiolytic and anticonvulsant at the lower dosage range, with sedation, amnesia and anaesthesia appearing as the dose is increased (Table 6.1).

Anxiolysis

Anxiolysis is one of the most useful therapeutic properties of the benzodiazepines, and since the introduction of chlorodiazepoxide in 1960 they have been used extensively for the treatment of anxiety and related disorders. There are no significant differences in the anxiolytic efficacy between the various benzodiazepines. Currently drugs with a shorter half-life, such as alprazolam, lorazepam, clonazepam or clorazepate, are preferred to the longer-acting diazepam. While some patients may experience drowsiness or other sedative effects after initiation of therapy, these symptoms often diminish with continued therapy. This may be due to adaptation or tolerance. Tolerance develops to the nonspecific sedative effects of benzodiazepines during long-term therapy, but is much less common to their anxiolytic effects. In most patients a daily dose can be found that results in substantial clinical improvement with few or no sedative side-effects.[4]

Some patients receiving benzodiazepines experience a paradoxical increased feeling of anger, irritability and aggression, opposite to the usual calming effects of the drug. Such effects are rare, and have been particularly associated with the ultra-short-acting triazolam. This led to its withdrawal in the UK and some other countries. Hyperexcitability has been described with alprazolam and lorazepam. The use of benzodiazepines with faster elimination, high binding activity and/or a triazolo structure is associated with a higher risk for the development of more severe psychiatric effects. Agitation, panic reactions and anxiety may be more severe with flunitrazepam than with other benzodiazepines.

Sedation and hypnosis

Benzodiazepines produce sedation and hypnosis at concentrations higher than those required for anxiolysis (Fig. 6.3). Because of their wide safety index, they have replaced barbiturates for the treatment of insomnia. Natural sleep is characterized by a cyclic pattern repeating itself four or five times over a period of 5–8 h During each cycle five different levels of sleep can be differentiated. To produce the beneficial effects of sleep pharmacologically, it is important that this cyclic pattern is minimally disturbed. Levels 3 and 4 are the deeper levels characterized by 'slow-wave sleep', with δ waves appearing in the electroencephalogram (EEG). Rapid eye movement (REM) sleep is part of the lighter sleep levels. Dreaming occurs during REM sleep. The periods of REM and slow-wave sleep are crucial for effective sleep.

Benzodiazepines increase the effective sleeping time by decreasing the awakening periods during the total sleeping time. Total sleeping time is increased, and especially light sleeping in level 2 is prolonged. The time spent in both REM sleep and in level 3 and 4 sleep is reduced. With short-acting benzodiazepines a rebound increase in REM sleep may occur, leading to unpleasant dreams. The effects of benzodiazepines on the awaking EEG resemble those of other sedative–hypnotic drugs. α Activity is reduced, but there is an increase in low-voltage β activity.

Tolerance, the reduction over time in one or more

Table 6.1 Relationship between effects of benzodiazepines, dose and receptor occupancy		
Benzodiazepine agonist	**Effect**	**Postulated receptor occupancy (%)**
Low dose	Anxiolysis	20–30
	Anticonvulsive effect	20–30
	Slight sedation	20–30
	Reduced attention	20–30
	Amnesia	50
	Intense sedation	50
	Muscle relaxation	60–90
High dose	Hypnosis	60–90

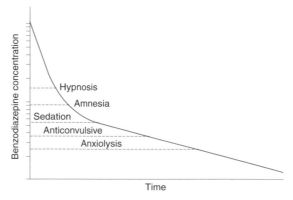

Fig. 6.3 General relationship between plasma benzodiazepine concentration (logarithmic scale) and pharmacological effect.

pharmacological effects as a consequence of prolonged administration of benzodiazepines, is well recognized. Tolerance develops to the nonspecific sedative effects, whereas tolerance to the anxiolytic effects of benzodiazepines is less common. Tolerance develops rapidly with the shorter-acting triazolam, alprazolam and temazepam.[5] Flurazepam, diazepam and clonazepam are slowly eliminated and remain efficacious even after prolonged use. With midazolam, tolerance is more likely to develop when the dose is increased progressively. Tolerance to benzodiazepines is not associated with abuse or dependence.

Withdrawal of a benzodiazepine can lead to rebound anxiety or insomnia. The duration of the rebound is usually short, lasting only a few days. This is more likely with drugs with a short half-life, and these drugs should therefore be stopped gradually rather than abruptly. In some patients true physical dependence develops. The probability of physical dependence increases as the daily dose and duration of treatment increase. Withdrawal symptoms are generally autonomic and include excessive sensitivity to light and sound, tremors, sweating, insomnia, tachycardia, mild hypertension and, rarely, convulsions. The withdrawal syndrome is generally mild and always self-limiting, and patients recover without residual sequelae.

Amnesia

Benzodiazepines have profound and specific effects on memory, and it is interesting that the structures most involved in learning and memory, the cerebellum, hippocampus and cerebral cortex, also contain the highest concentrations of $GABA_A$ receptors. Benzodiazepines do not impair short-term memory but impair acquisition or encoding of new information in long-term memory.[6] They have no effect upon either retention or retrieval of previously stored information. In other words, they cause anterograde but not retrograde amnesia. However, benzodiazepines can facilitate retention of material learned before their administration, an effect known as retrograde facilitation.[6]

The effects on memory appear to be specific and not secondary to drug-induced drowsiness or sedation. Amnesia is more marked when the drug is given intravenously, and reliable amnesia may not occur after oral or intramuscular administration, although a single oral dose of lorazepam produces dose-dependent impairment of information acquisition and recall.[7] A single intravenous dose of midazolam will produce a brief, but very intense, period of amnesia lasting 20–30 min. In contrast, the amnesic effects of intravenous lorazepam are slower in onset (peak effect about 60 min) and may last for several hours. Flumazenil does not restore memory already lost, but normal memory function is regained.

Anticonvulsant activity

Benzodiazepines inhibit seizure activity of the brain and given intravenously are effective in terminating the repeated convulsions of status epilepticus. Their rapid onset of action is an advantage over other intravenous antiepileptic drugs. With most benzodiazepines sedation limits their usefulness as chronic antiepileptic drugs, although clonazepam and clobazam are effective in doses that do not produce sedation, and are sometimes used to treat myoclonic seizures in children. However, the anticonvulsant effect of oral benzodiazepine therapy for epilepsy quickly becomes ineffective owing to the development of tolerance.

Muscle relaxation

Muscle relaxation by benzodiazepines is caused by central inhibition of glycine receptors in the cerebellum and spinal cord, and not to any action on muscles. This action is independent of their sedative effect. Some, for example clonzepam, produce muscle relaxation in nonsedative doses.

Cardiovascular effects

Benzodiazepines cause only minor haemodynamic effects. Under normal circumstances, the predominant effect is a dose-related decrease in systemic vascular resistance with a moderate reduction in systolic blood pressure and stroke volume. The haemodynamic effects are greater when given in combination with an opioid. The effects of midazolam on blood pressure are more pronounced than those of diazepam.

Respiratory effects

The response to both hypercapnia and hypoxia is depressed following intravenous benzodiazepines, and depending on the dose and speed of injection respiratory depression can vary from a slight decrease in tidal volume to apnoea. After intravenous administration of benzodiazepines, apnoea occurs in 25–30% of patients. The incidence of apnoea is related to dose, speed of injection, age of the patient and presence of debilitating disease. Midazolam produces the greatest respiratory depression, although differences between the benzodiazepines are small and probably not of clinical relevance. Patients with chronic obstructive pulmonary disease are prone to the depressant effects of benzodiazepines, which should be avoided or the dose should be carefully titrated.[8]

PHARMACOKINETICS

Physiochemical properties

The pharmacokinetic characteristics of the benzodiazepines are closely related to their physiochemical properties. The benzodiazepines are very lipophilic compounds and rapidly cross the blood–brain barrier and placenta. They are basic drugs with pK_a values ranging from 1.84 (flunitrazepam) to 6.1 (midazolam) so that they are extensively un-ionized in blood; this is responsible for their lipid solubility and, except for midazolam, poor water solubility (Table 6.2). At a pH of less than 4, midazolam exists as an open imidazole ring which is water soluble. At physiological pH, the ring closes yielding a highly lipid-soluble molecule (Fig. 6.4). The midazolam solution is acidified to pH 3 to make it water soluble.

The benzodiazepines are all extensively bound to plasma proteins, principally albumin (Table 6.2). Patients with hepatic or renal dysfunction, or other diseases associated with hypoalbuminaemia, will therefore have higher free (unbound) concentrations and thus an enhanced response compared with normal subjects. The ratio of cerebrospinal fluid (CSF) to plasma concentration increases almost linearly with increasing free fraction for benzodiazepines (Fig. 6.5). There is a significant correlation between plasma albumin concentration and the time required for induction of anaesthesia with midazolam. Valproic acid displaces diazepam from its protein binding and decreases its metabolism. Heparin displaces benzodiazepines from plasma binding sites, and the protein binding of midazolam is decreased by aspirin.

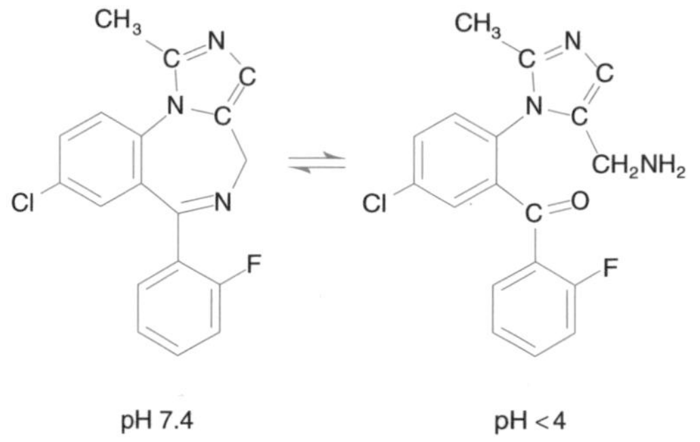

Fig. 6.4 pH-dependent structure of midazolam.

Absorption

Absorption of the benzodiazepines is high after oral administration and, for most, the bioavailability is also high (Table 6.2). An exception is midazolam (bioavailability 48%), reflecting its much higher hepatic clearance and thus first-pass metabolism. Peak plasma concentrations after oral intake vary from 30–80 min for diazepam to between 1 and 2.5 h for lorazepam, although clinical effects are usually seen within 20–30 min for most drugs. The onset of oral midazolam is more rapid, with peak effects as early as 20–30 min. Oral absorption is affected by gastric pH; an increase in pH leads to a greater concentration of un-ionized

Drug	Oral bioavailability (%)	pK_a	Percentage un-ionized at pH 7.4	Lipid solubility (λ_{ow})	Protein binding (%)	V_d (l kg^{-1})	Cl (ml kg^{-1} min^{-1})	$t_{1/2}$ (h)
Midazolam	42	6.2	94.1	475	95	0.5–1.5	6–8	1.5–3
Oxazepam	97	1.7	99.9	97	98	0.6	1.05	5–15
Temazepam	80	1.31	99.9	–	97	1.06	0.9	6–16
Lorazepam	93	1.3	99.9	73	91	1–3	0.8–1.3	10–20
Flunitrazepam	85	1.84	99.9	–	78	3.3	3.5	10–25
Nitrazepam	78	3.2	99.9	125	87	1.9	0.85	20–50
Diazepam	100	3.3	99.9	309	99	1–2	0.25–0.5	26–50
Clonazepam	98	1.5	99.9	250	86	3.2	1.6	24–56
Flumazenil	16	1.7	99.9	14	50	0.6–1.2	13–16	0.8–1.15

Table 6.2 Pharmacokinetics of benzodiazepines

λ_{ow}, Octanol–water partition coefficient at pH 7.4; $t_{1/2}$, elimination half-life.

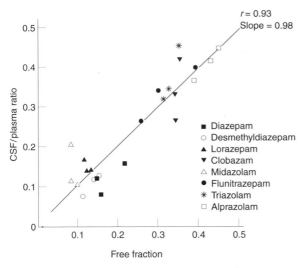

Fig. 6.5 Ratio of cerebrospinal fluid (CSF) to plasma concentration plotted against the free (unbound) fraction in plasma for various benzodiazepines following intravenous administration to cats. Higher free fractions (lower protein binding) is associated with enhanced entry of drug into the CSF. From Arendt RM *et al. J Pharmacol Exp Ther* 1983; **227**: 98–106.

benzodiazepines in the stomach, and this enhances absorption. The presence of food or aluminium-containing antacids will delay gastric emptying and absorption.

The uptake of intramuscular diazepam is slow and unpredictable, and because the injection is very painful this route is not recommended. Higher plasma diazepam concentrations are achieved after oral than intramuscular administration. The poor absorption of intramuscular diazepam is related to its low solubility at physiological pH and possible precipitation at the injection site. Following intramuscular administration of lorazepam and midazolam, absorption is rapid and complete. The onset of action for intramuscular lorazepam can take up to 40 min and the duration of action is 12–24 h. The onset of action after intramuscular administration of midazolam is 5–15 min; its effect lasts about 2 (range 1–6)h. Midazolam can also be given rectally and, although the bioavailability by this route is low (5–27%), the onset is fairly rapid. Midazolam can be administered via the nasal mucosa and this route has been used in children before induction of anaesthesia. A dose of 0.2–0.3 mg kg^{-1} produces good sedation within 10–15 min.

Metabolism

Benzodiazepines are metabolized in the liver and excreted as glucuronide conjugates in the urine. The presence of pharmacologically active metabolites is largely responsible for the variability in the duration of action among the different compounds. The major metabolite of diazepam is desmethyldiazepam, which is approximately as potent as diazepam. The half-life of desmethyldiazepam is about 90 h. Although desmethyldiazepam concentrations are relatively low after a single intravenous dose of diazepam, its contribution to the pharmacological effect becomes significant after repeated doses or with continuous infusions, when desmethyldiazepam plasma concentrations can become equal to or even greater than those of diazepam. Desmethyldiazepam is also an important metabolite of chloridazepoxide, ketazolam, medazepam and prazepam (Fig. 6.6).

The principal metabolite of midazolam is α-hydroxy-midazolam, which is nearly as potent as midazolam itself. After oral administration the substantial first-pass metabolism of midazolam results in relatively high concentrations of this metabolite, but due to rapid elimination it makes little contribution to the overall clinical effect. Oxazepam, lorazepam, temazepam and triazolam have no active metabolites. For oxazepam, temazepam and lorazepam, conjugation with glucuronic acid is the primary metabolic pathway.

Drug interactions

The phase I metabolism of the benzodiazepines is mediated predominantly by cytochrome P450 enzymes in the liver. For midazolam and triazolam this is by the CYP3A4 isoenzyme, whereas the enzymes involved in the metabolism of diazepam are CYP3A and CYP2C19. Substances that either inhibit or induce these enzymes can have a marked effect on the pharmacokinetics of benzodiazepines, sometimes with unpredictable effects, especially following oral administration.[9] After oral administration there is also significant CYP3A4 mediated first-pass metabolism in the intestinal epithelium. Inhibitors of CYP3A4 include erythromycin, ketoconazole, itraconazole, verapamil, diltiazem, cimetidine and the selective serotonin reuptake inhibitors fluvoxamine and fluoxetine. Rifampicin, carbamazepine and phenytoin are inducers of CYP3A4. The peak plasma concentration may be increased fourfold and the half-life prolonged by up to sixfold when oral midazolam or triazolam are coadministered with potent CYP3A inhibitors such as the azole antimycotics or erythromycin. The dual route of metabolism for diazepam makes it susceptible to inhibition and induction through either or both pathways. Inhibition of diazepam metabolism by omeprazole or fluvoxamine, both of which inhibit CYP2C19, can reduce the plasma clearance by up to 50% and prolong the elimination half-life to 118 h.[10]

Recently there has been considerable interest in the interaction between grapefruit juice and benzodia-

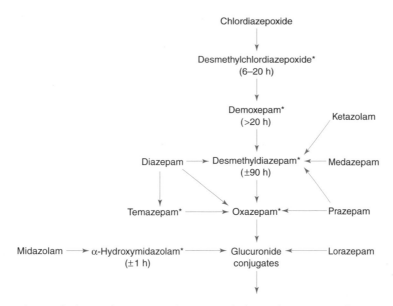

Fig. 6.6 Metabolic pathways for benzodiazepines. *Active metabolite. Values in parentheses are elimination half-lives.

zepines. Grapefruit juice inhibits CYP3A4 in the bowel wall and liver, and reduces the first-pass metabolism of benzodiazepines, resulting in decreased clearance and increased plasma concentrations. This effect is found only with grapefruit juice and not with other citrus fruits and is thought to be caused by flavinoids and other ingredients of the grapefruit.

Enzyme induction causes decreased plasma concentration and a reduction in pharmacological effect. Oral midazolam in combination with carbamazepine, phenytoin or rifampicin decreases the peak plasma midazolam concentration by more than 90%, with a large decrease in hypnotic and psychomotor effects.[11,12]

Intravenous administration bypasses both the CYP3A enzymes of the bowel wall and the first-pass hepatic metabolism, so that the effects of induction or inhibition of CYP3A will be of a lesser magnitude. Despite this the clearance of intravenous midazolam is significantly reduced after pretreatment with erythromycin, itraconazole or fluconazole.[9]

Distribution and elimination

Most benzodiazepines except for midazolam have relatively low clearances and volumes of distribution, so that the elimination half-lives are long (Table 6.2). Since many also have active metabolites, often with half-lives exceeding those of the parent drug, there is a poor correlation between plasma concentration and clinical effect. Diazepam and midazolam easily pass the blood–brain barrier, whereas lorazepam takes a considerable time to penetrate into the brain and peak effects may be delayed for up to 1 h after intravenous administration. This slow onset may be due to lower

lipophilicity and slow association with benzodiazepine receptors. Slow dissociation from the receptors may also explain the long duration of lorazepam. The half-life of lorazepam is shorter than that of diazepam.

Advanced age and liver disease impair the metabolism of diazepam and midazolam. Because lorazepam, oxazepam and temazepam undergo glucuronide conjugation, they are less influenced by these factors. Age tends to reduce the clearance of diazepam significantly, and to a lesser extent that of midazolam. The pharmacokinetics of all benzodiazepines are influenced by obesity. The volume of distribution is increased and, although plasma clearance is not altered, elimination half-lives are prolonged owing to delayed return of the drug into the plasma.

DIAZEPAM

Diazepam is used for premedication, as a sedative–hypnotic, anticonvulsant and for the treatment of alcohol withdrawal and panic attacks. Diazepam is widely considered the anticonvulsant of choice for the treatment of status epilepticus. It should be administered in incremental intravenous doses until fits are controlled and definitive therapy can be initiated. The use of diazepam in patients with tetanus has the advantage that, besides sedative effects, muscle relaxant properties are produced.

After intravenous administration diazepam rapidly passes the blood–brain barrier but, due to a small diffusible fraction in plasma and a high lipid solubility causing buffering in the brain itself, the pharmacological effect lags considerably behind the plasma concentration (hysteresis). This, together with the presence of an active metabolite, means that there is a poor correlation between plasma concentration and clinical effect. Redistribution is responsible for the disappearance of clinical effects within 10–15 min after bolus intravenous injection. Diazepam is insoluble in water and the drug was originally solubilized in propylene glycol, ethanol and sodium benzoate acid as Valium. This preparation causes pain on injection and venous damage. The preferred preparation for intravenous injection is diazepam solubilized in a soyabean emulsion (Diazemuls).

Delayed recovery and wide biological variations in response are the main disadvantages. Diazepam has a long elimination half-life of between 20 and 70 h. This, combined with an active metabolite with a very long half-life, may result in a prolonged recovery time and significantly decreased performance of psychomotor function for up to 24 h after its administration. In patients with renal failure the metabolite oxazepam may enter an enterohepatic cycle, and oxazepam glucuronide is regenerated back to oxazepam by intestinal bacteria. This will further delay recovery. Elderly patients may be more sensitive to diazepam, and the dose should be reduced by 50–75%.

MIDAZOLAM

Midazolam is the only water-soluble benzodiazepine. It is also available as a tablet and rectal suppository. Following a single intravenous bolus injection of midazolam in healthy patients, the time to peak sedation is 5–10 min and the duration of sedative effect ranges from 30 to 120 min. The onset of action is rapid owing to the high lipophilicity of midazolam, although slightly slower than that of diazepam. This may be due to the time necessary for the midazolam ring to close once the drug enters the blood. This closing process has a half-life of about 10 min. The short duration of action after bolus injection is due to rapid redistribution into peripheral tissues. The active metabolite of midazolam, a-hydroxymidazolam, is 60–80% as potent as midazolam, with an elimination half-life of about 1 h in patients with normal renal function.

When midazolam is administered for sedation as a continuous infusion for longer than 24 h to critically ill patients, the duration of clinical effect is often prolonged, owing to accumulation of midazolam and possibly also of a-hydroxymidazolam. The clinical effects of midazolam may be increased in patients with renal failure as a result of accumulation of a-hydroxymidazolam. Following a continuous infusion of midazolam for 7 days, the sedative effects of the drug may last for 2 days or longer after stopping the drug. The elimination half-life of midazolam is further increased in obese and elderly patients as a result of

larger volumes of distribution and decreased elimination clearance. Patients with significant liver disease have decreased midazolam clearance. However, considerable metabolic clearance has been described in patients with liver failure. This is probably due to extrahepatic biotransformation.

LORAZEPAM

Lorazepam, a long-acting benzodiazepine with no active metabolites, is five to ten times more potent than diazepam, and has a much slower onset of action than diazepam or midazolam. It is only moderately lipid soluble and is approximately 90% protein bound. The elimination half-life is 10–20 h. Compared with diazepam, the duration of action is three to four times longer. The time to peak sedation is 30 min after a single intravenous bolus injection of lorazepam to healthy individuals, and the duration of sedation is 10–20 h. The elimination half-life of lorazepam does not appear to be prolonged in elderly patients or in those with significant liver dysfunction when administered as a single bolus injection.

After long-term continuous infusion of lorazepam the residual sedative effects may persist for between two and several days after discontinuation of the infusion. Oral administration of 2–4 mg lorazepam results in sedation within 30 min, lasting for more than 4 h. Unlike diazepam, intramuscular absorption of lorazepam is reliable and produces similar effects to oral administration. After intravenous administration of 2–4 mg lorazepam, sedation emerges within 5 min and lasts for 4–6 h. The amnesic effects of lorazepam is dose dependent and increases from 50% to 70% of patients with doses of 2–4 mg. Two mg lorazepam has equipotent efficacy as 10 mg diazepam. Lorazepam causes fewer cardiovascular and respiratory side-effects than other benzodiazepines.

Midazolam is often used as a continuous infusion for long-term sedation of patients in the intensive care unit. However, prolonged recovery may result, notably in patients with renal and hepatic failure. Moreover tachyphylaxis occurs when midazolam is administered over several days. Lorazepam is a good alternative to midazolam for sedation in the intensive care unit. There is less development of tolerance, it has no active metabolites, and recovery time is not effected by hepatic or renal failure.

FLUNITRAZEPAM

Intravenous flunitrazepam produces pharmacological effects similar to those of diazepam but causes less complete amnesia, which lasts only about 20 min. It has been used as an alternative to diazepam for induction of anaesthesia in patients undergoing cardiac surgery. The onset of action is unpredictable and recovery may be prolonged owing to a long half-life and an active metabolite (desmethylflunitrazepam).

TEMAZEPAM

Temazepam (3-hydroxydiazepam) is one of the minor metabolites of diazepam used as a sedative and anxiolytic. It is a popular choice for premedication (adult dose 20–40 mg). It is insoluble in water and no intravenous preparation is available. Oral availability is high and it is rapidly absorbed, with peak concentrations being reached within 2–3 h. It is particularly suitable for the elderly and patients with hepatic dysfunction. Biotransformation is mainly by glucuronidation and there are no active metabolites.

FLUMAZENIL

Flumazenil is a pure competitive antagonist at the benzodiazepine receptor.[13] It has an elimination half-life of 1 h and a duration of action of approximately 30 min, shorter than that of midazolam (Table 6.2). Liver failure substantially increases the elimination half-life of flumazenil.

Flumazenil, in increments of 0.1–0.2 mg intravenously, is used to reverse benzodiazepine-induced sedation, for example with continuous infusion therapy in patients in intensive care. The dose needed seldom exceeds 1 mg. Because of its short duration, resedation may occur requiring repeated doses or administration by infusion (100–200 μg h^{-1}). Flumazenil is also used to treat comatose patients suspected of having overdosed with benzodiazepines. It should not be used in patients with closed head injuries since reversal of sedation may result in increased intracranial pressure.

Side-effects due to flumazenil are usually minor. Some patients may experience nausea and transient agitation. Arrhythmias and other adverse haemodynamic affects have been described. Convulsions may rarely occur, and are more common in patients receiving tricyclic antidepressants. Flumazenil should be used cautiously in patients on long-term benzodiazepine medication since an acute withdrawal syndrome may be provoked. If these patients become unmanageable, sedation should be continued with a nonbenzodiazepine such as haloperidol.

NONBENZODIAZEPINE SEDATIVES

ZOLPIDEM

Zolpidem is an imidazolopyridine compound that binds to a subgroup of the GABA$_A$ receptor. This specific binding results in selective sedative resembling that of the benzodiazepines. Zolpidem has only weak anticonvulsive activity and lacks anxiolytic and muscle relaxant effects. It is as effective as benzodiazepines in shortening sleep latency and prolonging total sleep time in patients with insomnia. Therapeutic doses range from 10–25 mg in the adult to 5–10 mg in geriatric patients. Oral zolpidem is rapidly absorbed, with an oral bioavailability of 70%. It is eliminated by conversion to inactive compounds in the liver, largely through oxidation. The plasma half-life is approximately 2.4 h. In patients with liver cirrhosis the plasma half-life may be prolonged more than twofold. In patients with renal failure elimination is prolonged owing to an increase in its volume of distribution.

ZOPICLONE

Zopiclone is the first representative of the cyclopyrrolones and binds to a subgroup of the GABA$_A$ receptor. Its pharmacological profile is comparable to that of the short-acting benzodiazepines. Oral absorption is fast and plasma peak levels are reached by 1.5–2 h. Biotransformation to inactive metabolites takes place in the liver. The elimination half-life is 5 h, increasing to 10 h in patients with liver cirrhosis.

The effects of zolpidem and zopiclone on sleeping patterns are not comparable with those of the benzodiazepines. They increase the time spent in deeper sleeping levels 3 and 4, and do not influence REM sleep and light sleeping levels. Side-effects and contraindications to its use are similar to those for the benzodiazepines.

BARBITURATES

The hypnotic and sedative effects of barbiturates were known long before they were used as intravenous anaesthetics. Barbiturates were widely used to treat insomnia before the introduction of the benzodiazepines. Their main disadvantages are a high degree of tolerance and dependence. The oxybarbiturates are used primarily for the production of sleep. Barbiturate-induced sleep resembles physiological sleep, but time spent in REM sleep is reduced. Drowsiness may last for only a few hours after a hypnotic dose of barbiturates, but subtle distortions of mood and impairment of judgement and fine motor skills may persist for many hours. When the drug is withdrawn, there is a rebound increase in nightly REM sleep, and this is associated with nightmares and reduced effectiveness of sleep. Barbiturates, especially phenobarbitone and mephobarbitone, are highly effective in the treatment of epilepsy, also when patients are refractory to other anticonvulsants.

After oral intake, absorption of barbiturates is complete. Biotransfomation is via the cytochrome P450 system, and this explains the interaction with many drugs metabolized by this system. Barbiturates induce cytochrome P450 enzymes, increasing the rate of biotransformation of a number of drugs.

BUTYROPHENONES

Haloperidol and droperidol are butyrophenones, classical antipsychotics which act by central dopaminergic blockade, although blocking of 5-hydroxytryptamine (5-HT), GABA and glutamate also are important. They were discovered accidentally when screening pethidine analogues for analgesic activity. Together with the phenothiazines, they belong to the neuroleptic group of drugs. Butyrophenones have little hypnotic effect and anxiolysis is due to environmental dissociation. They are indicated in the agitated restless patient. Some of the most distressing, although uncommon, adverse effects of these drugs are extrapyramidal side-effects, related to their binding to postsynaptic dopamine receptors. The effects of butyrophenones on respiration are minimal. The cardiovascular effects are due to a mild α-blocking effect, resulting in decreased vascular resistance and venous pooling of blood. In hypovolaemic patients these effects may result in profound hypotension.

DROPERIDOL

Droperidol is the only butyrophenone commonly used in anaesthesia. In combination with an opioid it was formerly used to produce neuroleptanalgesia. However, because of prolonged sedation, extrapyramidal side-effects and anxiety, this combination is now seldom used. Today the main indication is as an antiemetic.

Droperidol is a potent antiemetic in low doses (0.5–1.25 mg in adults), but is not effective in motion sickness. Although these doses produce little sedation, extrapyramidal side-effects, anxiety and restlessness may still occur.

After intravenous administration droperidol is rapidly distributed, and elimination is mainly by hepatic metabolism. The elimination half-life is 100–135 min. Droperidol readily crosses the blood–brain barrier, producing more sedative and antiemetic effects than haloperidol. Droperidol reduces the sensitivity to adrenaline and noradrenaline (α-blocking effect). It has mild quinidine-like antiarrhythmic activity and does not influence myocardial contractility.

HALOPERIDOL

Haloperidol is mainly used for the treatment of psychoses such as schizophrenia and to control severe agitation in patients with delirium tremens due to alcohol abuse. It is occasionally used in patients in intensive care who are unresponsive to conventional sedatives. Haloperidol has strong dopaminergic and weak anticholinergic activity. The drug may also inhibit catecholamine receptors and reuptake of various neurotransmitters in the midbrain. Because of first-pass metabolism, the oral bioavailability is 60%. Haloperidol is 92% bound to plasma proteins. The elimination half-life is 12–40 h. The α-blocking effects of haloperidol are weak compared with those of droperidol, and intravenous doses of up to 150 mg can be administered without untoward effects.

PHENOTHIAZINES

The name phenothiazine derives from the basic chemical structure common to these compounds (Fig. 6.7). The nature of the side-chain determines the potency and pharmacological specificity. Thus, the piperizine compounds are much more potent as dopamine D_2 antagonists and have relatively less α-adrenergic blocking activity. In addition to dopamine antagonism, the phenothiazines are also antagonists at α-adrenoceptors, histamine H_1, muscarinic and 5-HT_2 receptors. Not surprisingly, therefore, they have widely different therapeutic applications. They are used as anxiolytics, antipsychotics and antiemetics. Phenothiazines have an antipsychotic effect by antagonizing dopamine-mediated neurotransmission. At the level of the basal ganglia they produce extrapyramidal effects; these are more likely after high doses or in combination with monoamine oxidase inhibitors.

After intravenous injection arrhythmias and hypotension may occur, and phenothiazines should be used with caution in patients with cardiovascular disease. Arrhythmias resulting from phenothiazine

---

Summary box 6.2 Butrophenones

- Belong to neuroleptic class of drugs.

- Act primarily by central dopaminergic blockade, but also block 5-HT, GABA and glutamate.

- Have little hypnotic activity.

- Haloperidol is used in the treatment of schizophrenia and other psychoses.

- Droperidol was used formerly in combination with an opioid to produce neuroleptanaesthesia.

- Main indication for droperidol is now as a potent antiemetic.

- Side-effects:

  - hypotension due to α-adrenoceptor blockade

  - extrapyramidal effects – rigidity, tremor and akinesia.

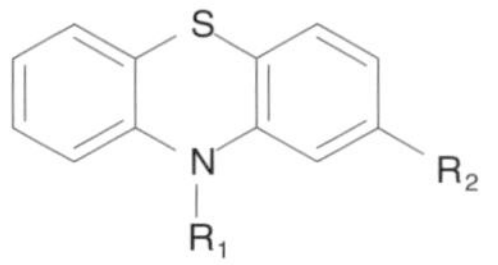

Fig. 6.7 General chemical structure of the phenothiazines.

administration should be treated with cardioversion; procainamide and quinidine are contraindicated. Promethazine should not be given to neonates and young children as the drug is associated with the 'sudden infant death syndrome'.

AZAPIRONES

These are a new class of anxiolytic drugs which are thought to act by reducing 5-HT neurotransmission by acting as partial agonists or antagonists at 5-HT_{1A} receptors. Azapirines do not interact with benzodiazepine receptors. Buspirone, the first drug of this class, combines anxiolytic activity with antidepressant effects. Other azapirones are ipsapirone and gepirone. They do not produce sedation, hypnosis or cognitive impairment. The anxiolytic effects of buspirone evolve gradually over 1–4 weeks, and it is therefore indicated only for long-term treatment. Absorption is fast and

Summary box 6.3 Azapirones

- Thought to act by reducing 5-HT neurotransmission by acting as partial agonists or antagonists at 5-HT_{1A} receptors.

- Do not interact with benzodiazepine receptors.

- Combine anxiolytic activity with antidepressant effects.

- Reduce anxiety without producing sedation, hypnosis or cognitive impairment.

- Anxiolytic effects take days or weeks to develop.

- Members of class include buspirone, ipsapirone and gepirone.

complete, but because of extensive first-pass effect the bioavailability is only 5%.

Biotransformation is by dealkylation and oxidation. The dealkylated metabolite is found in high concentrations in the brain and has α-adrenergic antagonistic activity. In combination with monoamine oxidase inhibitors, buspirone may produce hypertension.

REFERENCES

1. Ferrero P, Costa E, Conti-Tronconi B, Guidotti A. A diazepam binding inhibitor (DBI)-like neuropeptide is detected in human brain. *Brain Res* 1986; **399**: 136–142.
2. Rothstein JD, Garland W, Puia G, Guidotti A, Weber RJ, Costa E. Purification and characterization of neurally occurring benzodiazepine receptor ligands in rat and human brain. *J Neurochem* 1992; **6**: 2102–2115.
3. Olasmaa M, Guidotti A, Costa E et al. Endogenous benzodiazepines in hepatic encephalopathy. *Lancet* 1989; **i**: 491–492.
4. Shader RJ, Greenblatt DJ. Use of benzodiazepines in anxiety disorders. *N Engl J Med* 1993; **328**: 1398–1405.
5. Vgontzas AN, Kales A, Bixler EO. Benzodiazepine side effects: role of pharmacokinetics and pharmacodynamics. *Pharmacology* 1995; **51**: 205–233.
6. Ghonheim MM, Mewaldt SP. Benzodiazepines and human memory: a review. *Anesthesiology* 1990; **72**: 926–938.
7. Shader RI, Drefuss D, Gerrein JR et al. Sedative effects and impaired learning and recall after single oral doses of lorazepam. *Clin Pharmacol Ther* 1986; **39**: 526–530.

8. Smoller JD, Pollack MH, Otto MW et al. Panic anxiety, dyspnoea, and respiratory disease. Theoretical and clinical considerations. *Am J Respir Crit Care Med* 1996; **154**: 6–17.
9. Friedericy HJ, Bovill JG. The role of the cytochrome P450 system in drug interactions in anaesthesia. *Baillieres Clin Anaesthesiol* 1998; **12**: 213–228.
10. Perucca E, Gatti G, Cipolla G et al. Inhibition of diazepam metabolism by fluvoxamine: a pharmacokinetic study in normal volunteers. *Clin Pharmacol Ther* 1994; **56**: 471–476.
11. Backman JT, Olkkola KT, Neuvonen PJ. Rifampin drastically reduces plasma concentrations and effects of oral midazolam. *Clin Pharmacol Ther* 1996; **59**: 7–13.
12. Backman JT, Olkkola KT, Ojala M et al. Concentrations and effects of oral midazolam are greatly reduced in patients treated with carbamazepine or phenytoin. *Epilepsia* 1996; **37**: 253–257.
13. Withwam JG, Amrein R. Pharmacology of flumazenil. *Acta Anaesthesiol Scand* 1995; **39** (Suppl. 108): 3–14.

7

JG Bovill

OPIOIDS

Summary box 7.1 Pharmacological effects of opioids

- Analgesia, supraspinal and spinal.

- Respiratory depression.

- Sedation (in cats and horses causes excitation).

- Euphoria (in the presence of discomfort).

- Dysphoria (in the absence of discomfort).

- Nausea and vomiting.

- Miosis (mydriasis in cats).

- Inhibition of gastrointestinal peristalsis.

- Increased bile duct pressure.

- Urinary retention.

- Muscle rigidity.

- Antitussive.

- Tolerance and physical dependence.

Throughout history humans have used a wide variety of plants or plant extracts to alleviate the pain and suffering caused by disease and trauma. The most prominent of these has been opium, a resinous substance obtained by incising the unripe seed head of the opium poppy, *Papaver somniferum*. The word opium is derived from the Greek 'opos', meaning juice. In modern times opium has been replaced by morphine, the most abundant of the more than 50 alkaloids present in opium.

Morphine constitutes 10–20% of raw opium. It was isolated from opium in 1806 by the German pharmacist Sertürner, who named it after the Greek god of dreams, Morpheus. Other important alkaloids in opium are codeine (0.5%) and papaverine (1%). Morphine is still considered the prototype opioid agonist to which all opioids are compared. Today numerous drugs are available with pharmacological properties similar to those of morphine. Many semisynthetic derivatives, such as codeine (methylmorphine), hydromorphone, oxymorphone and hydrocodone, are made by simple modifications of the morphine molecule. For others (e.g. fentanyl) the relationship with morphine is less obvious. As a class these drugs are variously referred to as opiates or opioids. An opioid is defined as any substance having morphine-like actions that are competitively antagonized by naloxone.

Opioids interact with specific receptors, the opioid receptors, to produce a variety of pharmacological effects. In 1976 Martin and colleagues[1] found that morphine and allied drugs produced three distinct syndromes in chronic spinal dogs, which they attributed to separate receptors. They named these after the prototype agonist producing the distinct physiological effect: μ (mu) for morphine, κ (kappa) for keto-cyclazocine and σ (sigma) for SKF-10 047 (*N*-allylnormetazocine). However, the σ receptor, to which they attributed the dysphoric effects of nalorphine, is not an opioid receptor since actions mediated by it are not reversed by naloxone and it shows a preferential affinity for *dextro*- rather than *laevo*-isomers of some benzomorphans. The dysphoric symptoms produced by some of the partial opioid agonists such as nalorphine and pentazozine are, however, thought to be due to an interaction with the σ receptor.

Currently three distinct opioid receptor types, μ, δ and μ, are recognized and all have recently been cloned. The μ receptor has two subtypes, a high-affinity μ_1 receptor and a low-affinity μ_2 receptor. The supraspinal mechanisms of analgesia produced by μ-opioid agonist drugs is thought to involve the μ_1 receptor whereas spinal analgesia, respiratory depression and the effects of opioids on gastrointestinal function are associated with the μ_2 receptor. Recently a third subtype has been described which binds opioid alkaloids such as morphine, but has essentially no, or exceedingly low, affinity for the naturally occurring endogenous opioid peptides or nonalkaloid opioids such as fentanyl.[2] This alkaloid-selective peptide-insensitive receptor has been designated as a subtype of the μ receptor (μ_3) based on its affinity for morphine. The μ_3 receptor has a broad distribution in macrophages, astrocytes and endothelial cells. It may to be involved in immune processes. The endogenous ligand for this receptor may be morphine or codeine.[3] Morphine- and codeine-like substances have been isolated from the brain of several species, and biosynthetic pathways for morphine production have been demonstrated in mammals, similar to that used by the opium poppy.[4]

Two subtypes of the δ receptor and three subtypes of the κ receptor also have been described. Selective κ agonists may have therapeutic potential, lacking the adverse side-effects produced by the current μ-receptor agonists. Unfortunately, all of the κ agonists identified to date produce a spectrum of side-effects including locomotor impairment, sedation, central nervous system (CNS) disturbances and diuresis. One κ agonist, enadoline, has undergone clinical trials but with limited success.[5]

CELLULAR MECHANISMS

The opioid receptors are G protein-coupled receptors whose effects are primarily inhibitory. Opioids close N-type voltage-operated calcium channels and open calcium-dependent inwardly rectifying potassium channels. This results in hyperpolarization and a reduction in neuronal excitability.[6] κ receptors may act only on calcium channels.[7] Opioids also inhibit adenylyl cyclase, which converts adenosine triphosphate to cyclic adenosine 3',5'-monophosphate (cAMP), decreasing the concentration of cAMP. Changes in the level of cAMP may be responsible for modulation of neurotransmitter release (e.g. substance P). cAMP also activates and regulates protein kinase C (PKC), which alters the expression of intermediate early genes such as c-*fos*. C-*fos* is a marker of activity in neurons that are associated with nociception, and its expression is depressed by morphine.[8]

Opioids also have excitatory effects. Nanomolar con-

Summary box 7.2 Cellular mechanisms of opioid drugs

- Interact with μ, δ and κ opioid receptors.

- Mimic actions of the endogenous opioid peptides, β-endorphin, met- and leu-enkephalin, and dynorphin.

- Opioid receptors are G protein-coupled receptors. Primary effects of opioids are inhibitory but also produce excitatory effects.

Inhibitory mechanisms

- Close N-type calcium channels.

- Open inwardly rectifying potassium channels.

- Inhibit adenylyl cyclase, decreasing the concentration of cAMP.

- Inhibit release of nociceptive neurotransmitters (e.g. substance P and glutamate).

Excitatory mechanisms

- Nanomolar concentrations stimulate adenylyl cyclase.

- Cause transient increase in intracellular Ca^{2+} concentration.

- Open L-type calcium channels.

- Mobilize Ca^{2+} from intracellular stores.

- Increase intracellular level of protein kinase C.

---

centrations, acting via G_s proteins, stimulate adenylyl cyclase activity in certain neurons.[9] This may account for some responses to opioids, such as paradoxical hyperalgesia and pruritus. Another important stimulatory effect is a transient increase in cytoplasmic free Ca^{2+} concentration, $[Ca^{2+}]_i$, secondary to Ca^{2+} influx via L-type Ca^{2+} channel opening as well as mobilization of Ca^{2+} from inositol triphosphate-sensitive intracellular stores.[10] Changes in $[Ca^{2+}]_i$ may contribute to inhibition by opioids of the release of excitatory substances responsible for modulation of nociception, such as substance P and glutamate, from central and peripheral endings of primary afferents. Calcium channel blockers enhance morphine analgesia.[11]

ENDOGENOUS OPIOID PEPTIDES

The natural ligands for the opioid receptors are the endogenous opioid peptides, the endorphins, enkephalins and dynorphins. Each is derived from distinct precursors, proopiomelanocortin, proenkephalin and prodynorphin, which are the translation products of separate genes. The opioid peptides share a common N-terminal tetrapeptide fragment, Tyr-Gly-Gly-Phe-... extended with either methionine or leucine. This terminal appears to have a messenger or signal function, perhaps determining receptor selectivity. A Tyr-Gly-Gly-Phe-Met or -Leu core is necessary for μ and δ, but not μ binding, whereas the same core extended with Arg is necessary for κ binding (Fig. 7.1). β-Endorphin binds primarily to μ opioid receptors whereas met- and leu-enkephalin bind to both μ and δ receptors, although more so to δ than to μ receptors. The dynorphins are the natural ligand for the κ opioid receptors (Table 7.1). Although the endogenous opioids are analgesic, their clinical usefulness is severely limited by rapid biodegradation by peptidases. β-Endorphin is more resistant to enzymatic degradation than the smaller enkephalins but it does not penetrate the blood–brain barrier. When injected intrathecally β-endorphin produces potent, long-lasting analgesia. The endogenous opioids are neurotransmitters at postsynaptic receptors, modulating transsynaptic membrane potential. At presynaptic receptors they function as neuromodulators, modulating the release of other neurotransmitters, such as substance P and glutamate.

OPIOID PHARMACOLOGY

ANALGESIA

The CNS in mammals reacts to nociceptive stimuli at many levels that are involved in the transmission, modulation and sensation of pain. Endogenous opioids and opioid receptors are located at key points in the pain pathways (Fig. 7.2). Two anatomically distinct sites exist for opioid-mediated analgesia, supraspinal and spinal; systemically administered opioids produce analgesia at

Table 7.1 Binding characteristics of endogenous opioid peptides to opioid receptors			
	μ	δ	κ
β-Endorphin	55%	45%	–
Met-enkephalin	29%	70%	1%
Leu-enkephalin	40%	55%	5%
Dynorphin	10%	20%	70%

both sites. The μ receptor is most commonly associated with analgesia, but specific δ and κ agonists also mediate antinociception at spinal and supraspinal sites. In the dorsal horn the release of substance P, glutamate and other nociceptive neurotransmitters from the afferent terminals of sensory fibres is inhibited by activation of presynaptic μ, δ and κ receptors (Fig. 7.3). Opioids selectively modulate 'second pain' sensation carried by slowly conducting, unmyelinated C fibres but have little effect on 'first pain' carried by small, myelinated Aδ fibres. Opioids also interfere with the action of prostaglandins at peripheral sites; in particular, μ agonists inhibit prostaglandin E_2-induced hyperalgesia in a dose-dependent manner.[12]

Activation of supraspinal opioid receptors results in the transmission of descending impulses that block spinal nociceptive reflexes, inhibit spinal nociceptive neurons and produce analgesia. Supraspinally, the μ_1 receptor is primarily involved in antinociception. The periaqueductal grey contains a very high density of μ receptors and is the major site of the supraspinal component of opioid analgesia. It receives inhibitory projections from the hypothalamus and the nucleus raphe magnus in the reticular formation, and mediates descending inhibition of nociceptive transmission. Descending inhibitory pathways use noradrenaline and 5-hydroxytryptamine (5-HT) as neurotransmitters in the spinal cord rather than opioid peptides.

Recently, all three types of opioid receptor have been demonstrated on peripheral terminals of sensory nerves.[13] Activation of these receptors seems to require an inflammatory reaction since locally applied opioids do not produce analgesia in healthy tissue. This may be due to the disruption of the normally impermeable perineurium by inflammation, together with, in the later stages, an upregulation of the receptors by peripherally directed transport of opioid receptors from the dorsal horn. The inflammatory process also may render previously inactive receptors active. Intraarticular morphine (1–5 mg) provides good analgesia

Peptides	Sequence
β-Endorphin	Tyr-Gly-Gly-Phe-Met-Thr-Ser-Glu-Lys-Ser-Gln-Thr-Pro-Leu-Val-Thr-Leu-Phe-Lys-Asn-Ala-Ile-Ile-Lys-Asn-Ala-Tyr
Leu-Enkephalin	Tyr-Gly-Gly-Phe-Leu
Met-Enkaphalin	Tyr-Gly-Gly-Phe-Met
Dynorphin	Tyr-Gly-Gly-Phe-Leu-**Arg**-Arg-Ile-Arg-Pro-Lys-Trp-Asp-Asn-Gln

Fig. 7.1 Amino acid alignments of the endogenous opioid peptides illustrating their common tetrapeptide terminal fragment (underlined). The Arg in position 6 of dynorphin is shown in bold type to highlight its possible importance in κ-receptor binding.

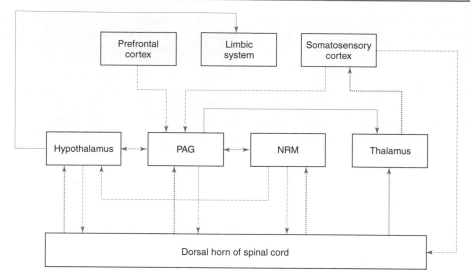

Fig. 7.2 Connections between the various parts of the central nervous system involved in nociceptive processing and pain recognition. PAG, periaqueductal grey; NRM, nucleus raphe magnus of the reticular activating system.

lasting 12 h or longer (sometimes up to 48 h) after arthroscopic surgery, without systemic side-effects.

RESPIRATORY DEPRESSION

All pure μ-agonist opioids produce dose-related depression of ventilation, which seems to be mediated by μ_2 receptors. Pure κ agonists have little effect on respiration. The primary respiratory effect of opioids is a reduction in the sensitivity of the respiratory centre to carbon dioxide. Morphine also depresses both medullary and peripheral chemoreceptors. In the medulla the effect involves inhibition of acetylcholine release, and a shift in the apnoeic threshold (Fig. 7.4).[14] This explains the ability of physostigmine to reverse opioid-induced respiratory depression. Initially respiratory rate is affected more than tidal volume, which may even increase. With increasing doses respiratory rhythmicity is disturbed, resulting in the irregular, gasping breathing characteristic of opioid overdose. In addition to retention of carbon dioxide, respiratory depression also may result in hypoxia. The hypoxic drive to ventilation is also depressed by opioids.

Other CNS depressants such as barbiturates, benzodiazepines and inhalational anaesthetics potenti-

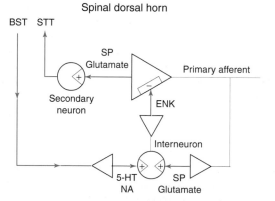

Fig. 7.3 Interconnections in the dorsal horn of the spinal cord between primary nociceptive afferent fibres, enkephalinergic interneurons, descending inhibitory fibres carried in the bulbospinal tracts (BST) and the secondary neurons that transmit nociceptive information to the brain via the spinothalamic tract (STT) and other ascending tracts. SP, substance P; 5-HT: 5, hydroxytryptamine (serotonin); NA, noradrenaline.

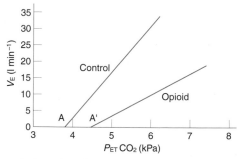

Fig. 7.4 Carbon dioxide response curves illustrating the effect of opioids. Administration of an opioid causes a parallel shift in the response curve to the right with an increase in the apnoeic threshold, i.e. the arterial partial pressure of carbon dioxide at which ventilation will cease, from A to A', and a decrease in the slope of the response curve. These two effects are mediated at different levels: the shift in the apnoeic threshold is a medullary effect whereas the change in slope is due to an action on the respiratory centre.

ate the respiratory effects of opioids. Stimulation, and especially pain, counteracts the depressant effects of opioids. A patient who has received intraoperative opioids may breathe satisfactorily at the end of anaesthesia, when subjected to external stimuli, but relapse into respiratory depression when these stimuli are absent. Elderly patients are more sensitive to the respiratory depressant effects of opioids than younger patients and the dosage needs to be adjusted accordingly.

MUSCLE RIGIDITY

Muscle rigidity is commonly associated with the administration of opioids; it seems to be associated primarily with central activation of the μ receptor (possibly the μ_1 isoreceptor), whereas supraspinal δ_1 and κ_1 receptors may attenuate this effect.[15] Rigidity involving the thoracic and abdominal muscles can sometimes interfere with ventilation to such an extent that manual ventilation is impossible without the use of a muscle relaxant. This is common when an opioid is given during induction of anaesthesia, but may also be manifest at other times including the postoperative period. Muscle rigidity is reversed by naloxone and neuromuscular blocking drugs, and is attenuated by barbiturates and benzodiazepines. The mechanism of opioid-induced muscle rigidity remains unresolved. It may be related to interactions between opioids and the dopaminergic system, involving inhibition of dopamine release in the striatum. Catatonic movements of the limbs are frequently observed in patients given high doses of opioids.

TOLERANCE AND PHYSICAL DEPENDENCE

Following prolonged or repeated exposure to opioids, a diminished responsiveness to their actions develops which can be seen at the cellular level. While tolerance is often associated with chronic exposure for days or weeks, it can develop after minutes to hours. Physical dependence is a state, sometimes associated with drug tolerance, that comes about as a consequence of sustained exposure to a drug whereby adaptive changes occur leading to the required presence of the drug for normal function. Withdrawal of the drug or antagonism of its action elicits various pathophysiological disturbances collectively known as a 'withdrawal syndrome'.

Opioid withdrawal initially results in restlessness and an intense craving for the drug, accompanied by yawning, running nose, lacrimation, perspiration, and aches and pains. The pupils become dilated and there are associated signs of hyperactivity of the sympathetic nervous system such as hypertension and pilomotor stimulation.

The exact mechanism underlying the development of tolerance remains uncertain and it is likely that several are involved. Studies following chronic opioid exposure in animals have failed to find consistent changes in binding affinity or receptor number, or the changes that are observed do not correlate with the development of tolerance. There is evidence that chronic exposure may involve an uncoupling of the receptor from a G protein with a resultant increase in adenylyl cyclase activity. Acute tolerance or desensitization may also involve the uncoupling of the receptor from the G protein–adenylyl cyclase cascade, and may represent an initial step in the development of chronic tolerance and dependence. Acute tolerance may also involve a change in the receptor itself such as receptor sequestration within the cell (i.e. receptor down-regulation). However, if uncoupling of the receptor from the G protein–adenylyl cyclase cascade is the main mechanism of tolerance, this can be only partial since administration of naloxone to tolerant animals and humans causes an acute rebound exaggerated response, indicating that a connection between receptor occupation and subcellular responses remains intact.

It is likely that as tolerance develops there is a cellular response to the continued presence of the opioid that compensates for its inhibitory effects. Chronic receptor stimulation may cause compensatory, slowly developing, increases in adenylyl cyclase activity and increases in cellular cAMP concentration. This in turn induces cAMP phosphodiesterase and an increase in the rate of degradation of cAMP, resulting in a negative feedback mechanism maintaining homeostasis of cAMP concentrations. The overshoot produced by naloxone in tolerant animals would then be a result of this compensatory response suddenly occurring in the absence of opioid inhibitory effects.

The biochemical events underlying the stimulatory, as opposed to the inhibitory, effects of opioids, such as increases in PKC, also are involved in the development of tolerance.[16] Activation of PKC can desensitize the K^+ channels normally opened by opioids. The increase in PKC activity may be associated with upregulation of L-type calcium channels. Block of these channels with diltiazem prevents both the increase in PKC activity and the development of tolerance in rats.

GASTROINTESTINAL TRACT

The gastrointestinal tract is the only system outside the CNS with significant concentrations of opioid receptors. This reflects their common embryonic origins. Opioids increase intestinal tone and decrease propulsive peristalsis, resulting in delayed gastric emptying and constipation or ileus. These effects appear to be mediated via μ_2 rather than μ_1 receptors. Opioids increase common bile duct pressure and decrease bile production and flow, primarily as a result of spasm of the sphincter of Oddi. The tone of the bile duct itself is also increased.

CARDIOVASCULAR SYSTEM

Most of the haemodynamic effects of opioids are related to decreased central sympathetic outflow, specific vagal effects or, in the case of morphine and pethidine, histamine release. Histamine release is reduced by slow administration. Pretreatment with a combination of H_1 and H_2 antagonists can block the effects of histamine release. Morphine may also have a direct action on vascular smooth muscle, independent of histamine release. Fentanyl and its analogues do not cause histamine release. All opioids, with the exception of pethidine, produce bradycardia by actions on the afferent fibres of the vagus and the nucleus tractus solitarius and nucleus commissuralis, which have very high densities of opioid receptors. Pethidine often produces tachycardia, possibly due to the structural similarities with atropine. Isolated heart or heart muscle studies have demonstrated dose-related negative inotropic effects for opioids. However, these occurred at concentrations 100 to several thousand times those found clinically, even with the high doses used in cardiac anaesthesia. Indeed, the lack of myocardial depression is one of the reasons that high doses of opioids are popular in cardiac anaesthesia.

There is considerable experimental and clinical evidence that endogenous opioids contribute to the pathophysiology of haemorrhagic and endotoxic shock. While naloxone has no significant cardiovascular effects in normal animals or humans, in haemorrhagic shock it produces a pressor response and a rise in cardiac output. Endogenous opioid peptides released during shock may impair the reflex vasoconstrictor response to haemorrhage, and this is reversed by naloxone.

EMETIC EFFECTS

Nausea and vomiting are common and undesirable side-effects of opioids. Opioids initiate the vomiting reflex by stimulating a specialized area of the brain located in the area postrema called the chemoreceptor trigger zone (CTZ). This in turn leads to activation of the 'vomiting centre' located in the reticular formation of the medulla, close to the area postrema. Nausea and vomiting are more common in ambulatory patients, due to vestibular stimulation of the CTZ, which is sensitized by opioids. Opioids depress the vomiting centre and, with increasing plasma concentrations, this effect overcomes the CTZ stimulant effect.

INDIVIDUAL DRUGS

MORPHINE

Morphine, the protptype μ agonist, is available as the sulphate or hydrochloride salt. It is poorly lipid soluble, owing to the presence of two hydroxyl groups that confer polar characteristics to the molecule (Fig. 7.5). The phenolic hydroxyl group on C3 is a very important functional group. It serves to amplify the van der Waal forces binding the aromatic ring to the opioid receptor through hydrogen bonding. Masking the hydroxyl group by acetylation or methylation, as in heroin or codeine, changes the pharmacological effect. Its low lipophilicity means that morphine cannot easily cross the blood–brain barrier. However, because of its low potency, with bolus intravenous administration influx to the brain may be almost as rapid as with more lipid-soluble drugs since it is forced down a steep concentration gradient. As the concentration gradient

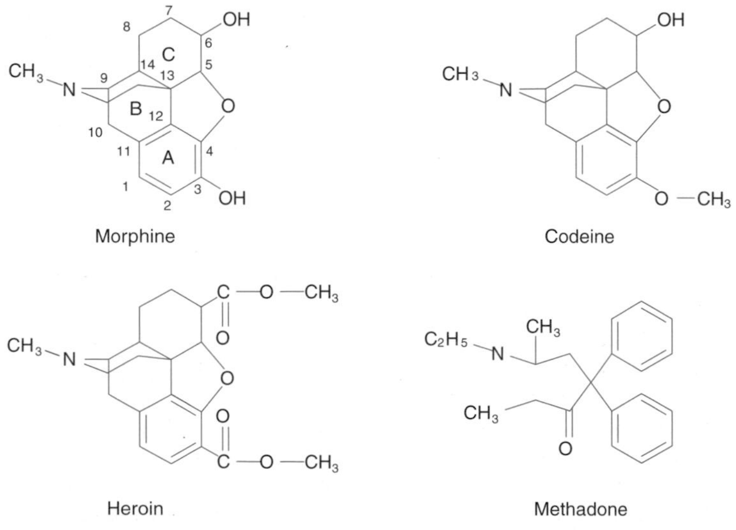

Fig. 7.5 Chemical structure of morphine and allied opioids.

dissipates, efflux from the brain becomes dependent on factors such as lipid solubility, and so will be slower than for more lipophilic opioids. Morphine is well absorbed from the gastrointestinal tract, although significant presystemic metabolism occurs. The usual adult intramuscular dose of 10–15 mg will produce analgesia, reaching a peak in about 30 min and lasting for 4–5 h. With larger doses the incidence of side-effects increases out of proportion to the increase in analgesia. For severe pain it is preferable to titrate small doses, for example 1–2 mg intravenously, until adequate analgesia is achieved. The oral dose is about 50% higher than the intramuscular dose.

CNS depression is the usual effect of morphine, and sedation and drowsiness are frequently observed with therapeutic doses. When given in the absence of pain, morphine may sometimes produce dysphora – an unpleasant sensation of fear and anxiety. The most important stimulatory effects of morphine in humans are emesis and miosis. Miosis, due to stimulation of the Edinger–Westphal nucleus of the third nerve, occurs with all morphine-like drugs. The combination of pinpoint pupils, coma and respiratory depression are classical signs of morphine overdosage. Stimulation of the solitary nuclei may also be responsible for depression of the cough reflex (antitussive effect).

Pharmacokinetics and metabolism

Morphine is an amphoteric molecule, with both basic and acidic properties. At physiological pH, however, it acts as a basic drug with pK_a 7.87. The pharmacokinetic parameters for morphine and other agonist opioids are given in Table 7.2. Morphine undergoes extensive hepatic biotransformation, principally by phase II conjugation to morphine-3-glucuronide (M3G), the major metabolite, 5–10% to morphine-6-glucuronide (M6G), and the remainder undergoes sulphate conjugation. Although the liver is the primary organ of conjugation, extrahepatic metabolism of morphine occurs in the kidney and possibly in the gut.

M3G has no analgesic activity but may antagonize the analgesic effects of morphine. M6G is pharmacologically active with a potency higher than morphine. The plasma concentration of M6G exceeds that of the parent drug by a factor of 9 within 30 min of intravenous administration (Fig. 7.6). Despite its polarity it crosses the blood–brain barrier and undoubtedly contributes to the analgesic effect.[17] Even allowing for its slower penetration into the brain, it may be that 50% or more of the respiratory depression observed by 1 h following systemic administration of morphine is due to this metabolite.[18] Patients with renal insufficiency have impaired elimination of morphine glucuronides, and M6G makes a significant contribution to morphine intoxication in these patients.

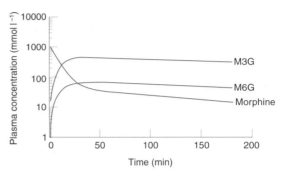

Fig. 7.6 Changes in the plasma concentrations of morphine, morphine-3-glucuronide (M3G) and morphine-6-glucuronide (M6G) following an intravenous bolus of morphine.

In neonates, and especially in premature infants, the mechanism for glucuronide conjugation is poorly developed. Renal function is also very inefficient. The pharmacokinetics of morphine in neonates is thus markedly different from that in older children and adults. This, together with age-related differences in the development of opioid receptors, may explain their increased sensitivity to morphine.

CODEINE PHOSPHATE

Codeine, one of the principal alkaloids of opium, has an analgesic efficacy much lower than that of other opioids, because of an extremely low affinity for opioid receptors. It is approximately one-sixth as potent as morphine. It has a low abuse potential. In contrast to other opioids, with the exception of oxycodone, codeine is relatively more effective when administered orally than parenterally. This is due to methylation at the C_3 site on the phenyl ring, which may protect it from conjugating enzymes.

Codeine is used in the management of mild to moderate pain, often in combination with nonopioid analgesics such as aspirin or paracetamol. It is valuable as an antitussive agent and for the treatment of diarrhoea. Side-effects are uncommon and respiratory depression, even with large doses, is seldom a problem.

DIAMORPHINE

Diamorphine (3,6-diacetylmorphine; heroin) is a semisynthetic derivative of morphine. It is a prodrug with no opioid activity itself. All its pharmacological activity derives from hydrolysis to monoacetylmorphine (MAM) and then to morphine in the plasma and tissues. Diamorphine also undergoes metabolism in the tissues, including the CNS, by esterases. Diamorphine and MAM are more lipid soluble than morphine and may act as carriers to facilitate the entry of morphine into the CNS. It is a potent analgesic with a high potential for addiction and its manufacture and use, even for medical

	pK_a	Un-ionized (%)	Lipid solubility*	Protein binding (%)	Oral availability (%)	Cl (l min⁻¹)	$V_{d_{ss}}$ (litres)	$t_{1/2}$ (h)
Morphine	7.9	24	1.4	35	25–50	1.2	200	1.7
Methadone	8.3	5.9	57	85	90	0.18	410	35
Pethidine	8.6	7.4	39	70	50–55	1.02	260	4–8
Diamorphine	7.63	37	280	40	–	–	–	–
Fentanyl	8.4	9.1	816	84	Negligible	1.53	335	3.6
Alfentanil	6.5	88.8	128	92	–	0.24	27	1.6
Sufentanil	8.0	19.7	1757	93	Negligible	0.9	123	2.8
Remifentanil	7.07	68	NA	92	–	3–4	25–62	10–20 min

Table 7.2 Pharmacokinetic parameters for the opioid agonists

* Lipid solubility is expressed as the octanol: water partition coefficient. NA, data not available.

purposes, is illegal in the USA and some other countries. Although it is claimed that diamorphine produces more sedation and less nausea and vomiting than morphine, it is likely that the incidence of side-effects with equianalgesic doses is similar to that of other opioids. A 5-mg dose of diamorphine is equipotent with 10 mg morphine, but the duration of action is shorter, about 2 h. Because diamorphine undergoes rapid deacetylation in solution, injections should always be freshly prepared. Interest in the use of diamorphine by the epidural or intrathecal routes has recently become more evident owing to its greater lipid solubility in comparison with morphine.

METHADONE
Methadone is a synthetic opioid commercially available as a racemic mixture. The R(–) isomer is 50 times more potent than the S(+) isomer. Methadone produces less sedation and euphoria but in other respects the side-effects are the same as those of morphine. Its high bioavailability after oral administration (80–90%) and its long half-life make it useful in the management of cancer pain. It is widely used in the treatment of withdrawal symptoms in opioid addicts. Methadone is equipotent with morphine when given orally or intramuscularly, but may be somewhat less potent when given intravenously. Athough the duration of a single dose is comparable to that following morphine administration, with repeated doses accumulation occurs so

that there needs to be either lower doses or longer intervals between doses to avoid overdosage.

THE PHENYLPIPERIDINES
Clinically important phenylpiperidines include pethidine (meperidine), phenoperidine, fentanyl, alfentanil, sufentanil and the recently introduced remifentanil. Pethidine was the first totally synthetic opioid. It is less potent than morphine, 75 mg pethidine being approximately equivalent to 10 mg morphine. The low potency may be related to the absence of a hydroxyl group on the phenyl ring. Although fentanyl and its congeners also lack this hydroxyl group, this is compensated for by groups on the piperidine nitrogen that confer markedly increased potency. Phenoperidine is an N-phenylpropyl derivative of norpethidine, a metabolite of pethidine. It is almost totally restricted to use as a supplement to inhalational anaesthesia and in patients requiring prolonged mechanical ventilation. As a supplement during anaesthesia, the usual dose is 0.5–1 mg intravenously in spontaneously breathing patients, and up to 5 mg in those in whom Intermittent Positive Pressure Ventilation (IPPV) is used. Remifentanil is a μ agonist with an analgesic potency similar to that of fentanyl, a rapid onset and a very short duration of action. In veterinary practice carfentanil is used to sedate large animals, but this is not used in humans.

The phenylpiperidines share a common chemical structure, a phenyl ring connected either directly (pethidine and phenoperidine) or by a nitrogen atom to a six-membered piperidine ring (Fig. 7.7). The structure is also found in morphine and related opioids, and piperidine derivatives represent the ultimate simplification of the morphine skeleton. The structure of pethidine is found in the morphine molecule, with only the piperidine and aromatic rings retained (compare Figs 7.5 and 7.7). Even in methadone, which has a two-dimensional structure that does not resemble that of other opioids, the remnants of the piperidine ring are discernible, and in three dimensions the molecule has an opioid-like pseudopiperidine configuration (see Fig. 7.5).

Delayed respiratory depression in the postoperative period has been reported following small intravenous doses of fentanyl given during anaesthesia. This has been attributed to enterohepatic recirculation, with sequestration of fentanyl in the stomach and subsequent reabsorption from small intestine. However, the pharmacokinetics of fentanyl make this very unlikely. A more probable explanation is release of fentanyl from body stores, especially muscle, as a result of increased patient activity in the postoperative period. Because of its large mass, muscle can store up to 55% of the fentanyl present in the body. Delayed respiratory depression has also been reported following continuous infusions of alfentanil. The decline in plasma concentration when an infusion is stopped is less rapid than from a comparable concentration following a single bolus injection, and administration of alfentanil by infusion can convert a short-acting drug into a relatively long-acting one.

The combination of pethidine with monoamine oxidase inhibitors (MAOIs) can cause a serious adverse reaction, which can present in two distinct forms. The excitatory form is characterized by sudden agitation, delirium, headache, hypotension or hypertension, rigidity, hyperpyrexia, convulsions and coma. It is thought to be caused by an increase in cerebral 5-HT concentrations as a result of inhibition of monoamine oxidase. This is potentiated by pethidine, which blocks neuronal uptake of 5-HT. The depressive form, which is frequently severe and fatal, consists of respiratory and cardiovascular depression and coma. It is the result of the inhibition of hepatic microsomal enzymes by MAOIs, leading to accumulation of pethidine. Phenoperidine should also be avoided in patients taking MAOIs, but other opioids appear to be safe.

Pharmacokinetics and metabolism

The phenylpiperidines are basic compounds, with pK_a values varying from 6.5 (alfentanil) to 8.4 (fentanyl). Owing to its low pK_a, 85% of alfentanil in blood is nonionized, resulting in rapid passage across the blood–

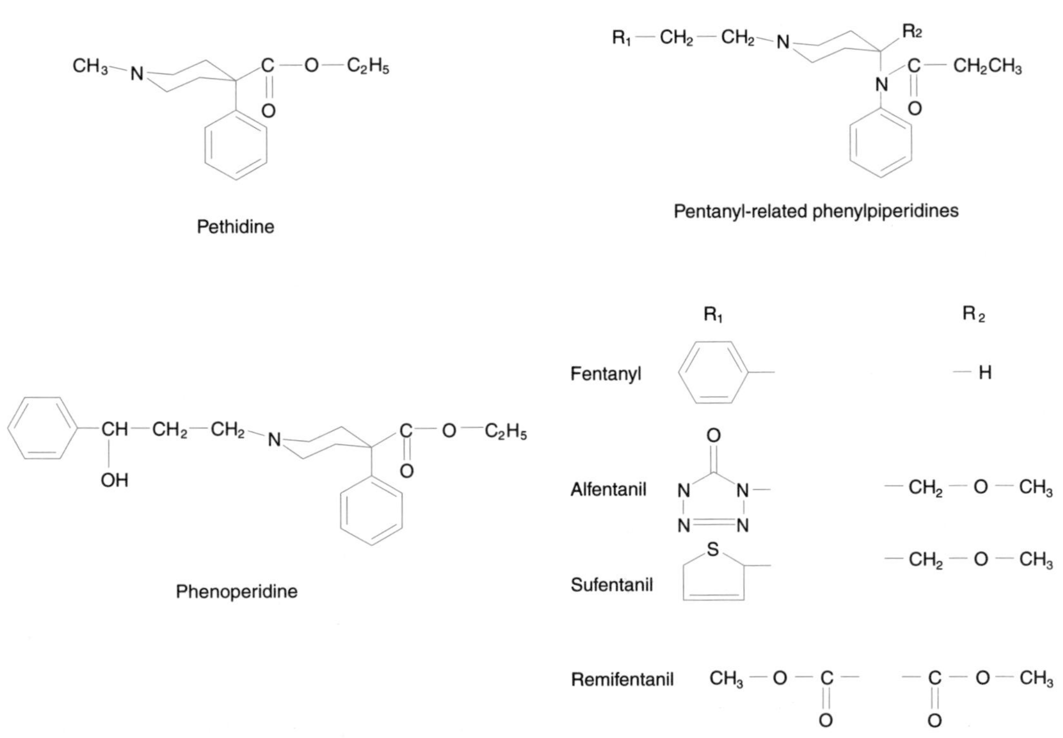

Fig. 7.7 Chemical structure of the phenylpiperidines.

brain barrier and a fast onset of action. Its blood–brain equilibration half-time $(t_{1/2}k_{eo})$ is about 1 min compared with 5–6 min for fentanyl and sufentanil. As with many basic drugs, the phenylpiperidines are highly protein bound, particularly to a_1-acid glycoprotein (AAG). The concentration of AAG is increased following trauma and surgery, and in patients with chronic inflammatory diseases or malignancy, and is decreased in neonates, during pregnancy and in women taking oral contraceptives. Although these changes affect the unbound opioid fraction, their consequences in clinical practice will be minimized by distribution processes so that the unbound concentration may only be marginally altered.

The phenyl ring confers high lipophilicity to the phenylpiperidine opioids. Lipophilicity, together with the un-ionized fraction, is an important determinant of the ability of a drug to cross the blood–brain barrier. Although the lipid solubility of alfentanil is lower than that of the other drugs (Table 7.2), the high un-ionized fraction allows rapid access to the CNS.[19] Indeed, the moderate lipophilicity of alfentanil may contribute to its rapid onset of action, since fewer molecules will be bound to nonspecific lipid sites within the brain and thus more will be available to interact with the receptors. The apparent volume of distribution of alfentanil in the brain is about 20 times less than that of fentanyl.[20] The properties that enable the phenylpiperidines to cross the blood–brain barrier also ensure rapid penetration across the placental barrier.

The biotransformation of the phenylpiperidines is primarily by hepatic phase I metabolism, catalysed by cytochrome P450 isoenzymes. Drugs that inhibit P450 activity, such as cimetidine and erythromycin, decrease the metabolism of these opioids. The elimination of alfentanil is significantly slowed in patients treated with erythromycin, with delayed recovery and prolonged postoperative respiratory depression.[21] Neither fentanyl nor alfentanil has metabolites that are pharmacologically active. Desmethyl sufentanil, a minor metabolite of sufentanil, is pharmacologically active but its contribution to the overall pharmacological effect is likely to be negligible. The hepatic intrinsic clearance of sufentanil is greater than liver blood flow so that the 'first-pass' effect will be almost total. The clearance of sufentanil in children is similar to that of young adults. However, clearance of sufentanil in neonates is only about 40% of the value in infants and older children, partly due to the low activity of cytochrome P450, which is only 25–50% of that in adults.

Pethidine undergoes extensive hepatic metabolism by N-demethylation to norpethidine and hydrolysis to pethidinic acid. Phenoperidine is metabolized to pethidine, norpethidine and pethidinic acid. Norpethidine has a long plasma half-life in normal patients (14–21 h) and even longer in those with diminished renal function. Pethidine and norpethidine can readily cross the placental barrier and accumulate in the fetus. Both compounds are weak bases and ion trapping occurs in the fetal plasma. The elimination of pethidine in neonates is slower than in adults, with the half-life prolonged for up to 6 days. Only about 7% of unchanged pethidine is excreted in the urine. This amount is, however, markedly influenced by urinary pH. Acidification of the urine reduces the excretion of unchanged pethidine to less than 1%, whereas with urinary alkalinization this is increased to 20–25%. With increasing doses of pethidine signs of CNS excitation (tremors, muscle twitching and eventually convulsions) predominate over CNS depression. Norpethidine, a major metabolite of pethidine, may be the principal mediator of these CNS excitatory effects. CNS toxicity is most likely to occur in patients with renal failure and where the oral route is used, owing to the significant presystemic metabolism, which results in rapid accumulation of norpethidine. It may take several days for normal neurological functions to return.

Remifentanil incorporates a methyl ester group attached to the nitrogen of the piperidine ring, making it susceptible to hydrolysis by nonspecific esterases in the blood and tissues, with very rapid degradation to inactive metabolites. The β-adrenoceptor antagonist esmolol is metabolized by a similar enzymatic mechanism. With infusions of $2\,\mu g\,kg^{-1}\,min^{-1}$ for 3 h, patients resumed spontaneous ventilation 4–10 min after stopping the remifentanil infusion.[22] Clearance is not affected by the presence of a cholinesterase inhibitor such as neostigmine. Remifentanil is not a good substrate for butyrylcholinesterase (pseudocholinesterase), so its pharmacokinetics will be not different in patients with cholinesterase deficiency.

For fentanyl and sufentanil, hepatic extraction is high and hepatic clearance is dependent on liver blood flow; factors decreasing this will slow elimination and prolong effect. Conversely, because the liver has such a large reserve capacity of metabolizing enzymes, their elimination is not significantly altered in patients with hepatic disease until liver function becomes severely compromised. In contrast, alfentanil has an intermediate hepatic extraction (0.3–0.5) and alfentanil clearance will be sensitive to changes in both liver blood flow and reduced enzyme capacity in patients with liver disease. Although the kidneys play a minor role in the elimination of most opioids, renal disease can influence their pharmacokinetic profile, secondary to alterations in plasma proteins and intravascular and extravascular volumes. Available evidence suggests that neither the pharmacokinetics nor the pharmacodynamics of remifentanil are altered significantly in patients with liver or renal disease.

EPIDURAL AND INTRATHECAL OPIOIDS

The discovery of opioid receptors in the spinal cord was quickly followed by the administration of morphine, and later other opioids, by the spinal route. Epidural and intrathecal administration of opioids is now widely used for postoperative and obstetric analgesia. In contrast to local anaesthetics, spinal opioids cause minimal sympathetic efferent and motor blockade. Pethidine, which has local anaesthetic activity, can produce sensory and motor blockade. Intrathecal pethidine 1 mg kg^{-1} is effective as a sole agent for spinal anaesthesia, and post-operative analgesia lasts for several hours. The intrathecal route has the advantage that the drug is deposited closer to its site of action, so that the onset is faster and smaller doses are needed compared with the epidural route. Details of epidural and intrathecal opioids are given in Tables 7.3 and 7.4. Because remifentanil is formulated with glycine as a vehicle, it should not be used epidurally or intrathecally. Glycine is an inhibitory neurotransmitter and can cause reversible motor dysfunction if given spinally.[23]

After epidural injection, an opioid may transfer into the cerebrospinal fluid (CSF), into the blood or bind to epidural fat which will act as a reservoir, the extent depending on the drug's lipophilicity. Lipid solubility is important in determining both transfer across the meninges and systemic absorption. Systemic absorption is not affected significantly by the volume in which a drug is administered, but it is significantly reduced by the addition of adrenaline. After epidural administration morphine passes slowly into the CSF with an absorption half-life of 22 min. Systemic uptake can result in blood morphine concentrations similar to those seen with intramuscular injections of the same dose. Sufentanil, which is highly lipid soluble, can be detected in the plasma within 2–5 min after epidural injection, and part of the analgesic effect of the more lipid-soluble opioids may be due to a supraspinal action amplifying the direct spinal action. Epidural fentanyl and sufentanil produce a more consistent and intense

---

Summary box 7.3 Factors contributing to respiratory depression after spinal opioids

- Advanced aged.

- High-risk patients.

- Large doses of opioids.

- Poorly lipid-soluble opioids.

- Intrathecal higher risk than epidural route.

- Concomitant administration of parenteral opioids or CNS depressants.

- Thoracic epidural opioids.

Table 7.3 Commonly used epidural opioids

		Analgesic effect			
	Bolus dose	Onset (min)	Peak effect (min)	Duration (h)	Continuous infusion
Morphine	2–5 mg	10–40	30–60	12–24	–
Pethidine	30–75 mg	5–10	12–30	2–4	10–15 mg h^{-1}
Methadone	5 mg	8–20	15–25	5–15	–
Diamorphine	5–7 mg	5–10	20–30	6–15	0.3–1 mg h^{-1}
Fentanyl	25–50 μg	5–10	10–20	2–4	0.5–1 μg kg^{-1} h^{-1}
Sufentanil	10–30 μg	5–10	10–20	4–6	0.15–0.3 μg kg^{-1} h^{-1}
Alfentanil	1–2 mg	5–10	10–15	1–2	–
Buprenorphine	0.15–0.3 mg	5–20	15–30	4–15	–

Table 7.4 **Commonly used intrathecal (subarachnoid) opioids**				
	Dose (mg)	**Onset (min)**	**Duration (h)**	**Comments**
Morphine	0.1–0.5	15–30	10–30	Dosage > 0.5 mg increases incidence of side-effects, especially respiratory depression
Pethidine	10–30	5–10	10–15	High doses (1 mg kg^{-1}) used for surgical anaesthesia, lasting 40–120 min
Diamorphine	1–2	5–10	10–20	Higher doses do not prolong analgesia but increase incidence of side-effects

analgesia than morphine, with a faster onset. However, the duration is short, although this can be overcome by giving these drugs as continuous epidural infusions.

Side-effects and complications tend to be higher with the intrathecal than the epidural route. A common side-effect is pruritus, the incidence of which is higher with morphine than with other opioids, and is higher with intrathecal than with epidural administration. It is dose dependent, with an incidence of about 10% after 5 mg epidural morphine. The risk of severe distressing itching is about 1%. Pruritus most commonly affects the head and trunk region initially, but may spread to all areas of the body, and begins about 3 h after injection. It may be related to cephalad spread of morphine within the CSF. Prophylactic naloxone infusion at a rate of 5 μg kg^{-1} h^{-1} will reduce the frequency of pruritus without reversing analgesia. A small (10 mg) intravenous dose of propofol may be equally effective.

Rostral spread is largely responsible for emetic symptoms and respiratory depression. Nausea and vomiting has a reported incidence of up to 75% and, again, is worse with intrathecal than epidural morphine administration. The incidence of respiratory depression is low (0.25–0.5%) with epidural morphine but is potentially the most serious complication with these routes and is frequently delayed until several hours after drug administration. It can be profound and long lasting. Although late-onset respiratory depression is rare with the more lipid-soluble opioids, early respiratory depression within 30 min of injection can occur due to extensive uptake into the systemic circulation. The other important side-effect is urinary retention, with an overall incidence of about 40%. This can develop insidiously and, since bladder sensation is partially or wholly lost, may not be reported by the patient until gross overdistension of the bladder has occurred. Although administration of parasympathetic agents has been recommended as the first line of treatment, there is a high failure rate. Naloxone, 0.4 mg intravenously, will immediately restore normal micturition but will also reverse analgesia.

Although epidural opioids will provide adequate analgesia during the early stages of labour, they are usually ineffective in controlling pain during the final stages. For this reason it has become common practice to combine low concentrations of an opioid such as fentanyl 2 μg ml^{-1} or sufentanil 1 μg ml^{-1} with the local anaesthetic bupivacaine 0.125%. An initial epidural bolus of 10 ml of this solution is followed by an epidural infusion at a rate of 8–10 ml h^{-1}. This provides good analgesia throughout labour, with minimal side-effects.

There has been speculation that epidural opioids may reactivate herpex simplex in pregnant patients. The aetiology is unclear. Herpes simplex after delivery is potentially dangerous because of the risk of herpes encephalitis in the infant. Spinal opioids should therefore be avoided in the parturient with a history of recurrent herpes simplex.

PURE ANTAGONISTS

NALOXONE

Naloxone is the *N*-allyl derivative of oxymorphone (Fig. 7.8). It is a competitive antagonist at μ, δ and κ receptors but is more potent at the μ receptor. By itself it is virtually devoid of pharmacological activity, but will precipitate withdrawal symptoms in opioid addicts and has been used for the detection of addiction. When given to patients who have had an excessive perioperative dose of an opioid, naloxone will reverse not only the respiratory depression but also analgesia. A dose of 0.2–0.4 mg is effective in reversing opioid-induced respiratory depression, although it is better to titrate naloxone in increments of 0.04 mg to avoid acute reversal of analgesia. There have been reports of intense pressor responses, tachycardia and severe pulmonary oedema occurring when naloxone has been used to reverse the effects of large doses of an opioid. The plasma half-life of naloxone (1.0–1.5 h) is considerably shorter than that of most opioids, and the clinical effects of a single injection last only 30–90 min. On occasions repeated doses or a continuous intravenous infusion may be

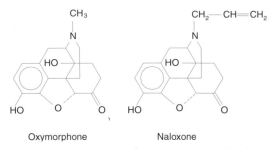

Oxymorphone   Naloxone

Fig. 7.8 Chemical structure of oxymorphone and naloxone.

required. An infusion of 0.2–0.4 mg h^{-1} will usually suffice to prevent opioid-induced respiratory depression without affecting analgesia.

Recently attention has focused on the therapeutic use of naloxone in patients with endotoxic shock. There is considerable animal evidence to support this therapeutic approach, which is thought to work by antagonizing the high levels of circulating β-endorphin produced by endotoxins. The results of naloxone treatment of shock in humans remains controversial.

NALTREXONE AND NALMEFENE

Naltrexone and nalmefene are structurally related to naloxone. Naltrexone is the N-cycloprophylmethyl analogue of oxymorphone, whereas nalmefene is the N-allyl analogue. They have similar pharmacological properties to naloxone but with longer durations of action, with elimination half-lives in excess of 8 h. They also have significant oral availability. Nalmefene, which is equipotent with naloxone, has been used in anaesthesia to reverse opioid-induced respiratory depression. Its prolonged effect could make it potentially useful when given prophylactically to prevent respiratory depression due to spinal opioids. Naltrexone is used mainly in the management of addicts.

PARTIAL AGONISTS

The history of this class of drugs dates from 1914 when Pohl, in an attempt to improve the analgesic properties of codeine, synthesized N-allylcodeine, which he found could antagonize the respiratory depression produced by morphine. This discovery remained almost unnoticed by the medical profession until Weijland and Erickson synthesized N-allylmorphine (nalorphine) in 1942. Nalorphine is an example of how minor structural changes to an existing opioid can give compounds with very different pharmacological properties. Nalorphine is equipotent with morphine as an analgesic and in causing respiratory depression. Unfortunately nalorphine's severe psychotomimetic activity, including unpleasant visual hallucinations, precludes its clinical use as an analgesic. Until the discovery of naloxone, nalorphine was widely used for its antagonist properties in the treatment of opioid overdose.

The term mixed agonist–antagonist drugs is often used to describe this class of drugs. It was thought that they were agonists or partial agonists at the κ receptor and antagonists at the μ receptor. Although this explained rather neatly the phenomenon that they could act as analgesics and yet antagonize the effects of morphine, it is now generally accepted that they are partial agonists at opioid receptors.[24] When a partial agonist is combined with a low concentration of a full agonist, so that few of the receptors are occupied by the agonist, the partial agonist can occupy the free receptors and complement the analgesic effect of the full agonist. However, when a partial agonist is introduced in the presence of a high concentration of full agonist, then the latter will be displaced from the receptor by the partial agonist, resulting in a reduction in the response. The dysphoric side-effects of some of this class of drugs are thought to be due to binding to the nonopioid σ receptor. The chemical structures of the drugs in this group are shown in Fig. 7.9.

PENTAZOCINE

Pentazocine, the N-dimethylallyl derivative of phenazocine, was the first member of the so-called agonist–antagonist opioids to be used with clinical success. Its analgesic potency is approximately one-third to one-fifth that of morphine. Pentazocine is a racemic mixture and analgesia resides exclusively in the L-isomer. In equianalgesic doses pentazocine causes the same degree of respiratory depression as morphine. However, as with other partial agonists, both the response curves for respiratory depression and analgesia are plateau shaped, with the plateau being reached at a dose of approximately 60 mg for the average adult. Peak blood concentrations after oral administration are reached by 1–3 h and between 15 and 45 min after intramuscular administration. The oral bioavailability is about 20%.

Pentazocine produces an increase in blood pressure, heart rate and plasma levels of catecholamines. This is associated with increased systemic vascular resistance, pulmonary artery pressure and myocardial workload, and decreased myocardial contractility. Pentazocine is contraindicated in the treatment of patients with acute myocardial infarction. Psychomimetic side-effects such as hallucinations, bizarre dreams and sensations of depersonalization occur in about 6–10% of patients; they are more common in elderly patients, in those who are ambulatory, and when doses above 60 mg are given. Nausea occurs in approximately 5% of patients, although vomiting is less common. Other commonly reported side-effects are dizziness and drowsiness. Euphoria is less common than with pure agonist drugs,

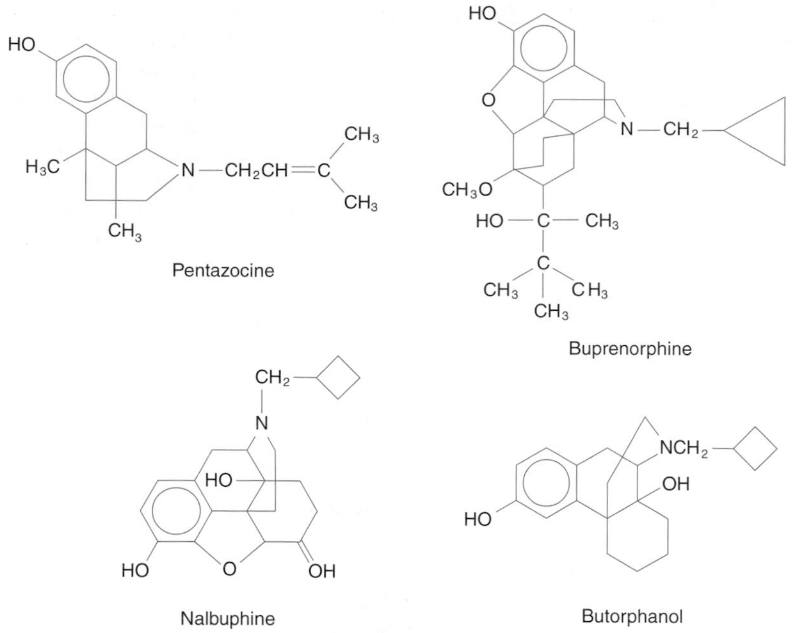

Fig. 7.9 Chemical structure of the partial opioid agonists.

which may account in part for the lower risk of physical dependence and 'drug-seeking' behaviour, although repeated use of pentazocine will result in physical dependence.

BUTORPHANOL TARTRATE

Butorphanol tartrate is a fully synthetic morphinan derivative, 3.5 to 5 times as potent as morphine. It is a weak partial μ-receptor agonist and is relatively ineffective at reversing the effects of full agonists. The relatively low incidence of psychomimetic effects in humans compared with pentazocine suggests a lack of significant σ-receptor action. The recommended doses are 1–4 mg intramuscularly every 3–4 h or 0.5–2 mg intravenously. The onset of analgesia occurs within 10 min after intramuscular administration, and peak analgesic activity is reached within 30–45 min. Given intravenously, peak analgesia is reached in less than 30 min. Butorphanol is metabolized mainly in the liver to inactive metabolites, hydroxybutorphanol and norbutorphanol. The terminal half-life is 2.5–3.5 h. Butorphanol is about 80% bound to plasma proteins.

Respiratory depression produced by butorphanol 2 mg intravenously is similar to that of 10 mg morphine. However, unlike morphine, there is a ceiling effect for respiratory depression with increasing doses of butorphanol. Clinically, near-maximal depression occurs after 4 mg in normal adults. In healthy volunteers, butorphanol 0.03–0.06 mg kg^{-1} produces no significant cardiovascular changes. However, in patients with cardiac disease, progressive increases in cardiac index and pulmonary artery pressure occur. These changes are similar to those produced by pentazocine, and butorphanol is therefore best avoided in patients with recent myocardial infarction.

NALBUPHINE HYDROCHLORIDE

Nalbuphine hydrochloride is structurally related to oxymorphone and naloxone. It is approximately equipotent with morphine. Nalbuphine is metabolized in the liver to inactive metabolites. About 7% of administered nalbuphine is excreted in the urine as unchanged drug or conjugates. The plasma terminal half-life is approximately 5 h. The onset of analgesia is within 2–3 min of intravenous administration and 15 min after intramuscular injection, and lasts 3–6 h with an adult dose of 10 mg. With equianalgesic doses, similar degrees of respiratory depression to that of morphine occur up to a dose of approximately 0.45 mg kg^{-1}. With higher doses a 'ceiling effect' occurs. Intravenous nalbuphine causes minimal haemodynamic changes in patients with cardiac disease. Nalbuphine does not increase cardiac workload or pulmonary artery pressure, and thus is safe in the management of patients after acute myocardial infarction.

Sedation, possibly mediated by κ-receptor activation, occurs in one-third of subjects given doses of 10–20 mg. The incidence of psychomimetic side-effects is lower than with pentazocine. Chronic administration can result in physical dependence which resembles that seen with pentazocine rather than morphine, although the abuse potential would seem to be low. Nalbuphine causes withdrawal symptoms in opioid-dependent subjects. In doses of up to 0.2 mg kg^{-1} it is an effective antagonist of opioid-induced respiratory depression. Its use is sometimes associated with a number of side-effects, including nausea, hypertension, tachycardia and confusion. Larger doses also tend to antagonize analgesia. However, by careful titration of small incremental doses, it is possible to achieve satisfactory reversal of respiratory depression without precipitating pain and haemodynamic side-effects.

BUPRENORPHINE

Buprenorphine is a semisynthetic derivative of thebaine, one of the most chemically reactive of the opium alkaloids. It has significant μ-receptor agonist activity, although its intrinsic activity is low. Buprenorphine binds to and dissociates from the μ receptor very slowly, which may account for its low potential for physical abuse. This stable interaction with the μ receptor is also likely to be the explanation for the difficulty with which naloxone will reverse the agonist effects of buprenorphine once these have been established, although the agonist effects can be blocked by naloxone given before buprenorphine.

Buprenorphine is approximately 30 times as potent as morphine. A dose of 0.3 mg intramuscularly has a duration of analgesic action of 6–18 h. Buprenorphine is also effective sublingually. The average bioavailability by this route is about 55%, but absorption is slow and the time to achieve peak plasma concentrations is variable, with a range of 90–360 min. The onset of action is rather slow (5–15 min) after both intramuscular and intravenous administration, possibly due to slow receptor association.

In animals there is a bell-shaped response curve for respiratory depression with buprenorphine, rather than the typical flattened dose–response curve of the partial antagonists. There is some evidence for a similar effect in humans, with the response curve peaking at doses between 0.3 and 0.6 mg intramuscularly. When respiratory depression occurs, it is important to realize that no satisfactory antagonist exists: naloxone, even in a dose as large as 14–16 mg, may only partially reverse this side-effect. Doxapram may in some situations prove a useful alternative. Drowsiness and dizziness are the most common side-effects, although they rarely constitute a major problem. In comparison with other opioids, buprenorphine appears to have a very low abuse potential. This may be due to the lack of euphoria and the nature of the drug interaction with the opioid receptor.

Buprenorphine is lipophilic and extensively bound to plasma proteins: protein binding is 95–98%. Its pK_a is 9.24. There are no data on oral bioavailability in humans, but in the dog bioavailability is only 3–6% . In humans the hepatic extraction ratio is 0.85 so that oral systemic availability would be expected to be about 15% or less. Buprenorphine is almost completely metabolized in the liver by N-dealkylation and conjugation. The terminal half-life is approximately 5 h. Because of slow receptor binding there is no direct relationship between plasma concentration and clinical effect.

MISCELLANEOUS DRUGS

MEPTAZINOL

Meptazinol is a hexahydroazepine derivative structurally related to pethidine. It is approximately equipotent with pethidine. It is moderately selective for the μ_1 receptor and clinically it behaves as a partial μ agonist. It has low affinity for κ receptors. Meptazinol-induced analgesia can be reversed almost completely by naloxone, although higher doses are needed than for pure opioid agonists. Meptazinol will also reverse the signs of acute morphine overdosage and precipitate withdrawal symptoms in morphine-dependent animals. A component of meptazinol's analgesic activity is mediated by an effect at central cholinergic synapses, a mode of action different from that of all other conventional analgesics. Unlike opioids, each of the isomers of meptazinol possesses equal analgesic potency, although its cholinergically mediated analgesia is stereospecific.

Meptazinol in clinically effective analgesic doses appears to be almost devoid of respiratory side-effects. It has a minimal effect on haemodynamics after intramuscular administration. It may have mild positive inotropic activity, and increases in blood pressure and heart rate lasting up to 20 min have been reported after meptazinol 1.6 mg kg^{-1} intravenously. Meptazinol is a basic lipophilic drug with low (23%) protein binding. It is rapidly conjugated in the liver to the glucuronide. The terminal half-life in adults is approximately 2 h.

DEZOCINE

Dezocine is a partial μ agonist approximately equipotent to morphine with respect to analgesia. It is as effective as morphine for moderate to severe postoperative pain. It produces sedation and dysphoria in humans, suggesting that it has κ-receptor activity. In single doses, however, dezocine is a slightly more potent respiratory depressant than morphine, although a 'ceiling' effect to dezocine-induced respiratory depression occurs with increasing dose. Maximum depression occurs at about 2.3 mg kg^{-1} intravenously. Clinically important haemodynamic changes have not been observed with usual analgesic doses. Dezocine produces euphoria and increased drug-liking scores in individuals without a history of drug abuse, and produces subjective effects in human ex-addicts that are similar to those of morphine. The drug can produce substantial cardiovascular depression in dogs, but cardiovascular effects are not found in humans given analgesic doses.

TRAMADOL HYDROCHLORIDE

Tramadol is a centrally acting analgesic that acts at opioid receptors and also modifies nociceptive transmission by inhibition of noradrenaline and serotonin. It has a low affinity for opioid receptors, comparable to that of codeine. It is approximately equipotent to pethidine. It may be administered orally, rectally or intravenously. Oral tramadol has proved effective for the treatment of patients with cancer pain.

The tolerance and dependence potential of tramadol is low, even during treatment for up to 6 months. Tramadol can cause respiratory depression, although this is considerably less than with the classical opioid agonists, when it is given in the recommended dose. It is generally well tolerated; dizziness, nausea, sedation, dry mouth and sweating are the most common side-effects.

The mean oral availability of tramadol is 68%, with peak plasma concentrations achieved by 1.5–2 h. Tramadol is extensively metabolized by the liver and the elimination half-life is about 5–6 h. The metabolite O-desmethyl tramadol has two to four times the analgesic potency of tramadol in mice and rats. Tramadol should not be given to patients taking MAOIs.

REFERENCES

1. Martin WR, Eades CG. The effects of morphine- and nalorphine-like drugs in the nondependent and morphine-dependent chronic spinal dog. *J Pharmacol Exp Ther* 1976; **197**: 517–532.
2. Lambert DG. Opioid receptors. *Curr Opin Anaesthesiol* 1995; **8**: 317–322.
3. Hosztafi S, Furst Z. Endogenous morphine. *Pharmacol Res* 1995; **32**: 15–20.
4. Kodaira H, Spector S. Transformation of thebaine to oripavine, codeine, and morphine by rat liver, kidney, and brain microsomes. *Proc Natl Acad Sci USA* 1988; **85**: 1267–1271.
5. Pande AC, Pyke RE, Greiner M *et al*. Analgesic efficacy of enadoline versus placebo or morphine in postsurgical pain. *Clin Neuropharmacol* 1996; **19**: 451–456.
6. McFadzean DF. The ionic mechanisms underlying opioid actions. *Neuropeptides* 1988; **11**: 173–180.
7. North RA. Opioid receptor types and membranes on ion channels. *Trends Neurosci* 1986; **9**: 174–176.
8. Abbadie C, Besson J-M. Effects of morphine and naloxone on basal and evoked Fos-like immunoreactivity in lumbar spinal cord neurons of arthritic rats. *Pain* 1993; **52**: 29–39.
9. Crain SM, Shen K-F. Opioids can evoke direct receptor-mediated excitatory effects on sensory neurons. *Trends Pharmacol Sci* 1990; **11**: 77–81.
10. Smart D, Smith G, Lambert DG. Mu-opioids activate phospholipase C in SH-SY5Y human neuroblastoma cells via calcium-channel opening. *Biochem J* 1995; **305**: 577–581.
11. Santillan R, Maestre JM, Hurle MA, Florez J. Enhancement of opiate analgesia by nimodipine in cancer patients chronically treated with morphine: a preliminary report. *Pain* 1994; **58**: 129–132.
12. Ferreira SH, Nakamura M. II – Prostaglandin hyperalgesia: the peripheral analgesic activity of morphine, enkephalins and opioid antagonists. *Prostaglandins* 1979; **18**: 191–200.
13. Stein C. Peripheral mechanisms of opioid analgesia. *Anesth Analg* 1993; **76**: 182–191.
14. Berkenbosch A, Olievier CN, Wolsink JG *et al*. Effects of morphine and physostigmine on the ventilatory response to carbon dioxide. *Anesthesiology* 1994; **80**: 1303–1310.
15. Vankova ME, Weinger MB, Chen DY *et al*. Role of central mu, delta-1, and kappa-1 opioid receptors in opioid induced muscle rigidity in the rat. *Anesthesiology* 1996; **85**: 574–583.
16. Smart D, Lambert DG. The stimulatory effects of opioids and their possible role in the development of tolerance. *Trends Pharmacol Sci* 1996; **17**: 264–269.
17. Osborne R, Joel S, Trew P, Slevin M. Morphine and metabolite behaviour after different routes of morphine administration: demonstration of the importance of the active metabolite morphine-6-glucuronide. *Clin Pharmacol Ther* 1990; **47**: 12–19.
18. Hasselstrom J, Berg V, Löfgren A, Säwe J. Long lasting respiratory depression induced by morphine-6-glucuronide. *Br J Clin Pharmacol* 1989; **27**: 515–518.
19. Bernards CM, Hill HF. Physical and chemical properties of drug molecules governing their diffusion through the meninges. *Anesthesiology* 1992; **77**: 750–756.
20. Björkman S, Stanski DR, Verotta D, Harashima H. Comparative tissue concentration profiles of fentanyl and alfentanil in humans predicted from tissue/blood partition data obtained in rats. *Anesthesiology* 1990; **72**: 865–873.
21. Bartkowski RR, McDonnell TE. Prolonged alfentanil effect following erythromycin administration. *Anesthesiology* 1990; **73**: 566–568.
22. Dershwitz M, Randel GI, Rosow CE *et al*. Initial clinical experience with remifentanil, a new opioid metabolized by esterases. *Anesth Analg* 1995; **81**: 619–623.
23. Buerkle H, Yaksh TL. Studies in continuous intrathecal administration of short lasting μ-opioids, remifentanil and alfentanil, in the rat. *Anesthesiology* 1996; **84**: 926–935.
24. Bowdle TA. Partial agonist and agonist–antagonist opioids: basic pharmacology and clinical applications. *Anaesth Pharmacol Review* 1993; **2**: 135–151.

8

RP Woda, A Reeves

DRUGS FOR PSYCHIATRIC DISORDERS AND EPILEPSY

Psychotropic drugs may be associated with unpredictable drug interactions during anaesthesia. The anaesthetist should, therefore, have a good understanding of the pharmacology of these drugs and their potential interactions. As new psychotropic drugs are developed, and are prescribed to patients who require surgery, this will become increasingly important.

ANTIPSYCHOTIC AGENTS

The use of these drugs dates from the early nineteenth century with the introduction of promethazine, which is still used in psychiatric practice. Later, in 1949–1950, chlorpromazine, another phenothiazine, was developed. Antipsychotic drugs can be divided into three groups, based on their chemical structure: phenothiazines, thioxanthenes, and other heterocyclic compounds including the butyrophenones (haloperidol). They are known as neuroleptic agents. More recently developed agents, such as the dibenzodiazepines, diphenyl-butylpiperazines and benzamides, which produce less motor disturbance than the classical neuroleptics, are often referred to as atypical neuroleptics.

Neuroleptic drugs preserve spinal reflexes and unconditioned nociceptive avoidance behaviours, while spontaneous movements and complex behaviour are suppressed. They also reduce initiative and interest in the environment, with a flattening of the affect and less display of emotions. Psychotic patients become less agitated and restless, and have fewer hallucinations, delusions, and disorganized or incoherent thought processes. All these drugs have sedative as well as antipsychotic effects. Tolerance to their sedative effects is often seen in extremely agitated psychotic patients.

Phenothiazines are three-ringed structures in which two benzene rings are connected by a sulphur and a nitrogen atom. If the nitrogen at position 10 is replaced by a carbon with a double bond, the compound becomes a thioxanthene. The phenothiazines are subdivided according to the their side-chain constituents into aliphatic derivatives (e.g. chlorpromazine), piperazine derivatives (e.g. perphenazine) and piperidine derivatives (e.g. thioridazine). The piperazine compounds are the most potent drugs with a greater risk of producing extrapyramidal side-effects, but cause less sedation or autonomic effects such as hypotension. The aliphatic derivatives are the least potent, but are clinically effective. Thioxanthenes closely resemble the aliphatic phenothiazines, both chemically and pharmacologically. The butyrophenones are chemically unrelated to other neuroleptics, but resemble the piperazine-type phenothiazines in their pharmacological activity.

The mechanism of action of antipsychotics is due mainly to antagonism of dopamine in the basal ganglia and limbic portions of the forebrain (Figs 8.1 and 8.2). Neuroleptic drugs block presynaptic and postsynaptic dopamine D_2 receptors, and some (particularly phenothiazines, thioxanthenes and clozapine) also block D_1 receptors. Postsynaptic D_2 receptors stimulate phospholipase C to convert phosphatidylinositol bisphosphate to inositol triphosphate and diacylglycerol, which activate intracellular protein kinases. This pathway is inhibited by neuroleptics acting via D_2 receptors and by lithium, which inhibits the phosphatase that liberates inositol from inositol phosphate. Lithium also inhibits the exocytotic release of dopamine (and noradrenaline) from the nerve terminal. Clozapine is relatively nonselective between D_1 and D_2 receptors, but has a high affinity for D_4.

Because it takes days or weeks for the antipsychotic effects to become apparent, an increase in the number of dopamine receptors, or other indirect actions, may be more important than direct receptor antagonism. Dopamine antagonism by phenothiazines in the basal ganglia probably explains their neurological side-effects including extrapyramidal signs, acute dystonia, akathisia and the neuroleptic malignant syndrome. This syndrome, although rare, is characterized by tremor, signs of autonomic instability, hyperthermia, stupor and raised levels of creatine kinase. Management is immediate cessation of the offending drug and supportive care. Administration of dantrolene and

Summary box 8.1 Neuroleptic antipsychotic drugs

- Phenothiazines:

  - aliphatic derivatives (e.g. chlorpromazine)

    - very sedative, moderate anticholinergic, moderate extrapyramidal effects.

  - piperidine derivatives (e.g. thioridazine)

    - moderately sedative, very anticholinergic, fewer extrapyramidal effects.

  - piperazine derivatives (e.g. fluphenazine)

    - less sedative, less anticholinergic, pronounced extrapyramidal effects.

- Thioxanthenes (e.g. flupenthixol):

  - chemically related to phenothiazines

  - side-effects similar to those of aliphatic phenothiazines.

- Butyrophenones (e.g. haloperidol):

  - chemically unrelated to other neuroleptics

  - resemble piperazine phenothiazines in activity and side-effects.

- Atypical drugs (e.g. clozapine, risperidone, sulpiride):

  - much lower incidence of extrapyramidal effects

  - useful in patients resistant to other neuroleptics.

  - clozapine:

    - causes neutropenia and agranulocytosis in 1–3% of patients

    - blocks D_4 receptors in limbic areas but little effect on striatal D_2 receptors.

  - risperidone:

    - nonsedative

    - lacks anticholinergic and α-blocking activity.

  - sulpiride:

    - very specific D_2 antagonist

    - moderately sedating

    - low doses do not cause extrapyramidal effects, but this advantage is lost at high doses.

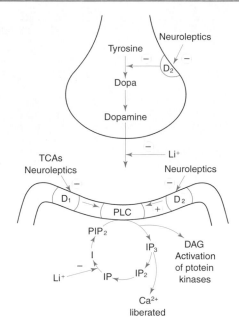

Fig. 8.1 Sites and mechanisms of action of antipsychotic drugs and lithium. Neuroleptic drugs block presynaptic and postsynaptic dopamine D_2 receptors, and some also block D_1 receptors. TCAs, tricyclic antidepressants; PLC, phospholipase C; PIP_2, phosphatidylinositol bisphosphate; IP_3, inositol triphosphate; DAG, diacylglycerol; IP, inositol phosphate; I, inositol.

bromocriptine, a dopaminergic agonist, may be useful. Although this syndrome appears similar to malignant hyperthermia, it is not associated with a known defect in calcium metabolism in skeletal muscle. Phenothiazines lower the seizure threshold and reduce discharge patterns in the electroencephalogram (EEG). They also affect temperature control causing hypothermia or hyperthermia, depending on the ambient temperature.

Many neuroleptic drugs have antiemetic properties, partly related to the antagonism of dopamine in the chemoreceptor trigger zone. They also block muscarinic cholinergic and α-adrenergic receptors, which results in side-effects such as dry mouth, blurred vision and postural hypotension (Fig. 8.2). In the pituitary gland dopamine acting on D_2 receptors inhibits the release of prolactin. The blocking of this effect by neuroleptics results in increased prolactin release, which can cause endocrine side-effects such as gynaecomastia, menstrual irregularities, impotence and weight gain. Chlorpromazine is a significant α-adrenergic blocking drug with some ability to block cholinergic receptors. Blocking α-adrenergic receptors results in postural hypotension and reflex tachycardia. Chlorpromazine has direct negative inotropic actions on the heart and a quinidine-like antiarrhythmic effect. Electrocardiographic (ECG)

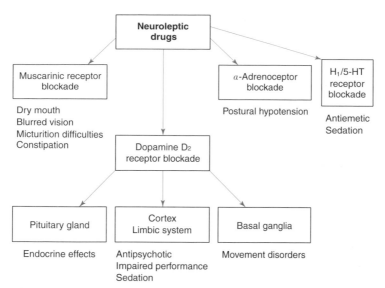

Fig. 8.2 Consequences of dopamine D_2 receptor blockade. 5-HT, 5-hydroxytryptamine (serotonin).

changes include prolongation of the Q-T and P-R intervals, blunting of T waves and S-T segment depression. ECG changes are particularly common with thioridazine, which has been associated with ventricular arrhythmias and sudden death. Apart from clozapine, an atypical neuroleptic drug, most nonphenothiazine neuroleptics do not cause significant hypotension.

Antagonism of muscarinic receptors causes side-effects such as blurred vision, increased intraocular pressure, dry mouth and eyes, constipation and urinary retention. Since acetylcholine opposes the actions of dopamine in the basal ganglia, drugs with high antimuscarinic activity, such as clozapine and thioridazine, cause fewer extrapyramidal side-effects than other neuroleptics. Many phenothiazines and some other neuroleptics (e.g. thioridazine) are histamine H_1 antagonists. This partly accounts for their sedative and antiemetic activity.

The neuroleptic drugs are highly lipophilic and highly membrane and protein bound. They accumulate in the brain, lung and other tissues with a high blood supply. Elimination half-lives of these drugs are around 20–40 h, and the duration of action can be as long as 24 h for some formulations. They undergo mainly oxidative metabolism in the liver, the metabolites being conjugated with glucuronic acid. Most metabolites are biologically inactive. The metabolism of the phenothiazines, and of chlorpromazine in particular, is complex and there is a highly variable correlation between plasma concentrations and clinical effect. In part this is due to large and variable tissue binding but also to induction of their own hepatic metabolism. Table 8.1

summarizes the doses and side-effect profiles of a selected list of antipsychotic agents.

ANTIANXIETY DRUGS

Benzodiazepines are widely used to treat anxiety. Their use for other indications is discussed in Chapter 6, so this chapter will focus on their use in psychiatric practice. Benzodiazepines block EEG arousal from stimulation of brainstem reticular formation. They also cause depression of spinal reflexes that are mediated by the brainstem reticular system. They raise the seizure threshold and act as anticonvulsants. Their mechanism of action, via the γ-aminobutyric acid (GABA)–chloride ion channel receptor complex, occurs in the limbic system, amygdala, hippocampus and hypothalamus.

The most common side-effects of the benzodiazepines are drowsiness and ataxia. There can be an increased incidence of irritability and hostility with chronic use. Teratogenic effects, resulting in midline cleft deformities of the lip and palate, have been reported but remain controversial.[1] Benzodiazepines, however, are a safe class of drugs and patients on long-term therapy present few anaesthetic problems.

Other drugs used to treat anxiety disorders are the barbiturates and antihistamines such as hydroxyzine. A newer anxiolytic drug, buspirone, does not appear to work through the GABA system but is a 5-hydroxy-tryptamine $(5\text{-HT})_{1A}$ receptor antagonist. Unlike benzodiazepines, buspirone produces little tolerance or dependence. (See Chapters 6 and 7 for detailed pharmacology of these drugs.)

	Adult dose (mg)		Side-effects			Half-life (h)	Antagonism[*]		
Drug	Oral	IM	Sedation	Extra-pyramidal	Hypotension		NA	ACh	5-HT$_2$
Chlorpromazine	200–800	25–50	+++	++	+++IM ++ oral	30	++	=	=
Triflupromazine		20–60	++	+++	++	11	n/a	n/a	n/a
Mesoridazine	75–300	25	+++	−	+++		n/a	n/a	n/a
Thioridazine	150–600		+++	+	++	17	+	=	=
Fluphenazine	2–20	1.25–2.5	+	+++	+	20	=	−	−
Perphenazine	8–32	5–10	++	++	+	9	−	−	−
Trifluoperazine	5–20	1–2	+	+++	+	11	−	−	−
Chlorprothixene	50–400	25–50	+++	++	++	9	+	=	+
Thiothixene	5–30	2–4	+	++	++	34	−	−	−
Haloperidol	2–20	2–5	+	+++	+	20	−	−	+
Loxapine	60–100	1.25–50	+	++	+	3.5	=	−	+
Molindone	20–225		++	+	+		n/a	n/a	n/a
Pimozide	2–6		+	+++	+	54	−	++	−

Table 8.1 Antipsychotic Drugs

[*] Role of antagonism of noradrenaline (NA), acetylcholine (ACh) and serotonin (5-HT) in comparison with the antagonism of dopamine for pharmacological effects; ++, more important; +, important; =, equally important; −, less important; n/a, no data available; IM, intramuscular.

ANTIDEPRESSANTS

Depression is one of the most common psychiatric illnesses. Its presentation varies in severity from intense sadness and despair to mental slowing and loss of concentration. Some 10–15% of depressed patients display suicidal behaviour. Drugs used in the management of depression fall into four categories: tricyclic antidepressants, monoamine oxidase inhibitors (MAOIs), lithium and selective serotonin-reuptake inhibitors.

Summary box 8.2 Antidepressant drugs

- Most are thought to work by inhibiting the neuronal reuptake of adrenaline and 5-HT.

- All antidepressant drugs can provoke seizures and are not safe in depressive epileptic patients.

- Benefits do not become apparent for 2–3 weeks. This may be related to gradual changes in the sensitivity of 5-HT and adrenergic receptors.

TRICYCLIC ANTIDEPRESSANTS

These are the most common agents used to treat depression. The first drug in this class was imipramine, a dibenzazepine structurally very similar to the phenothiazines. The name 'tricyclic antidepressants' derives from of the three-ringed configuration of these substances. Tricyclic antidepressants are basic drugs and are not well absorbed from the stomach but are very

Summary box 8.3 Tricyclic antidepressants

- Related to phenothiazines.

- Sedative and autonomic side-effects limit their use.

- Overdosage causes cardiotoxicity, but convulsions also are common.

well absorbed from the duodenum. They are highly plasma protein bound and have long half-lives of 1–5 days (Table 8.2). Metabolism is by hepatic microsomal enzymes followed by conjugation with glucuronic acid. Metabolism is slower in patients aged over 60 years and faster in children.

Tricyclic antidepressants potentiate noradrenaline, 5-HT and dopamine in the central nervous system by blocking their reuptake by nerve terminals (Fig. 8.3). Synthesis, storage and release are not affected. Most tricyclic antidepressants have much less effect on dopamine uptake than on noradrenaline or 5-HT. Blockade of dopamine reuptake is associated with stimulant activity, whereas blockade of noradrenaline and 5-HT are associated with antidepressive effects. Tricyclic antidepressants also reduce the number of cerebral β-adrenergic receptors and brain responsiveness to β-adrenergic agonists. In addition, they are antagonists at muscarinic cholinergic, α-adrenergic and H_1 and H_2 histamine receptors. These actions do not contribute to their antidepressive effects but are responsible for several of their side-effects.

The clinical effects of tricyclic antidepressants are divided into an early and late response. In the first

Table 8.2 Antidepressant drugs

Drug	Amines affected	Half-life (h)	Sedation	Anticholinergic activity	Hypotension	Cardiac effects	Convulsions
Tricyclics							
Amitriptyline	NA, 5-HT	21	+++	+++	+++	+++	++
Imipramine	NA, 5-HT	18	++	++	++	+++	++
Doxepin	NA, 5-HT	17	+++	++	+++	++	++
Desipramine	NA	22	±	+	+	++	+
Nortriptyline	NA	31	+	+	+	++	+
Protriptyline	NA	78	±	++	+	+++	++
MAOIs							
Isocarboxazid	NA, 5-HT, DA	6	±	++	+	++	+
Phenelzine	NA, 5-HT, DA	± 1	+	−	−	−	−
Tranylcypromine	NA, 5-HT, DA	± 2	+	−	++	−	−
SSRIs							
Fluoxetine	5-HT	84	±	−	−	−	±
Paroxetine	5-HT	24	±	−	−	−	−
Sertraline	5-HT	25	±	−	−	−	−

NA, noradrenaline; 5-HT, 5-hydroxytryptamine (serotonin); DA, dopamine; +++, marked effect; ++, moderate effect; +, mild effect; ±, minimal or no effect.

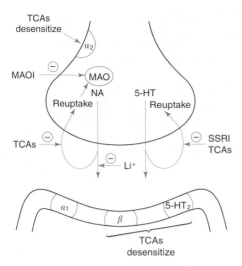

Fig. 8.3 Sites and mechanisms of action of antidepressant drugs. Tricyclic antidepressants (TCAs) block the reuptake of noradrenaline and 5-hydroxytryptamine (5-HT) and desensitize presynaptic a_2 and postsynaptic β adrenoceptors and 5-HT$_2$ receptors. MAOI, monoamine oxidase inhibitor; NA, noradrenaline; SSRI, selective serotonin-reuptake inhibitor.

weeks of drug administration, sleepiness, light headedness and difficulty in concentration can occur. Decreases in blood pressure, dry mouth, blurred vision and gait disturbances are also common. The antidepressant effects are not evident until after about 2–3 weeks. With time, the antidepressant effects become more obvious and these early symptoms are less evident. With chronic therapy, sleep disturbances are lessened as there are fewer awakenings, an increase in stage 4 sleep and a general decrease in time spent in rapid eye movement (REM) sleep. Urinary retention, constipation, blurred vision, dry mouth and mild sinus tachycardia result from the drugs' anticholinergic properties. Other cardiovascular effects include postural hypertension, flattening or inversion of the T waves on the ECG, and direct myocardial depression. These are due to a combination of α-adrenergic antagonism, antimuscarinic effects and inhibition of noradrenaline reuptake. The tricyclic antidepressants also can cause slowing of cardiac conduction, resulting in ventricular arrhythmias, and enhancement of the effects of other cardiac depressant drugs.

With overdoses of these drugs there is reduced reuptake of catecholamines, resulting in arrhythmias and hypertension. Tricyclic compounds have a high affinity for cardiac muscle. There is a quinidine-like action on the ECG and depressed myocardial contractility. The severity of the poisoning can be estimated from the degree of QRS widening. Once catecholamine reserves are depleted, severe cardio-

respiratory depression and coma develop. Treatment includes gastric lavage, as the anticholinergic effects delay gastric emptying by 12 h or longer. Supportive therapy should be aimed at correcting any electrolyte and acid–base disturbances as these contribute to arrhythmias. Pharmacological treatment of arrhythmias should be resisted if possible, as this may potentiate the cardiotoxicity. Life-threatening arrhythmias may develop even after the patient has apparently recovered from the overdose, and ECG monitoring should be continued for several days. Because of their large volume of distribution, dialysis is not helpful in reducing plasma concentrations of tricyclic antidepressants.

Tricyclic antidepressants have efficacy in other disorders besides depression. They are useful in the management of chronic pain syndromes, migraine headaches, sleep disorders, neuralgias, irritable bowel syndrome and peptic ulcer disease. There has also been some benefit observed in the treatment of bulimia, obsessive–compulsive disorders and alcoholism. In children, tricyclic antidepressants have been used in the management of enuresis.

The toxicity of the tricyclic antidepressants related to anaesthesia is largely due to their anticholinergic and adrenergic antagonist properties. Blocking of noradrenaline reuptake will enhance the action of direct-acting sympathomimetic drugs. Their anticholinergic properties lead to potentiation of atropine-like drugs, and ST–T wave and conduction abnormalities may occur during neostigmine reversal of neuromuscular block. Severe ventricular arrhythmias have been reported following administration of pancuronium to dogs chronically receiving imipramine and anaesthetized with halothane.[2] This suggests that pancuronium should be given with caution to patients taking tricyclic antidepressant drugs who are anaesthetized with volatile anaesthetics that sensitize the myocardium to catecholamines.

MONOAMINE OXIDASE INHIBITORS

The use of MAOIs in the management of depressive disorders is associated with considerable controversy, related to the complications associated with these drugs. They are, however, indicated when other agents, such as tricyclic antidepressants, give an unsatisfactory therapeutic result, or when electroconvulsive therapy is contraindicated or refused. Their introduction to psychiatry arose from the development of drugs used to treat tuberculosis. In 1951, isoniazid was developed and its derivative iproniazid, also effective in the management of tuberculosis, was found to have mood-elevating properties. Further investigation revealed that the mechanism of this action was inhibition of monoamine oxidase (MAO). Iproniazid, phenelzine and isocarboxazid are derivatives of hydrazine, a substance

---

Summary box 8.4 Monoamine oxidase inhibitors

- The older MAOIs are irreversible, nonselective inhibitors of MAO.

- Usefulness is limited by adverse side-effects: postural hypotension, anticholinergic effects and liver toxicity.

- Potentially dangerous interactions with foods containing tyramine, indirectly acting sympathomimetics (e.g. ephedrine) and pethidine.

- Newer drugs such as moclobemide are reversible inhibitors that are relatively selective for MAO-A.

---

that is extremely toxic to the liver. Tranylcypromine, pargyline, clorgyline and deprenyl are not hydrazine derivatives, but are derived from the cyclization of the side-chains of amphetamines.

MAOIs are readily absorbed after oral ingestion. There are no parenteral preparations. Maximum inhibition of MAO takes 5–10 days to develop, with a peak therapeutic effect in 2 weeks. MAOIs are metabolized to an active metabolite and acetylated in the liver.

MAOIs act by inhibition of MAO located in mitrochondrial membranes in nerve terminals, the liver and other organs. MAO, which is present in nearly all tissues, catalyses the oxidative deamination of multiple monoamines, including the catecholamines and 5-HT. There are two subtypes of MAO: MAO-A has a substrate preference for 5-HT and is the main target for the anti-depressive MAOIs, and MAO-B preferentially catalyses phenylethylamine and other nonpolar aromatic amines. Both subtypes deaminate noradrenaline and dopamine. Most of the current drugs inhibit both subtypes. The first generation of MAOIs (e.g. phenelazine, tranyl-cypromanine and iproniazid) irreversibly inhibit MAO-A and, because the formation of new enzyme is a slow process, their actions persist for up to 2 weeks after they are stopped. Newer drugs such as clorgyline are reversible, MAO-A-selective, inhibitors. The increased concentration of monoamines in the central nervous system is thought to be responsible for the elevation in mood. MAOIs also cause a decrease in REM sleep and have been used for the management of narcolepsy.

Side-effects of MAOIs include agitation, hallucinations, constipation, fatigue, dry mouth, blurred vision, dizziness, vertigo, tremors, insomnia, hyper-reflexia, hyperpyrexia, hyperhidrosis and convulsions. The hydrazine derivatives can cause hepatotoxicity. The side-effects associated with anaesthesia are largely associated with the cardiovascular toxicity.[3,4] The most common cardiovascular side-effect is orthostatic hypo-tension. Hypertensive crisis has also been reported during anaesthesia. This is largely associated with the concomitant administration of exogenous catecholamines. The administration of indirectly acting amines such as amphetamines, tyramine or ephedrine are the most unpredictable in their response as degradation of monoamines at the nerve terminal is inhibited. Directly acting catecholamines are inactivated by catechol-α-methyltransferase and are more predictable in their response than the indirectly acting catecholamines.

Historically in anaesthesia the recommendations have been to discontinue MAOIs for 2–3 weeks before elective surgery. This recommendation was based on a concern regarding hypertensive crisis and the possible need for indirectly acting catecholamines during anaesthesia. Hyperpyrexia and hypertension have been observed with the use of pethidine and MAOIs. Although anaesthetics have been administered successfully to patients receiving MAOIs[5] and preoperative recommendations have become relative rather than absolute, concern and controversy persist regarding this topic.

SELECTIVE SEROTONIN-REUPTAKE INHIBITORS

The selective serotonin-reuptake inhibitors (SSRIs) act by inhibition of neuronal serotonin (5-HT) reuptake, resulting in an increased concentration of synaptic 5-HT. These drugs are not necessarily more effective than tricyclic antidepressants or MAOIs, but are better tolerated by patients as they have fewer anticholinergic and cardiovascular side-effects.

The toxicity and side-effects of the SSRI antidepressants have not been described fully, as experience with them is limited. Detailed reports regarding interactions with general anaesthetics are not available. Administration of methohexitone for electroconvulsive therapy to a patient on paroxetine therapy has been reported to cause a spontaneous seizure.[6] This finding, if supported by other studies, may indicate caution with the concomitant use of other drugs that lower the seizure threshold, or neurosurgical procedures that increase seizure activity, in patients receiving SSRIs.

Summary box 8.5 Selective serotonin-reuptake inhibitors

- Lack autonomic side-effects of tricyclics.

- Main side-effects are gastrointestinal: nausea, vomiting, diarrhoea and constipation.

- Especially useful in patients with cardiovascular disease.

SSRIs and their metabolites are inhibitors of the CYP3A subgroup of human cytochrome P450 enzymes.[7] CYP3A enzymes metabolize several drugs used in anaesthesia, including midazolam and the fentanyl group of opioids. An increased pharmacological effect may be expected when these drugs are given to patients on SSRIs. Fluvoxamine and paroxetine are also potent inhibitors of CYP2D6.[8] Formation of the hepatotoxic metabolite after paracetamol overdose is mediated by CYP2D6 and administration of fluvoxamine has been proposed as treatment of this condition.

LITHIUM SALTS

The lithium salts, lithium carbonate and lithium citrate, are used in the management of manic disorders. Lithium is a monovalent cation and is readily absorbed from the gastrointestinal tract. The drug is almost completely eliminated by the kidneys with an elimination half-life of 20–24 h. Interestingly, little if any effect is observed when lithium is administered to a normal human, although its effects on agitation and mania are well established. The mechanism of its action is poorly understood. Lithium inhibits neuronal release of noradrenaline and dopamine (Figs 8.1 and 8.2), and alters the reuptake and presynaptic storage mechanisms. It also inhibits the hydrolysis of inositol-1-phosphate, resulting in a decrease in the second messengers inositol triphosphate and diacylglyceride and a decreased responsiveness of neurons to muscarinic–cholinergic, α-adrenergic and other stimuli.

Lithium causes a number of toxic effects. These include vomiting and diarrhoea, tremors, ataxia, confusion, seizure, cardiac arrhythmias, coma and death. Long-term administration of lithium has a renal effect which begins with sodium and water retention with an associated oedematous state. Later, polydipsia and polyuraemia develop and appear to be similar to nephrogenic diabetes. This is probably related to inhibition of antidiuretic hormone or adenylyl cyclase, enhancing reabsorption of water from the distal convoluted tubules and collecting ducts. Because of the narrow therapeutic window and the risk of toxicity, it is essential to monitor peak and trough plasma concentrations routinely to ensure nontoxic levels. The effective plasma concentration is 0.75–1.25 mEq l^{-1}, with toxicity occurring at peak levels.

Lithium has been associated with delayed recovery from neuromuscular blocking agents used during general anaesthesia,[9] possibly due to inhibition of acetylcholine synthesis and release. Lithium is chemically similar to sodium, but is removed from the cell very slowly compared with sodium, and by replacing sodium during cellular depolarization it may interfere with the action potential by inhibiting the reestablishment of the membrane potential. Cardiac arrhythmias, including conduction abnormalities and ST segment and T-wave changes, may occur during general anaesthesia in patients taking lithium salts.

ANTIEPILEPTIC DRUGS

The incidence of epilepsy is approximately 1 in 150, making these heterogeneous disorders rather common. However, the antiepileptic drugs are useful medications for a variety of other disorders, and many patients taking antiepileptic drugs do not have epilepsy. Some common indications are trigeminal neuralgia, bipolar affective disorder, tremor, peripheral pain disorders (e.g. neuropathies), central pain disorders (e.g. spinal cord injury) and migraine.

Although a number of epilepsy syndromes are much more common in the early years of life, the incidence of epilepsy begins to rise dramatically at about age 65 years, and as the population ages the segment of the population at risk expands. In addition, as the usefulness of these drugs for nonepileptic conditions increases, it is reasonable to expect that 1% or more of the population may be taking these drugs.

The implications for anaesthetic care of patients with epilepsy necessarily revolve around the medications they are taking. The direct effects of antiepileptic drugs on anaesthetic care, regardless of the aetiology of the epilepsy, range from the mild and inconsequential to the life threatening.

Toxicity associated with antiepileptic drugs is most frequently manifest by mild, subjective, cognitive impairment. Patients may complain of memory difficulties, poor concentration, fatigue or lethargy. After general anaesthesia, a patient already partially impaired by an antiepileptic drug may be slightly slower to return to cognitive baseline than other patients. None the less, it is not recommended to discontinue antiepileptic drugs before anaesthesia. It takes days or weeks, and occasionally months, to taper off antiepileptic drugs safely. In addition to the time required, stopping or reducing the dose of these drugs puts the patient at risk of increased seizures.

Summary box 8.6 Lithium

- Used in manic-depressive illness.

- Therapeutic and toxic concentrations are similar; plasma concentrations must be measured (therapeutic range 0.4–1.0 mmol l^{-1}).

- Signs of lithium toxicity include drowsiness, ataxia and confusion, and ultimately coma.

SPECIFIC ANTIEPILEPTIC DRUGS

Summary box 8.7 Antiepilepsy drugs

Phenytoin

- Effective in many forms of epilepsy except absence seizures

- Saturable kinetics

- Potent inducer of P450 enzymes – drug interactions are common

- Also used as class 1B antiarrhythmic agents

- Acute administration potentiates nondepolarizing muscle relaxants; chronic administration reduces their action.

Carbamazepine

- Similar profile to phenytoin but fewer unwanted side-effects

- Widely used for disorders other than epilepsy (e.g. trigeminal neuralgia)

- Potent inducer of P450 enzymes; drug interactions are common.

Valproate

- Relatively few serious side-effects; liver damage rare but serious

- May affect platelet aggregation and cause thrombocytopenia

- Can be given intravenously.

Ethosuximide

- Main drug for treatment of absence seizures, but may exacerbate other forms

- Interactions with nondepolarizing muscle relaxants similar to phenytoin

- Relatively few side-effects, mainly nausea and vomiting.

Phenobarbitone

- Mainly used as secondary drug

- Highly sedative

- Potent inducer of P450 enzymes.

Benzodiazepines

- Not used for primary treatment

- Used to treat status epilepticus.

Barbiturates

The most widely used barbituric acid derivatives for the treatment of epilepsy are phenobarbitone and primidone. Owing to prominent sedative effects, their use is declining, as equally efficacious, less sedating drugs become widely available. Although primidone has anticonvulsant effects of its own, it is metabolized to phenobarbitone and a weakly active metabolite, phenylethylmalonamide. The efficacy and toxicity profiles of the drugs are similar. Primidone has no clear advantage over phenobarbitone and, because it is liable to produce hypersensitivity reactions, it is now seldom used.

Acute administration of phenobarbitone potentiates nondepolarizing neuromuscular blockade while chronic administration (typically the case in clinical practice) may induce resistance to block.[10] Phenobarbitone may increase the rate of liver injury in patients anaesthetized with halothane.[11] This may be related to induction of cytochrome P450 enzymes. Patients started on phenobarbitone acutely before surgery are more likely to be sedated, and recovery from anaesthesia may be expected to be somewhat prolonged.

Hydantoins

Introduced in 1938, phenytoin remains one of the mainstays of therapy for epilepsy. Related compounds are mephenytoin and ethotoin, but their use is very limited. Phenytoin is indicated for the treatment of partial epilepsy. Although oral bioavailability is high (about 90%), occasional patients are either poor absorbers or rapid metabolizers (or both). Phenytoin has a narrow therapeutic window, with effective plasma concentrations in the range 10–20 mg l^{-1}; some patients may manifest signs of toxicity with concentrations as low as 5–6 mg l^{-1}. Phenytoin hepatic metabolism is readily saturable so that pharmacokinetics can become nonlinear in the therapeutic concentration range, and elimination follows Michaelis–Menton kinetics. This means that small increments in the dose can produce unexpectedly high plasma concentrations, since the half-life increases as the dose is increased. Failure to appreciate this can easily lead to overdose. The metabolism of phenytoin can be induced by other anticonvulsants and is inhibited by a large number of drugs, including the tricyclic antidepressants and isoniazid. Phenytoin itself is a potent inducer of cytochrome P450 enzymes and thus increases the metabolism of other drugs, such as oral anticoagulants and contraceptives.

Like phenobarbitone, acute administration of phenytoin may potentiate nondepolarizing muscle relaxants,[12] while chronic ingestion may reduce their action.[13] Patients 'prophylactically loaded' with phenytoin before surgery (e.g. neurosurgical patients) may have an unexpectedly prolonged response to muscle relaxants. These effects are probably related to the membrane-stabilizing properties of the drug, inhibiting voltage-sensitive Na^+ channels and possibly also an effect on Ca^{2+} channels. These properties account for its class 1B antiarrhythmic actions (see Chapter 14). Inhibition of Na^+ and Ca^{2+} channels is also responsible for its anticonvulsant actions.

Orally administered phenytoin generally causes few cardiovascular effects unless the patient has severe underlying cardiac disease. Intravenous administration, however, can have potentially catastrophic haemodynamic results. Phenytoin is almost insoluble in water and intravenous formulations contain propylene glycol, sodium hydroxide and ethanol. Intravenous phenytoin should be given slowly, under ECG control. Because of the high pH of the solution (pH 12) it must be diluted with physiological saline, not glucose or dextrose. Phenytoin solutions must not be mixed with other drugs because of the risk of precipitation of phenytoin crystals. While hypotension is the most likely potential complication of intravenous phenytoin infusion, especially at rates above 50 mg min^{-1}, severe cardiac electrical disturbances may occur. Local phlebitis may occur at the site of injection, and if extravasation into perivascular tissues occurs the patient may suffer ischaemic compromise of the distal limb. When this local reaction causes limb vascular insult, it has been termed the 'purple glove syndrome'. Treatment of the purple glove syndrome begins with evaluation of the adequacy of distal circulation, warming and slight elevation of the limb, and consultation with an orthopaedic surgeon; rarely fasciotomy may be required to reduce the risk of ischaemic tissue necrosis due to a compartment syndrome.

Because of the many problems of intravenous phenytoin, fosphenytoin, a phosphorylated ester prodrug, has been developed. Esterification of a phosphate group increases solubility, causes fewer side-effects and permits intramuscular administration. The phosphorus-containing group is cleaved to yield phenytoin in the blood; the half-life of this process is 8–12 min on intravenous administration, and about twice that on intramuscular administration.[14] Serious side-effects of fosphenytoin are much less common, but do include mild hypotension and transient itching, especially in the perineal area.

Carbamazepine

Carbamazepine is chemically related to the tricyclic antidepressants, being structurally similar to imipramine. It is widely used for partial epilepsy, and is generally well tolerated and effective. It is also widely used for its mood-stabilizing effects. Of all the antiepileptic drugs, carbamazepine is the most frequently used for disorders other than epilepsy. Carbamazepine is a mainstay of treatment for trigeminal neuralgia, and is also used in a variety of painful central and peripheral neurological disorders. In general, the anticonvulsant profile of carbamazepine is similar to that of phenytoin. It is currently available only in oral formulation, although attempts have been made to develop a parenteral formulation. Two oral forms are available: a rapid absorption formulation and a newer sustained-release formulation.

Carbamazepine's mechanism of action is not entirely understood. Modulation of Na^+ channel function, particularly rapid repetitive firing, possibly accounts for a portion of its anticonvulsant effect. Recent studies have linked carbamazepine to the so-called peripheral-type benzodiazepine receptor.[15] Action at a benzodiazepine receptor may explain the occasionally prominent withdrawal effects on abrupt cessation of carbamazepine. This may be important in patients who have been switched abruptly from carbamazepine to another antiepileptic drug (usually one with a parenteral formulation) before operation.

A significant portion of carbamazepine is metabolized to carbamazepine-10, 11-epoxide, which is thought to cause a disproportionate number of side-effects, although it does possess anticonvulsant properties. Oxcarbazepine, a carbamazepine derivative, is not metabolized to carbamazepine-10, 1 l-epoxide. Clinical effectiveness, side-effects and toxicity are otherwise similar to those of carbamazepine. The half-life is about 20 h after starting medication, but drops to about 12 h after 2–4 weeks of administration, due largely to induction of hepatic microsomal enzymes.

Like the tricyclic antidepressants, carbamazepine can interfere with intracardiac conduction, and even modest doses may cause sinus bradycardia, sinus pauses, Stokes–Adams attacks and total atrioventricular block. Hence, patients taking carbamazepine should be considered at higher risk than average for developing cardiac conduction abnormalities during anaesthesia. Like other antiepileptic drugs, carbamazepine interacts with nondepolarizing muscle relaxants, although mivacurium does not seem to be affected.[16,17]

Carbamazepine can induce hyponatraemia and water retention. This is more prominent in the elderly and with higher doses, but can occur even with modest doses. Evidence suggests that both central (hypothalamic) and peripheral (renal) processes may cause this. Fluid management of the patient taking carbamazepine during anaesthesia should be undertaken with the understanding that the patient is essentially taking an antidiuretic.

Valproate

Valproate (valproic acid) is widely used for both partial onset and primary generalized onset epilepsy. It is also used for prophylaxis of migraine headache and bipolar affective disorder. Like many antiepileptic drugs, its mechanism of action is incompletely understood.

Although it is a branched-chain fatty acid, valproate is 90% protein bound to albumin, keeping most of the drug in the vascular compartment (Table 8.3). Metabolism is mainly hepatic and thus valproate should be used cautiously in patients with impaired hepatic function. Like many other antiepileptic drugs, it can induce its own metabolism. An intravenous formulation is available which can be used before surgery, or in patients receiving the oral drug but in whom oral administration is temporarily not indicated. It can be given either as a single injection or as a continuous intravenous infusion at a dose comparable to that used orally. For other patients in whom intravenous administration is indicated, the recommended intravenous dose is 400–800 mg (approximately 10 mg kg^{-1}) injected slowly over 3–5 min followed by either repeated injections or continuous infusion to a maximum dose of 2500 mg per day. Intravenous valproate

does not cause significant hypotension or cardiac arrhythmias.

Valproate may affect platelet aggregation in some patients, and thrombocytopenia has been reported in children. However, significant alteration in haemostasis or intraoperative blood loss due to valproate has not been demonstrated.[18,19] Current data do not support withdrawal of valproate before surgery as a putative prophylaxis against excessive bleeding. Like the other antiepileptic drugs, valproate appears to hasten recovery from neuromuscular blockade when administered chronically, and to delay recovery when administered acutely.[20]

Ethosuximide

Ethosuximide is most frequently used for so-called 'typical absence epilepsy', which is seen in children, usually before the age of 12 years. The drug, available only as an oral formulation, is well absorbed. The main side-effects are gastrointestinal, especially nausea, but sedation and headaches also occur. There are no clear reports of unusual interactions or toxicity with anaesthetic agents. As with many of the other antiepileptic drugs, chronic treatment appears to hasten recovery from neuromuscular blockade, whereas acute treatment has the opposite effect.

Newer antiepileptic drugs

In recent years a number of newer antiepileptic drugs

Table 8.3 Pharmacology of commonly used antiepileptic drugs						
Drug	Parenteral formulation	Half-life (h)	V_d (l kg^{-1})	Protein bound (%)	Effect on neuromuscular blockade	Special precautions
Phenobarbitone	Yes	80–120	0.75	50	Chronic ↓ Acute ↑	Respiratory depression. Increased risk of halothane hepatotoxicity
Primidone	No	5–15	0.75	Minimal	Chronic ↓ Acute ↑	Metabolized to phenobarbitone
Phenytoin	Yes	18–22	0.8	90	Chronic ↓ Acute ↑	Consider use of fosphenytoin to avoid haemodynamic and local complications
Carbamazepine	No	12–20	0.8–2	75	Chronic ↓ Acute ↑	Affects cardiac conduction. May lower plasma Na$^+$ concentration. Can have marked withdrawal syndrome
Valproate	Yes	9	0.15	90	Chronic ↓ Acute ↑	P450 enzyme inhibitor; increased risk of hepatotoxicity
Ethosuximide	No	29	0.6	Minimal	Chronic: effect not well known Acute ↑	Used primarily for absence seizures (petit mal)

has become available. These include felbamate, lamotrigine, gabapentin, topiramate, zonisamide and vigabatrin. In addition, tiagabine, flunarizine, remacemide, rufinamide, losigamone, ganaxolone and progabide may become available for use in epilepsy. Cinnarizine and its fluorinated derivative, flunarizine, block excessive calcium flux in muscle cells and neurons, and are used primarily to treat vertigo and migraine. There is little information about the effects of these newer drugs in relation to anaesthesia. Until further work is done, it is safest to assume that they will have detrimental effects on anaesthesia. Specifically, it is probably prudent to assume that they will enhance neuromuscular blockade with acute administration; reduce blockade with chronic administration; enhance recovery from general anaesthesia with chronic administration; and increase the likelihood of toxic anaesthetic reactions (e.g. hepatic toxicity).

OTHER CONSIDERATIONS IN ANAESTHESIA

Care of the patient with epilepsy includes consideration of the possibility of a seizure before, during or after anaesthesia. The expected motor manifestations will appear in the absence of neuromuscular block. However, if neuromuscular blocking agents have been used, one may observe only the autonomic manifestations of the seizure, typically abrupt tachycardia and hypertension. In some patients, however, seizures may present with bradycardia, asystole or other cardiac rhythm disturbances.[21] Because the average seizure lasts approximately 2 min, it is wisest to wait and observe for a period of time, rather than administer drugs to reduce blood pressure or heart rate.

REFERENCES

1. Safra MJ, Oakley GP Jr. Association between cleft lip with or without cleft palate and prenatal exposure to diazepam. *Lancet* 1975; **ii**: 478–480.

2. Edwards RP, Miller RD, Roizen MF *et al*. Cardiac responses to imipramine and pancuronium during anesthesia with halothane or enflurane. *Anesthesiology* 1979; **50**: 421–425.

3. Stack CG, Rogers P, Linter SPK. Monoamine oxidase inhibitors and anaesthesia. *Br J Anaesth* 1988; **60**: 222–227.

4. Wells DG, Bjorksten AR. Monoamine oxidase inhibitors revisited. *Can J Anaesth* 1989; **36**: 64–74.

5. O'Hara JF, Maurer WG, Smith MP. Sufentanil–isoflurane–nitrous oxide anesthesia for a patient treated with monoamine oxidase inhibitor and tricyclic antidepressant. *J Clin Anesth* 1995; **7**: 148–150.

6. Folkerts H. Spontaneous seizure after concurrent use of methohexital anesthesia for electroconvulsive therapy and paroxetine: a case report. *J Nerv Ment Dis* 1995; **183**: 115–116.

7. von Moltke LL, Greenblatt DJ, Schmider J, Harmatz JS, Shader RI. Metabolism of drugs by cytochrome P450 3A isoforms. Implications for drug interactions in psychopharmacology. *Clin Pharmacokinet* 1995; **29** (Suppl. 1): 33–44.

8. Brøsen K. Drug interactions and the cytochrome P450 system. The role of cytochrome P450 1A2. *Clin Pharmacokinet* 1995; **29** (Suppl. 1): 20–25.

9. Hill GE, Wong KC, Hodges MR. Lithium carbonate and neuromuscular blocking agents. *Anesthesiology* 1977; **46**: 122–126.

10. Hans P, Ledoux D, Bonhomme V, Brichant JF. Effect of plasma anticonvulsant level on pipecuronium-induced neuromuscular blockade: preliminary results. *J Neurosurg Anesth* 1995; **7**: 254–258.

11. Nomura F, Hatano H, Ohnishi K, Akikusa B, Okuda K. Effects of anticonvulsant agents on halothane-induced liver injury in human subjects and experimental animals. *Hepatology* 1986; **6**: 952–956.

12. Gray HS, Slater RM, Pollard BJ. The effect of acutely administered phenytoin on vecuronium-induced neuromuscular blockade. *Anaesthesia* 1989; **44**: 379–381.

13. Ornstein E, Matteo RS, Weinstein JA *et al*. Accelerated recovery from doxacurium-induced neuromuscular blockade in patients receiving chronic anticonvulsant therapy. *J Clin Anesth* 1991; **3**: 108–111.

14. Boucher BA. Fosphenytoin: a novel phenytoin prodrug. *Pharmacotherapy* 1996; **16**: 777–792.

15. Weiss SRB, Post RM. Contingent tolerance to carbamazepine: a peripheral-type benzodiazepine mechanism. *Eur J Pharmacol* 1991; **193**: 159–163.

16. Alloul K, Whalley DG, Shutway F, Ebrahim Z, Varin F. Pharmacokinetic origin of carbamazepine-induced resistance to vecuronium neuromuscular blockade in anesthetized patients. *Anesthesiology* 1996; **84**: 330–339.

17. Spacek A, Neiger FX, Spiss CK, Kress HG. Chronic carbamazepine therapy does not influence mivacurium-induced neuromuscular block. *Br J Anaesth* 1996; **77**: 500–502.

18. Winter SL, Kriel RL, Novacheck TF *et al*. Perioperative blood loss: the effect of valproate. *Pediatr Neurol* 1996; **15**: 19–22.

19. Ward MW, Barbaro NM, Laxer KD, Rampil IJ. Preoperative valproate administration does not increase blood loss during temporal lobectomy. *Epilepsia* 1996; **37**: 98–101.

20. Jellish WS, Modica PA, Tempelhoff R. Accelerated recovery from pipecuronium in patients treated with chronic anticonvulsant therapy. *J Clin Anesth* 1993; **5**: 105–108.

21. Reeves AL, Nollet KE, Klass DW, Sharbrough FW, So EL. The ictal bradycardia syndrome. *Epilepsia* 1996; **37**: 983–987.

Section 3
DRUGS ACTING ON THE PERIPHERAL NERVOUS SYSTEM

9

E Samain, J Marty

PHARMACOLOGY OF THE AUTONOMIC NERVOUS SYSTEM

The autonomic nervous system (ANS) is involved in the regulation of a wide variety of automatic functions and plays a major role in the physiological adaptation of the body to stress and exercise. The ANS is divided into the sympathetic and parasympathetic nervous systems, which act as physiological counterbalances. Consequently, the functioning of organs controlled by the ANS represents the balance of the influence of each component. Understanding the physiology and the pharmacology of the ANS is essential for anaesthetists.[1]

AUTONOMIC NERVOUS SYSTEM ANATOMY

Afferent pathways to the ANS provide sensory information from nociceptors, chemoreceptors and mecanoreceptors in organs or in vascular walls, to sympathetic and parasympathetic integration centres located along the cerebrospinal axis. The cerebral cortex represents the highest level of ANS integration, and autonomic function can be modulated by cortical influences. The hypothalamus contains most of the integration centres of the ANS, and hypothalamic nuclei are involved in long-term regulation of blood pressure and the reaction to stress, and water regulation, through connections to the pituitary. The nucleus tractus solitarius, located in the medulla, is a primary integration area for information coming from baroreceptors and the hypothalamus. It is involved in the short-term regulation of blood pressure, through adjustments of vascular tone.

Both sympathetic and parasympathetic efferent pathways comprise two-neuron chains: a preganglionic myelinated neuron from the ANS centres relays in an ANS ganglion with a postganglionic unmyelinated neuron. Sympathetic ganglia are close to the central integration centres. In contrast, body cells of parasympathetic postganglionic neurons are located near or within effector organs (Fig. 9.1). Thus, each preganglionic sympathetic neuron can influence 10 times more postganglionic neurons than its parasympathetic counterpart. This is consistent with the diffuse physiological response produced by sympathetic activation compared with the limited and discrete effect of parasympathetic function (Table 9.1).

SYMPATHETIC NERVOUS SYSTEM ANATOMY

Fig. 9.2 shows the organization of the sympathetic nervous system and its innervation of effector organs. Cell bodies of preganglionic sympathetic neurons are located in the intermediolateral grey horn of the thoracic (T1–T12) and the first three lumbar (L1–L3) segments of the spinal cord. Myelinated axons of these cells leave the spinal cord and enter one of the 22 pairs of ganglia of the paravertebral sympathetic chain. In the paravertebral chain, preganglionic axons can: (1) synapse with postganglionic neurons; (2) exit without synapsing in the paravertebral chain and terminate in a collateral ganglion, such as the coeliac and inferior mesenteric ganglia; and (3) pass upward or downward in the chain to synapse with postganglionic neurons at another level. Postganglionic unmyelinated C-type fibres exit from paravertebral ganglia to innervate blood vessels, sweat glands and piloerector muscles. Their distribution is similar to somatic sensory distribution but, because of significant overlap in distribution, a sensitive dermatome can receive sympathetic

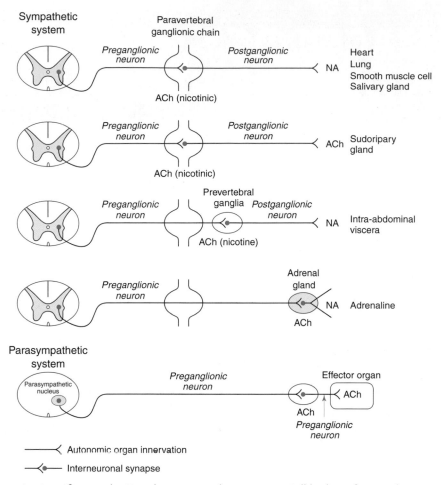

Fig. 9.1 Bipolar organization of sympathetic and parasympathetic system. Cell bodies of sympathetic preganglionic neurons are located in the intermediolateral grey horn of the spinal cord. Parasympathetic nuclei are located in the brainstem and in the second to fourth sacral segments of spinal cord. ACh, acetylcholine; NA, noradrenaline.

innervation from three or four spinal cord segments. Each postganglionic neuron has several nerve endings and thus can release noradrenaline at numerous different sites. The adrenal glands, however, receive direct innervation from preganglionic neurons originating from the fifth to ninth thoracic segments.

PARASYMPATHETIC NERVOUS SYSTEM ANATOMY

Parasympathetic preganglionic fibres arise from nuclei located in the brainstem and from the second to fourth sacral segments of the spinal cord. The third, seventh and ninth cranial nerves supply parasympathetic innervation for the eyes, lacrymal and salivary glands. The vagus nerve innervates the heart, tracheobronchial tree and intraabdominal organs, except for the distal part of the colon. The sacral preganglionic fibres provide parasympathetic innervation of the distal colon and genitourinary organs.

NEUROTRANSMITTERS IN THE ANS

Acetylcholine (ACh) is the neurotransmitter of all parasympathetic nerves and of preganglionic sympathetic nerves, including fibres innervating the adrenal glands, by stimulation of nicotinic and not muscarinic receptors (Fig. 9.1). Postganglionic sympathetic nerves release noradrenaline, except for fibres innervating sweat glands which secrete ACh. Chromaffin cells in the adrenal medulla synthesize noradrenaline and adrenaline. Stimulation of the preganglionic nerves to the adrenal glands induces the release of large amounts of a mixture of adrenaline and noradrenaline, which act as neurotransmitter hormones.

Table 9.1 Effects of sympathetic and parasympathetic nervous system activation and type of receptor involved in the observed effect

Effector	Location	Sympathetic stimulation (adrenergic receptor)	Parasympathetic stimulation (muscarinic receptors)
Heart	Sinus node Atrioventricular node His–Purkinje Cardiomyocytes Coronary arteries	Increase in automaticity (β_1) Increase in conduction (β_1) Increase in conduction and automaticity (β_1) Increase in contractility (β_1) Increase in conduction, automaticity (β_1) Arteriolar vasodilatation (β_1) Arteriolar vasoconstriction (α_1)	Decreased automaticity (M_2) Decreased conduction (M_2) Minimal effect Slight decrease in contractility (M_2) ?
Blood vessels	Systemic circulation Pulmonary circulation	Vasoconstriction (α_1) Vasodilatation (β_2) Vasoconstriction (α_1)	Vasodilatation (M_3) Vasodilatation?
Bronchial tree	Bronchial muscles Bronchial secretion	Relaxation (β_2) Decrease (β_2)	Constriction (M_3) Increase (M_3)
Gut	Gallbladder Gastrointestinal tract	Relaxation (β_2) Decrease in motility (β_2) Sphincter constriction (α_1)	Contraction (M_3) Increase in motility (M_3) Sphincter relaxation (M_3)
Bladder	Detrusor Sphincter – trigone	Relaxation (β_2) Contraction (α_1)	Contraction (M_3) Relaxation (M_3)
Glands	Sweat Lacrimal Gastrointestinal glands	Increase secretions (neurotransmitter: ACh) Decrease secretions (α_1) Decrease secretions (α_1)	0 Increase secretions (M_3) Increase secretions (M_3)
Eye	Iris	Mydriasis	Myosis
Uterus	Uterine muscle	Contraction (α_1), relaxation (β_2)	0

ADRENERGIC NEUROTRANSMISSION: CATECHOLAMINES

Catecholamine synthesis

Catecholamines are composed of a catechol nucleus and an amine-containing side chain (Fig. 9.3). The endogenous catecholamines involved in sympathetic neurotransmission in humans are noradrenaline, the transmitter of most sympathetic postganglionic fibres, and adrenaline, the major hormone of the adrenal gland. Dopamine, also an endogenous catecholamine, is the neurotransmitter of the extrapyramidal system and other mesolimbic and mesocortical neurons. Some of the chromaffin cells of the adrenal medulla, the physiological 'equivalent' of postganglionic neurons, secrete noradrenaline but most (80%) secrete adrenaline.

Synthesis of noradrenaline occurs in the sympathetic nerve endings or in vesicles near the cell body that subsequently move to the nerve endings (Fig. 9.3). Briefly, L-phenylalanine is hydroxylated to L-tyrosine, which is then converted to L-3,4-dihydroxyphenylalanine (L-Dopa). This reaction is the rate-limiting step in the synthesis of noradrenaline. Stimulation of adrenergic nerves or adrenal glands activates tyrosine hydroxylase through a kinase-catalysed phosphorylation, and gene expression of the enzyme is increased. These two mechanisms maintain the catecholamine content of the vesicles constant during adrenergic stimulation. L-Dopa and the following molecules in the synthesis cascade are catecholamines. L-Dopa is decarboxylated to dopamine, the precursor of noradrenaline and adrenaline.

Noradrenaline is stored in synaptic vesicles for subsequent release in response to membrane depolarization by an action potential. The entry of calcium into the cell is important in coupling the electrical impulse to migration of the synaptic vesicles to the surface and their exocytosis into the extracellular

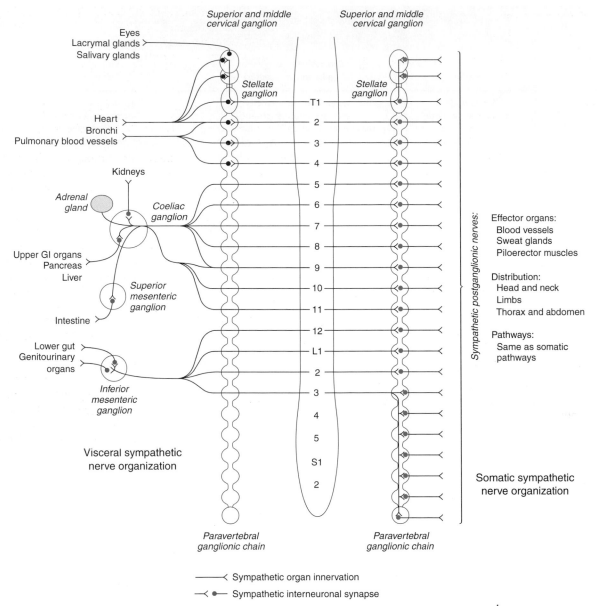

Fig. 9.2 Schematic representation of the organization of the peripheral sympathetic nervous system. Nerves innervating blood vessels, sweat glands and piloerector muscles that pass in the somatic skeletal muscle nerves (right side) have been separated from nerves innervating the head, intrathoracic and intraabdominal organs (left side). GI, gastrointestinal.

fluid (Fig. 9.4). The action of noradrenaline released into the synaptic cleft is very brief, reflecting the efficiency of termination pathways. Much of noradrenaline is taken up into the nerve terminal for recycling; the remainder diffuses from sympathetic receptors and is then diluted in the junctional fluid or is catabolized.

Two active transport systems are responsible for the reuptake of noradrenaline: one is involved in reuptake into the cytoplasm of the nerve ending and the second

in transporting noradrenaline into the synaptic vesicle. This reuptake provides a major source of noradrenaline to the nerve ending in addition to synthesis. It can be blocked by several compounds, namely cocaine and tricyclic antidepressants. Noradrenaline can also be taken up into non-neuronal tissue (heart, blood vessels). Enzymatic breakdown and diffusion of noradrenaline are of minor importance in terminating its action. Noradrenaline is metabolized by catechol-O-methyltransferase (COMT) and monoamine oxidase (MAO).

Molecules structures   Enzymatic cascade

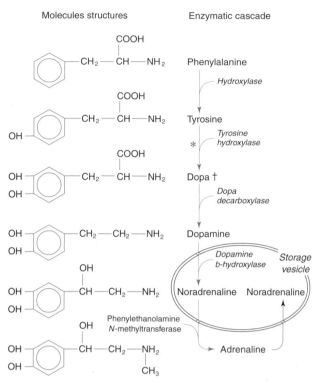

Fig. 9.3 Molecular structures and enzymatic cascade of catecholamine synthesis. *Rate-limiting step; †Dopa: L-3,4-dihydroxyphenylalanine.

The primary metabolite of MAO and COMT, 3-methoxy-4-hydroxymandelic acid, is excreted in the urine. Inhibition of MAO causes an increase in tissue concentrations of noradrenaline and produces an antidepressant effect. Inhibition of COMT does not have significant pharmacological effects.

CHOLINERGIC NEUROTRANSMISSION

ACh is the neurotransmitter for all preganglionic autonomic fibres, all postganglionic parasympathetic nerves and the postganglionic sympathetic fibres that innervate sweat glands. It is synthesized in cholinergic nerve endings by acetylation of choline with acetyl coenzyme A and stored in presynaptic vesicles, each containing approximately 10^4 molecules of ACh. An action potential triggers a massive release of ACh. The shape of the synapse is such that most ACh comes into contact with acetylcholinesterase (AChE), the enzyme responsible for its hydrolysis, before reaching the postsynaptic receptor sites. In 'fast' cholinergic synapses such as in autonomic ganglia, where AChE is concentrated in the presynaptic terminals, ACh is hydrolysed within 1 ms by AChE, so that a presynaptic action potential produces only one postsynaptic action potential. In contrast, transmission mediated at nicotinic receptors, such as the neuromuscular junction, is much slower. ACh which is not degraded by AChE binds to the postsynaptic receptors, generating an excitatory postsynaptic potential. The transient nature of this event is caused by the rapid degradation of ACh by AChE.

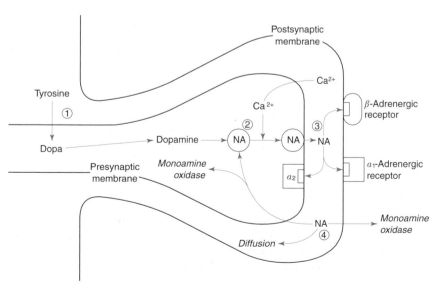

Fig. 9.4 Functional representation of an adrenergic synapse. 1, Noradrenaline (NA) synthesis and storage in synaptic vesicles; 2, NA is released in synaptic cleft in response to electrical depolarization of the cell membrane; 3, coupling of NA with the receptors; 4, NA reuptake or metabolism (see text for further details).

ANS RECEPTORS

ADRENERGIC RECEPTORS

Adrenergic receptors are classified into two main classes: α and β adrenoceptors, each with several subclasses. The rank order of potency of agonists for α receptors is adrenaline $\geq$ noradrenaline >> isoprenaline, and for β receptors isoprenaline > adrenaline $\geq$ noradrenaline.[2] Adrenaline is equipotent with noradrenaline at β_1 receptors but 10–50-fold more potent than noradrenaline at β_2 receptors. Stimulation of postsynaptic α_1 receptors is excitatory. In contrast, stimulation of presynaptic α_2 receptors inhibits noradrenaline release.[3] Some α-adrenergic agonists such as phenylephrine, methoxamine and metaraminol selectively stimulate α_1 receptors and others such as clonidine or mivazerol are more potent agonists at α_2 than α_1 receptors. While α_1 and β_1 receptors located on postsynaptic sympathetic junctions are responsible for activating sympathetic nerve responses, α_2 and β_2 receptors, which are more sensitive to circulating catecholamines, are considered autoreceptors, participating in the autofeedback loop to regulate release of noradrenaline.

Distribution of adrenergic receptors

Molecular cloning techniques have identified nine subtypes of adrenergic receptors (α_{1A}, α_{1B}, α_{1D}, α_{2A}, α_{2B}, α_{2C} and β_1, β_2, β_3), although the function of all these subtypes is not yet known.[2] Individual response to β-adrenergic stimulation depends on the distribution and density of β_1 and β_2 receptors. β_1 Receptors are located mainly on the heart where they are involved in the cardiac effect of adrenergic stimulation. β_2 Receptors are located mainly on the smooth muscle cells and other sites (Table 9.2). Recent studies with radiolabelled ligand have shown that both types of β receptor may coexist on each tissue. β_3 Receptors, tenfold more sensitive to noradrenaline than to adrenaline, have been isolated and the gene encoding them has been identified. They are found at unique sites such as in brown adipose tissue and the gall-

	α_1-Adrenergic	**α_2-Adrenergic**	**β_1-Adrenergic**	**β_2-Adrenergic**
Location	Ganglionic synapses Smooth muscle cells of vascular tree GI tract, urinary bladder Lacrimal and GI glands	Heart Platelets Adipose tissue CNS	Heart Adipose tissue Liver	Smooth muscle cells of vascular tree GI tract Bronchial tree Urinary bladder
Agonist	Noradrenaline Adrenaline Isoprenaline Dopamine Ephedrine (indirect) Phenylephrine Methoxamine	Noradrenaline Adrenaline Clonidine Dexmetomidine Mivazerol Lofexidine	Noradrenaline Adrenaline Isoprenaline Dopamine Ephedrine (indirect) Dobutamine Salbutamol (weak) Prenalterol	Adrenaline Isoprenaline Dopamine Ephedrine (indirect) Dobutamine Salbutamol Terbutaline Isoxyme Ritodrine Fenoterol
Antagonist	Phenoxybenzamine Phentolamine Tolazoline Piperoxan Labetalol Bucindolol Prazosin Doxazosin Indoranium Urapidil (also 5-HT agonist)	Phenoxybenzamine Phentolamine Tolazoline Piperoxan Yohimbine Idazoxam Rauwolscine	Propranodol Oxprenolol (ISA) Sotalol Alprenolol (ISA) Labetalol Bucindolol Metoprolol Esmolol (ultrashort-acting) Atenolol	Propranodol Oxprenolol (ISA) Sotalol Alprenolol (ISA) Labetalol

GI, gastrointestinal; CNS, central nervous system; 5-HT, 5-hydroxytryptamine; ISA, intrinsic sympathetic activity.

bladder. Their precise role remains unclear, but they may mediate responses to adrenergic stimulation in adipose tissue, promoting lipolysis and heat generation.

Molecular basis of adrenergic receptor function

Adrenergic receptors belong to the large superfamily of receptors coupled to guanine nucleotide-binding proteins (G proteins). Even though catecholamines are hydrophilic molecules, they do not bind to the extracellular terminal of the receptor but instead to the more hydrophobic membrane-spanning domains, forming a ligand-binding pocket. Binding produces a conformational change in the receptor, especially the third intracellular loop that interacts with the G protein (Fig.

9.5). β-Adrenergic receptors couple to a G_s protein, activating adenylyl cyclase, and calcium ion channels in some cells. a_1-Receptors couple to a G_q protein, activating phospholipases, especially phospholipase C_β. G_i proteins linked to a_2 receptors inhibit adenylyl cyclase and also regulate some ion channels.

Regulation of adrenergic receptors

Chronic administration of β-adrenoceptor antagonists without intrinsic sympathetic activity to normal subjects can increase the number of β-adrenergic receptors (receptor upregulation).[4] Discontinuation of treatment can lead to a withdrawal syndrome characterized by systemic and cardiac hyperactivity. Patients with

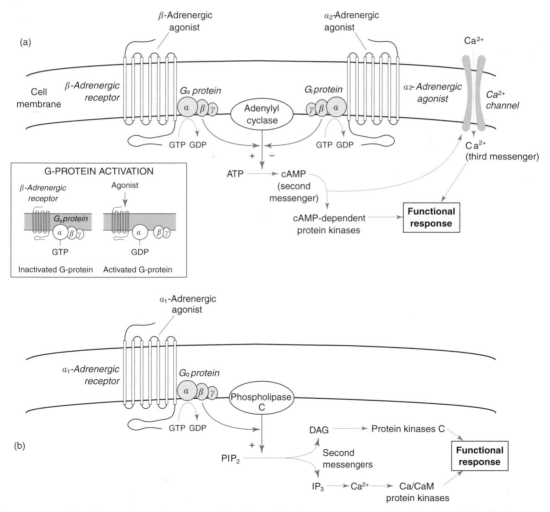

Fig. 9.5 G protein-mediated signal transduction mediated by adrenergic receptors. (a) Occupation of the β-adrenergic receptor coupled to a G_s protein activates adenylyl cyclase and increases production of cyclic adenosine monophosphate (cAMP), whereas activated a_2-adrenergic receptors associate with G_i proteins and inhibit adenylyl cyclase. (b) Activation of a_1-adrenergic receptors induces stimulation of phospholipase C, leading to hydrolysis of phosphatidylinositol biphosphate (PIP$_2$) to diacylglycerol (DAG) and 1,4,5-inositol triphosphate (IP$_3$). GDP, guanosine diphosphate; GTP, guanosine triphosphate; ATP, adenosine triphosphate.

congestive heart failure have increased plasma noradrenaline concentrations and a subsequent reduction in β-adrenoceptor density.[5] β_1 Receptors are selectively downregulated and consequently β_2 receptors become more responsive for the inotropic effects of catecholamines. In these circumstances a_1 receptors may also mediate a positive inotropic effect.[6] Desensitization of adrenergic receptors by agonist administration has been demonstrated for β_2 agonists in asthma and for a agonists during circulatory shock. It is a multistep process, including: (a) phosphorylation of receptors; (b) sequestration of receptors in intracellular compartments; (c) uncoupling of the receptor (decreased formation of second messenger despite persistent binding of the agonist to the receptor); and (d) internalization of the receptor to intracellular sites. A slow decrease in the number of receptors through receptor degradation is also possible after prolonged stimulation by agonists.

DOPAMINE RECEPTORS

Dopamine is a neurotransmitter of major importance in the central nervous system (CNS), and peripheral dopaminergic nerves and dopamine receptors are involved in the regulation of regional blood flow, especially renal blood flow. Dopamine receptors are classified into two subtypes: DA_1 and DA_2. DA_1 Receptors are postsynaptic and are located on arterial smooth muscle cells of the kidney and gastrointestinal tract. Stimulation of DA_1 receptors mediates vasodilatation of renal and mesenteric vessels. DA_2 Receptors are presynaptic and their stimulation may inhibit

peripheral release of noradrenaline and perhaps ACh at sympathetic nerve endings.

CHOLINERGIC RECEPTORS

Cholinergic receptors, present on many ANS synapses, were classified pharmacologically in 1914 by Sir Henry Dale into muscarinic and nicotinic receptors. Nicotinic receptors, sensitive to nicotine and ACh, are located in postganglionic sympathetic and parasympathetic synapses (see Fig. 9.1). Muscarinic receptors are activated selectively by muscarine, the active substance of the poisonous mushroom, *Amanita muscaria*, and blocked by atropine. Five muscarinic receptors subtypes, M_1–M_5, have been identified, encoded by different cellular genes (Table 9.3).[7] They are G protein-coupled receptors. The second messenger of M_1, M_3 and M_5 receptors is phospholipase, while M_2 and M_4 receptors couple negatively to adenylyl cyclase to decrease intracellular cyclic adenosine monophosphate (cAMP) concentration. Stimulation of M_3 receptors located on vascular smooth muscle cells induce an endothelium-dependent vasodilatation, mediated by nitric oxide. Anticholinergic drugs antagonize the effect of ACh at muscarinic postganglionic receptors.

PHARMACOLOGICAL ACTIONS MEDIATED BY ANS RECEPTORS

a_1 Receptors

a_1 Receptors are implicated in constriction of arterial and venular vessels (Table 9.1).[6] They also mediate myocardial contractility, particularly in patients with

Table 9.3 Location and clinical effect of stimulation of muscarinic receptor subtypes					
	M_1	M_2	M_3	M_4	M_5
Receptor sequence	m1	m2	m3	m4	m5
Second messenger	PLC (+)	cAMP (−)	PLC (+)	cAMP (−)	PLC (+)
Location	ANS ganglia Stomach Brainstem, hippocampus	Preganglionic synapses Heart CNS	Smooth muscle cell Secretory gland CNS cortex	Adrenal gland Brainstem, striatum	CNS
Clinical effect	Gastric acid production	Bradycardia	Secretion, constriction	?	?
Agonists	Oxotremorine	Pilocarpine	Piperidine	?	
Selective antagonists	Pirenzepine	Methoctramine	4-DAMP, HHS	?	?

PLC (+), stimulation of phospholipase C and phosphoinositide metabolism; cAMP (−), inhibition of adenylyl cyclase and reduction of cyclic adenosine monophosphate production; ANS, autonomic nervous system; CNS, central nervous system; 4-DAMP, 4-diphenylacetoxy-*N*-methylpiperidine; Hexahydra-sila-diferidol, HHS.

heart failure when there is desensitization of β_1 receptors. This inotropic effect involves calcium rather than cAMP.[5] a_1 Receptors are also involved in myocardial stunning and in arrhythmias related to myocardial ischaemia.

β_1 and β_2 Receptors

Stimulation of cardiac β_1 receptors increases heart rate, the force of myocardial contraction, conduction and excitability (Table 9.1). β_1 Receptors are also involved in renin secretion. The main effect of β_2 receptors is relaxation of smooth muscles (bronchial, intestinal, uterine and arterial vessels). Their stimulation also produces cardiac effects (chronotropic, inotropic, dromotropic and bathmotropic), and they are involved in glycoregulation.

SYMPATHETIC NERVOUS SYSTEM PHARMACOLOGY

SYMPATHOMIMETIC AGENTS

ADRENALINE

Summary box 9.1 Adrenaline

- Endogenous catecholamine produced mainly by the adrenal medulla.

- Acts on a_1, β_1 and β_2 adrenoceptors.

- Causes arteriolar and venous vasoconstriction (a_1 effect).

- Increases force of myocardial contraction and tachycardia (β_1 effect).

- Relaxes bronchial smooth muscle (β_1 effect).

- Used in cardiogenic and anaphylactic shock, and severe bronchospasm.

Pharmacological properties

Adrenaline (epinephrine) is a potent stimulant of a-, β_1- and β_2-adrenergic receptors (see Table 9.2). The most prominent actions of adrenaline are on the heart and smooth muscle cells.

Cardiovascular Effects

The cardiovascular effects of adrenaline are the result of arteriolar and venous vasoconstriction by an a_1 action, arterial vasodilatation, especially in skeletal and pulmonary vascular beds due to β_2-receptor stimulation,

and a positive inotropic action due to β_1 stimulation. At low concentrations vasodilatation and positive inotropic actions predominate, but with high concentrations, as after an intravenous bolus dose, the predominant effect is vasoconstriction (Table 9.4). Blood pressure rises rapidly to a peak, proportional to the dose and heart rate increases, although reflex bradycardia may occur in response to a rapid increase in blood pressure. This can increase myocardial oxygen consumption and decreases cardiac efficiency (work done relative to oxygen consumption). Low intravenous infusion rates ($< 0.2\,\mu g$ kg^{-1} min^{-1}) decrease peripheral resistance, increase cardiac output, and mean arterial pressure is moderately increased, with a greater increase in systolic than in diastolic pressure so that the pulse pressure increases. At infusion rates above $0.2\,\mu g$ kg^{-1} min^{-1}, a-adrenergic stimulation becomes prominent, although β_2-adrenergic stimulation persists.

The main vascular effect of adrenaline is exerted on the smaller arterioles and veins. Reactivity varies between different vascular beds, so that there is redistribution of blood flow. Cutaneous and mucosal blood flow is decreased, although mesenteric and muscle skeletal blood flow are preserved or increased during adrenaline infusion. Renal blood flow is decreased even with infusion rates as low as $0.035\,\mu g$ kg^{-1} min^{-1}. Excretion of Na^+ is reduced, but when adrenaline is administered to treat low cardiac output or arterial hypotension, renal blood flow and diuresis may increase due to improved renal perfusion pressure.

Stimulation of cardiac β_1 and a_2 receptors increases heart rate as spontaneous diastolic depolarization of the sinoatrial node is accelerated and intracardiac conduction time is reduced. Systole is shortened although duration of diastole is not altered. A positive inotropic effect is observed and the rate of ventricular muscle relaxation is enhanced. Adrenaline may cause arrhythmias by accelerating ectopic foci and decreasing the ventricular refractory period. Changes in the transmembrane potential that occur following full repolarization of the action potential can induce ventricular tachycardia.

Miscellaneous Effects

β_2-Adrenergic receptor stimulation induces a potent bronchodilatation.[8] This effect is most evident when bronchial muscle cells are constricted by disease. Adrenaline is a potent mydriatic; it decreases gastrointestinal motility and increases sphincter tonic activity. In the nonpregnant uterus a-receptor stimulation causes contraction. However, during the last month of pregnancy adrenaline inhibits uterine contractions. Adrenaline relaxes the detrusor muscle and contracts the sphincters of the bladder. This effect may lead to retention of urine. Infusion of adrenaline causes plasma

Table 9.4 Pharmacology of some adrenergic agonists

Drug	Catecholamine	Mechanism of action	Dosage IV bolus	Dosage IV infusion	Myocardial function $\beta_1(\beta_2?)$	Heart rate β_1	Arrhythmogenic effect β_1	Vasoconstriction α_1	Vasodilatation β_2
Receptor					$\beta_1(\beta_2?)$	β_1	β_1	α_1	β_2
Noradrenaline	Yes (natural)	Direct	NR	$0.01-1.5$ $\mu g\,kg^{-1}\,min^{-1}$	++ to +++	– (reflex) to ++	++++	++++++	0 to +
Adrenaline	Yes (natural)	Direct	$0.1-0.5$ mg	$0.01-0.5$ $\mu g\,kg^{-1}\,min^{-1}$	+++++	++++	++++	++ to ++++	0
Dopamine	Yes (natural)	Direct (indirect)	NR	$3-20$ $\mu g\,kg^{-1}\,min^{-1}$	+++	+++	++++	+++	+++++
Isoprenaline	Yes (synthetic)	Direct	0.4 mg	$0.015\,\mu g\,kg^{-1}\,min^{-1}$ to desired effect	+++++	+++++	+++++	0	+++++
Dobutamine	Yes (synthetic)	Direct	NR	$3-20$ $\mu g\,kg^{-1}\,min^{-1}$	+++++	+++++	++++	0	++
Ephedrine	No (synthetic)	Indirect	3–6 mg	NR*	++	++	+	++++	0
Phenylephrine	No (synthetic)	Direct	50–150 mg	$0.15-0.75$ $\mu g\,kg^{-1}\,min^{-1}$	(0)	– (reflex) or 0	0	++++++	0

IV, intravenous; NR, not recommended. * May be used for short-duration IV infusion only because of tachyphylaxis.

glucose, lactate, free fatty acid concentrations to increase. Serum phosphorus and potassium levels decrease during adrenaline administration as β_2-adrenergic stimulation favours an intracellular entry of these anions.

Indications and therapeutic use

Intravenous adrenaline 0.1–0.5 mg is the drug of choice for the treatment of cardiocirculatory arrest and of anaphylactic shock. The efficiency of adrenaline in these situations is related mainly to the α-adrenergic-induced vasoconstriction but in anaphylactic shock β_2-induced bronchodilatation is also valuable. For the treatment of acute asthma adrenaline has largely been replaced by more selective β_2-adrenergic bronchodilators.[8] In cardiac arrest, endotracheal administration may be a useful alternative when intravenous access is not readily available although the plasma concentration after endotracheal administration is only one-tenth of that obtained after intravenous administration. For the treatment of circulatory shock, adrenaline is given as an infusion at a rate of 0.1–3 μg kg^{-1} min^{-1}. Lower rates, 0.01–0.1 μg kg^{-1} min^{-1} are used for an inotropic effect in cardiac surgery.

Adrenaline is not stable in alkaline solutions and must be protected from light.

NORADRENALINE

Summary box 9.2 Noradrenaline
• Endogenous neurotransmitter at postganglionic sympathetic neurons.
• Potent α_1-adrenoceptor agonist.
• Increases peripheral resistance and blood pressure.
• Minimal inotropic action.
• Useful to treat severe hypotension due to low peripheral vascular resistance (e.g. sepsis).

Pharmacological properties

Noradrenaline is the endogenous neurotransmitter at postganglionic sympathetic neurons. It constitutes approximately 10–20% of the catecholamines in the adrenal gland. It is a potent α-adrenergic agonist, although it has some β-agonist activity (Table 9.2).

Cardiovascular effect

α-Adrenergic stimulation produces a rise in total peripheral resistance and an increase in both systolic and diastolic pressure. Regional blood flows are decreased in most vascular beds, especially skin, skeletal muscle, kidney and liver. Glomerular filtration is maintained unless the decrease in renal blood flow is marked, but when noradrenaline is administered to treat profound hypotension, it may improve renal perfusion pressure and renal blood flow. Noradrenaline induces marked venoconstriction, leading to a shift of blood from peripheral to central vascular compartments, producing an increase in cardiac preload. The effect of noradrenaline on cardiac output is therefore variable, depending mainly on the alteration in ventricular loading condition, as noradrenaline exerts minimum positive inotropic effect (Table 9.4).

When administered intravenously during aortocoronary bypass grafting to treat arterial hypotension, noradrenaline allows a rapid return of blood pressure to baseline values and does not significantly alter left ventricular end systolic and end diastolic area or ejection fraction. Changes in heart rate are moderate during noradrenaline infusion. However, reflex bradycardia may occur when noradrenaline is administered as an intravenous bolus. Ventricular arrhythmias are less frequent with noradrenaline than with adrenaline, but nodal rhythm, atrioventricular dissociation, bigeminal rhythm, and ventricular tachycardia or fibrillation have been recorded. Despite direct stimulation of α-adrenoceptors located on coronary arteries, coronary blood flow is substantially increased during noradrenaline infusion, in response to the increase in myocardial oxygen consumption. Thus, because of myocardial oxygen imbalance, patients with coronary artery disease may develop myocardial ischaemia.

Pulmonary artery resistance and pulmonary arterial pressure increase during noradrenaline infusion. This increase is usually moderate, except in patients with pulmonary hypertension in whom the increase in pulmonary pressure may be critical and induce right ventricular failure.

Indications and therapeutic use

Noradrenaline is indicated when the haemodynamic goal is to increase total peripheral resistance and blood pressure with minimal positive chronotropic effect. It is therefore widely used in the early stage of septic shock, which is associated with profound abnormalities in vascular tone and adrenergic responsiveness. Noradrenaline bitartrate is available for intravenous infusion. Continuous infusion by an infusion pump is necessary because of its very short half-life. It should be given through a central vein, since extravasation may produce local skin necrosis. Noradrenaline should not be mixed with alkaline solutions. The initial infusion rate is between 0.01 and 0.1 μg kg^{-1} min^{-1}, and subsequently increased up to 1–1.5 μg kg^{-1} min^{-1} until the haemodynamic goal is achieved. Arterial pressure, heart rate and cardiac rhythm must be monitored carefully, and organ perfusion, especially renal perfusion, and the effect on cardiac output should also be monitored.

DOPAMINE

Summary box 9.3 Dopamine

- Major neurotransmitter in the CNS.

- Precursor of noradrenaline.

- Used for its cardiovascular effects, which are dose-dependent.

- Low doses ($< 2 \mu g\, kg^{-1}\, min^{-1}$): main action on DA_1 receptors, increasing renal blood flow and urine output.

- Intermediate doses ($2-10 \mu g\, kg^{-1}\, min^{-1}$): stimulates β_1-adrenoceptors, producing an inotropic effect.

- High doses ($> 10 \mu g\, kg^{-1}\, min^{-1}$): effect is mainly α_1-mediated vasoconstriction.

- α_1-Mediated pulmonary vasoconstriction can increase pulmonary shunting, resulting in hypoxaemia.

Pharmacological properties
Dopamine is the precursor of noradrenaline in the synthesis cascade of endogenous catecholamines and differs from noradrenaline in the absence of a β-hydroxyl group (see Fig. 9.3). Dopamine, a major neurotransmitter in the central nervous system, can modulate the activity of some sympathetic ganglia. It also has some extraneuronal actions; it decreases gut motility, decreases the synthesis and secretion of aldosterone, and increases renal blood flow and sodium excretion.

Cardiovascular and Renal Effects
Dopamine produces a direct and dose-dependent stimulation of α- and β-adrenoceptors and of dopaminergic DA_1 receptors, and an indirect release of noradrenaline from sympathetic nerve endings. As the affinity of the different types of receptors for the catecholamine varies, the observed result depends on the dose administered. Very low doses of intravenous dopamine ($0.5-2 \mu g\; kg^{-1}\; min^{-1}$) do not produce significant systemic haemodynamic effects, but are sufficient to stimulate vascular and renal dopaminergic DA_1 and DA_2 receptors. Renal blood flow and glomerular filtration rate increase and proximal tubular

reabsorption of sodium is partially inhibited, leading to an increase in urinary sodium output. Low doses ($2-5 \mu g\; kg^{-1}\; min^{-1}$) stimulate β_1-adrenergic receptors and release noradrenaline from nerve terminals. Myocardial contractility, cardiac output and systolic blood pressure are increased, whereas increases in heart rate and diastolic blood pressure are less pronounced. Significant redistribution of blood flow is observed and total peripheral resistance is usually unchanged.

With doses above $10 \mu g\; kg^{-1}\; min^{-1}$, stimulation of α_1-adrenergic receptors becomes prominent and produces a significant arteriolar and venous vasoconstriction. Blood pressure is increased and the effect on cardiac output is variable. The beneficial effect on renal and mesenteric blood flow is lost progressively as the infusion rate is increased. Tachycardia and arrhythmias are frequent. As with noradrenaline, high doses of dopamine increase myocardial oxygen consumption. Metabolic regulation increases coronary blood flow despite stimulation of coronary artery α_1 receptors but ischaemia may occur in patients with coronary artery stenosis. Pulmonary vasoconstriction in well-ventilated zones increases intrapulmonary shunting and may lead to hypoxaemia.

Miscellaneous Effects
Nonhaemodynamic effects of intravenous dopamine are minimal. It does not cross the blood–brain barrier and has no significant central effect. Stimulation of renal cortical receptors decreases secretion of aldosterone. Secretion of prolactin and thyroid stimulating hormone are partially inhibited.

Metabolism
When administered intravenously, dopamine is rapidly removed from plasma by enzymatic metabolism (COMT and MAO). Elimination half-life is 6–9 min, but important variability exists between individuals. Renal or hepatic failure is responsible for a significant decrease in dopamine plasma clearance. It is ineffective orally. Dopamine infusion rates should be reduced progressively because the exogenous dopamine is taken up into the presynaptic vesicles of the sympathetic nervous system and synthesis of endogenous dopamine is thus decreased.

Indications and therapeutic uses
Dopamine is widely used at low to intermediate doses to increase renal blood flow in patients with oliguria and low or normal peripheral vascular resistance, as in cardiogenic or septic shock, after cardiac or aortic surgery, or renal and hepatic transplantation. However, the beneficial effect of dopamine in these circumstances remains unproven. At higher doses, it is useful as an inotrope when increased myocardial contractility

combined with a pressor effect is required, such as in cardiogenic shock or sepsis. However, the marked vasopressor effects at high doses limits its usefulness and when infusion rates above about $10 \mu g \ kg^{-1} \ min^{-1}$ are reached it is probably preferable to switch to another inotrope such as dobutamine, or to use combinations of these drugs.

Dopamine should not be mixed with alkaline solution. As dopamine causes a release of noradrenaline at terminal nerve endings, it should not be administered to patients treated with MAO inhibitors. As response may vary widely, careful adjustment of dose is also necessary in patients treated with tricyclic antidepressant drugs.

EPHEDRINE

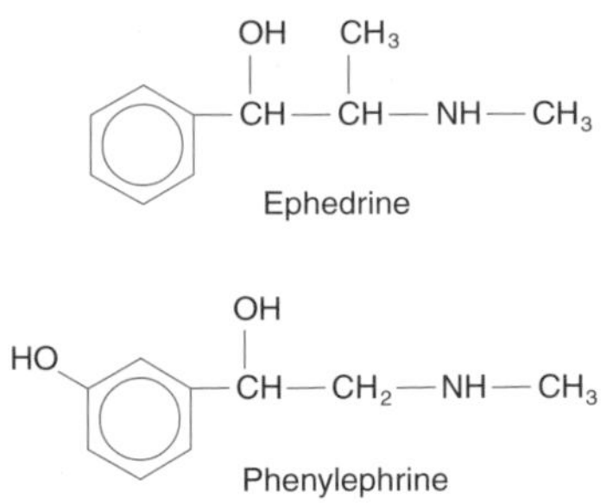

Fig. 9.6 Structure of ephedrine and phenylephrine.

> **Summary box 9.4 Ephedrine**
>
> - Noncatecholamine sympathomimetic.
>
> - Polar lipid-soluble compound.
>
> - Cardiovascular effects similar to those of adrenaline, but ephedrine is less potent and longer acting.
>
> - Indirect action by release of noradrenaline from sympathetic nerve terminals.
>
> - Useful in preventing and treating hypotension associated with epidural and spinal anaesthesia.
>
> - In obstetric patients preserves uterine blood flow better than other vasoconstricters.

Pharmacological properties

Ephedrine is a natural plant alkaloid. Its chemical structure is related to adrenaline but it lacks the two hydroxyl groups on the benzene ring (i.e. it is not a catechol) and it has a methyl substitution on the α carbon (Fig. 9.6). As a consequence it is not a substrate for either COMT or MAO and thus has a longer duration of action than adrenaline. The absence of the hydroxyl groups also makes it less polar and more lipid soluble than adrenaline and so it readily crosses cell membranes and the blood–brain barrier. These properties also mean that it is effective orally. The ephedrine molecule has two chiral centres and thus four isomers are possible, L- and D-ephedrine and L- and D-pseudoephedrine. Only L-ephedrine, the most potent sympathomimetic isomer, and racemic pseudoephedrine are used clinically. Pseudoephedrine is used in over-the-counter oral nasal decongestants. Ephedrine exerts its sympathomimetic effects indirectly by releasing noradrenaline from sympathetic nerve terminals and also by a direct action on β_2-adrenoceptors. It is not metabolized and is excreted unchanged by the kidney.

Cardiovascular Effects

Cardiovascular effects of ephedrine differ from those of adrenaline mainly in their much lower potency and longer duration of action (see Table 9.1). When administered intravenously, the main effect of ephedrine is related to α-adrenergic stimulation, which produces arterial and venous vasoconstriction. Ephedrine also weakly stimulates cardiac β-adrenoceptors, producing a slight positive inotropic and chronotropic action. The net haemodynamic effect of intravenous ephedrine is an increase in arterial pressure, heart rate and cardiac output.

Distribution of blood flow is altered after ephedrine administration: coronary, cerebral and muscle blood flow are increased, whereas renal and splanchnic blood flows are decreased. Ephedrine is widely used as a sympathomimetic agent during regional anaesthesia, because of its ability to counteract the increase in venous capacitance caused by sympathetic block. Historically, ephedrine has been the preferred vasoconstrictor for the treatment of hypotension after epidural and spinal anaesthesia in obstetrics because it preserves uterine perfusion better than pure α-adrenergic agonists such as phenylephrine.[9] In vitro studies have suggested that direct uterine vasoconstriction by ephedrine is reduced during pregnancy. Prophylactic ephedrine either improved or maintained intervillous blood flow in women undergoing caesarean section during regional anaesthesia.[10] This beneficial effect may be related to the increase in cardiac output secondary to ephedrine's β-receptor stimulation, compensating for uterine arterial vasoconstriction due to α-adrenergic receptor stimulation. Alternatively the action of ephedrine may be due to release of nitric oxide. Nitric oxide synthase (NOS) is upregulated in uterine arteries during pregnancy, and ephedrine stimulates NOS to release nitric oxide and diminish direct vasoconstriction.[11]

Miscellaneous Effect

Bronchial muscle relaxation is less prominent but more sustained with ephedrine than with adrenaline. Mydriasis occurs after topical application of the drug. Ephedrine is less effective than adrenaline in raising blood glucose concentration. The CNS effect of ephedrine is similar to the stimulation induced by amphetamines, but is considerably less pronounced.

Indications and therapeutic use

Ephedrine is indicated to treat arterial hypotension during regional and general anaesthesia. When hypotension is secondary to hypovolaemia, ephedrine is useful because its fast onset of action allows a rapid return of blood pressure to normal values, and its relatively long duration of action gives time for fluid loading. A rapid decrease in efficiency is observed during repeated intravenous boluses or continuous infusion, because of depletion of noradrenaline in presynaptic nerve endings. Ephedrine should therefore be administered as intravenous boluses of 5–10 mg or by short-duration intravenous infusion only. As with dopamine and other indirect sympathetic agonists, interactions with MAO inhibitors may produce a dramatic increase in blood pressure. Care is also indicated in patients who are taking tricyclic antidepressants.

PHENYLEPHRINE

Summary box 9.5 Phenylephrine

- Potent a_1-adrenoceptor agonist.

- Causes vasoconstriction in both resistive and capitance vessels.

- May have detrimental effects in patients with poor left ventricular function due to ischaemic heart disease.

- Drug of choice to treat hypotension in patients with aortic stenosis.

Pharmacological properties

Phenylephrine is a synthetic sympathomimetic agent that differs from adrenaline in the absence of a hydroxyl group at position 4 on the benzene ring (Fig. 9.6). It is a powerful a_1-adrenoceptor agonist used widely in anaesthesia to treat hypotension. Its ability to release noradrenaline accounts for only a small part of its action.

Cardiovascular Actions

The predominant action of phenylephrine is potent vasoconstriction in resistive and capacitive vascular beds (Table 9.4). Although high concentrations can stimulate β receptors in the heart, phenylephrine has minimal positive inotropic effects in the doses used clinically. However, in situations where cardiac β_1 receptors are desensitized, phenylephrine can mediate a positive inotropic effect through a-adrenergic stimulation. After intravenous administration there is an increase in systolic and diastolic arterial blood pressure. Peripheral resistance is considerably increased and cardiac output is slightly decreased due to transient alteration in left ventricular filling dynamics.[12] Heart rate remains unchanged or is slightly decreased as a result of reflex bradycardia. This lack of tachycardia could be an advantage in patients with ischaemic heart disease. However, there is evidence that ephedrine can cause a significant alteration in left ventricular function which can be detrimental to patients with coronary artery disease.[12,13] In contrast, phenylephrine is the drug of choice for patients with valvular aortic stenosis as it is effective in treating arterial hypotension, induces no deleterious effect on left ventricular function and improves left ventricular filling dynamics.[12]

The effect of phenylephrine on uterine haemodynamics has been investigated extensively. Experimentally, phenylephrine is efficient in restoring arterial blood pressure during epidural anaesthesia, but fails to improve fetal oxygenation and is less efficient than ephedrine at restoring uterine blood flow.[9]

Indications and therapeutic use

Phenylephrine should be diluted before administration to obtain a final concentration of 100 μg ml^{-1}. Because of its very rapid onset and short duration of action, arterial hypotension during general anaesthesia can be treated efficiently with intravenous phenylephrine given as a bolus of 50–100 μg or by infusion at 10–20 μg min^{-1}. The absence of positive chronotropic and inotropic action must be taken into account, especially in patients with hypotension associated with bradycardia and in those with left ventricular dysfunction.[12]

β-ADRENERGIC BRONCHODILATORS

Pharmacological properties

β_2-Adrenergic receptor agonists have gained popularity over catecholamines, methylaxanthines and anticholinergic agents as bronchodilators in the treatment of bronchial asthma.[8] The recently developed β_2-adrenergic agonists, which are not degraded by the enzyme COMT, are of particular interest because of their long duration of action. They can be divided into intermediate-acting bronchodilators (3–6 h) such as orciprenaline (metaproterenol), salbutamol, terbutaline, fenoterol and long-acting (more than 12 h) agents, salmeterol and formoterol. The latter are highly lipophilic compounds with extended side-chains and possess a high affinity for the β_2-adrenoceptor. The mechanism of the prolongation of action differs between the agents: formoterol enters the cell membrane from which it progressively leaches out; the side-chain of salmeterol binds to a highly specific domain of the β_2 receptor allowing prolonged receptor stimulation.

Respiratory Effects

β_2-Adrenergic agonists produce bronchodilatation by interaction with β_2-adrenoceptors located on bronchial smooth muscle cells. They are effective for the relief of acute symptoms and the prevention of exercise-induced bronchoconstriction. The inhalation route is preferred as, for any given degree of bronchodilatation, it produces fewer side-effects than oral or parenteral routes. Parenteral therapy is useful in patients with severe obstruction and the oral route can be used in children too young to use a metered-dose inhaler correctly. β_2-Adrenergic stimulation also produces an increase in mucociliary clearance, inhibition of cholinergic neurotransmission and an inhibition of histamine, leukotriene and prostaglandin release from lung mast cells. However, the role of this last action on chronic inflammation of the tracheobronchial tree is uncertain.

Miscellaneous Effects

Systemic absorption of β_2-adrenergic agonists may induce adverse reactions. Tremor is frequently observed, due to stimulation of adrenergic receptors in skeletal muscle. Stimulation of vascular smooth muscle produces vasodilatation and a decrease in arterial blood pressure. Heart rate increases as a result of the reflex response to hypotension and direct stimulation of cardiac β_2-adrenoceptors. The QTc interval on the electrocardiogram is increased. β_2-Adrenergic agonist-induced arterial pulmonary vasodilatation may suppress compensatory vasoconstriction in areas of decreased ventilation in patients with severe asthma and may decrease arterial oxygen tension. Metabolic responses include hyperglycaemia, hypokalaemia and hypomagnesaemia.

Side-effects Related to Long-term Administration

Regular administration of β_2-adrenergic agonists may lead to the development of tolerance, with a decrease in duration of action of bronchodilatation, which occurs in the first few weeks of treatment and remains stable thereafter. Loss of protection against bronchoconstrictor stimuli may also occur and there may be rebound

effects when prolonged treatment with intermediate-acting β_2 bronchodilator is stopped abruptly. This is, however, usually minimal and transient and is not observed with the long-acting agents.

Indications and uses

Inhaled β_2 bronchodilators are available as wet aerosol from a jet nebulizer or as dry aerosol from a metered-dose inhaler (gas propellant aerosol or breath-propelled dry powder). They are indicated for the treatment of acute episodes of bronchoconstriction and for prevention of exercise-induced asthma. A long duration of protection against nocturnal and exercise-induced crises can be achieved with long-acting β_2-adrenergic agonists prescribed at regular intervals. Intermediate-acting β_2 bronchodilators should be given to relieve bronchoconstriction occurring between administrations of a long-acting agent.

ADRENOCEPTOR ANTAGONISTS

Adrenoceptor antagonists inhibit the interaction of noradrenaline, adrenaline and other sympathomimetic drugs with adrenoreceptors. Except for phenoxybenzamine, which binds covalently to α-adrenergic receptors, all agents interact competitively with the adrenergic receptors and are therefore reversible antagonists.

α-ADRENERGIC ANTAGONISTS

Pharmacological properties

α-Adrenergic antagonists are chemically heterogeneous compounds that exhibit significant differences in affinity for α_1- and α_2-adrenoceptors (see Table 9.2). The most important action of α-adrenoceptors antagonists is inhibition of the vasoconstriction induced by endogenous catecholamines. The observed effect depends on the activity of the adrenergic system at the time of drug administration and the relative affinity of the antagonist for α_1- and α_2-adrenoceptors. When the sympathetic tone is high (i.e. during hypovolaemia), vasodilatation occurs and a marked fall in blood pressure may occur. The effect on blood pressure is much less when sympathetic tone is low, as in resting supine subjects.

The decrease in blood pressure triggers a baroreflex response that induces an increase in cardiac output and heart rate, and fluid retention. Furthermore, sympathetic outflow and release of neurotransmitter by sympathetic nerve endings can be potentiated by α_2-adrenoceptor blockade. Selective α_2-adrenoceptor antagonists such as yohimbine can therefore induce activation of adrenergic receptors located in the heart and vascular bed, and thus an increase in heart rate and blood pressure. With nonselective α_1/α_2-adrenoceptor antagonists the increase in sympathetic outflow to the vascular bed is blunted by vascular a_1 blockade, resulting in inhibition of vasoconstriction.

a-Adrenoceptor antagonists can impair contraction of the trigone and sphincter muscles of the urinary bladder, leading to decreased resistance to urine outflow. The potential effect of a_2-adrenoceptor antagonism on insulin release, platelet aggregation and bronchial smooth muscle contraction, although poorly documented, seems to be minimal in clinical use.

Nonselective a-adrenoceptor antagonists

Phentolamine, an imidazoline, is a nonselective competitive a-adrenoceptor antagonist that also blocks 5-hydroxytryptamine (5-HT) receptors and K^+ channels. Phentolamine administration in normal subjects produces a decrease in systemic peripheral resistances and blood pressure, and an increase in heart rate and cardiac output. Pressor response to catecholamines and the ability to respond to hypovolaemia is impaired. Phentolamine still has a place in the short-term control of hypertension in patients with phaeochromocytoma.

Tolazoline is related to phentolamine but is less potent. It has been used in the treatment of pulmonary hypertension in the newborn.

a_1-Adrenoceptor antagonists

Prazosin is a potent and selective a_1-adrenoceptor antagonist that has been used for the control of blood pressure in hypertensive patients. Administration of prazosin generally does not induce any significant increase in heart rate because of its lack of activity on a_2-adrenoceptors and its direct effect on the CNS to suppress sympathetic outflow. Cardiac output is not increased despite reduced afterload because of the marked effect of prazosin on venous tone. The main adverse effects of prazosin are syncopal reactions that may follow the first administration, and postural hypotension during chronic administration.

Doxazosin and terazosin are compounds related to prazosin that retain high specificity for a_1-adrenergic receptors but possess different pharmacological profiles, with longer elimination half-lives that allow once-daily oral treatment. Doxazosin has also been proposed for the preoperative management of hypertension in patients with phaeochromocytoma.

Urapidil is a selective, although weak, a_1-adrenoceptor antagonist which also acts as an agonist–antagonist of serotonin 5-HT$_{1A}$ receptors in the CNS. Urapidil is extensively metabolized and has an elimination half-life of 3 h. In Europe urapidil is available in oral formulation for treatment of hypertension and in intravenous formulation for the management of acute hypertension in the perioperative period.

β-ADRENOCEPTOR ANTAGONIST DRUGS

β-Adrenoceptor antagonists, often referred to as β blockers, are an important group of drugs used mainly in cardiovascular diseases. The first compound of this class to be developed was dichlorisoprenaline, a partial antagonist with a low potency. It was soon replaced by the more potent propranolol, a pure antagonist. Propranolol is nonselective, with an equal blocking effect on β_1 and β_2 receptors. Other β-adrenoceptor antagonists (e.g. oxprenolol and alprenolol) are nonselective with considerable partial agonist activity. The agonistic effects are often referred to as intrinsic sympathomimetic activity. Propranolol is also a potent local anaesthetic because of its ability to block sodium channels in excitable tissue and thus alter the action potential of nerves and cardiac muscle. This property, unrelated to β-adrenergic blockade, is described as membrane stabilizing or quinidine-like, and is present equally in both enantiomers of propranolol. Many of the newer drugs, such as atenolol, are selective for β_1 receptors with no agonist activity. Selective β_1-adrenergic receptor antagonists have received considerable clinical attention in cardiology and anaesthesiology

---

Summary box 9.6 β-Adrenoceptor antagonists

- Used mainly to treat:

  - hypertension

  - cardiac arrhythmias

  - angina pectoris.

- Important hazards are:

  - bronchoconstriction

  - bradycardia

  - cardiac failure (possibly less with partial agonists).

- Side-effects include:

  - cold extremities

  - insomnia

  - depression.

- Many show rapid first-pass metabolism, hence poor bioavailability.

- Labetalol blocks both a and β receptors; it is used in hypertension.

because of their efficiency in the treatment of hypertension, coronary artery disease and some types of arrhythmias. Labetalol combines α- and β-blocking activity, but its effect on β receptors predominates at low doses.

The chemical structures of the various β blockers vary widely, but they have one general feature in common: an aminopropanol moiety linked to an aromatic system (Fig. 9.7). All β-adrenoreceptor antagonists have chiral centres and exist as two optical isomers (enantiomers). The β-adrenergic blocking properties reside predominantly in one enantiomer, which in the case of propranolol is the S-(−) isomer, commonly called l-propranolol. Most, including propranolol, are marketed as the racemate.

Haemodynamics

The cardiovascular effects depend on the degree of sympathetic activity. In a subject at rest there is little change in heart rate, cardiac output or arterial pressure, but these are reduced during exercise or excitement. Drugs with partial agonist activity, such as oxprenolol, increase the heart rate at rest but reduce it during exercise. Maximum exercise tolerance is considerably reduced in normal subjects, partly because of the limitation of the cardiac response, and partly because the β-mediated vasodilatation in skeletal muscle is

reduced. Coronary blood flow is reduced, but relatively less than the myocardial oxygen consumption, so the oxygen supply–demand ratio is improved, an effect of importance in the treatment of angina pectoris. In normal subjects, the reduction of the force of contraction of the heart is of no importance, but it may have serious consequences for patients with heart disease.

β-Adrenoceptor antagonists have long been used for the treatment of hypertension. The antihypertensive effect seems to be due mainly to a persisting reduction in cardiac output. Acute intravenous administration causes a rapid reduction in heart rate and cardiac output, but no acute fall in blood pressure. The decrease in cardiac output is due mainly to a fall in heart rate in hypertensive patients but to a reduction in stroke volume in normotensive subjects. During prolonged oral administration in hypertensive patients, the significant reduction in cardiac output remains, whereas the total peripheral resistance falls from an initially raised level. β-Adrenoceptor antagonists shift the dose–response curve for the heart rate increase produced by isoprenaline to the right (Fig. 9.8). There is a clear dissociation between the β-blocking effect, evident from the reduced heart rate and cardiac output, and the antihypertensive effect, which appears hours or days later. This has been called the delayed vasodilating effect. Dissociation is also evident when treatment is stopped; heart rate returns to the initial untreated level, sometimes with a temporary overshoot, whereas blood pressure returns only gradually to the initial level. In addition to the reduction in cardiac output, reduction of

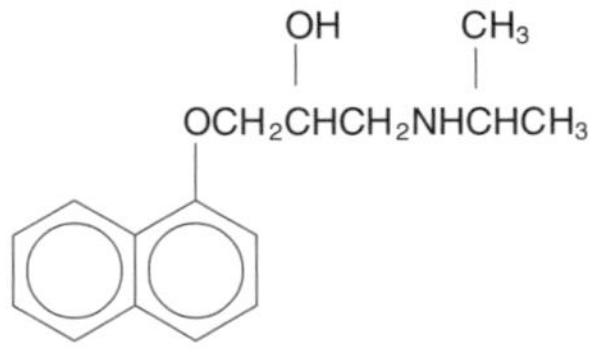

$OH \quad CH_3$

$OCH_2CHCH_2NHCHCH_3$

Propranolol

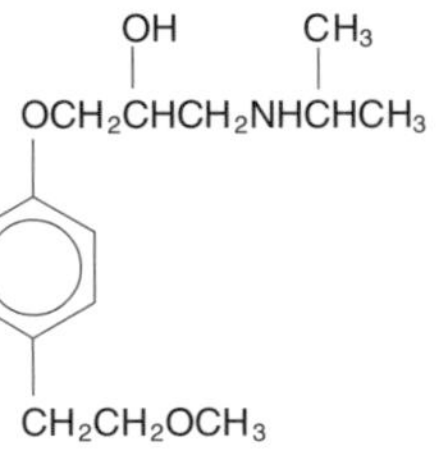

$OH \quad CH_3$

$OCH_2CHCH_2NHCHCH_3$

$CH_2CH_2OCH_3$

Metoprolol

$OH \quad CH_3$

$OCH_2CHCH_2NHCHCH_3$

O

$CH_2CH_2COCH_3$

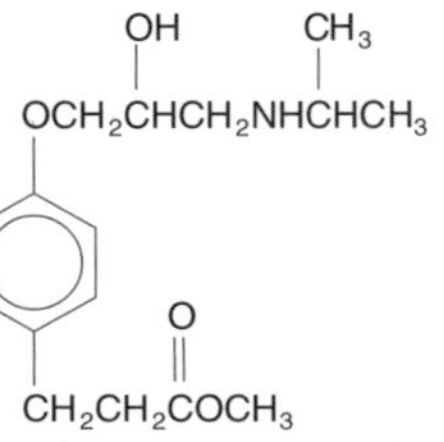

Esmolol

Fig. 9.7 Structure of propranolol, metoprolol and esmolol.

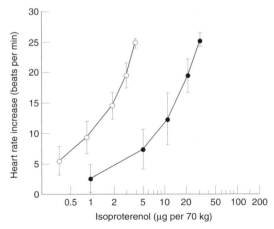

Fig. 9.8 Log dose–response curves for the increase in heart rate produced by isoprenaline (isoproterenol) in patients receiving β-adrenoceptor antagonists (●) and a drug-free control group (○). From Tarnow J, Komar K. Altered hemodynamic response to dobutamine in relation to the degree of preoperative beta-adrenoceptor blockade. *Anesthesiology* 1988; **68**: 912–919, with permission.

renin release from the juxtaglomerular cells of the kidney and a reduction in central sympathetic activity may also contribute to the antihypertensive effect. Because reflex vasoconstriction is preserved, postural and exercise-induced hypotension are much less troublesome than with many other antihypertensive drugs. Many β-adrenoceptor antagonists have an anti-dysrhythmic effect which is of clinical importance.

Pharmacokinetics

The pharmacokinetic profile of the β blockers is closely related to their lipophilicity. Propranolol is the most lipid soluble of the β-adrenoceptor antagonists. The extent of systemic bioavailability varies considerably, depending mainly on the lipophilicity of the drug, although plasma–protein binding appears to play a role as well. Compounds such as propranolol, oxpranolol and pindolol are rapidly and completely absorbed when given orally, whereas the absorption of nadolol and the β_1-selective agent atenolol varies widely. The elimination half-life of most agents is 3–6 h, and elimination is mainly by metabolism of the lipophilic agents, whereas the hydrophilic ones are excreted mainly by the kidneys.

Adverse effects

Airway resistance in normal subjects is only slightly increased by β-receptor antagonists, and this is of no consequence. In asthmatic subjects, however, the effect of nonselective β-receptor antagonists (such as propranolol) can be dramatic with severe, life-threatening bronchoconstriction. It is also of clinical importance in patients with other forms of obstructive lung disease (e.g. chronic bronchitis, emphysema). The danger is less with β_1-selective antagonists, but none is so selective that this danger can be ignored.

In spite of the involvement of β-receptors in the hyperglycaemic actions of adrenaline, β-receptor antagonists cause only minor metabolic changes in normal subjects. They do not affect the onset of hypoglycaemia following an injection of insulin, but somewhat delay the recovery of blood glucose concentration. In diabetic patients, the use of β-receptor antagonists increases the likelihood of exercise-induced hypoglycaemia because the normal adrenaline-induced release of glucose from the liver is diminished. Also, sympathetic reflexes are an important cue by which hypoglycaemia is recognized; these symptoms are reduced by β-receptor antagonists, so hypoglycaemia is less likely to be noticed by the patient.

Patients taking β-receptor blocking drugs often complain of fatigue, which is probably due to reduced cardiac output and reduced muscle perfusion during exercise. Cold extremities is a common side-effect, possibly caused by a loss of β receptor-mediated vaso-dilatation in cutaneous vessels. Other side-effects asso-ciated with β-receptor antagonists are not obviously the result of β-receptor blockade. One is bad dreams, which occur mainly with highly lipid-soluble drugs (e.g. pro-pranolol) that enter the brain easily.

ESMOLOL

Esmolol differs from the other β-adrenoceptor antagonists because it can be rapidly titrated and its pharmacological effects dissipate within 30 min after the drug is discontinued. The chemical structure of esmolol is similar to that of metoprolol and propranolol (see Fig. 9.7). However, it differs from these agents in that it has an ethylene-extended methyl ester group in the para position of the phenyl ring. The addition of the ester group makes the molecule susceptible to rapid hydrolysis by plasma and erythrocyte esterases, resulting in a drug with a short duration of action (terminal half-life 9.2 min). In this respect esmolol is similar to the opioid remifentanil. Unlike most ester-containing drugs (e.g. suxamethonium), esmolol is not metabolized by plasma cholinesterase. The hydrolysis of esmolol results in the formation of a weakly active carboxylic acid metabolite (1/1500 the potency of esmolol). The pharmacokinetic properties of esmolol in patients with end-stage renal and hepatic diseases do not differ significantly from those observed in normal subjects. In animal studies, esmolol has been found to be 50 times less potent than propranolol. However, in humans, esmolol appears to be 1/15 as potent as propranolol. Esmolol is relatively β_1 selective, is devoid of intrinsic sympathomimetic activity, and has 1/100 the local anaesthetic effect of propranolol.

The main indication in anaesthesia is to control tachycardia, for example during controlled hypotension. It is given intravenously; the recommended dose by infusion is $500\,\mu g\,kg^{-1}\,min^{-1}$ over 4 min followed by a maintenance infusion of $50\,\mu g\,kg^{-1}\,min^{-1}$. If the desired effect is not achieved, the loading dose can be repeated and the infusion rate increased to $100\,\mu g\,kg^{-1}\,min^{-1}$ to a maximum rate of $300\,\mu g\,kg^{-1}\,min^{-1}$. Blood pressure should be carefully monitored as esmolol can cause hypotension.

LABETALOL

Labetalol is a competitive, nonselective antagonist of α_1, β_1 and β_2 adrenoceptors. The α-receptor antagonist activity is much less pronounced than the β-receptor antagonist action.

Pharmacokinetics

Oral labetalol is absorbed rapidly with peak blood levels 1–2 h after administration. Due to extensive first-pass metabolism, the bioavailability is 30–40%, with marked intersubject variability. Labetalol is distributed exten-sively to the liver, lungs and kidneys, but not to the brain. The plasma half-life is up to 4 h. Labetalol is about 50% bound to plasma protein. It is metabolized extensively in the liver with less than 5% of the drug appearing unchanged in the urine.

Uses

Labetalol is used orally to treat severe hypertension in patients with phaeochromocytoma and during clonidine withdrawal reactions. In anaesthesia it is a useful drug for the induction of controlled hypotension because of the absence, at clinical doses, of tachycardia. It is especially effective in conjunction with potent inhalational anaesthetics. Labetalol is also used to control acute rises in blood pressure, especially in patients with phaeochromocytoma, and to prevent further rises of blood pressure during intubation in hypertensive patients, for example in preeclamptic women. The advantages of labetalol are a lesser degree of pulmonary shunting, absence of tachycardia, and absence of rebound hypertension and tachyphylaxis compared with other commonly used agents. Labetalol should be avoided in asthmatics as it can precipitate bronchospasm in these patients.

Dosage

Intravenous injections of 0.5–2.0 mg kg^{-1} may be given for severe hypertension. Small, frequent boluses or slow incremental infusions, beginning with 0.5–1.0 mg kg^{-1} h^{-1} may produce fewer hypotensive episodes than single injections. During anaesthesia in adult patients, in the absence of potent inhalational anaesthetic agents, an initial dose of 25–30 mg is required to achieve a significant blood pressure reduction. Further increments of 5–10 mg may be given. In the presence of inhalational agents the initial dose should be not more than 20 mg.

PARASYMPATHETIC SYSTEM PHARMACOLOGY

CHOLINERGIC AGONISTS

ACh has no therapeutic application because of its lack of specificity as a cholinergic agonist and its short half-life. However, numerous derivatives have been synthesized to obtain drugs with more selective and prolonged action. Two classes of compounds have muscarinic agonist properties: (1) ACh and choline esters, and (2) cholinomimetic natural alkaloids and synthetic analogues.

ACETYLCHOLINE AND CHOLINE ESTERS

Of the several hundred synthetic choline derivatives, only three are of clinical interest: methacholine, carbachol and bethanechol. The pharmacological effects of ACh and choline esters are complex as they result from the variable ability of these compounds to stimulate many of the effector organs innervated by postganglionic parasympathetic nerves, sympathetic and parasympathetic ganglia innervated by preganglionic fibres and motor endplates of skeletal muscle. These effects are summarized in Table 9.1.

Pharmacological properties

ACh has significant cardiovascular actions. After intravenous administration there is a decrease in arterial blood pressure due to vasodilatation in all vascular beds caused by stimulation of muscarinic receptors. Stimulation of these receptors by ACh induces the release of nitric oxide, which causes the vascular smooth muscle cells to relax. When endothelial cells are damaged, ACh stimulation of the muscarinic receptors located on smooth muscle cells induces vasoconstriction.

ACh decreases the slope of the spontaneous diastolic depolarization of the sinoatrial node, slowing heart rate. However, the baroreflex response to hypotension may dampen the direct effect of ACh on heart rate so that intravenous administration may result in a tachycardia. The rate of conduction in the atrioventricular node and to a lesser extent in the Purkinje conduction system is decreased and the refractory period is increased. This may lead to complete heart block when a large dose of a cholinergic agonist is administered intravenously. Finally, ACh exerts a moderate negative inotropic effect on ventricular myocytes. This effect is more marked when contractility is enhanced by adrenergic stimulation. Selective stimulation of M$_2$ receptors may have a beneficial effect on myocardial oxygen balance by decreasing myocardial consumption, and this may be a potential treatment of myocardial ischaemia.

Miscellaneous Effects

ACh and choline esters increase peristaltic activity and secretory activity of the gastrointestinal tract. This may be accompanied by nausea, vomiting and intestinal cramps. Ureteral peristalsis, contraction of the detrusor muscle and maximal voluntary voiding pressure are increased. In contrast, the trigone and external sphincter are relaxed. ACh and choline esters cause bronchoconstriction in addition to increased secretion of all glands receiving innervation from parasympathetic nerves. When administered topically to the eye they produce miosis.

Indication and uses

Bethanechol chloride is used to stimulate the smooth muscle of the gastrointestinal tract, to facilitate bladder evacuation when organic obstruction is absent, and to increase salivation in cases of xerostomia. Methacholine chloride may be administered by inhalation for the diagnosis of bronchial hyperreactivity.

CHOLINOMIMETIC ALKALOIDS

Pilocarpine, muscarine and arecoline are the three most important natural alkaloids with cholinomimetic action. Muscarine, which stimulates almost exclusively muscarinic receptors, and arecoline, which also acts at nicotinic receptors, have no therapeutic use. Pilocarpine is a tertiary amine obtained from *Pilocarpus* plants. It is used as a sialagogue and myotic agent. Pilocarpine 5–10 mg orally is used for the treatment of xerostomia in Sjögren syndrome or after neck irradiation. When instilled into the eye as 0.5–4.0% drops, pilocarpine causes a prolonged miosis, spasms of the muscles of accommodation, and a transient and moderate increase in intraocular pressure, followed by a prolonged decrease. It is used for the treatment of open-angle glaucoma.

MUSCARINIC ANTAGONISTS

Naturally occurring anticholinergic drugs such as atropine and hyoscine (scopolamine) are the alkaloids of the belladonna plants, and have been in clinical use for more than a century. Their antimuscarinic action

---

Summary box 9.7 Musacarinic antagonists

- Compete with ACh for muscarinic receptors.

- Either tertiary or quaternary amines.

- Tertiary amines readily cross the blood–brain barrier and can cause CNS effects; quaternary amines do not cross the blood–brain barrier.

- Tertiary amines are:

  - atropine

  - hyoscine

  - homatropine.

- Quaternary amines are:

  - methylatropine

  - ipratropine

  - glycopyrronium.

---

results from competitive antagonism of muscarinic receptors in peripheral tissues, blocking the effects of ACh. In general, they do not cause significant antagonism at nicotinic receptors.

Atropine and hyoscine are tertiary amines which easily cross the blood–brain barrier and thus can have an effect on the CNS (Table 9.5). The more recently developed quaternary muscarinic receptor antagonists have some different pharmacological properties; they are unreliably absorbed after oral administration and they penetrate the blood–brain barrier poorly. As a result, central effects are generally lacking.

Pharmacological properties

Central Nervous System

Atropine can stimulate the medulla and higher cerebral centres, but in doses used clinically to treat vagal bradycardia the CNS effects are minimal. With higher doses, such as may be used when atropine is administered in combination with an anticholinesterase for muscle relaxant reversal, central excitation becomes more prominent, leading to restlessness, irritation, disorientation or even delirium. Scopolamine in therapeutic doses normally causes drowsiness, amnesia, euphoria and fatigue. The sedative effects of scopolamine are still used for patient premedication. However, in some patients CNS excitation may be seen with therapeutic doses. Glycopyrronium and other quaternary compounds are devoid of CNS effect.

Cardiovascular System

Intravenous doses of atropine greater than about 0.5 mg cause progressive tachycardia by an interaction with M_2 receptors and by blocking vagal effects on the sinoatrial pacemaker. These doses can abolish many types of vagal bradycardia or asystole, such as those produced by stimulation of carotid glomus, eyeball pressure or peritoneal traction. They also antagonize the cardiac slowing induced by AChE inhibitors or by some intravenous anaesthetic agents with parasympathomimetic action. The blockade of vagal influence on the atrioventricular (AV) node can lessen the degree of some second-degree AV block, i.e. AV block induced by digitalis toxicity. In patients with a high degree of AV block, atropine may accelerate idioventricular rate. However, smaller doses of atropine (below 0.5 mg) or glycopyrronium (0.1–0.2 mg) can induce bradycardia, even if the drugs are administered following bilateral vagotomy. This effect suggests that anticholinergic drugs are not pure muscarinic receptor antagonists and that a weak peripheral muscarinic agonist activity occurs. This is mediated by increased release of ACh in the heart due to stimulation of M_1 receptors.

Table 9.5 Muscarinic anticholinergic agents			
	Atropine	Hyoscine	Glycopyrronium
Duration of action Intravenous Intramuscular	 15–30 min 2–4 h	 30–60 min 4–6 h	 2–4 h 6–8 h
Tachycardia	++++*	±*	±
Bronchial secretions	–	– – – –	– – –
Salivary and gastric secretions	–	–	– – –
Gut motility	– –	–	– – –
Central nervous system	++	+++†	o

* Bradycardia at low doses; † sedation followed by central excitation.

Eye

Atropine-like drugs dilate the pupil (mydriasis) and paralyse accommodation. They abolish the normal pupillary reflex constriction to light or upon convergence of the eyes. When administered parenterally, they have little effect on intraocular pressure, except in patients with narrow-angle glaucoma in whom intraocular pressure may occasionally rise. In wide-angle glaucoma, a significant rise in pressure is unusual. Penetration of the conjunctiva by quaternary ammonium is very low and these compounds are not of use in ophthalmology.

Respiratory Tract

Secretions of the nose, mouth, pharynx and bronchi are inhibited by antimuscarinic agents. This action is more pronounced where there is excessive secretion, as in chronic bronchitis. They also have a potent bronchodilator effect, mediated by blockade of ACh action on muscarinic M_3 receptors on the airway smooth muscle cells. The use of muscarinic antagonists in the therapy of respiratory disease has recently regained interest with the development of quaternary ammonium compounds, such as ipratropium, oxitropium and tiotropium bromide. Unexpectedly, these anticholinergic agents produce bronchodilatation without any effect on ciliary clearance. When administered by inhalation, the effects of ipratropium are confined exclusively to the mouth and respiratory tract, because of the very low absorption rate. The main therapeutic use of inhaled ipratropium is in chronic bronchitis.

Miscellaneous Effects

Muscarinic antagonists cause marked inhibition of gastrointestinal motility and secretions, through an action on M_3 receptors. However, selective histamine H_2-receptor antagonists have largely replaced these agents as inhibitors of acid secretion. Pirenzepine is a tricyclic compound that is selective for M_1 relative to M_2 and M_3 muscarinic receptors. It inhibits gastric acid secretion and can block vagally mediated bronchoconstriction. It is devoid of CNS effects because of low penetration of the blood–brain barrier. It is used in the treatment of peptic ulcers.

ANTICHOLINESTERASES

Anticholinesterase drugs exert their pharmacological action mainly by inhibition of acetylcholinesterase (AChE), the enzyme responsible for the hydrolysis of ACh to choline and acetic acid. AChE is located mainly in ANS cholinergic synapses and in motor endplates of skeletal muscle. Anticholinesterases inhibits hydrolysis by binding to the AChE and forming relatively stable complexes that prevent ACh reaching the catalytic site of the enzyme. AChE inhibition results in accumulation of ACh in the synapses, and postsynaptic cholinergic transmission is prolonged. Therapeutic doses of anticholinesterase drugs produce stimulation of muscarinic receptors at ANS effector organs and stimulation followed by depression of all ANS ganglia and skeletal muscle nicotinic receptors. Toxic doses of anticholinesterases may also produce stimulation followed by depression of CNS cholinergic receptors, which may be fatal.

Anticholinesterase may be divided into reversible and irreversible inhibitors. Hydrolysis of ACh is only inhibited for several hours by reversible anticholinesterase, as the inhibition is related to competition at the catalytic site between ACh and the inhibitor. In contrast, AChE is inhibited for a much longer period with irreversible inhibitors, as the enzyme becomes firmly and sometimes irreversibly phosphorylated in the process, and recovery of the enzyme can take from 60 min up to several weeks, depending on the compound involved. Most of the irreversible anticholinesterase drugs are organophosphate compounds.

REVERSIBLE ANTICHOLINESTERASES

Physostigmine (eserine), the first reversible anticholinesterase to be developed, was obtained from the Calabar bean, the seed of *Physostigma venenosum*. The quaternary derivatives, neostigmine and pyridostigmine, are compounds of greater stability and equal or greater potency. Edrophonium, an analogue of neostigmine that lacks the carbamoyl group, has a lower potency and shorter duration of action.

Pharmacological properties

Skeletal Neuromuscular Junction

The physiology of cholinergic transmission at the skeletal neuromuscular junction is considered elsewhere in this book, and will only be summarized here. Normally the ACh released in a motor axon ending is hydrolysed so rapidly by AChE that its concentration falls below the threshold concentration during the refractory period of the muscle fibre. After partial inhibition of AChE, the ACh released may persist long enough to set up repetitive muscle action potential and to diffuse to other muscle fibres, resulting in their asynchronous contraction (fibrillation). Furthermore, persistent action of ACh on the axon terminal can initiate the synchronous contraction of an entire motor unit (fasciculation). Finally, when ACh catabolism is sufficiently inhibited by cholinesterase antagonists, a depolarizing block of the neuromuscular junction occurs.

Gastrointestinal Tract

In humans, anticholinesterase drugs enhance gastric contraction and secretion of gastric acid. The lower portion of the oesophagus is stimulated by neostigmine, and motor activity of the bowel, particularly the colon, is increased. Anticholinesterases are used occasionally in the treatment of gastrointestinal atony.

Miscellaneous Effects

Low doses of anticholinesterase drugs increase the secretory response of secretory glands innervated by cholinergic nerves, including the bronchial, lacrymal, sweat, salivary, intestinal and pancreatic glands. Higher doses produce an increase in the resting rate of secretion. Smooth muscle fibres of bronchioles and ureters are contracted. The cardiovascular effects of these drugs reflect both ganglionic and postganglionic effects of an excess of ACh. Bradycardia occurs and, at higher doses, a decrease in arterial blood pressure.

Indication and use of cholinesterase inhibitors

AChE inhibitors are used for the treatment of gastrointestinal tract and urinary bladder atony, glaucoma and myasthenia gravis. In anaesthesia, neostigmine and edrophonium are used for reversing dopolarizing neuromuscular block. At doses used to obtain the therapeutic nicotinic action, muscarinic effects are always present. To prevent muscarinic effects (hypotension, bradycardia and bronchospasm), they must be combined with a muscarinic inhibitor of acetylcholine such as atropine or glycopyrronium. Physostigmine, unlike neostigmine and edrophonium, crosses the blood–brain barrier and is used to treat the anticholinergic syndrome, which can be caused by overdose of tricyclic antidepressants. This syndrome is also occasionally seen after general anaesthesia, and manifests as a patient in whom recovery from anaesthesia is excessively prolonged. In this situation, when other possible causes have been excluded, physostigmine, 1 mg intravenously, can sometimes produce a dramatic improvement.[14,15]

ORGANOPHOSPHORUS COMPOUNDS

Organophosphorus compounds are irreversible inhibitors of AChE. They are the most widely used insecticides in the world, and some are potential chemical warfare agents.[16] Organophosphorus insecticides are usually esters, amides or thiol derivatives of phosphoric or phosphonic acids. These agents have no therapeutic use, but are of particular interest to anaesthetists as patients with organophosphorus poisoning may present with severe cardiorespiratory distress requiring intensive care.

Mechanisms of action

Organophosphorus compounds exert their action by inhibition of several enzymes, the most important being AChE. Interaction between organophosphorus and AChE leads to a stable and sometimes irreversible phosphorylation of the enzyme, which becomes inactivated. Reactivation of the inhibited enzyme is possible, depending on the tissue and the compound. The process of reactivation may be induced by some oxime reagents. However, response to reactivating agents decreases with time, a process described as ageing of the inhibited enzyme. Other toxic effects of organophosphorus compounds are related to: (1) phosphorylation of a specific esteratic enzyme in the nervous system, responsible for delayed neuropathy; (2) abnormally high concentrations of ACh at the muscular endplate responsible for prolonged depolarization and myopathic changes; and (3) phosphorylation of numerous other enzymes; however, the clinical relevance of these reactions is not known.

Acute clinical signs of organophosphorus poisoning

Cholinergic Phase

Cholinergic manifestations are related to ACh accumulation in all postganglionic nerve endings (muscarinic signs), autonomic ganglia, skeletal muscle endplates (nicotinic signs) and CNS synapses. The symptoms may arise in various combinations and the time of onset may extend from a few minutes, after massive intoxication, to several hours. Nicotinic receptor stimulation results in muscle twitching, fasciculation, cramp and muscle weakness. Weakness of respiratory muscles associated with depression of respiratory centres, bronchospasm and tracheobronchial hypersecretion are responsible for respiratory distress. Bradycardia is often present and may progress to heart block. Vomiting is frequent and loss of consciousness may precipitate pulmonary aspiration. Muscarinic stimulation also leads to increased sweating, salivation, lacrimation and blurring of vision. Some 1–4 days after organophosphorus intoxication, some patients may develop a myopathic state referred to as the 'intermediate syndrome'. The main symptom is muscle weakness, which affects predominantly proximal limb muscles, neck flexors and muscles innervated by cranial motor nerves. Paralysis of respiratory muscle can lead to respiratory distress. A delayed polyneuropathy also has been described after poisoning with noninsecticide organophosphorus agents. The neuropathy develops 2–4 weeks after intoxication and produces distal weakness of the hands and feet, sometimes preceded by paraesthesia and calf pain. Wasting of the involved muscles occurs and recovery is uncommon.

GANGLION-BLOCKING DRUGS

The physiological changes induced by autonomic ganglionic blockade can be predicted if it is known which part of the ANS is predominantly involved in the regulation of a particular organ (Table 9.6). After the discovery that tetraethylammonium compounds acted on ANS ganglia, several structurally different chemical compounds were found to be ganglion blockers: *cis*-quaternary ammonium (hexamethonium and pentolinium), sulphonium derivatives (trimetaphan) and, more recently, secondary amines (mecamylamine).

Pharmacological properties

Cardiovascular Effects

The cardiovascular effects of ganglion-blocking drugs result predominantly from their vasodilator action on arterioles, causing a decrease in peripheral resistance, and on veins, leading to distal pooling of blood and a decrease in cardiac preload. Blood pressure and cardiac output are decreased, and this effect is more marked when sympathetic tone is high. Postural hypotension is therefore frequently observed in hypertensive patients treated with these drugs. Because of differences in autonomic innervation between organs, regional blood flows are usually redistributed after ganglionic blockade. Skin blood flow is increased, skeletal blood flow usually remains unchanged, and splanchnic and renal blood flows are decreased. As a consequence of

Table 9.6 Predominant tone of autonomic nervous system on effector organs and clinical effect of ganglionic blockade						
	Predominant tone					
	Sympathetic		**Parasympathetic**			
Organ	Vessel	Sweat gland	Heart	Eye	Urinary bladder GI tract	Salivary gland
Neurotransmission	Adrenergic	Cholinergic	Cholinergic	Cholinergic	Cholinergic	Cholinergic
Ganglionic blockade	Vasodilatation	Secretion decrease	Heart rate increase	Mydriasis Focus impairment	Urinary retention	Secretion and motility decrease

parasympathetic block to the heart, an increase in heart rate is the rule in normal subjects treated with ganglion blockers. However, in patients with preexisting tachycardia, reflecting high sympathetic outflow to the heart, a decrease in heart rate may occur.

Miscellaneous Effects

Ganglion blockers decrease salivary, gastrointestinal and sweat gland secretions, and gastrointestinal tract motility is impaired, resulting in constipation. The urinary bladder capacity is increased and voiding of the bladder is often incomplete. Penile erection and ejaculation are also frequently impaired.

Indication and therapeutic uses

The main indication for ganglion-blocking drugs such as mecamylamine and trimetaphan is hypertension. Because of the frequency and intensity of adverse reactions, they have been replaced by more effective and better tolerated agents. Ganglion-blocking drugs may be indicated for the control of hypertension in patients with acute aortic dissection or as additional agents to induce controlled hypotension during surgery. Trimetaphan is also used in patients with spinal cord injury who develop autonomic hyperreflexia.

REFERENCES

1. Marty J. Adrenergic function and reflexes during anaesthesia. *Curr Opin Anaesthesiol* 1989; **2**: 60–63.
2. Insel PA. Adrenergic receptors – evolving concepts and clinical implications. *N Engl J Med* 1996; **334**: 580–585.
3. Starke K. Alpha-adrenoceptor subclassification. *Rev Physiol Biochem Pharmacol* 1981; **88**: 198–236.
4. Aarons RD, Nies AS, Gal J et al. Elevation of β-adrenergic receptor density in human lymphocytes after propranolol administration. *J Clin Invest* 1980; **65**: 949–957.
5. Ungerer M, Bohm M, Elce JS, Erdmann E, Lohse MJ. Altered expression of beta-adrenergic receptor kinase and beta₁-adrenergic receptors in the failing human heart. *Circulation* 1993; **87**: 4543–4563.
6. Ruffolo RR Jr, Nichols AJ, Stadel JM, Hieble JP. Structure and function of alpha-adrenoceptors. *Pharmacol Rev* 1991; **43**: 475–505.
7. Lambert DG, Appadu BL. Muscarinic receptor subtypes: do they have a place in clinical anaesthesia? *Br J Anaesth* 1995; **74**: 497–498.
8. Nelson HS. β-Adrenergic bronchodilators. *N Engl J Med* 1995; **333**: 499–506.
9. McGrath JM, Chesnut DH, Vincent RD et al. Ephedrine remains the vasopressor of choice for treatment of hypotension during ritodrine infusion and epidural anesthesia. *Anesthesiology* 1994; **80**: 1073–1081.
10. Hollmen AI, Jouppila R, Albright GA et al. Intervillous blood flow during caesarean section with prophylactic ephedrine and epidural anaesthesia. *Acta Anaesthesiol Scand* 1984; **28**: 396–400.
11. Li P, Tong C, Eisenach JC. Pregnancy and ephedrine increase the release of nitric oxide in ovine uterine arteries. *Anesth Analg* 1996; **82**: 288–293.
12. Goertz AW, Lindner KH, Schhtz W et al. Influence of phenylephrine bolus administration on left ventricular filling dynamics in patients with coronary artery disease and patients with valvular aortic stenosis. *Anesthesiology* 1994; **81**: 49–58.
13. Schwinn DA, Reves JG. Time course and hemodynamic effects of alpha-1-adrenergic bolus administration in anesthetized patients with myocardial disease. *Anesth Analg* 1989; **68**: 571–578.
14. Martin B, Howell-PR. Physostigmine: going ... going ... gone? Two cases of central anticholinergic syndrome following anaesthesia and its treatment with physostigmine. *Eur J Anaesthesiol* 1997; **14**: 467–470.
15. Link J, Papadopoulos G, Dopjans D et al. Distinct central anticholinergic syndrome following general anaesthesia. *Eur J Anaesthesiol* 1997; **14**: 15–23.
16. Karalliedde L, Senanayake N. Organophosphorus insecticide poisoning. *Br J Anaesth* 1989; **63**: 736–750.

10 C Meistelman, B Plaud

NEUROMUSCULAR BLOCKING DRUGS

When muscle relaxants were introduced in 1942, they changed the practice of anaesthesia and made possible the development of balanced anaesthesia. The first relaxant was intoconstrin, obtained from the plant *Chondodendrum tomentosum*. Since then numerous compounds have been synthesized and introduced into clinical practice.

PHYSIOLOGY OF NEUROMUSCULAR TRANSMISSION

Each muscle fibre is served by, at the most, three neuromuscular junctions. The nerve cell together with the muscle fibre it innervates is called the 'motor unit'. The axon forms intimate contact with a single muscle fibre, looses its myelin sheath and then branches to form the neuromuscular junction. There is no direct contact between the nerve terminal and the muscle fibre; they are separated by a narrow (0.02–0.05 μm) gap, the synaptic cleft (Fig. 10.1). There are two types of muscle fibres: slow-twitch fibres such as the soleus muscle, which have slow contraction times and are resistant to fatigue, and fast-twitch fibres, which have fast contraction times and are less resistant to fatigue (e.g. the diaphragm). The nerve terminal contains vesicles of acetylcholine and mitochondria and cisternae, which are involved in the recycling of the vesicles. The enzyme acetylcholinesterase is present in the synaptic cleft and is concentrated in the folds of the synaptic cleft. Neuromuscular transmission starts with the arrival of a nerve action potential at the nerve terminal and concludes with depolarization of the postjunctional membrane. The whole process takes only a few milliseconds.

RELEASE OF ACETYLCHOLINE

Acetylcholine, the neurotransmitter of the neuromuscular junction, is synthesized from choline and acetyl coenzyme A by choline acetyltransferase. About half of the acetylcholine present in each nerve terminal is contained in vesicles, each containing about 12 000 molecules of acetylcholine, which are concentrated at the active zone near the cell membrane opposite the crests of the junctional folds of the endplate (Fig. 10.1). The rest is present in the axoplasm.

In the absence of nerve impulses, acetylcholine is spontaneously released as packets or quanta from the nerve endings. Each quantum, thought to be the content of one vesicle, contains about 5000–10 000 molecules. This release causes a slight depolarization (0.5–1.0 mV) of the postjunctional motor endplate, the miniature endplate potential (MEPP). The MEPP is too small to generate an action potential and muscle contraction. When acetylcholine is released by an action potential, more than 100 quanta are released simultaneously and produce the full endplate potential (EPP). When the EPP reaches threshold (−50 mV), it triggers a muscle action potential. Release of acetylcholine is strongly dependent on extracellular calcium,

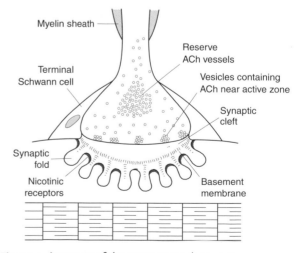

Fig. 10.1 Anatomy of the neuromuscular junction.

which enters through voltage-gated calcium channels and binds to synaptotagmin, an integral membrane protein of synaptic vesicles.[1] Synaptotagmin, which is essential for fast neurotransmitter release, combines with syntaxin, a plasma membrane docking protein, leading to fusion and exocytosis of synaptic vesicles docked at the active zone and discharge of acetylcholine into the synaptic cleft.

POSTJUNCTIONAL EVENTS

Following release and diffusion across the synaptic cleft, acetylcholine interacts with the cholinergic nicotinic receptors clustered on the crests of the junctional folds. The receptor density in this area is 10 000–30 000 μm^{-2}. Two molecules of acetylcholine must bind to the α subunits of the receptor to induce the conformational changes that allow Na^+ to enter the cell, making the inside less negative. If a large number of receptors opens simultaneously, the cells become sufficiently depolarized to trigger an action potential. The propagation of the action potential to the whole muscle is then independent of acetylcholine receptors. The action potential causes voltage-sensitive calcium channels to open, and intracellular Ca^{2+} concentration increases rapidly. The calcium binds with troponin, removing the inhibition by troponin of actin and myosin, and muscle contraction follows. The influx of Ca^{2+} also mobilizes reserve vesicles by an action on synapsin I, a complex phosphoprotein which forms part of the vesicle.

PREJUNCTIONAL EVENTS

During high-frequency stimulation, under physiological conditions, the release of acetylcholine decreases but is sufficient to depolarize the endplate above threshold. Low concentrations of acetylcholine may facilitate further release of acetylcholine. The decrease in acetylcholine release during high-frequency stimulation (train-of-four (TOF), tetanus) in the presence of nondepolarizing muscle relaxants explains the progressive decrease in muscle response, i.e. fade. This effect may be mediated through prejunctional receptors, which mobilize reserve acetylcholine into the readily releasable store.[2]

EFFECTS OF MUSCLE RELAXANTS AT THE NEUROMUSCULAR JUNCTION

DEPOLARIZING MUSCLE RELAXANTS: SUXAMETHONIUM (SUCCINYLCHOLINE)

Suxamethonium produces depolarization of the postsynaptic membrane which is similar to, but more persistent than, that achieved by acetylcholine. The onset of neuromuscular block is characterized by fasciculations of muscles fibres thought to represent

---

Summary box 10.1 Depolarizing muscle relaxants

- Suxamethonium is the only one used clinically.

- Structure of suxamethonium is similar to two acetylcholine molecules back to back.

- Block is not associated with fade on repetitive muscle stimulation.

- Not antagonized by anticholinesterases, which can increase the degree of block.

- Repeated doses or administration by continuous intravenous infusion can lead to phase II block.

- Metabolized in blood by plasma cholinesterase:

  - patients with decreased plasma cholinesterase concentrations or those with genetically determined defect of the enzyme may have prolonged block following suxamethonium.

- Risk of severe hyperkalaemia with patients with burn injuries or with massive tissue trauma.

- Can cause bradycardia, especially in children.

- Trigger for malignant hyperthermia.

---

random repetitive neuronal firing. It could also be due to the depolarization of prejunctional receptors, and the abolition of fasciculations by *d*-tubocurarine may represent an action at the presynaptic receptor. The neuromuscular block is characterized by a twitch response to indirect stimulation, which is diminished but sustained with repetitive stimulation (i.e. absence of fade) (Fig. 10.2). It is associated with endplate depolarization and development of a surrounding zone of inexcitability through which a muscle action potential evoked by direct stimulation cannot propagate. During prolonged depolarization, the muscle may gain sodium and chloride and lose significant amounts of potassium, sufficient to raise serum levels of this ion. With continuous administration a 'phase II block' develops, characterized by fade and post-tetanic facilitation. One of the mechanisms for this could be excessive activation of presynaptic nicotinic receptors, leading to reduced transmitter output. It could also be due to desensitization of the endplate, which then becomes refractory to chemical stimulation.

NONDEPOLARIZING MUSCLE RELAXANTS

Nondepolarizing muscle relaxants (NDMRs) bind competitively at the same site as acetylcholine on the α

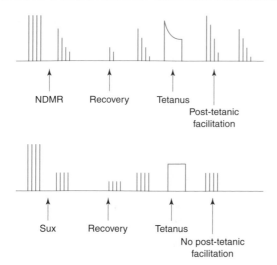

Fig. 10.2 Response to train-of-four and tetanus for depolarizing and nondepolarizing and (upper) muscle relaxants (NDMR). Sux, suxamethonium.

subunit of the nicotinic postjunctional receptor. The binding of one nicotinic antagonist molecule to one of the two a subunits of the receptor prevents opening of the channel because both a subunits need to bind acetylcholine for activation of the channel. In a given situation, the proportion of receptors occupied by the agonist depends on the affinity of the binding site for the agonist, on its affinity for the antagonist, and the concentration of agonist and antagonist. Non-NDMR drugs may also be able to block the open receptor because they can access the mouth of the open channel

---

Summary box 10.2 Nondepolarizing muscle relaxants

- Competitive antagonists of acetylcholine at nicotinic receptors.

- Reversed by anticholinesterases, e.g. neostigmine, edrophonium.

- Block characterized by fade and post-tetanic facilitation.

- Bulky molecules belonging to two main chemical groups:

  - isoquinoline based – tubocurarine, atracurium, cisatracurium, doxacurium, mivacurium

  - steroid based – pancuronium, vecuronium, rocuronium, pipecuronium, rapacuronium.

- Speed of onset inversely proportional to potency.

---

but cannot pass through, thus preventing further ionic movement. This type of block is noncompetitive but its role is probably marginal.

Only a small fraction of receptors needs to bind acetylcholine to produce depolarization. This has been referred as the 'margin of safety' of neuromuscular transmission. About 75% of receptors need to be occupied by the muscle relaxant before a decrease in twitch height becomes apparent. Block is usually complete in peripheral muscles when 92% of receptors are occupied. Peripheral muscles have a smaller margin of safety than the diaphragm. The block produced by NDMRs is characterized by fade to repetitive stimulation and tetanus. Following tetanic stimulation, synthesis of acetylcholine is increased, which continues for some time after cessation of stimulation. This results in post-tetanic facilitation where a muscle response to a single stimulus or TOF is enhanced (Fig. 10.2).

Structure

The currently available NDMRs belong to one of two chemical classes: bis-quaternary diester derivatives of benzylisoquinolinium compounds and the 2, 16-bisamino steroidal compounds. These are bulky molecules with two cationic centres formed by quaternary nitrogens or, at physiological pH, protonated tertiary nitrogens, separated by a distance of 1.2–1.4 nm. This interionic distance is optimal for neuromuscular blocking potency.

Onset and potency

An inverse relationship between potency and the speed of onset for NDMRs has been demonstrated by Bowman et al.[3] (Fig. 10.3). The neuromuscular junction has a very high concentration of nicotinic receptors, and up to 75% of receptors must be occupied by a relaxant before neuromuscular block can be detected. With a low-potency NDMR, more molecules are administered than in the case of a more potent drug, and the receptors at the neuromuscular junction will be occupied more rapidly as a result of a greater concentration gradient between the synaptic cleft and the receptors. This high concentration gradient encourages a faster onset of action.

Priming

Priming, by which a small dose of relaxant (generally 10–30% of the effective dose $(ED)_{95}$) (dose producing 95% of maximum neuromuscular block) is administered 2–4 min before the intubating dose, has been used in an attempt to speed the onset of action of NDMRs. It is thought that priming works by partial filling of excess receptors, requiring only a small additional increment in receptor occupancy to achieve neuromuscular block. However, the effect of priming is small and may be associated with symptoms in sensitive muscles such as the eyes and upper airway muscles. Swallowing reflexes are also likely to be depressed, increasing the risk of regurgitation and aspiration.[4]

MONITORING OF NEUROMUSCULAR BLOCKADE

Visual or tactile evaluation of muscular responses following nerve stimulation is the easiest way to assess neuromuscular block during anaesthesia. However, fade can be difficult to detect manually or visually, and can lead to underestimation of neuromuscular block. Measurement of muscular strength using a force transducer is a more accurate method. Unfortunately, the force transducers available limit this technique to monitoring of the adductor pollicis.

Summary box 10.3 Terminology of neuromuscular block
• Onset time: time from drug administration to maximum effect. • Clinical duration: time from drug administration to 25% recovery of the twitch response. • Total duration of action: time from drug administration to 90% recovery of twitch response. • Recovery index: time from 25% to 75% recovery of the twitch response.

STIMULUS PATTERN

Train-of-four
TOF consists of four stimulations at a frequency of 2 Hz, which can be repeated at 10–12-s intervals. No control value is needed for TOF measurement. The TOF ratio is the ratio of the height of the first and the fourth response. A TOF ratio of at least 0.8 is necessary to guarantee adequate recovery of respiratory function after neuromuscular block. However, visual or tactile evaluation of the TOF ratio can be misleading, because it is not always possible to detect fade until the TOF ratio is as low as 0.4–0.5, even for experienced observers.

Tetanus, post-tetanic count
Although tetanic stimulation has been used in the past to detect fade during recovery, it offers little advantage compared with the TOF. The main indication for tetanic stimulation is in performing a post-tetanic count (PTC)

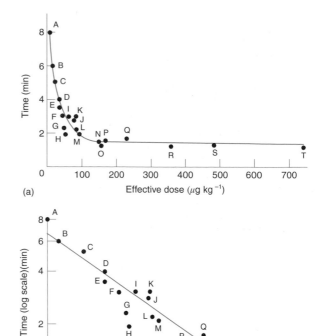

Fig. 10.3 Relationship between effective dose and onset time for 20 chemically related aminosteroidal neuromuscular blocking drugs. The effective dose (abscissa) is the mean dose to produce 50% twitch depression at the tibialis anterior. From Bowman et al.[3]

when profound neuromuscular block exists and no responses to TOF are detectable. PTC consists of a 50-Hz tetanic stimulation applied for 5 s, followed after a 3-s pause by single twitch stimulations at 1 Hz. For a given drug, the number of detectable responses correlates inversely with the time for spontaneous recovery of TOF (Fig. 10.4).[5] PTC should not be tested more often than every 5 min.

Double-burst stimulation
Double-burst stimulation (DBS) was introduced to improve the detection of fade during visual or tactile evaluation. DBS consists of two, very short, 50-Hz tetanic bursts (two to four pulses) separated by 750 ms. $DBS_{3,3}$ consists of two bursts of three impulses. The two contractions induced by a DBS are of greater amplitude than the contractions after a TOF, and visual or manual assessment of fade is easier.[6]

Accelerography
Accelerography is based on the principle that acceleration, recorded by a piezoelectric transducer, is

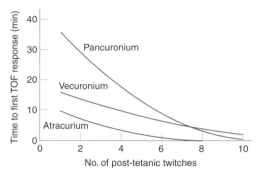

Fig. 10.4 Relationship between post-tetanic count and the predicted time until appearance of the first response of the train-of-four (TOF) for pancuronium, vecuronium and atracurium. Compiled using data from Viby-Morgensen *et al.*[5] (pancuronium), Bonsu *et al.*[16] (atracurium) and Eriksson *et al.*[17] (vecuronium).

proportional to force if mass remains unchanged. The advantages of accelerography is an easy set-up of the transducer and the possibility of monitoring muscles other than the adductor pollicis. The accelerographic T4 : T1 ratio can be greater than 1.0 in the absence of neuromuscular block. It has reduced sensitivity and a greater variability at low twitch heights.

Electromyography
Electromyography (EMG) uses the electrical activity obtained from surface electrodes placed over a contracting muscle as an index of neuromuscular transmission. An advantage is that it does not require bulky equipment and can be used in children. The accuracy depends on the muscle monitored. EMG monitoring of the hypothenar muscles overestimates the degree of recovery from neuromuscular block.

ACTION OF RELAXANTS ON DIFFERENT BODY MUSCLES
The laryngeal adductor muscles and the diaphragm are more resistant to the effects of NDMRs than peripheral muscles such as the adductor pollicis, possibly due to the larger number of acetylcholine receptors present on respiratory muscles.[7,8] Thus a clinical block of the adductor pollicis may not result in complete paralysis of the respiratory muscles. The duration of effect of pancuronium at the adductor pollicis is approximately twice that at the diaphragm. Surprisingly the onset of neuromuscular block is significantly more rapid at the respiratory muscles than at the adductor pollicis (Fig. 10.5). This is because of the much greater blood supply to the laryngeal muscles and the diaphragm than to peripheral muscles, so that after a bolus dose peak plasma concentrations occur earlier in these muscles than in skeletal muscles. Conversely, plasma concentrations decrease more rapidly, and because the laryngeal adductor muscles and the diaphragm recover at higher plasma concentrations, recovery from neuromuscular block occurs sooner than for the adductor pollicis.

The muscles of the upper airway are particularly sensitive to the effects of muscle relaxants. The masseter is approximately 15% more sensitive to NDMRs than the adductor pollicis. Small doses of pancuronium (0.02 mg kg^{-1}) depress the swallowing reflex to a greater extent than the strength of peripheral muscles.

CLINICAL APPLICATIONS

Onset
Because paralysis of the adductor pollicis lags behind onset at the laryngeal adductor muscles and the

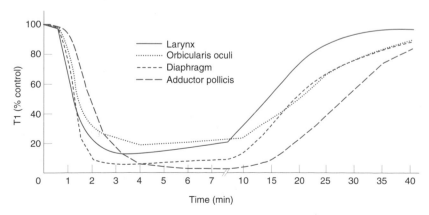

Fig. 10.5 Onset and recovery of neuromuscular blockade after injection of vecuronium 0.07 mg kg^{-1} at four muscles. Data from Donati *et al.*[7]

diaphragm, monitoring the adductor pollicis to determine the time for good intubating conditions could be misleading. Since the sensitivity of the orbicularis oculi is close to that of the respiratory and laryngeal muscles, monitoring this muscle may reliably detect when respiratory muscles and vocal cords are paralysed (Fig. 10.6).[8]

Surgical relaxation

When profound neuromuscular block is required, absence of the TOF response at the adductor pollicis cannot be relied upon to avoid hiccups, cough or extrusion of the abdominal contents, which can occur for the reasons discussed above. In this situation the PTC techniques described above can be used. The major drawback of this technique is that it cannot be repeated more often than every 5 min. Alternatively the TOF can be monitored at the orbicularis oculi, since there is good agreement between the response of the orbicularis oculi and diaphragmatic paralysis.[7] When profound block is not essential, monitoring of the adductor pollicis, using TOF, is sufficient.

Recovery

The adductor pollicis is the preferred muscle for monitoring recovery since, when it has almost completely recovered, it can be assumed that there is no residual paralysis of either the diaphragm or the laryngeal muscles. A TOF ratio of at least 0.8–0.9 is needed to avoid any respiratory problem secondary to residual neuromuscular block. However, because some muscles of the upper airway are very sensitive to the effects of relaxants, monitoring of the adductor pollicis should be used in conjunction with clinical tests of recovery, such as the patient's ability to lift the head for

5 s, to stick out the tongue or to swallow, because they indicate a sufficient degree of recovery to protect the upper airway against obstruction or aspiration. Recovery depends, among other factors, on the pharmacokinetics of the different drugs (Fig. 10.7).

INDIVIDUAL DRUGS

SUXAMETHONIUM (SUCCINYLCHOLINE)

Pharmacology

Suxamethonium is a bisquaternary ammonium compound with a chemical structure resembling two molecules of acetylcholine back to back (Fig. 10.8), which explains many of its actions. However, it is removed from the neuromuscular junction 1000 times more slowly than acetylcholine, by plasma cholinesterase (pseudocholinesterase or butyrylcholinesterase) (Table 10.1). Suxamethonium is not a substrate for acetylcholinesterase. The mean doses producing 50% block (ED_{50}) and 95% block (ED_{95}) at the adductor pollicis are 0.3 and 0.5–0.6 mg kg^{-1} respectively. Suxamethonium is rapidly hydrolysed by plasma cholinesterase to choline and succinylmonocholine. Following suxamethonium 0.5 mg kg^{-1}, onset time is 60–90 s at the adductor pollicis and within 60 s at the laryngeal adductor muscles and the diaphragm. Suxamethonium 1.0 mg kg^{-1} produces complete neuromuscular block in about 60 s, and recovery is 90% complete within 6–12 min. When a small dose of NDMR is given before suxamethonium, the onset time is increased by about 30% and, with the exception of pancuronium, which inhibits cholinesterase, the duration of action is decreased by 30–50%. The dose of suxamethonium must be increased by 50–100% to achieve comparable paralysis. Prolonged administration of suxamethonium

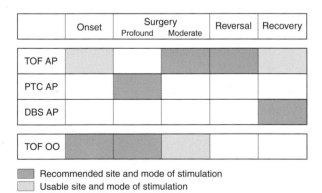

	Onset	Surgery		Reversal	Recovery
		Profound	Moderate		
TOF AP					
PTC AP					
DBS AP					
TOF OO					

■ Recommended site and mode of stimulation
□ Usable site and mode of stimulation

Fig. 10.6 Different modes and sites of stimulation suggested for monitoring of neuromuscular blockade during anaesthesia. TOF, train-of-four; PTC, post-tetanic count; DBS, double-burst stimulation; AP, adductor pollicis; OO, orbicularis oculi. From Meistelman C. *Curr Opin Anaesthesiol* 1993; **6**: 720–726.

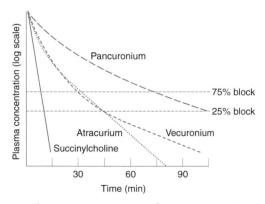

Fig. 10.7 Plasma concentrations after equipotent doses of pancuronium, vecuronium, atracurium and succinylcholine as a function of time. From Donati F. *Semin Anesth* 1994; **13**: 310–320.

Table 10.1 Metabolism and excretion of muscle relaxants			
		Excretion (%)	
Muscle relaxant	**Metabolism**	**Kidney**	**Liver**
Succinylcholine	Plasma cholinesterases (90%)	1–2	–
Atracurium	Hofmann elimination and ester hydrolysis (60–90%)	10–40	–
Cisatracurium	Hofmann elimination (80%)	10–15	–
Doxacurium	Plasma cholinesterases (< 10%)	60–80	10–20
Metocurine	–	40	2
Mivacurium	Plasma cholinesterases (95–99%)	< 5	–
Pancuronium	Liver (10–20%)	70	30
Pipecuronium	Liver (10%)	70	20
Rocuronium	Liver (10%)	30	70
Tubocurarine	–	40–60	10–40
Vecuronium	Liver (40%)	20–30	70–80

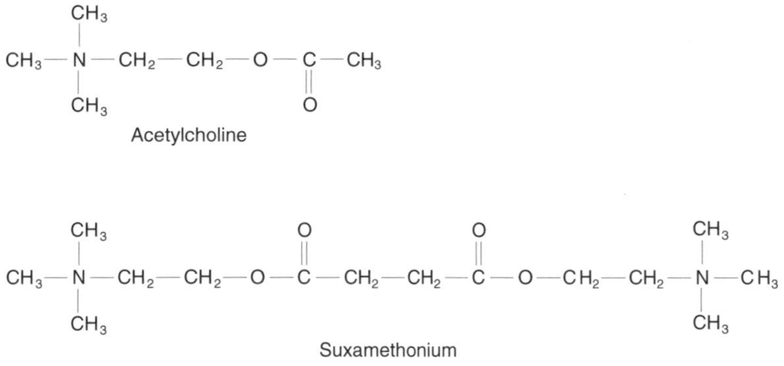

Acetylcholine

Suxamethonium

Fig. 10.8 Structure of acetylcholine and suxamethonium. Suxamethonium can be considered as two molecules of acetylcholine joined back to back.

leads to a change in the nature of the block to one resembling that of NDMR (phase II block).

Side-effects
Suxamethonium can produce a number of side-effects, although these are usually of minor clinical importance. The life-threatening complications malignant hyperthermia, anaphylaxis and extreme hyperkalaemia are rare but may arise without warning.

The incidence of muscle fasciculation is high, especially in adults. It can be prevented by giving a small dose of NDMR before suxamethonium but care must be taken to avoid partial paralysis in awake patients. The reported incidence of muscle pain varies from 1.5 to 89%. Early postoperative mobility may be a factor in determining the severity of muscle pain. A relationship between fasciculations and muscle pain has not been established. Administration of suxamethonium is followed by a transient increase in serum potassium concentration, which is usually clinically insignificant. Severe hyperkalaemia producing arrhythmias or cardiac arrest may occur in patients with burns, trauma, sepsis, neurological and muscular disorders. The mechanism is thought to be the extrajunctional spread of acetylcholine receptors. In burn patients, suxamethonium should be avoided for several weeks to months after complete healing, when the patient reverts to a normal metabolic state.

Because of its structural similarity to acetylcholine, suxamethonium can produce sinus bradycardia with nodal or ventricular escape beats, especially in children and infants when vagal tone is predominant. These can be prevented by previous administration of atropine or glycopyrronium. Suxamethonium-induced catecholamine release can cause tachycardia in adults, although this is seldom pronounced following a single dose. In contrast a second dose may cause bradycardia by a mechanism that is poorly understood.

Suxamethonium is associated with a mean increase in intraocular pressure of about 8 mmHg, lasting for up to 10 min. This may be due to a sustained contraction of the extraocular muscles and is not reliably prevented by pretreatment with NDMRs. Suxamethonium has traditionally been avoided in patients with a penetrating eye injury. However, there is a greater increase in intraocular pressure during laryngoscopy and intubation in lightly anaesthetized, poorly paralysed patients.

Suxamethonium causes an increase in intragastric pressure which may be as high as 40 cmH$_2$O and is related to the severity of the fasciculations. The pressure in the lower oesophageal sphincter increases during fasciculations by more than the intragastric pressure, and this may lessen the risk of aspiration. There is also an increase in intracranial pressure, possibly related to an increase in the partial pressure of carbon dioxide during fasciculations. It can be prevented by precurarization.

Masseter muscle rigidity (MMR) is a contracture of the masseter to a degree that interferes with tracheal intubation, despite an adequate concentration of suxamethonium. Indeed, an increase in masseter muscle tone of up to 500 g lasting 1–2 min is a normal finding.[9] Traditionally MMR has been taken to herald the development of malignant hyperthermia. However, although occasionally MMR may precede malignant hyperthermia, most cases of MMR may simply represent the extreme of a spectrum of tension changes in response to suxamethonium. The incidence of MMR is within 0.5–1%, whereas the incidence of malignant hyperthermia is about 1:12 000 in children and 1:30 000 in adults. None the less, patients developing MMR should be monitored carefully for evidence of hypermetabolism (hypercapnia, metabolic acidosis, tachycardia, increased oxygen consumption, hyperthermia), and possible triggers of malignant hyperthermia such as anaesthetic vapours should be avoided if treatment is continued.

The incidence of anaphylactic reactions may be close to 0.06%, and, of all muscle relaxants, suxamethonium was associated with the greatest number of serious reactions.[10] Almost all the cases of anaphylaxis have been reported in Europe or Australia. Anaphylactic reactions are more frequent than anaphylactoid ones. Patients with a history of anaphylactic reaction to suxamethonium may exhibit a cross-reaction, at least in vitro, with NDMRs. The cross-reactivity is related to the common structural features of these drugs, all of which contain quaternary ammonium ions.

About 3–5% of patients have a genetically determined deficiency of plasma cholinesterase, the enzyme responsible for the metabolic breakdown of suxamethonium (see Chapter 2). There are several types of abnormal cholinesterase, the most common being those associated with the atypical, fluoride-resistant and silent genes.[11] In patients with the atypical gene mutation, pseudocholinesterase is often present in normal amounts, but its affinity for suxamethonium is reduced compared with the normal form of the enzyme. The duration of action of suxamethonium is slightly increased (10–20 min) in patients heterozygous for this gene. Neuromuscular block may be very prolonged (45–360 min) in patients homozygous for either the atypical or silent genes.[12] Homozygotes for the silent gene have little or no cholinesterase activity and are extremely sensitive to suxamethonium.

The *atypical* gene mutation is diagnosed on the basis of inhibition of cholinesterase by the local anaesthetic dibucaine (cinchocaine). Dibucaine inhibits normal pseudocholinesterase whereas the abnormal form is approximately 20 times less sensitive to such inhibition. The percentage inhibition is called the 'dibucaine number'. Based on the dibucaine number, individuals can be classified into three groups: normal individuals (dibucaine number between 71% and 85%), intermediate (dibucaine number approximately 60) and atypical (dibucaine number approximately 20). Those in the intermediate group are heterozygous with a frequency of about 1 in 25 and do not normally show significant sensitivity to suxamethonium or ester drugs. The frequency of the atypical homozygotes is 1 in 3000 to 1 in 10 000 and they are sensitive to suxamethonium. These are the patients who develop 'scoline apnoea'. The fluoride-resistant gene results in the production of cholinesterase that is resistant to inhibition by fluoride ion. Patients who are homozygote for this gene are moderately sensitive to suxamethonium.

The concentration of plasma cholinesterase may be decreased during pregnancy, hepatic disease, burns, sepsis, malnutrition, treatment by cyclophosphamide or ecothiopate eye drops. This may increase the duration of action of suxamethonium by 25–50%.

LONG-ACTING NDMRs

d-Tubocurarine; Metocurine

Tubocurarine is a monoquaternary benzylisoquolinium compound. It is eliminated unchanged in the urine and bile (Table 10.1). In patients with renal failure the action is prolonged due to changes in its pharmacokinetics, as the sensitivity to *d*-tubocurarine remains unchanged. The onset of action is slow (4–7 min with once the ED_{95}) and the clinical duration is 80–100 min.

d-Tubocurarine is the only benzylisoquolinium to block transmission in autonomic ganglions at doses of less than 10 times the ED_{95} (Table 10.2). A dose of 0.3–0.5 mg kg^{-1} can induce histamine release, and this may be more important than ganglionic block in the production of hypotension and tachycardia. Because of the long duration of action and the cardiovascular side-effects *d*-tubocurarine has been replaced by other NDMRs.

Metocurine (dimethyltubocurarine) is a methylated derivative of *d*-tubocurarine. The ED_{95} is 0.3 mg kg^{-1}. Histamine release is less than with *d*-tubocurarine. Pharmacokinetic parameters are close to those of

Table 10.2 Autonomic effects and histamine release of muscle relaxants			
Muscle relaxant	Autonomic ganglion	Cardiac muscarinic receptors	Histamine release
Succinylcholine	Stimulation	Modest stimulation	Slight
Atracurium	o	o	Moderate
Cisatracurium	o	o	None to slight
Doxacurium	o	o	Slight
Metocurine	Weak block	o	Slight
Mivacurium	o	o	Moderate
Pancuronium	o	Weak block	o
Pipecuronium	o	o	o
Rocuronium	o	Weak block	o
Tubocurarine	Block	o	Strong
Vecuronium	o	o	o

d-tubocurarine, but metocurine is more dependent on renal function for excretion. It has been used in association with pancuronium because their cardiovascular effects counteract each other. However, the use of metocurine has diminished with the introduction of NDMRs free from cardiovascular side-effects.

Pancuronium

Pancuronium is a synthetic bisquaternary aminosteroid compound (Fig. 10.9). It is metabolized mainly by acetylation in the liver to 3-OH and 17-OH derivatives which are excreted in the urine. The 3-OH metabolite, which is 40–50% as potent as pancuronium, is the only one detected in humans. The 17-OH metabolite has about one-fiftieth the potency of pancuronium. Elimination is mainly by the kidney (Table 10.1) and in renal failure clearance is decreased, resulting in a prolonged duration of action, because biliary excretion cannot compensate for the decrease in glomerular filtration rate. Plasma clearance is also reduced in patients with hepatic disease. However, resistance to the initial dose is frequently observed in patients with liver cirrhosis, owing to a larger distribution volume. Pharmacokinetics (Table 10.3) are similar between adults and children. In the elderly, the plasma clearance is lower than in young adults because the glomerular filtration rate decreases with age.

Onset time of maximum neuromuscular block is about 3.5 min after twice the ED_{95}. Following administration of twice the ED_{95}, the clinical duration of action and total duration of action are close to 70–80 and 120 min respectively (Table 10.4). Accumulation occurs with a progressive increase in the duration of action after repeated doses. When reversing pancuronium, the fourth response of the TOF should be detected before giving neostigmine. The halogenated inhalational anaesthetic agents shift the dose–response curve to the left, an effect that is dependent on the concentration and duration of administration. The potentiating effects of enflurane are greater than those of isoflurane or halothane.

Pancuronium increases heart rate, arterial blood pressure and cardiac output. These cardiovascular effects are related to vagolytic and sympathomimetic effects. Pancuronium blocks muscarinic M_2 receptors in the heart, sympathetic nerve endings and dopaminergic interneurons in sympathetic ganglia in doses within the clinical range. It also increases the release of

Table 10.3 Pharmacokinetic parameters of muscle relaxants				
Drug	V_{dss} (ml kg^{-1})	Clearance (ml kg^{-1} min^{-1})	Elimination half-life (min)	Protein bound (%)
Suxamethonium	6–16	200–500	2–8	30
Tubocurarine	450	2–4	200	40–50
Metocurine	400–470	1.2	220–360	35
Pancuronium	260–280	1.9	110–135	30
Pipecuronium	340–425	1.6–3.4	100	–
Doxacurium	230	2.7	99	28–34
Vecuronium	180–250	3.6–5.3	50–53	30–57
Rocuronium	170–210	3.4	70–80	25
Atracurium	180–280	5.5–10.8	17–20	51
Cisatracurium	110–200	4–7	18–27	–
Mivacurium cis-trans	146–588	26–147	1–5	–
trans-trans	123–338	18–79	2–8	–
cis-cis	191–346	2–5	41–200	–

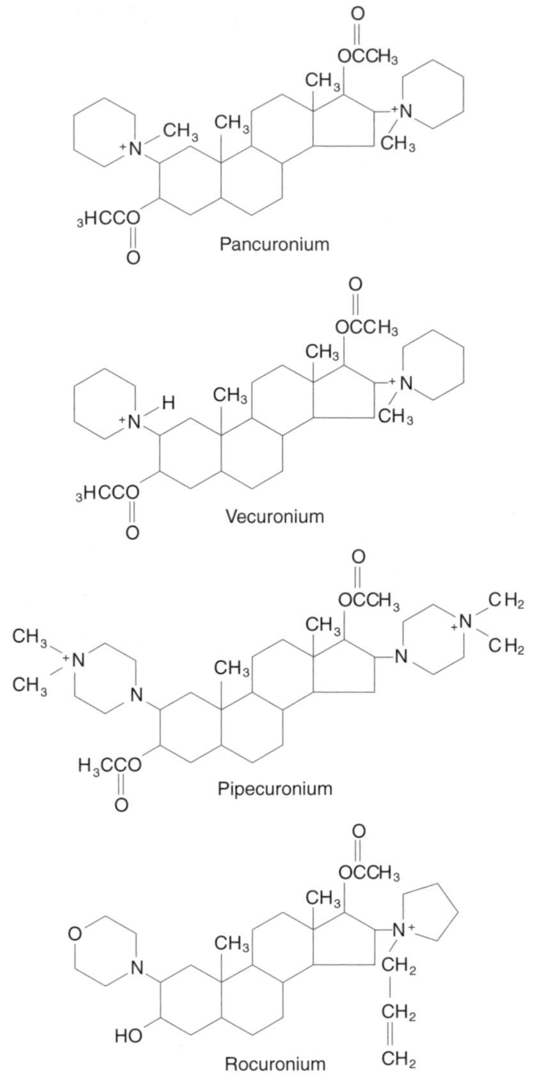

Fig. 10.9 Structures of aminosteroid muscle relaxants.

noradrenaline and decreases its reuptake from the sympathetic nerve endings in the atria and vascular smooth muscle. Unlike tubocurarine, pancuronium does not cause histamine release.

Pipecuronium

Pipecuronium bromide is a steroidal NDMR (Fig. 10.9) which resembles pancuronium in potency and duration of action. It is metabolized in the liver to a 3-OH derivative which has 40–50% the potency of the parent drug. Renal elimination accounts for 37–41% of elimination; biliary excretion is negligible (2%). Plasma clearance is decreased in patients with renal failure, leading to a marked prolongation of the elimination half-life. In patients with cholestasis, neither the pharmacokinetics nor the time course of action are significantly different from those of normal patients.

A dose of twice the ED_{95} results in complete block in 3.0–3.5 min, with a clinical duration of action of 70–110 min. Like other NDMRs, a bolus of pipecuronium exerts greater effect in adults and infants than in children. The onset of action is slower in patients older than 70 years, but the duration of action is not significantly prolonged provided renal function is normal. Pipecuronium is comparable to other long-acting relaxants in terms of potentiation of neuro-muscular block by halogenated agents and reversal by anticholinesterase drugs. Edrophonium is relatively ineffective against pipecuronium-induced neuro-muscular block, even when almost complete recovery has taken place.

Pipecuronium is devoid of cardiovascular side-effects, and doses of up to three times the ED_{95} do not produce significant changes in heart rate or blood pressure. It lacks the autonomic effects of pancuronium and does not cause histamine release. Because of its long duration of action and interindividual variability in response, the use of pipecuronium is limited to long surgical procedures.

Doxacurium

Doxacurium, a benzylisoquinolinum compound (Fig. 10.10), is the most potent NDMR currently available (Table 10.4). It is hydrolysed by cholinesterase. Doxacurium is largely cleared unchanged primarily in the urine and to a lesser degree in the bile. Its pharma-cokinetics resembles those of pancuronium (see Table 10.1). Plasma clearance typically decreases by 50% in severe renal disease, resulting in a 20% increase in the clinical duration of action. Hepatic failure does not affect doxacurium pharmacokinetics. The steady-state volume of distribution is the only parameter significantly altered in the elderly.

The time to maximum block is 10 min at 0.03 mg kg^{-1}, decreasing to 6 and 3.5 min after a bolus of 0.05 and 0.08 mg kg^{-1} respectively, and the clinical duration of action varies between 46 and 337 min. The duration of action is increased in the elderly but the ED_{95} remains unchanged when compared with that in young adults. The speed of recovery, following neostigmine adminis-tration, is highly variable but more than 30 min may be required to obtain a TOF ratio above 0.7.

Doxacurium is devoid of cardiovascular effects. At doses up to three times the ED_{95} it does not produce any significant increase of plasma histamine concentration, even when administered rapidly. Like pipecuronium, it was introduced to provide relaxation for long surgical procedures without side-effects such as tachycardia. Its slow onset of action makes it unsuitable for facilitating tracheal intubation.

Table 10.4 Pharmacology of nondeloparizing muscle relaxants					
	ED_{95} (mg kg^{-1})	Intubating dose (mg kg^{-1})	Onset time (min)	Total duration of action (min)	Recovery index (min)
Suxamethonium	0.5	1.0	1.0	6–12	–
Atracurium	0.230	0.5	3–4	50–60	11–12
Cisatracurium	0.048	0.150	4–5	70–80	12–15
Doxacurium	0.03	0.05	6	120	40
Mivacurium	0.08	0.2	3	30	6–7
Pancuronium	0.05	0.07–0.1	3.5–4	120	30–40
Pipecuronium	0.045	0.08	3.5–4	120	30–40
Rocuronium	0.3	0.6	1.5	60–70	14
Vecuronium	0.04	0.08–0.1	3	50–60	12
Tubocurarine	0.3	0.6	4–5	80–100	40–60

INTERMEDIATE-ACTING NDMRs

Vecuronium

Vecuronium is a synthetic, steroid-based, mono-quaternary compound (see Fig. 10.9) derived from the demethylation of pancuronium. It undergoes spontaneous deacetylation to 3-OH, 17-OH and 3, 17-dihydroxy metabolites, although some of these metabolites are also formed in the liver. The most potent metabolite is the 3-OH derivative which is half as potent as vecuronium. The 17-OH and the two dihydroxy metabolites have almost no neuromuscular blocking activity. Vecuronium and the 3-OH derivative are eliminated by the kidneys.

Although the elimination half-life of vecuronium is longer than that of atracurium (see Table 10.3), the duration of action and rate of recovery are similar (Table 10.4) because of its more rapid distribution, so that plasma concentrations decrease rapidly. This also explains why larger doses are associated with a longer recovery index. In cases of repeated doses, accumulation may occur, especially in patients with renal failure. The elimination half-life of vecuronium is increased in patients with liver cirrhosis or cholestasis as the result of a decreased clearance, the volume of distribution being unchanged.

The dose–response of vecuronium is similar in elderly and young adults. The clinical duration of action is shorter in children than in adults and infants. Even at doses eight times the ED_{95}, vecuronium has no significant cardiovascular effects and does not induce histamine release. The intermediate duration of action following vecuronium administration makes it useful for most surgical procedures, including day-care surgery. The onset of action after administration of once the ED_{95} is within 5–6 min. An initial dose of 0.07–0.1 mg kg^{-1} provides good intubating conditions within 2–3 min and a clinical duration of action of about 25–40 min (Table 10.4). A continuous intravenous infusion of 1–2 µg kg^{-1} min^{-1} will maintain a 90% block at the adductor pollicis. Large doses (0.2–0.4 mg kg^{-1}) have been used to provide rapid intubating conditions in place of suxamethonium. However, the duration of action will be prolonged to 90–120 min.

Rocuronium

Rocuronium is the latest steroid-based muscle relaxant to be introduced into clinical practice. It has a shorter onset of action than vecuronium or atracurium. The pharmacokinetics of rocuronium and vecuronium are similar (see Table 10.3). The pharmacodynamics of rocuronium do not appear to be significantly altered in patients with renal failure, although there is decreased plasma clearance and an increased mean residence time in patients with renal failure. The duration of action is increased two- to threefold in patients with hepatic

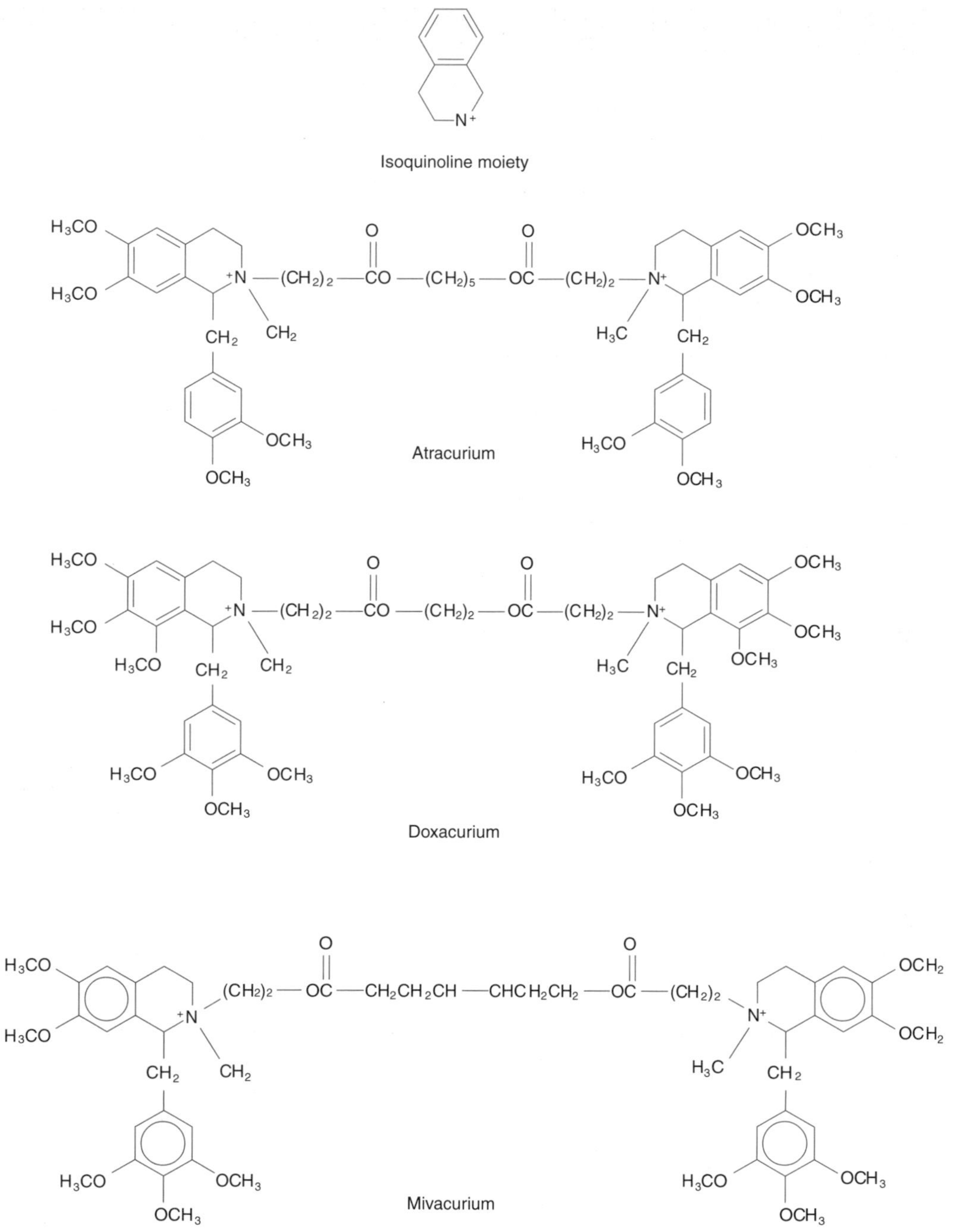

Fig. 10.10 Structures of the isoquinoline moiety and the benzylisoquinolinium muscle relaxants.

dysfunction, possibly due to an increase in the volume of distribution.

Rocuronium is about one-seventh as potent as vecuronium (Table 10.4). The low potency may explain its rapid onset of action when compared with other NDMRs. The onset of action after a dose of 0.6 mg kg^{-1} is close to 90 s at the adductor pollicis. Follow-ing equipotent doses, the duration of action of rocuronium is similar to that of atracurium and vecuronium. Minimal cumulative effects have been observed with up to three repeated doses under halothane anaesthesia.

Rocuronium has minimal vagolytic properties, and haemodynamic changes are clinically insignificant. Like

153

other steroidal NDMRs, it does not cause histamine release. The main advantage of rocuronium is its short onset of action, which provides good intubating conditions 60–90 s after a bolus of 0.6 mg kg^{-1}. Rocuronium can be used when rapid tracheal intubation is indicated and suxamethonium is contraindicated. However, remember that an intubating dose will result in paralysis for 30–40 min.

Atracurium

Atracurium is a benzylisoquinolinium compound (Fig. 10.10) with four asymmetrical centres so that there are 16 possible stereoisomers. Commercial atracurium contains ten isomers. It is metabolized by ester hydrolysis and Hofmann elimination. The latter, which involves the conversion of an amide to an amine under alkaline conditions, results in atracurium being unstable at body temperature and pH. For this reason it is stored at 4°C and pH 3. Breakdown products of atracurium include laudanosine, acrylates and quaternary organic acids. High laudanosine plasma concentrations (17 μg ml^{-1}) cause convulsions in the dog but have never been implicated in humans. The acrylates are highly reactive substances which may be hepatotoxic but there have been no reported problems in humans. The ratio of ester hydrolysis to Hofmann elimination differs from species to species, but in humans up to about 60% probably undergoes ester hydrolysis in the liver. The breakdown of atracurium is independent of plasma cholinesterase.

The pharmacokinetics and pharmacodynamics are not significantly altered in patients with renal failure. However, recovery may be prolonged following repeated doses in these patients. Laudanosine may accumulate in patients with renal failure, but the concentration reached when administered by continuous infusion is ten times less than the toxic plasma level. In patients with fulminant hepatic failure, the volume of distribution is significantly increased but the elimination half-life remains unchanged.

Doses above three times the ED$_{95}$ can induce histamine release with a decrease in blood pressure. Histamine release can be reduced by slow intravenous injection. The duration of action depends on the dose administered; an intubating dose (0.5 mg kg^{-1}) provides muscle relaxation for 25–40 min in adults. Atracurium pharmacodynamics are little affected in the elderly, probably because atracurium elimination is organ independent. The onset time is more rapid and the duration of action slightly shorter in children than in adults. The breakdown of atracurium is decreased by hypothermia.

Atracurium is indicated for procedures necessitating an intermediate to long duration of action, and in day-case surgery. Due to its lack of accumulation,

maintenance can be obtained by a continuous infusion of 5–10 μg kg^{-1} min^{-1}.

Cisatracurium

Cisatracurium is one of the 10 isomers of atracurium. Hofmann elimination is the predominant elimination pathway, ester hydrolysis playing a limited role in humans. The two metabolites are laudanosine and a monoquaternary alcohol. Urinary excretion is a minor elimination pathway for cisatracurium but a major pathway for the elimination of laudanosine. Because of a greater potency than atracurium, both the dose administered and the production of laudanosine are lower.

At twice the ED$_{95}$ the pharmacodynamic profile of cisatracurium is similar to that of an equipotent dose of atracurium, apart from a slower onset of action. A more rapid onset is produced by increasing the dose (2.7 min at 0.2 mg kg^{-1}). The clinical duration of action ranges from 45 min after twice the ED$_{95}$ to approximately 90 min at eight times the ED$_{95}$. The recovery index is constant after repeated bolus doses or continuous infusions, suggesting a lack of cumulation.[13] When neostigmine is given at 10% of T1, complete recovery from neuromuscular block is obtained in 7 min. The intensity of block and the clinical duration of action are not modified by renal or hepatic failure, although in patients with hepatic dysfunction the onset of action is significantly shorter. In contrast to atracurium, cisatracurium does not produce histamine release at doses up to eight times the ED$_{95}$.

SHORT-ACTING NDMRs

Mivacurium

Mivacurium is a benzylquinolinium diester (Fig. 10.10) consisting of three isomers. It is hydrolysed by plasma cholinesterase. Clearance of the *cis-trans* and *trans-trans* isomers correlates with plasma pseudocholinesterase activity.[14] The *cis-cis* isomer is more slowly hydrolysed but its potency is only one-tenth that of the two other isomers. Mivacurium is hydrolysed at 70–88% the rate of suxamethonium. There is little accumulation; the recovery index is 6–7 min and does not change over a wide dose range nor after infusions lasting up to 5 h. Administration of neostigmine or edrophonium after the start of spontaneous recovery reduces the recovery index by approximately 50%.

Prolonged block has been reported following the use of mivacurium in patients with low or abnormal levels of plasma cholinesterase. In patients heterozygous for the *atypical* gene, the duration of action is prolonged by about 50%. Mivacurium is four to five times more potent in homozygous abnormal patients than in those with the normal phenotype. In these patients the duration of action following 0.2 mg kg^{-1} may be very prolonged (6–8 h). Anticholinesterases should not be administered. Patients must be ventilated and sedated until spontaneous recovery occurs. Renal failure may reduce cholinesterase activity by 30–50%, prolonging the duration of action. There is an inverse correlation between plasma cholinesterase activity and the duration of action of mivacurium in patients with hepatic dysfunction. Mivacurium may induce histamine release which is dependent on dose and rate of administration.

The main advantage of mivacurium is a short duration of action, which makes it suitable for short surgical procedures requiring tracheal intubation. A dose of 0.2 mg kg^{-1} is necessary to obtain good intubating conditions. Maintenance of neuromuscular block can be obtained by a continuous infusion at a rate of 5–10 μg kg^{-1} min^{-1}. Monitoring is mandatory during continuous administration to detect recovery or prolonged duration of action in patients with unrecognized abnormal pseudocholinesterases.

ULTRASHORT-ACTING NDMRs

Rapacuronium (ORG 9487)

Rapacuronium is a new steroidal muscle relaxant with a rapid onset of action and the possibility of early reversal. Rapacuronium is metabolized to the 3-OH metabolite, which has half the potency of the parent compound. Plasma clearance (8.5 ml kg^{-1} min^{-1}) is greater than that of other NDMRs. The volume of distribution at steady state is 293 ml kg^{-1}. In plasma the 3-OH metabolite is rapidly detectable and could contribute to neuromuscular block following repeated doses.

Rapacuronium has a very low potency, the ED$_{90}$ being 1.15 mg kg^{-1}. Onset time at the adductor pollicis is 83 s after 1.5 mg kg^{-1} and good intubating conditions are obtained within 1 min after injection.[15] Complete spontaneous recovery occurs within 24 min; however, if neostigmine is given 2 min after drug administration, the TOF ratio returns to 0.7 in less than 12 min. Rapacuronium can produce a slight tachycardia owing to its vagolytic properties. The main advantage of this

new compound is a pharmacodynamic profile very similar to that of suxamethonium.[16] Further studies are necessary to demonstrate whether it can be used safely during rapid sequence induction.

REVERSAL OF NDMRs

The action of NDMRs is reversed by anticholinesterase drugs, which temporarily inactivate acetylcholinesterase and increase the amount of acetylcholine at the postsynaptic membrane. Because anticholinesterases act not only at the motor endplate, but at all muscarinic receptors, they cause excessive salivation, increased bowel activity and bradycardia. They are therefore combined with an anticholinergic agent such as atropine or glycopyrronium, which block the muscarinic but not the nicotinic effects of acetylcholine. Neostigmine and pyridostigmine, but not edrophonium, are hydrolysed by acetylcholinesterase. Edrophonium binds with the esteratic site on acetylcholinesterase, forming a loose electrostatic bond, and there is competition between it and acetylcholine for this site; the action of edrophonium is terminated as it simply diffuses away from the synaptic cleft. Neostigmine binds more strongly to both the anionic and esteratic sites on acetylcholinesterase. The durations of action of neostigmine, edrophonium and pyridostigmine are similar but the onset times differ considerably; the peak effect of edrophonium occurs at 1–2 min, neostigmine at 7–11 min and pyridostigmine at greater than 16 min. The onset of pyridostigmine is too slow for clinical purposes.[17]

The time to recovery depends on the intensity of the block when the reversal agent is given. It is recommended that at least one visible twitch of a TOF be visible before reversing. Reversal with edrophonium is superior to neostigmine only if significant spontaneous recovery has occurred. Intense blocks are better reversed with neostigmine. The chances of return of block in the recovery room after apparent complete reversal is greater with the long-acting NDMRs such as pancuronium when neostigmine has been administered at a deep level of neuromuscular block.

REFERENCES

1. Littleton JT, Bellen HJ. Synaptotagmin controls and modulates synaptic–vesicle fusion in a Ca^{2+}-dependent manner. *Trends Neurosci* 1995; **18**: 177–183.
2. Bowman WC, Prior C, Marshall IG. Presynaptic receptors in the neuromuscular junction. *Ann N Y Acad Sci* 1990; **604**: 69–81.
3. Bowman WC, Rodger W, Houston J, Marshall RJ, McIndewar I. Structure: action relationships among some desacetoxy analogues of pancuronium and vecuronium in the anesthetized cat. *Anesthesiology* 1988; **69**: 57–62.
4. D'Honneur G, Gall O, Gerard A, Rimaniol JM, Lambert Y, Duvaldestin P. Priming doses of atracurium and vecuronium depress swallowing in humans. *Anesthesiology* 1992; **77**: 1070–1073.
5. Viby-Morgensen J, Howardy-Hensen P, Chraemmer-Jorgensen B, Ording H, Engbaek J, Nielsen A. Posttetanic count (PTC): a new method of evaluating an intense nondepolarizing neuromuscular block. *Anesthesiology* 1981; **55**: 458–461.
6. Engbaek J, Ostergaard D, Viby-Mogensen J. Double burst stimulation (DBS): a new pattern of nerve stimulation to identify residual neuromuscular block. *Br J Anaesth* 1989; **62**: 274–278.

7. Donati F, Meistelman C, Plaud B. Vecuronium neuromuscular blockade at the diaphragm, the orbicularis oculi, and adductor pollicis muscles. *Anesthesiology* 1990; **73**: 870–875.

8. Donati F, Meistelman C, Plaud B. Vecuronium neuromuscular blockade at the adductor muscles of the larynx and adductor pollicis. *Anesthesiology* 1991; **74**: 833–837.

9. Plumley MH, Bevan JC, Saddler JM, Donati F, Bevan DR. Dose-related effects of succinylcholine on the adductor pollicis and masseter muscles in children. *Can J Anaesth* 1990; **37**: 15–20.

10. Laxenaire MC. Drugs and other agents involved in anaphylactic shock occurring during anaesthesia. A French multicenter epidemiological inquiry. *Ann Fr Anesth Reanim* 1993; **12**: 91–96.

11. Davis L, Britten JJ, Morgan M. Cholinesterase. Its significance in anaesthetic practice. *Anaesthesia* 1997; **52**: 244–260.

12. Jensen FS, Viby-Mogensen J. Plasma cholinesterase and abnormal reaction to succinylcholine: twenty years' experience with the Danish Cholinesterase Research Unit. *Acta Anaesthesiol Scand* 1995; **39**: 150–156.

13. Belmont MR, Lien CA, Quessy S *et al*. The clinical neuromuscular pharmacology of 51W89 in patients receiving nitrous oxide/opioid/barbiturate anesthesia. *Anesthesiology* 1995; **82**: 1139–1145.

14. Lien CA, Schmith VD, Embree PB, Belmont MR, Wargin WA, Savarese JJ. The pharmacokinetics a7nd pharmacodynamics of the stereoisomers of mivacurium in patients receiving nitrous oxide/opioid/barbiturate anesthesia. *Anesthesiology* 1994; **80**: 1296–1302.

15. Wierda JM, van den Broek L, Proost JH, Verbaan BW, Hennis PJ. Time course of action and endotracheal intubating conditions of Org 9487, a new short-acting steroidal muscle relaxant; a comparison with succinylcholine. *Anesth Analg* 1993; **77**: 579–584.

16. Bonsu AK, Viby-Mogensen J, Fernando PUE, *et al*. Relationship of post-tetanic count and train-of-four response during intense neuromuscular blockade caused by atracurium. *Br J Anaesth* 1987; **59**: 1089–1092.

17. Eriksson LI, Lennmahen C, Stain P, Viby-Mogernsen J. Use of post-tetanic count in assessment of a repetitive vecuronium-induced neuromuscular block. *Br J Anaesth* 1990; **65**: 487–493.

11 AGL Burm, JW van Kleef

LOCAL ANAESTHETICS

CHEMICAL STRUCTURES AND PHYSICOCHEMICAL PROPERTIES

The local anaesthetics used clinically are either amino esters or amino amides, composed of a lipophilic moiety, connected to a hydrophilic amine by an intermediate chain containing the ester or amide bond (Fig. 11.1). Most amino amide-type agents contain a stereocentre (chiral centre) in the form of a carbon atom with four different substituents (atoms or atomic groups) attached to it. Consequently, these molecules exist in two stereoisomeric forms, called enantiomers. These are distinguished by the prefixes R (from the Latin

Local anaesthetics are frequently used to provide surgical anaesthesia, for acute and chronic pain relief and for diagnostic procedures. The first local anaesthetic that found clinical application was cocaine, which was introduced in ophthalmology by Freud and Koller in 1894. Procaine, the first synthetic local anaesthetic, was introduced in 1905. Since then, several other synthetic local anaesthetics have been developed. A major milestone was the development of lignocaine. Introduced in 1944, it is still the most widely used local anaesthetic.

Although used clinically primarily to prevent pain transmission, local anaesthetics do not selectively block pain fibres, but affect all types of nerve fibre, irrespective of their function. The extent to which different fibres are affected varies with the local anaesthetic, dose, concentration and site of injection. Furthermore, the onset and duration of action vary between agents. Knowledge of their clinical pharmacology may help in selecting the most appropriate agent and dosage regimen for any particular application.

As local anaesthetics are applied close to the target nerve structures, they are not dependent on the general circulation to reach these targets. However, once deposited, they are taken up into the general circulation, and excessively high blood concentrations can cause systemic toxicity. Therefore, appreciation of the clinical pharmacology of local anaesthetics is also essential from a safety point of view.

Summary box 11.1 Local anaesthetics: classification based on chemical structure

Esters

- Cocaine.

- Procaine.

- Chloroprocaine.

- Amethocaine (tetracaine).

- Benzocaine.

Amides

- Cinchocaine (dibucaine).

- Lignocaine (lidocaine).

- Mepivacaine.

- Prilocaine.

- Bupivacaine.

- Ropivacaine.

- Etidocaine.

- Articaine.

rectus) and *S* (from the Latin sinister), reflecting their configuration in space. Another prefix reflects the direction in which they rotate plane-polarized light, which is always opposite for enantiomers: (–) represents the laevorotatory and (+) the dextrorotatory enantiomer. Most chiral local anaesthetics are used as racemates, containing equal amounts of the enantiomers. For example, bupivacaine is a 50/50 mixture of *S*(–)-bupivacaine and *R*(+)-bupivacaine. An exception is ropivacaine, which is a pure *S*(–)-enantiomer. Although enantiomers have identical physicochemical properties, they may differ in their pharmacokinetics, pharmacodynamics and toxicity.[1,2]

Because of the amino group, most local anaesthetics are weak bases with pK_a values ranging from 7.9 to 9.3 (Table 11.1). In the physiological pH range they consequently exist partially in the un-ionized form (B) and partially in the ionized form (BH$^+$), according to the reaction equation:

$$B + H^+ \rightleftharpoons BH^+$$

The distinction between ionized and un-ionized drug is important because only the un-ionized form can pass lipoprotein barriers between the site of injection and the site of action on the nerves. Ionization is, however, important when considering local anaesthetic activity. The ratio of the un-ionized and ionized forms can be calculated using the Henderson–Hasselbalch equation:

$$\log \frac{[BH^+]}{[B]} = pK_a - pH$$

Structural changes in the aromatic or amine part of the molecules are accompanied by profound changes in lipophilicity and protein binding (Table 11.1), and consequently in the pharmacokinetics as well as in the potency and duration of action (pharmacodynamics). In general, the substitution of longer aliphatic chains renders a molecule more lipophilic and increases the degree of protein binding. For example, the substitution of a butyl group for the methyl group in the amine part of mepivacaine gives bupivacaine, which has a 16-fold higher partition coefficient and a markedly greater degree of protein binding. In addition, bupivacaine is approximately four times more potent than mepivacaine and has a considerably longer duration of action.

PHARMACOKINETICS

When considering the pharmacokinetics of local anaesthetics, a distinction can be made between local disposition (distribution and elimination) and systemic disposition. Local distribution involves several

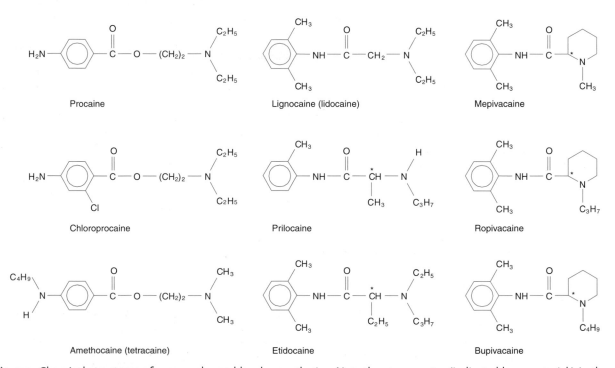

Fig. 11.1 Chemical structures of commonly used local anaesthetics. Note the stereocentre (indicated by an asterisk) in the molecular structures of prilocaine, etidocaine, mepivacaine, ropivacaine and bupivacaine.

Table 11.1 **Physiocochemical properties of commonly used local anaesthetics**				
Agent	pK$_a$ (25°C)	Partition coefficient[*] (25°C)	Serum protein binding[†] (%)	Blood : plasma concentration ratio[†]
Esters				
Procaine	9.1	1.7	–	–
Chloroprocaine	9.3	9	–	–
Amethocaine	8.6	221	–	–
Amides				
Lignocaine	8.2	43	70	0.84
Prilocaine	8	25	40	1
Etidocaine	8.1	800	95	0.61
Mepivacaine	7.9	21	75 (75/64)[‡]	0.92
Ropivacaine	8.2	115	95	0.69
Bupivacaine	8.2	346	95 (96/93)[‡]	0.73

[*] Octanol/buffer (pH 7.4); [†] protein binding and blood : plasma concentration ratios based on measurements of mixed enantiomers; [‡] plasma protein binding of individual enantiomers (S-enantiomer/R-enantiomer).

processes, including spread of the local anaesthetic by bulk flow, diffusion, transport via local blood vessels, and binding to local tissues. Local elimination is in all likelihood synonymous with systemic absorption (i.e. the uptake of local anaesthetic into the blood draining the area and subsequent transfer into the general circulation).

Local disposition determines the time course of the concentration of local anaesthetic at the sites of action. However, the current knowledge on local distribution is mainly theoretical, and real data are scarce. Therefore, this aspect will not be considered further.

SYSTEMIC ABSORPTION

Systemic absorption reduces the amount of local anaesthetic that is available for anaesthetic effect and thereby ultimately limits the duration of nerve block. In addition, it is of importance with respect to the systemic side-effects of local anaesthetics. Systemic absorption is dependent on the binding of local anaesthetic to tissues at and near the site of injection, and on local perfusion. Both vary with the site of injection. Furthermore, local anesthetics may alter local perfusion, both by affecting vasomotor tone and by producing sympathetic blockade.

Systemic absorption is generally biphasic, with an initial rapid phase followed by a much slower absorption phase.[3,4] The rapid absorption phase is related to the initial high concentration gradient between the drug in the injected solution and the blood. The slow phase probably reflects absorption after local tissue distribution has been completed and is therefore highly dependent on tissue–blood partitioning. The

initial absorption rates of lignocaine and bupivacaine after epidural injection are similar (Table 11.2). However, the secondary absorption of lignocaine is much faster than that of bupivacaine. This reflects the lower tissue affinity of lignocaine and is in keeping with its shorter duration of action.

Initial absorption rates after subarachnoid injection of lignocaine and bupivacaine are considerably slower than after epidural injection (Table 11.2). Indeed, with lignocaine the initial absorption is delayed to the extent that a biphasic absorption pattern is no longer identifiable. The slower initial absorption rates after subarachnoid injection are probably related to poorer perfusion of the subarachnoid space and less vasodilatation because of the lower doses. Slow absorption half-lives after epidural and subarachnoid administration are very similar. This suggests that secondary absorption occurs from a common tissue, possibly epidural fat. Absorption kinetics following other routes of administration have not been determined. Inspection of the concentration–time profiles suggests a biphasic absorption pattern following most procedures.

DISTRIBUTION

Being lipophilic drugs, local anaesthetics readily cross diffusion barriers, such as cell membranes, the blood–brain barrier and the placenta. Consequently, the tissue distribution of these drugs is likely to be highly dependent on tissue perfusion, and distribution at equilibrium probably involves the total volume of body fluid. Furthermore, local anaesthetics show significant, although widely varying, degrees of tissue binding.

Table 11.2 Systemic absorption kinetics of lignocaine and bupivacaine[*] following epidural and subarachnoid administration, ropivacaine

Parameter	Epidural lignocaine	Epidural bupivacaine	Epidural ropivacaine	Subarachnoid lignocaine	Subarachnoid bupivacaine
F1	0.38	0.28	0.52	–	0.35
$t_{1/2a1}$ (h)	0.16	0.12	0.23	–	0.83
F2	0.58	0.66	0.48	–	0.61
$t_{1/2a2}$ (h)	1.36	6.03	4.2	1.18	6.8
F (F1 + F2)	0.96	0.94	1.00	1.03	0.96

[*] Bupivacaine data are based on measurements of mixed enantiomers (a recent study indicated that systemic absorption kinetics are not enantioselective).
Abbreviations: F1 and F2 – fractions of the dose characterizing the fast and slow absorption phases; $t_{1/2a1}$ and $t_{1/2a2}$ – half-lives characterizing the fast and slow absorption phases; F – estimated total fraction of the dose that is ultimately absorbed into the general circulation (values of F do not differ significantly from 1, indicating 100% systemic availability).
Data are from Burm[3] and Emanuelsson et al.[4]

Lung uptake

Before entering the arterial circulation local anaesthetics pass through the lungs, where significant uptake may occur. For example, the first-pass lung uptake of lignocaine is approximately 60%. The implications of lung uptake vary with the input rate. When drug input is rapid, such as after inadvertent intravenous injection or following accidental premature cuff release during intravenous regional anaesthesia, peak arterial blood concentrations will be delayed and markedly lower than those in the pulmonary arterial blood. When drug input is slower, such as after most correctly performed blocks, the dampening effect of lung uptake on the arterial concentrations will be much smaller. With high doses, resulting in saturation of lung uptake, this effect will also be reduced.

Uptake into the brain and heart

The brain and heart are the main target organs for systemic toxicity. Rich perfusion, moderate tissue–blood partition coefficients and the lack of serious diffusion limitations ensure rapid uptake of local anaesthetics in these tissues and rapid tissue–blood equilibration. Tissue uptake is affected by changes in tissue–blood pH gradients.[5] Respiratory acidosis may not alter tissue–blood partitioning when it is accompanied by similar changes in tissue and blood pH. Metabolic acidosis increases the uptake into the tissues where it is generated, due to larger decreases in intracellular pH than in blood pH, resulting in ion trapping. On the other hand, metabolic acidosis

induced elsewhere will have the opposite effect. However, even though brain–blood and heart–blood partition coefficients may remain unchanged or be decreased, toxicity may still be increased, owing to an absolute decrease in intracellular pH, resulting in an increase in the fraction of ionized local anaesthetic, which is probably the most active form.

Placental transfer

The placenta is not a major barrier for the diffusion of local anaesthetics, and equilibration between fetal and maternal blood concentrations is extremely rapid. Nevertheless, total blood or plasma concentrations in umbilical cord blood are significantly lower than in maternal blood, in particular with highly protein-bound drugs such as bupivacaine and etidocaine. This reflects differences in protein binding, secondary to differences in protein concentrations, on either side of the placenta. Unbound concentrations are likely to be very similar in fetal and maternal blood, or possibly somewhat higher in the acidotic fetus due to ion trapping. Therefore, low fetal : maternal concentration ratios do not guarantee a wide safety margin for the fetus.

Volumes of distribution

The extensive tissue distribution of local anaesthetics may not be obvious when examining the volumes of distribution based on total plasma concentrations (Table 11.3). This is because extensive plasma protein binding masks extensive tissue binding. Volumes of distribution based on unbound plasma concentrations, however,

Table 11.3 Mean pharmacokinetic data, characterizing the disposition of amide-type local anaesthetics following intravenous administration in adult male volunteers

	V_{ss} (litres)	$V_{u_{ss}}$ (litres)	Cl (l min^{-1})	$t_{1/2}$ (h)
Lignocaine	76	255	0.8	1.6
Prilocaine	268	447	2.44	1.6
Etidocaine	81	1623	0.68	2.7
$S(+)$-mepivacaine	57	232	0.35	2.1
$R(-)$-mepivacaine	103	290	0.79	1.9
Ropivacaine	42	742	0.5	1.9
$S(-)$-bupivacaine	54	1498	0.32	2.6
$R(+)$-bupivacaine	84	1576	0.4	3.5

Data are reported or estimated using protein binding data and blood : plasma concentration ratios as reported in Table 11.1 and are specified with respect to venous plasma concentrations, except lignocaine and etidocaine data, which are with respect to arterial plasma concentrations. Data for individual enantiomers were obtained after intravenous administration of the racemates.
Abbreviations: V_{ss} and $V_{u_{ss}}$, volumes of distribution based on total and unbound plasma concentrations respectively; Cl, total plasma clearance; $t_{1/2}$, terminal (elimination) half-life.

demonstrate the greater tissue affinity of the more lipophilic agents.

The distribution of local anaesthetics is to some extent enantioselective. As shown in Table 11.3, the steady-state volume of distribution (V_{ss}) of $R(-)$-mepivacaine is approximately twice that of $S(+)$-mepivacaine, and the V_{ss} of $R(+)$-bupivacaine is 50% larger than that of $S(-)$-bupivacaine. Because the protein binding of these agents is also enantioselective, the corresponding volumes based on unbound concentrations of the enantiomers of mepivacaine ($V_{u_{ss}}$) differ less, and values of $V_{u_{ss}}$ for the enantiomers of bupivacaine are actually similar.

BIOTRANSFORMATION, CLEARANCES AND HALF-LIVES

Local anaesthetics are removed from the blood mainly by biotransformation; renal excretion of unchanged drug is minimal, at least in adults. Ester-type agents undergo rapid hydrolysis by plasma cholinesterase, red cell esterases and esterases in the liver. Hydrolysis rates decrease in the order: chloroprocaine > procaine > amethocaine. Biotransformation of amide-type agents occurs predominantly in the liver and involves several pathways, as is demonstrated by the metabolic breakdown of lignocaine (Fig. 11.2).

Clearances of the ester-type agents are normally very high, but may be lowered when the hydrolysis is depressed, such as when the esterases become saturated or when the enzymes are atypical. Plasma clearances of the amide-type agents vary considerably and are enantioselective (Table 11.3). The clearance of prilocaine exceeds normal liver blood flow, indicating significant extrahepatic clearance.

In vitro half-lives following intravenous administration of procaine and chloroprocaine are less than 1 min. The half-lives of the amide-type agents are considerably longer and vary approximately twofold (Table 11.3). Half-lives following perineural administration may be considerably longer than those after intravenous administration because slow systemic absorption rate limits the elimination following perineural administration.

Role of metabolites

Although most metabolites are pharmacologically inactive, some have pharmacological activity. This holds in particular for dealkylation products. Monoethylglycine

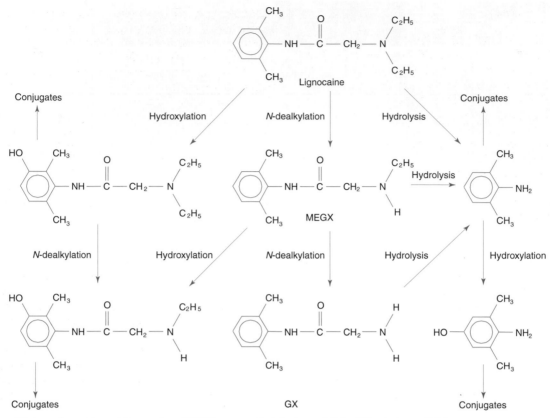

Fig. 11.2 Biotransformation of lignocaine. MEGX, monoethylglycine xylidide; GX, glycine xylidide.

xylidide (MEGX), a metabolite of lignocaine (Fig. 11.2) retains much of the activity of the parent drug and may contribute to the systemic effects during prolonged infusion or upon repeated dosing. Other metabolites that are pharmacologically active are glycine xylidide (GX), another metabolite of lignocaine, and pipecoloxylidide (PPX), an N-dealkylation product from mepivacaine, ropivacaine and bupivacaine.

Aminobenzoic acid derivatives, formed by hydrolysis of the ester-type agents, are responsible for the allergic reactions that may occur with these agents. The hydroxylation of o-toluidine, formed by amide hydrolysis of prilocaine, is believed to be responsible for the methaemoglobinaemia that is associated with higher doses of this agent.

CONCENTRATIONS FOLLOWING PERINEURAL ADMINISTRATION

Concentrations of ester-type agents have not been determined to any appreciable extent, but should be very low, because of rapid hydrolysis. Following single injections of the amide-type agents, the highest concentrations occur after intercostal and interpleural administration, irrespective of the agent. Peak concen-

trations are usually reached in 5–60 min, depending primarily on the route of administration.

In general, plasma or blood concentrations are independent of the concentration of the local anaesthetic in the administered solution and proportional to the dose. However, occasionally, disproportionately higher concentrations have been observed with more concentrated solutions and higher doses. This probably reflects saturation of local binding sites and/or more rapid systemic absorption secondary to more pronounced vasodilatation with the more concentrated solutions or higher doses. The speed of injection, alkalinization and carbonation have little or no effect on the peak plasma concentrations. Addition of adrenaline or phenylephrine usually reduces the peak plasma concentrations, but the effect varies with the local anaesthetic and route of administration.

Peak plasma concentrations in elderly patients are similar to those in younger adults. Similarly, peak concentrations in paediatric patients are broadly comparable to those in adults given similar doses on a milligram per kilogram basis. Peak concentrations in pregnant women are generally comparable to or somewhat higher than those in healthy nonpregnant women.

MODE OF ACTION

ANATOMICAL CONSIDERATIONS

Peripheral nerves are mixed nerves containing both sensory afferent fibres and autonomic and motor efferent fibres. Each individual axon or nerve fibre is surrounded by a connective tissue sheath (endoneurium; Fig. 11.3). Groups of axons are enclosed in an additional connective tissue sheath (perineurium). Finally, a number of axonal groups are encased in an external connective tissue sheath (epineurium). The endoneurium that surrounds the individual axon consists of a Schwann cell in the unmyelinated axon. In myelinated axons the Schwann cells have deposited myelin around the axon. This myelin sheath is interrupted at intervals by constrictions (nodes of Ranvier).

Functionally, the cell membrane or axolemma is the most important part of the nerve fibre. This semipermeable membrane, which separates a potassium-rich ionic solution (axoplasm) on the inside from a sodium-rich ionic solution on the outside, plays a crucial role in the transmission of electrical impulses.

TRANSMISSION OF NERVE IMPULSES

At rest, the nerve membrane is polarized: a voltage difference of approximately −70 to −80 mV exists between its inner and outer aspects.[7] This results from the relative impermeability of the membrane for Na^+ and selective permeability for K^+. This state is maintained by an energy-dependent active transport mechanism, the Na^+–K^+ pump, which constantly extrudes Na^+ from the inside in exchange for net uptake of K^+ against the concentration gradients.

A small depolarization of the membrane activates both sodium and potassium channels to an open conformation, increasing their conductance (Fig. 11.4). Since sodium channels open faster, the inward Na^+ current initially exceeds the outward K^+ current. Sodium ions entering the axoplasm further depolarize the membrane, opening more sodium channels and further increasing the current. This process continues until some sodium channels become inactivated and sufficient potassium channels are opened, which results in a net outward current and repolarization. Finally, the very small amounts of sodium that entered and potassium that left the axoplasm are restored by the Na^+–K^+ pump. Directly after a depolarization, when some sodium channels are still inactivated, the membrane is refractory to stimulation.

Ionic currents that enter the axon in a depolarized region flow down the axoplasm and exit through the membrane in adjacent regions, passively depolarizing these regions. As a consequence, action potentials are

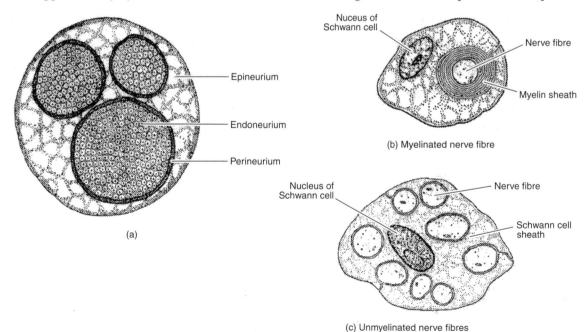

(a)

(b) Myelinated nerve fibre

(c) Unmyelinated nerve fibres

Fig. 11.3 (a) Cross-sectional diagram of a peripheral nerve. (b) Myelinated fibres are encased in myelin wrappings formed by one Schwann cell, which stretches longitudinally over approximately 100 times the diameter of the axon. The narrow gaps between the myelinated segments (i.e. the nodes of Ranvier) contain the ion channels. (c) Unmyelinated fibres are enclosed in bundles of five to ten axons by a chain of Schwann cells which embrace each axon with only one layer of membrane. From Covino and Vassallo.[6]

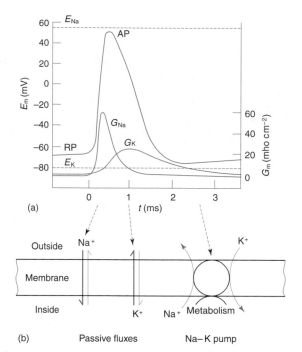

Fig. 11.4 *Action potential generation. (a) Changes in sodium and potassium conductances (G_{Na} and G_K, scale to the right) during an action potential (AP). The membrane potential (E_m) changes from the resting potential (RP) which is close to the potassium equilibrium potential (E_K), reaching a peak that is close to the sodium equilibrium potential (E_{Na}). (b) Sodium and potassium fluxes during and after the AP. From Narahashi.[8]*

propagated along the axon. This propagation is unidirectional, because the region behind the excited zone, which has just encountered a depolarization, is refractory to stimulation. Whereas in unmyelinated fibres action potentials are propagated relatively slowly between adjacent regions, the propagation in myelinated fibres is much faster, because the ionic currents spread rapidly along the insulated internodal regions between the nodes of Ranvier. This does not mean that individual depolarizations jump from one node to the next one in sequence. Active depolarization occurs simultaneously at several successive nodes of Ranvier, and depolarizations may actually skip past two inexcitable nodes to stimulate a third.

MECHANISM OF ACTION OF LOCAL ANAESTHETICS

Local anaesthetics primarily block nerve conduction by modifying the voltage-gated sodium channel activities without affecting the resting membrane potential.[7] Binding of a local anaesthetic to the sodium channels inhibits the conformational changes that underlie channel activation and thereby prevent the opening of the channels. As a consequence the sodium ion permeability of a stimulated membrane, and thereby the rate and degree of depolarization, decreases progressively with increasing local anaesthetic concentrations. When depolarization is insufficient to reach the excitability threshold, full action potentials do not develop and conduction block occurs.

Repetitive stimulation at high frequencies markedly enhances local anaesthetic blocks. This phenomenon, referred to as use-dependent, frequency-dependent or phasic block, is caused by channel activation accelerating local anaesthetic binding and/or a tighter binding when channels are in the activated or inactivated state compared with the resting state.

Both the un-ionized lipophilic (neutral base) and the ionized hydrophilic (cationic) forms are involved in local anaesthetic binding, whereby the cationic form has access to the local anaesthetic binding site via a hydrophilic route from the axoplasm, whereas the neutral base form may reach the binding sites via hydrophobic routes in the axonal membrane.

Although conduction block results primarily from inhibition of sodium channels, potassium and calcium channels are also inhibited by local anaesthetics. The greater the inhibition of potassium channels, the more the potency is reduced.

NERVE BLOCK IN CLINICAL PRACTICE

Association and dissociation of local anaesthetics with sodium channels are very fast processes and as such are not the major determinants of the time course of a nerve block. Instead the onset, intensity and duration of block depend directly on the changes in the concentration of local anaesthetic at the axonal membrane, which are dependent on pharmacokinetic factors.

Onset of action

Transport of local anaesthetic from the site of injection to the sites of action occurs by passive diffusion, although transport via blood vessels may contribute. For example, epidurally administered local anaesthetics may be transported to the spinal cord via the spinal radicular arteries.

To reach their sites of action local anaesthetics have to pass through several diffusion barriers, i.e. the epineurium, perineurium, endoneurium, myelin sheath and nonneural tissues. This diffusion is highly dependent on the lipophilicity of the drug and, since only un-ionized drug readily diffuses through biological membranes, on its pK_a and local pH. Consequently, one might expect the onset time to be shorter with more lipophilic agents, such as bupivacaine and etidocaine, than with less lipophilic agents, such as lignocaine, mepivacaine and prilocaine. However, this is offset by the more extensive tissue binding of the former agents. Therefore, onset times vary less between local anaesthetics than would be expected on the basis of their lipophilicity and diffusability.

Duration of action

The duration of nerve block depends primarily on the dose and the rate of systemic absorption of local anaesthetic. Extensive binding to local tissues delays systemic absorption and maintains the concentration near the sites of action. Consequently, the duration of action of the more lipophilic agents, which show the highest tissue affinities, is considerably longer than that of the less lipophilic agents.

Addition of a vasoconstrictor (commonly adrenaline) delays systemic absorption and increases the amount available for anaesthetic action. This would be expected to result in a faster onset, more intense block and a longer duration of action. The faster onset and more intense block is not always manifested clinically. The effect of adrenaline generally prolongs the duration, but this varies with the site of injection and the local anaesthetic.

Differential block

An important clinical consideration is the existence of differential blocks. Local anaesthetics are capable of blocking all types of nerve fibres. However, the rate of block, and also the concentration of local anaesthetic that is necessary to block the nerve fibres, varies with the fibre type. A marked degree of sensory–motor block dissociation is usually observed upon epidural administration of diluted bupivacaine (e.g. 0.125%) or ropivacaine (e.g. 0.2%) solutions. This makes these drugs particularly useful where analgesia with minimal muscle weakness is required, such as in obstetrics and for postoperative analgesia. A possible explanation for this sensory–motor dissociation is that the length of nerve in the dural root sleeves exposed to local anaesthetic is not sufficient to allow block of three consecutive nodes of Ranvier in the myelinated motor fibres because of the large internodal distances, but sufficient to block unmyelinated C pain fibres and produce a three-node block in myelinated A_δ pain fibres, which have smaller internodal distances.[9] Differential sympathetic–sensory block is observed during spinal anaesthesia as the final level of sympathetic block extends several segments higher than corresponding levels of sensory block. Consequently, high spinal blocks may be associated with profound cardiovascular effects.

SIDE-EFFECTS AND TOXICITY

REGIONAL SIDE-EFFECTS AND TISSUE TOXICITY

Since local anaesthetics do not selectively block fibres involved in pain transmission or motor function, regional side-effects are not uncommon.[10] These vary with the site of injection and include hypotension, hypoventilation, Horner syndrome, hypoglycaemia and urinary retention.

Clinically used local anaesthetics rarely produce localized nerve damage. Local nerve damage, in so far as this has been attributed to the local anaesthetic (solution), appears to be related to the use of inappropriate formulations or excessively concentrated solutions. For example, the combination of a low pH and the antioxidant sodium bisulphite is generally held responsible for the severe neurotoxic reactions that have occurred following epidural or subarachnoid injection of large doses of chloroprocaine. Chloroprocaine itself does not appear to be neurotoxic. Recently, several reports of cauda equina syndrome and transient radicular irritation, associated with the use of hyperbaric 5% lignocaine solutions for spinal anaesthesia, have raised concern with respect to the neurotoxic potential of this agent. The available evidence suggests, however, that the use of concentrated solutions rather than the agent *per se* is responsible for these phenomena, especially when the solutions are injected through narrow-bore needles or microbore catheters, which can result in very high local concentrations in the cerebrospinal fluid.

It should be emphasized that nerve damage associated with local or regional anaesthetic procedures may also be caused by other factors, such as faulty patient positioning, trauma from the needle or catheter, or from the operative procedure. Following central block, spinal cord ischaemia, secondary to a period of severe hypotension, must also be considered.

SYSTEMIC SIDE-EFFECTS AND TOXICITY

Systemic effects associated with correctly performed nerve blocks are usually benign and some are of therapeutic value, such as the antiarrhythmic effects of lignocaine. However, high blood concentrations will cause toxic reactions, primarily involving the central nervous system (CNS) and the cardiovascular system (CVS).[10] Causes may be an inadvertent intravascular (mostly intravenous) injection, premature tourniquet release during intravenous regional anaesthesia, overdosing with procedures that require relatively large doses, such as epidural or brachial plexus blocks, or as may occur during repeated administration or prolonged infusion. Occasionally toxic reactions follow administration of relatively small doses. This may occur, for

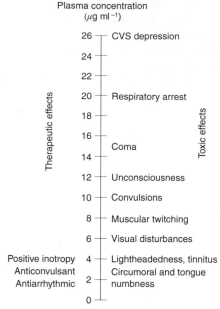

Fig. 11.5 Relationship between the plasma concentration of lignocaine and various therapeutic and toxic effects. From Mather and Cousins.[11]

example, with injections in the head or neck area, when the local anaesthetic gains access to the brain via alternative routes, such as upon direct injection into the carotid or vertebral arteries, or by retrograde spread along nerves or veins.

When drug input is gradual, subjective CNS symptoms, such as feelings of lightheadedness and dizziness, visual and auditory disturbances, such as tinnitus, disorientation and drowsiness may be followed by objective signs such as shivering, muscular twitching, tremors involving muscles of the face and distal parts of the extremities, and ultimately generalized convulsions (Fig. 11.5). These may be followed by a state of generalized CNS depression, manifested by unconsciousness, coma, respiratory depression and finally respiratory arrest. When drug input is rapid, such as after accidental intravascular injection, convulsions and CNS depression may occur rapidly and without preceding premonitory signs. CNS depression may also occur without preceding excitation, in particular when other CNS depressants have been administered.

Cardiovascular effects are primarily the result of a direct action of local anaesthetics on both the heart and peripheral blood vessels, but in part are mediated by the sympathetic nervous system. Direct effects include a decreased myocardial contractility, decreased cardiac conduction velocity and peripheral vasodilatation. The primary cardiac effects are electrophysiological, due to inhibition of sodium channels, resulting in a decrease in the maximum rate of depolarization (V_{max}) of the Purkinje fibres and ventricular muscle, and decreases in the action potential duration and effective refractory period. Lignocaine rapidly blocks inactivated and open sodium channels during the action potential, whereas a bupivacaine block develops slowly at low concentrations but rapidly at high concentrations. Recovery from a bupivacaine block is significantly slower than that from lignocaine. Lignocaine blocks channels in a 'fast-in–fast-out' fashion, whereas bupivacaine does so in a 'slow-in–slow-out' manner. Bupivacaine also is more potent at depressing ventricular V_{max}, resulting in slowed conduction of action potentials. This effect, which may be responsible for reentry arrhythmias such as ectopic ventricular beats and ventricular tachycardia, is manifested on the electrocardiogram by a prolonged PR interval and a widened QRS complex.

Local anaesthetics have a negative inotropic action on myocardial contractility. A distinct relationship exists between local anaesthetic potency and myocardial depression: the more potent agents (bupivacaine, etidocaine and amethocaine) depress cardiac contractility at the lowest concentrations. In addition, bupivacaine and etidocaine, but not amethocaine, have a far greater propensity to induce severe cardiac arrhythmias, including ventricular fibrillation, than the shorter-acting agents lignocaine and mepivacaine. These effects are believed to be due primarily to a direct cardiac effect, but may also be mediated through the CNS.

Summary box 11.4 Cardiovascular toxicity of bupivacaine

- Due to inhibition of cardiac sodium channels.

- Marked depression of the rapid phase of depolarization (V_{max}) of the cardiac action potential.

- Slow conduction leads to unidirectional block and reentry arrhythmias.

- Increased effective refractory period can result in ventricular tachycardia similar to torsades de pointes.

- Cardiotoxicity increased by acidosis and hypoxia.

- Pregnancy may increase potential for toxicity.

- With cardiac arrest, heart arrests in diastole.

- Resuscitation can be extremely difficult; cardiac arrest may require prolonged heart massage due to very prolonged recovery of the sodium channels from bupivacaine-induced inhibition.

Fortunately, the CVS is less susceptible to local anaesthetic toxicity than the CNS, because CVS toxicity is more likely to result in morbidity and mortality than CNS toxicity. Reports of cardiac arrests following administration of bupivacaine and etidocaine have raised concern in this respect. Studies, initiated because of this, have shown that the ratio of the doses or blood levels that are required to produce irreversible cardiovascular collapse and the doses or blood levels that produce convulsions is considerably smaller for both bupivacaine and etidocaine than for lignocaine. Another factor of concern with respect to the cardiotoxicity of bupivacaine and etidocaine is the propensity to produce ventricular arrhythmias. Finally, the cardiotoxicity of bupivacaine is potentiated markedly by acidosis and hypoxia, and enhanced in pregnancy. Pregnant women are believed to be more sensitive to the toxic effects of bupivacaine, but probably not of other local anaesthetics. This may be related to the hormonal changes in pregnancy which alter membrane excitability in nerves and the heart. It may also be related to reduced protein binding of bupivacaine during pregnancy, so that more drug is available to block sodium channels.

Prevention and treatment of systemic toxicity

The most important consideration with respect to the prevention of systemic toxicity is to avoid intravascular injections. In this respect, aspiration may be helpful to detect an intravascular location of the needle or catheter. Aspiration should be done gently and carefully in order to avoid collapse of the vessel walls, resulting in a false-negative test result. Injection of a test dose, generally consisting of a small volume of the local anaesthetic solution, to which adrenaline has been added to detect cardiovascular responses in the event of an intravascular injection, is also frequently applied. With procedures requiring higher doses, fractionated administration is also recommended, so that in the event of a (mild) toxic reaction the administration can be terminated before the full dose has been administered. Another consideration is that excessive doses have to be avoided.

When early signs of a systemic toxic reaction appear, the injection of the local anaesthetic should be stopped immediately and oxygen administered by face mask. By doing so, subtle signs and symptoms will vanish. The occurrence of seizures necessitates the use of anticonvulsant drugs (intravenous benzodiazepines or barbiturates) before cerebral hypoxia and (respiratory) acidosis complicate the situation. When short-acting local anaesthetics are the cause, seizures are usually of short duration and, if adequate treatment is instituted, are seldom life threatening. Convulsions induced by the longer-acting agents (bupivacaine) are more resistant to therapy. Arrhythmias and cardiovascular depression should be treated, depending on the clinical picture. Cardiovascular toxicity from bupivacaine, especially in obstetrics, may be refractory to conventional therapy. Cardiopulmonary resuscitation following bupivacaine-induced cardiovascular collapse can be extremely difficult. Hypoxia and acidosis can develop very rapidly, even in previously well-ventilated patients, and will further inhibit attempts at resuscitation. Massive doses of inotropic drugs and prolonged heart massage are often necessary. Isoprenaline at rates of $1-2\,\mu g\,min^{-1}$ may be useful in treating bradycardia and the depression of cardiac conduction caused by bupivacaine.

Phosphodiesterase inhibitors have been shown to increase survival in animal models. Bretylium has been advocated for the treatment of bupivacaine-induced arrhythmias.

ALLERGIC REACTIONS

True allergic reaction to local anaesthetics are rare and occur most frequently with the ester-type agents. Allergic reactions to the latter agents are due to the formation of para-aminobenzoic acid or derivatives thereof that are allergenic. Allergic reactions to amide-type agents are extremely rare and probably mostly caused by preservatives such as methylparaben, which is structurally related to para-aminobenzoic acid.

METHAEMOGLOBINAEMIA

Large doses of prilocaine (generally > 600 mg) can cause methaemoglobinaemia. This is believed to be related to the hydroxylation of o-toluidine, which is formed by the amide hydrolysis of prilocaine. Methaemoglobinaemia is spontaneously reversible or may be treated by intravenous administration of methylene blue.

CLINICAL APPLICATIONS

TOPICAL ANAESTHESIA

In general, onset of anaesthesia occurs most rapidly upon topical application to the mucous membranes. A relatively concentrated solution of a local anaesthetic is applied to the mucous membrane (nose, mouth, trachea, larynx, urethra, bladder, rectum). Cocaine and lignocaine are used frequently for topical anaesthesia (see individual agents). The absorption of the local anaesthetic from mucous membranes is usually very fast, particularly when applied in infected areas, and plasma concentrations can be reached comparable with those after direct intravenous administration.

Local anaesthetics are unable to penetrate intact skin in sufficient quantities to produce reliable anaesthesia. Efficient skin penetration requires the combination of a high water content and a high concentration of the water-insoluble base form of the local anaesthetic. This combination has been achieved by mixing lignocaine and prilocaine in their base forms (EMLA – Emulsion of Local Anaesthetics).[12] The melting points of these drugs are well above room temperature, but when mixed in a 1:1 ratio the melting point of the combination is lowered to approximately 18°C. Thus, when mixed in this ratio, lignocaine and prilocaine form a eutectic mixture, i.e. one that melts and solidifies without separation of its constituents. When crystals of lignocaine and prilocaine are mixed in equal amounts at room temperature, they melt to form an oil. When the oil is emulsified in water, the requirement of a high water content is fulfilled. Since the oil droplets in the emulsion contain a high concentration of local anaesthetics (EMLA 80%; conventional lignocaine in oil 20%), the second requirement is also fulfilled. After local application (application time 60–70 min), EMLA permits pain-free invasive procedures to be carried out on the skin, a property that is especially useful in children.

INFILTRATION ANAESTHESIA

With infiltration anaesthesia nerves are blocked at the peripheral nerve endings. Infiltration of the gingival mucosa is frequently performed for many routine dental procedures. Onset of action is almost immediate with all agents.

In intradermal and subcutaneous infiltration anaesthesia, very thin pain conducting nerves are easily blocked and therefore relatively diluted solutions may be used (e.g. lignocaine 0.5–1%, mepivacaine 0.5–1%, bupivacaine 0.125–0.25%). Any of the available agents can be used, the choice depending on the desired duration of anaesthesia. Lignocaine, mepivacaine and prilocaine are agents of moderate duration, whereas bupivacaine and ropivacaine are long-acting agents. The duration of infiltration blocks can be prolonged by the addition of adrenaline (optimum concentration $5 \mu g$ $ml^{-1} = 1 : 200\,000$), phenylephrine or noradrenaline.

PERIPHERAL NERVE BLOCK

Regional anaesthetic procedures involving the nerves of the peripheral nervous system are called peripheral nerve blocks. The most commonly used peripheral regional block techniques are brachial plexus block (interscalene, supraclavicular and axillary approach) of the upper extremity and psoas compartment, and sciatic nerve block of the lower extremity. Other techniques are: intercostal block, cervical plexus block and isolated peripheral nerve (e.g. median, ulnar, femoral) blocks.

To reach the neural target (i.e. the axolemma), the local anaesthetic must diffuse through a number of tissue layers. Of these the perineurium is the greatest diffusion barrier, delaying the onset of action. Other factors of importance with respect to the onset are the anatomical arrangement of different fibres within the nerves and the fact that different fibres may be blocked at different rates. Diffusion of the local anaesthetics proceeds from the outer surface of mixed nerves to the centre of the nerve. Consequently, 'mantle' fibres located near the outer surface will be blocked first. Usually, these fibres serve more proximal structures, whereas the more distal structures are served by 'core' fibres located near the centre of the nerve.

Because diffusion occurs from mantle to core, motor blockade may precede sensory blockade when motor fibres are located peripheral to sensory fibres.

This holds only when the concentration of local anaesthetic is greater than the minimal blocking concentration for the thickest motor fibres. However, if the concentration of the local anaesthetic solution is not quite sufficient to block the thickest fibres, the anatomical relationship will play no significant part in the blocking sequence and the motor fibres will always be the last to be blocked.

Most local anaesthetics can be used for peripheral nerve blocks. The most appropriate agent is usually selected on the basis of the duration of action and systemic safety. In general, the duration of action can better be prolonged by adding a vasoconstrictor than by increasing the dose.

INTRAVENOUS REGIONAL ANAESTHESIA

During intravenous regional anaesthesia a low concentration of local anaesthetic is injected in a limb vein that is separated from the general circulation by tourniquet occlusion. In general, both sensory and motor block will result if the limb involved is exsanguinated before the tourniquet is applied. However, the primary site of action is at the peripheral sensory nerve endings. Prilocaine 0.5% (40–80 ml; 200–400 mg) is currently the drug of choice because of its low toxicity.

In contrast to diffusion in peripheral nerve block, during intravenous regional anaesthesia the local anaesthetic diffusion proceeds from core to mantle. This is probably due to the fact that the local anaesthetic containing blood vessels are located in or near the core of the nerve(s). In intravenous regional anaesthesia, the ischaemia caused by the tourniquet that is inflated to 20–40 mmHg above the systolic pressure may also contribute to the numbing effect.

After tourniquet release the local anaesthetic effect of the agents with short or intermediate duration vanishes swiftly. Bupivacaine is contraindicated for intravenous regional anaesthesia owing to serious systemic toxicity after sudden (unwanted) cuff release.

CENTRAL BLOCKS

Epidural anaesthesia (analgesia)

Solutions injected into the epidural space will spread in all directions since there are no firm barriers to bulk flow in this so-called potential space, which is filled with loose adipose tissue, blood vessels and lymphatics. The suggested sites of action of local anaesthetics that are administered in the epidural space are the paravertebral nerve trunks, the dorsal root ganglia, the spinal nerve roots and the spinal cord. The dermatomal progression of anaesthesia following epidural administration suggests primarily blockade of the spinal roots. The dermatomal onset pattern, and other differences between spinal and epidural anaesthesia, suggests that the spinal cord itself is not the primary site of action during the initial phases of epidural anaesthesia.

Although most agents are useful for epidural anaesthesia, the most commonly used agents are lignocaine, mepivacaine and bupivacaine. In some countries chloroprocaine and etidocaine are also available. The choice of local anaesthetic varies with the required duration of action. For continuous procedures bupivacaine and ropivacaine are the drugs of choice.

Epidural anaesthesia is a technique whereby the degree of sensory and motor block can be adjusted to the clinical need. By changing the concentration of the local anaesthetic, or even the local anaesthetic itself, the clinical picture may change from sensory analgesia with little motor block to anaesthesia with intense motor blockade.

Spinal anaesthesia

Spinal anaesthesia is a very efficient technique in that a small amount of a local anaesthetic, injected into the subarachnoid space, results in a dense and widespread blockade. Because the amount of local anaesthetic required is so small, systemic toxicity is of little or no concern. The most commonly used agents are lignocaine, bupivacaine and tetracaine. Both hyperbaric solutions (by addition of glucose 5–9%) with a specific gravity greater than that of the cerebrospinal fluid (1.003 at 37°C) and hypobaric solutions are used. Specific gravities and, consequently, the clinical effects change considerably in the temperature range from 18 to 37°C.

The effects of an injection of a local anaesthetic solution into the lumbar subarachnoid space are the result of penetration of the local anaesthetic into the spinal nerve roots, the dorsal root ganglia and (superficial) layers of the spinal cord. Nerve roots in the subarachnoid space are devoid of epineural sheaths and the spinal cord itself is much like a desheathed peripheral nerve. This lack of diffusion barriers explains the fast onset and deep intensity of spinal anaesthesia.

INDIVIDUAL DRUGS

ESTERS

Cocaine is rarely used because of its systemic toxicity, addictive properties and tendency to produce allergic reactions. It is, however, an excellent topical agent and the only local anaesthetic that consistently produces vasoconstriction in clinically useful concentrations. As such, it is still used during ear, nose and throat surgery.

Procaine, the first synthetic local anaesthetic, is a relatively weak local anaesthetic with a slow onset and short duration of action. Rapid hydrolysis of procaine accounts for its low systemic toxicity.

Chloroprocaine differs from procaine by the addition of a chlorine atom to the aromatic ring. Like procaine, it has a low potency and short duration of action. In practice its onset of action is rapid if high doses are used. This is justified by the wide systemic safety margin of chloroprocaine, which is hydrolysed even faster than procaine. In addition, the allergic potential of chloroprocaine appears to be less than that of procaine. Because of these properties, chloroprocaine is used in some countries for epidural anaesthesia and in obstetric practice, as well as for peripheral nerve blocks requiring a short duration of action. Furthermore, chloroprocaine has been used in combination with bupivacaine to compensate the slow onset of the latter agent. However, the use of such a combination is controversial.

Amethocaine (tetracaine) is also structurally related to procaine, but is considerably more potent and has a longer duration of action. Because of its relatively slow hydrolysis, it is quite toxic; therefore its use is limited mainly to spinal anaesthesia.

Benzocaine differs from all other currently used local anaesthetics in that it lacks an amine group. Consequently, the agent does not exist in the un-ionized form and therefore is insoluble in water, and can be used only topically. Very rapid hydrolysis ensures a low systemic toxicity, but the formation of para-aminobenzoic acid may result in allergic reactions.

AMIDES

Cinchocaine (dibucaine), the first synthetic amide-type local anaesthetic, is nowadays rarely, if at all, used clinically.

Lignocaine (lidocaine), introduced more than 50 years ago, is still the most popular local anaesthetic today. Its relatively fast onset of action, intermediate potency and moderate duration of action, along with a reasonable safety margin, warrant its use for virtually all local and regional anaesthetic procedures. To prolong the duration of action of lignocaine and to enhance its systemic safety, a vasconstrictor (commonly adrenaline) is frequently added. Being an effective topical anaesthetic, lignocaine is also available in ointment, jelly, viscous and aerosol preparations. A eutectic mixture of lignocaine and prilocaine (EMLA cream) is available for dermal anaesthesia and analgesia. A hyperbaric 5% solution, containing 7.5% glucose, is available for spinal anaesthesia. The latter, however, has recently been blamed for causing problems when it is administered via narrow-bore needles or microcatheters. Therefore it is recommended to dilute the solution with an equal volume of cerebrospinal fluid before the injection.

Mepivacaine has an anaesthetic profile similar to that of lignocaine, but is not effective as a topical agent. It is used mainly for infiltration, peripheral nerve blocks and epidural anaesthesia, but is rarely used in obstetrics, because of its slow metabolism in the fetus. In some countries hyperbaric solutions are available for spinal anaesthesia. The duration of action of mepivacaine is usually somewhat longer than that of lignocaine.

Prilocaine has a similar potency to lignocaine but a somewhat longer duration of action. This is probably related to its less profound vasodilator activity. Because of this, prilocaine can be used for most applications without addition of a vasoconstrictor. Used as such, its duration of action is broadly comparable to that of lignocaine with adrenaline. Therefore, prilocaine is indicated in patients in whom adrenaline is contraindicated. Prilocaine is used mainly for infiltration, peripheral nerve block and intravenous regional anaesthesia (Bier block). In the latter application, advantage is taken of its low systemic toxicity. With prilocaine, toxic effects following tourniquet release are rarely seen, even in the event of accidental early release. A disadvantage of prilocaine is that higher doses result in methaemoglobinaemia. Because of this its use is limited to single-injection procedures. For the same reason it is generally avoided in obstetrics.

Bupivacaine is approximately four times more potent than lignocaine and has a long duration of action. Although the onset of action is slower with bupivacaine, it is still considered acceptable for most applications. It is used in concentrations varying from 0.125% up to 0.75% for various procedures, including infiltration anaesthesia, peripheral nerve blocks, epidural and spinal anaesthesia. For the latter application both glucose-free solutions and glucose-containing (hyperbaric) solutions are available. A major advantage of this agent is that, when dilute solutions are used, effective analgesia can be obtained with little or no motor block. As such, bupivacaine is frequently used, either as the sole agent or in combination with an opioid, for pain relief in obstetrics and for postoperative analgesia.

Ropivacaine is structurally closely related to both mepivacaine and bupivacaine. However, whereas mepivacaine and bupivacaine are available as racemates, ropivacaine is a pure S(−) enantiomer. It is broadly comparable to bupivacaine, but is somewhat faster in onset, slightly less potent and somewhat shorter acting in most procedures. Its major advantages, compared with bupivacaine, are that it is less cardiotoxic and has an even greater sensory–motor dissociation.[13]

Etidocaine is a long-acting local anaesthetic that differs from bupivacaine by its faster onset of action and its ability to produce profound motor block. Because of this it is used mainly in situations where intense motor block is required. The agent, however, is not available in many countries.

Articaine, a thiophene derivative, is commonly used in dentistry in some countries. It has undergone limited clinical evaluation as an epidural agent, but does not appear to have great advantages over other local anaesthetics.

REFERENCES

1. Burm AGL, van der Meer AD, van Kleef JW *et al.* Pharmacokinetics of the enantiomers of bupivacaine following intravenous administration of the racemate. *Br J Clin Pharmacol* 1994; **38**: 125–129.
2. Burm AGL, Cohen IMC, Van Kleef JW *et al.* Pharmacokinetics of the enantiomers of mepivacaine after intravenous administration of the racemate in volunteers. *Anesth Analg* 1997; **84**: 85–89.
3. Burm AGL. Clinical pharmacokinetics of epidural and spinal anaesthesia. *Clin Pharmacokinet* 1989; **16**: 283–311.
4. Emanuelsson B-MK, Persson J, Alm C *et al.* Systemic absorption and block after epidural injection of ropivacaine in healthy volunteers. *Anesthesiology* 1997; **87**: 1309–1317.
5. Nancarrow C, Runciman WB, Mather LE *et al.* The influence of acidosis on the distribution of lidocaine and bupivacaine into the myocardium and brain of the sheep. *Anesth Analg* 1987; **66**: 925–935.
6. Covino BG, Vassallo HG. *Local Anesthetics: Mechanisms of Action and Clinical Use.* New York: Grune and Stratton, 1976.
7. Butterworth JF, Strichartz GR. Molecular mechanisms of local anesthesia: a review. *Anesthesiology* 1990; **72**: 711–734.
8. Narahashi T. Drug-ionic channel interactions: single-channel measurements. *Ann Neurol* 1984; **16** (Suppl.): S39–S51.
9. Fink BR. Mechanisms of differential axial blockade in epidural and subarachnoid anesthesia. *Anesthesiology* 1989; **70**: 851–858.
10. Hogan Q. Local anesthetic toxicity: an update. *Reg Anesth* 1996; **21** (Suppl. 6S): 43–50.
11. Mather LE, Cousins MJ. Local anaesthetics and their current clinical use. *Drugs* 1979; **18**: 185–205.
12. Buckley MM, Benfield P. Eutectic lidocaine/prilocaine cream: a review of the topical anaesthetic/analgesic efficacy of a eutectic mixture of local anaesthetics (EMLA). *Drugs* 1993; **46**: 126–151.
13. Markham A, Faulds D. Ropivacaine: a review of its pharmacology and therapeutic use in regional anaesthesia. *Drugs* 1996; **52**: 429–449.

12 AJ Souter, PF White

NONSTEROIDAL ANTIINFLAMMATORY DRUGS

The nonsteroidal antiinflammatory drugs (NSAIDs) are a ubiquitous group of drugs with a long history in medicine (Fig. 12.1). For centuries, the extract of willow bark (containing the active ingredient salicin) was used for its antipyretic and pain-relieving properties. Aspirin (acetylsalicylic acid), a derivative of salicylic acid produced from salicin, was introduced by the pharmaceutical company Bayer in 1899, and has become one of the most widely used medicines in the world. NSAIDs are a heterogeneous group of compounds with analgesic, antiinflammatory and antipyretic properties. Many, for example phenylbutazone, have a high toxicity that restricts their use to the treatment of chronic inflammatory conditions such as rheumatoid arthritis. Over the past decade, the appearance of injectable preparations of NSAIDs has led to a resurgence of interest in their perioperative use as effective analgesics with fewer associated adverse effects than opioids.[1,2]

PHARMACOKINETICS OF NSAIDs

ABSORPTION

The NSAIDs are rapidly absorbed from the upper gastrointestinal tract. Rapid absorption of the non-ionized form of these drugs occurs in the low pH environment of the stomach. This absorption is dependent on the pK_a of the specific drug (i.e. the lower the pK_a the greater the proportion of the drug existing in its un-ionized, absorbable form). Both aspirin and paracetamol are well absorbed across the gastric mucosa. For most NSAIDs, however, the majority of uptake occurs in the small intestine. They also readily cross mucous membranes and can be administered in a rectal suppository form.

BIOTRANSFORMATION

NSAIDs are weak organic acids (pK_a 3–5) that bind extensively to plasma albumin (Table 12.1). An exception is paracetamol, which has a pK_a of 9.3 and negligible protein binding. NSAIDs are extensively metabolized in the liver, mainly undergoing phase II conjugation reactions. The high level of protein binding results in higher plasma than tissue levels, as well as a low volume of distribution.

ELIMINATION

As with most water-soluble drugs, NSAIDs are excreted primarily in the urine. The ratio of conjugated to free drug and their rate of elimination varies with the drug and the pH of the urine. The majority of these drugs

> **Summary box 12.1 Nonsteroidal antiinflammatory drugs**
>
> - NSAIDs are a heterogeneous group of compounds with analgesic antiinflammatory and antipyretic properties.
>
> - Most of the pharmacological effects and all of the side-effects of these drugs are the result of inhibition of the enzyme, cyclooxygenase, which converts arachidonic acid to various prostaglandins, prostacyclin (PGI_2) and thromboxanes.
>
> - Cyclooxygenase is inhibited irreversibly by aspirin and reversibly by other NSAIDs.
>
> - Two isoforms of cyclooxygenase exist:
>
>   - COX-1 is the constitutive form responsible for the production of prostaglandins involved in cellular 'housekeeping' functions.
>
>   - COX-2 is induced in cells activated by exposure to mediators of inflammation such as cytokines and endotoxin.
>
> - Most available NSAIDs are nonselective for these isoforms. Drugs with COX-2 selectivity have more antiinflammatory activity and fewer gastrointestinal or renal side-effects.

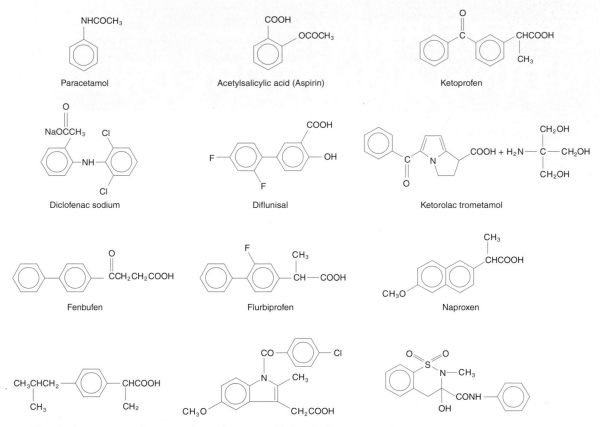

Fig. 12.1 Chemical structures of commonly used nonsteroidal antiinflammatory drugs.

and their metabolites are more highly ionized and, therefore, more readily excreted when the urine is alkaline. Small amounts are eliminated via the bile and excreted in faeces.

MECHANISMS OF ACTION

ANALGESIA

The NSAIDs are prostaglandin synthetase (cyclo-oxygenase) inhibitors that exert their analgesic effect in part by reducing prostaglandin production in inflamed or damaged tissue, thereby modulating inflammation and nociception (Fig. 12.2). Tissue trauma results in an inflammatory response mediated by a release of kinins, histamine, 5-hydroxytryptamine and substance P. These activate phospholipase A_2, which catalyses the production of arachidonic acid. Arachidonic acid, a major component of cell membrane phospholipids, is converted by cyclooxygenase (prostaglandin endoperoxide synthase) to the cyclic endoperoxides prostaglandin (PG) G_2 and PGH_2, which are in turn metabolized to various prostaglandins, prostacyclin (PGI_2) and thromboxanes (Fig. 12.3). These are responsible for nociception, in-

flammation and hyperalgesia.[2] Free nerve endings become sensitized and send a barrage of nociceptive impulses to the dorsal horn of the spinal cord where persistent nociceptive input can cause a so-called 'wind-up' phenomenon. This is a positive feedback mechanism, mediated in part via N-methyl-D-aspartate (NMDA) receptors, which exhibit enlargement of their receptive field and a reduction in the neural firing threshold. These mechanisms modulate the response to painful stimuli and can give rise to a state of hyperalgesia, where the perception of pain is greater than would normally be produced by a given stimulus.

Inhibition of prostaglandin synthesis by cyclooxygenase is the principal mode of action of NSAIDs in the relief of pain secondary to tissue injury or chronic inflammation. Cyclooxygenase is inhibited irreversibly by aspirin and reversibly by other NSAIDs. In addition to inhibition of cyclooxygenase, an additional mode of antiinflammatory activity of piroxicam and other oxicams is modulation of various cytokines, including interleukin (IL) 2, IL-6 and tumour necrosis factor a.[3] The effect on prostaglandin synthesis is not selective for inflamed tissue, and the widespread inhibition of

Table 12.1 Pharmacokinetics of commonly used nonsteroidal antiinflammatory drugs

Drug	Daily dose (mg)	Dosing interval (h)	Elimination half-life (h)	Volume of distribution (l kg^{-1})	Clearance (l kg^{-1}/h^{-1})	Metabolism (%)
Aspirin	4000	4–6	2–30	0.15	3.9	90
Paracetamol	4000	4–6	2.8	0.94	19.3	99
Ibuprofen	3200	4–6	2.5	0.14	3.5	99
Piroxicam	20	12–24	45	0.14	0.14	99
Ketorolac tromethamine	90	4–8	5.4	0.11–0.25	0.02–0.03	40
Diclofenac sodium	150	8–12	1–2	0.12	0.04–0.08	99
Ketoprofen	200	4–12	1.5–2	0.11	0.07	99
Tenoxicam	20	24	72	0.14	0.0017	99
Meloxicam	15	24	20	–	0.42–0.48	99

cyclooxygenase is responsible for several of the adverse effects of these drugs. In addition, the lipoxygenase pathway, which converts arachidonic acid to leukotrienes, is inhibited by indomethacin and diclofenac but not by salicylates.

Cyclooxygenase (COX) exists in at least two isoforms, COX-1 and COX-2. A third isoform, COX-3, has recently been described. COX-1 is the constitutive form responsible for the production of prostaglandins involved in cellular 'housekeeping' functions such as the regulation of vascular homeostasis and coordinating the actions of circulating hormones. COX-2 is induced in cells activated by exposure to mediators of inflammation such as cytokines and endotoxin, and may be responsible for the production of prostanoids that mediate inflammation, pain and fever. COX-1 is localized on the inner surface of the endoplasmic reticulum and COX-2 on the nuclear membrane. This puts restrictions on the properties of NSAIDs, which must be amphilic and lipid soluble to transverse intercellular barriers. COX-2 is upregulated by up to 50% in many colorectal adenocarcinomas, and treatment of patients with these cancers by NSAIDs has resulted in regression of the tumour.[4]

There are wide differences in the selectivity of NSAIDs for the isoforms. Some, such as aspirin, indomethacin and ibuprofen, are more potent inhibitors of COX-1 than of COX-2. Diclofenac, paracetamol and naproxen are equipotent inhibitors of both types. The therapeutic effects of the NSAIDs may be due to their ability to inhibit COX-2, whereas the side-effects, such as gastric and renal damage, correlate with inhibition of COX-1. Drugs with selectivity for COX-2 will have more antiinflammatory activity and fewer gastrointestinal or renal side-effects. Several COX-2-selective drugs are currently being developed. One of these, meloxicam, is undergoing investigation for the treatment of rheumatoid arthritis and osteoarthritis.[5]

Traditionally, the primary mechanism of NSAID activity was thought to be at peripheral sites.[6] However,

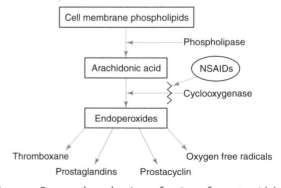

Fig. 12.2 Proposed mechanism of action of nonsteroidal antiinflammatory drugs (NSAIDs) on prostaglandin synthetase activity. From Souter *et al.*[1]

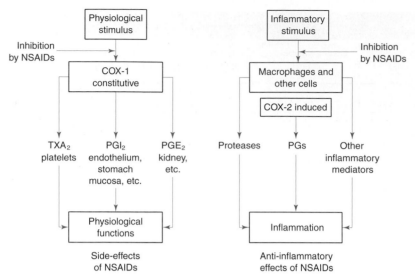

Fig. 12.3 Relationship between the pathways leading to the generation of prostaglandins by cyclooxygenase-1 (COX-1) and COX-2. NSAIDs, nonsteroidal antiinflammatory drugs; TXA$_2$, thromboxane A$_2$; PG, prostaglandin. From Vane JR, Botting RM. Overview – mechanisms of action of anti-inflammatory drugs. In: Vane JR, Botting J, Botting RM (eds). *Improved Non-steroidal Anti-inflammatory Drugs. COX-2 Enzyme Inhibitors*. London: Kluwer Academic Publishers, 1996, Figure 2, with kind permission from Kluwer Academic Publishers.

recent in vivo animal experiments suggest NSAIDs may also produce analgesia by a centrally mediated mechanism. Centrally administered NSAIDs reduce the thalamic response to peripheral nociceptive input and prevent the rise in prostaglandin concentrations in cerebrospinal fluid (CSF) following NMDA receptor activation.[7] NSAIDs inhibit both the immediate pain and the delayed hyperalgesia in response to formalin injection in the rat.[8] They also have significant actions on the dorsal horn, and these contribute to their analgesic and antiinflammatory actions. Several NSAIDs, including ketoprofen, indomethacin and diclofenac, appear in the CSF of humans at concentrations that equal or exceed the free fraction in plasma. An exception is ketorolac; the CSF : plasma concentration ratios of ketorolac are 1 : 1000.[9]

ANTIPYRETIC EFFECT

The antipyretic effect of the NSAIDs is also a consequence of central prostaglandin inhibition. Temperature regulation is controlled by the hypothalamus, which sets the point at which body temperature is maintained. In fever this is adjusted upwards, under the influence of pyrogens and prostaglandins released by the inflammatory process. Aspirin also prevents the release of endogenous pyrogens from white cells. NSAIDs in normal doses have no effect on temperature regulation in subjects with normal body temperature. However, toxic doses of salicylates produce hyperpyrexia as a result of intracellular uncoupling of oxidative phos-

phorylation, which inhibits a number of adenosine triphosphate (ATP)-dependent reactions. The increased energy released by this abnormal cellular respiration is dissipated as heat instead of being used to convert inorganic phosphate and adenosine diphosphate to ATP.

PLATELET FUNCTION

Platelets occupy a primary role in haemostasis, maintaining vascular integrity and contributing to the complex process of coagulation. They have also been implicated in the promotion of arteriosclerotic lesions. NSAIDs can interfere with platelet function by several mechanisms involving inhibition of cyclooxygenase. This blocks the formation not only of platelet-activating eicosanoids, such as PGG$_2$, PGH$_2$ and thromboxane A$_2$, but also of the platelet inhibitors PGD$_2$ and PGI$_2$. Aspirin is the only NSAID that is used therapeutically for its antiplatelet effects. Aspirin in low doses is used widely in patients with cardiovascular disease to reduce the incidence of myocardial infarction and stroke. Doses as low as 40 mg daily can produce maximum inhibition of thromboxane and prostacyclin synthesis. The use of aspirin can reduce the risk of myocardial infarction by 25% and reduce the risk of a fatal infarction significantly.

For most NSAIDs, except aspirin, the antiplatelet effect is present only while the drug is present in the body in sufficient concentration. In the case of aspirin the effect lasts for the 5–11 days of the life of the platelet because of the irreversible acetylation of platelet and megakaryocyte cyclooxygenase, coupled with the inability of platelets to synthesize new enzyme. With the exception of the therapeutic antiplatelet effect of the NSAIDs in patients with cardiovascular disease, the antiplatelet effect is of no or minimal clinical significance in haematologically normal patients. Despite numerous studies on NSAIDs and surgical bleeding, no firm conclusions can be drawn regarding an increased risk of haemorrhage in patients taking NSAIDs. Even the impact of peroperatively administered NSAIDs on blood loss is unclear. Aspirin and other NSAIDs should be avoided where possible during pregnancy. NSAIDs can cross the placenta and have been associated with significant neonatal bleeding. The mother may also have excessive intrapartum blood loss. In some pregnancies aspirin may, however, have a therapeutic indication, specifically in the prevention of preeclampsia.

ADVERSE EFFECTS OF NSAIDs

The effect of NSAIDs on prostaglandin synthesis is not selective for inflamed tissue, and the widespread inhibition of cyclooxygenase is responsible for several of the adverse effects of these drugs. The more insidious but potentially dangerous effects of NSAIDs are on the renal, clotting and gastrointestinal systems. Indeed in

---

Summary box 12.2 Adverse effects of NSAIDs

- Inhibition of cyclooxygenase (COX-1) is responsible for most of the adverse effects of these drugs.

- NSAIDs have little effect on renal function under normal circumstances, but in the presence of hypovolaemia or diminished renal blood flow cyclooxygenase inhibition may result in renal damage.

- Bleeding and ulceration of the gastric mucosa is a major limitation to the use of NSAIDs. This is due mainly to suppression of gastric prostaglandins. Several NSAIDs, including aspirin, also produce direct mucosal injury.

- Cyclooxygenase inhibition by NSAIDs depresses platelet function, producing an increase in bleeding time.

- In susceptible individuals NSAIDs may precipitate acute bronchospasm (aspirin-induced asthma).

- Rare haematological reactions, such as aplastic anaemia, agranulocytosis and thrombocytopenia, probably have an immunological basis.

---

some European countries (e.g. Germany), these concerns have led to their withdrawal as perioperative analgesics.

RENAL SYSTEM

Prostaglandins autoregulate renal blood flow locally, although they are not essential for maintaining renal function in the unstressed kidney. Any reduction in the renal circulation causes an increased production of catecholamines and activation of the renin–angiotensin system. The resulting renal vasoconstriction is counterbalanced by a compensatory release of prostaglandins to maintain adequate renal perfusion. In this situation inhibition of prostaglandin synthesis by NSAIDs can adversely affect renal function. Adverse reactions are, however, uncommon in patients with normal kidneys.

Renal toxicity associated with NSAIDs usually occurs when other risk factors are present (e.g. hypovolaemia, concurrent use of nephrotoxic drugs) and can present as life-threatening acute renal failure. In the presence of adequate hydration, inhibition of prostaglandin synthesis should not adversely affect renal function since renal blood is not dependent on prostaglandins in that situation. However, in the presence of hypovolaemia and cardiac failure, low cardiac output or liver disease, cyclooxygenase inhibition may result in renal vasoconstriction and deterioration of renal function. This is reversible if the NSAID is discontinued, but if not recognized can lead to prolonged renal ischaemia, acute tubular necrosis and permanent renal damage. While administration of NSAIDs to healthy patients will reduce renal blood flow by less than 10%, in patients in whom the renin–angiotensin system has been activated (e.g. congestive heart failure) the reduction may be up to 60% and may lead to clinical renal failure.

NSAIDs can also cause acute renal insufficiency in patients with preexisting chronic renal insufficiency since in these patients prostaglandins are essential to maintain renal function. Some diuretics (e.g. thiazides) stimulate prostaglandin production and the action of loop diuretics such as frusemide is prostaglandin dependent. Interactions between these agents and NSAIDs are common. All NSAIDs, and indomethacin in particular, can interfere with the pharmacological control of hypertension and congestive heart failure in patients receiving β-adrenoceptor antagonists, diuretics or angiotensin-converting enzyme inhibitors. Inhibition of the renal excretion of digoxin and lithium may increase the plasma concentrations of these drugs and increase the risk of toxicity.

NSAIDs administered to healthy patients for a short time after operation (e.g. for less than 72 h) are not associated with alterations in renal function. However, large doses of ketorolac (> 100 mg daily) administered to patients older than 65 years for more than 5 days can result in transient decreases in creatinine clearance. NSAIDs should therefore be used with caution in elderly patients and the duration of administration restricted to 72 h. They should also be avoided in the presence of preexisting renal disease, or where other nephrotoxic drugs are being administered and/or when conditions of hypovolaemia, low cardiac output or liver disease exist. In the absence of these contraindications, the perioperative administration of NSAIDs appears to be safe.

HAEMATOLOGICAL SYSTEM

Thromboxanes are endoperoxides closely related to the prostaglandins. These compounds are required for platelet aggregation. Prostacyclin, another endoperoxide, also depends on cyclooxygenase for its production and it has well characterized inhibitory effects on platelet aggregation (Fig. 12.2). However, cyclooxygenase inhibition by NSAIDs decreases platelet function, causing an increase in bleeding time. The antiplatelet effect of the NSAID compounds is the therapeutic rationale for the use of aspirin in reducing the risk of coronary thrombosis and transient cerebral ischaemic attacks.

Depressed platelet function is of obvious concern in the perioperative period.[10] When used perioperatively, NSAIDs do cause an increase in bleeding time, but do not act synergistically with anticoagulant drugs. Where bleeding is a recognized and relatively common complication of surgery (e.g. post-tonsillectomy), the administration of NSAIDs during operation has been associated with increase blood loss *per se*, as well as an increased need for surgical reexploration because of bleeding.[11] However, in patients undergoing transurethral prostatectomy and knee replacement surgery, blood loss is not affected by the perioperative use of NSAIDs.

One area of particular concern is in microvascular reconstructive plastic surgery where meticulous haemostasis is necessary to ensure flap survival. Currently, there are several anecdotal reports of increased haematoma formation associated with the perioperative use of NSAIDs. Nevertheless, NSAIDs have been promoted to increase microvascular blood flow by decreasing thrombosis in small blood vessels. Although studies in animal models have reported a short-term beneficial effect, the therapeutic efficacy of this approach is still highly questionable.

CARDIOVASCULAR SYSTEM

Prostaglandins are potent local regulators of vascular tone and, therefore, the NSAIDs can indirectly affect local tissue blood flow. More specifically, prostacyclin is a potent vasodilator, while PGE_2 and PGF_2 are potent vasoconstrictors and can induce coronary vasoconstriction. It is interesting that, despite their abilities to affect vascular tone, NSAIDs appear to have little effect on cardiovascular parameters including arterial blood pressure, systemic vascular resistance and cardiac output.[12] These findings may be due to a balanced reduction in prostaglandins with 'opposing' actions on vascular smooth muscle. Despite their limited effects, NSAIDs should be used with caution in patients with coronary ischaemia and/or hypertension.

GASTROINTESTINAL TRACT

Bleeding and ulceration of the mucosa of the gastrointestinal tract, in particular the stomach, are a major limitation to the use of NSAIDs. These effects in the stomach are linked to suppression of gastric prostaglandins, although other factors also play a role. A particularly troublesome feature of NSAID gastropathy is that the ulceration is often asymptomatic, the initial presentation frequently being severe haemorrhage or perforation. Bleeding ulcers and perforations are more common in patients aged over 60 years. Conventional antiulcer therapy, such as antacids, histamine H_2-receptor antagonists or proton pump inhibitors, is relatively ineffective in preventing NSAID-induced ulceration. The concomitant administration of the PGE_1 analogue, misoprostol, is more effective but is expensive and associated with an appreciable incidence of side-effects, notably diarrhoea.

Aspirin, in particular, undergoes ion trapping within the cells of the gastric mucosa. In the acid medium of the stomach, aspirin is non-ionized and is rapidly absorbed by passive diffusion. However, in the more alkaline milieu of the cell, salicylate ions are released. Salicylates inhibit cellular energy production by impairing mitochondrial phosphorylation, leading to increased cell membrane permeability and a cascade of events that results ultimately in cell death, focal erosions and bleeding. Other NSAIDs, especially indomethacin, can also cause focal lesions by increasing the permeability of the cell membrane, but the mechanism is not fully understood. Several NSAIDs, including aspirin, also produce direct mucosal injury and alter the structure of the gastric mucosa. At a pH below its pK_a (3.5), aspirin greatly reduces the surface hydrophobic, nonwettable layer of surface-active phospholipids that cover the gastric mucosa and prevent the passage of H^+ ions, to the point where cellular injury can occur. This hydrophobic layer is maintained by prostaglandins. NSAIDs reduce gastric mucosal blood flow at sites that eventually ulcerate, and injury to the vascular endothelium of the gastric mucosa occurs early after their administration.

The perioperative use of NSAIDs appears to be associated with a low incidence of gastrointestinal adverse effects. Gastrointestinal mucosal injury by NSAIDs in the perioperative period appears to be most common when the drugs are given for prolonged periods in situations where the mucosal blood flow is compromised, for example in sepsis or shock. It would seem prudent, therefore, to limit the dose and duration of administration of these drugs, and to avoid their use altogether when known risk factors for gastrointestinal bleeding are present. For ketorolac the dose should be limited to less than 100 mg per day and the duration to less than 5 days.

HYPERSENSITIVITY REACTIONS

In susceptible individuals NSAIDs may precipitate acute bronchospasm, a clinical syndrome referred to as aspirin-induced asthma. This affects between 10 and 20% of adults but is rare in children. The mechanism is related to cyclooxygenase inhibition, with shunting of arachidonic acid metabolism from the prostaglandin pathway to the biosynthesis of leukotrienes with resulting bronchospasm, increased mucosal permeability and secretion, and neutrophil influx to the tissues. True type I allergic reactions to NSAIDs, with specific immunoglobulin, IgE, are rare but anaphylactoid reactions with cardiovascular collapse have occasionally been described. This is more likely to occur in patients with a history of allergy or atopy, bronchial asthma, or with nasal polyps. Many of the rare but serious haematological reactions to NSAIDs, such as aplastic anaemia, agranulocytosis and thrombocytopenia, are likely to have an immunological basis.

PHARMACOLOGY OF INDIVIDUAL NSAIDs

ASPIRIN

Aspirin (acetylsalicylic acid) is the original and most widely used NSAID in clinical practice (Fig. 12.1). It is well absorbed in the stomach and upper intestine. In the low pH of the stomach, aspirin exists largely in its non-ionized form due to its low pK_a (3.5) and thus readily crosses into the gastric mucosal cells. It has been suggested that the drug is concentrated there in its ionized form, and this concentration effect may be an important factor in the production of gastric mucosal damage. Following absorption, aspirin is widely distributed throughout the body, readily crossing all cellular barriers. Aspirin is rapidly hydrolysed in the plasma, liver and erythrocytes to salicylate, which is eliminated more slowly than aspirin. The latter is responsible for some, but not all, of the analgesic activity. Approximately 70% of an oral dose of aspirin is absorbed into the systemic circulation intact, the remainder being absorbed as salicylate. Both the unchanged drug and its metabolites are excreted in the urine: in normal circumstances 10% appears as free salicylic acid and 75% as salicyluric acid. Excretion is facilitated by alkalinization of the urine, when up to 85% of the ingested drug is eliminated as salicylate. In acidic urine this propor-

tion may be as low as 5%. Metabolism is normally very rapid and aspirin has a plasma half-life of only 2–3 h. However, liver enzymes that form salicyluric acid and phenolic glucuronide are easily saturated and after multiple doses the terminal half-life may increase to 10 h.

In addition to its effects on prostaglandin synthesis, aspirin exerts other physiological effects. In high doses it affects cellular respiration by uncoupling oxidative phosphorylation, producing the metabolic acidosis commonly observed with an overdose. As the pH of the CSF falls and salicylate levels rise, the central medullary centres are stimulated to produce a compensatory respiratory alkalosis mediated by hyperventilation. Aspirin also affects renal urate secretion. At low doses, it can cause retention of uric acid by inhibiting renal tubular secretion, whereas higher doses exert a uricosuric effect by inhibiting tubular reabsorption. Salicylate has very weak activity against either COX isoform. Recent studies indicate that part of its antiinflammatory actions may be through suppression of the expression of genes involved in inflammation.

Aspirin is indicated for the treatment of mild pain, as an antipyretic, and for the pain and inflammation of arthritis. Aspirin is also used to reduce the risk of thrombotic conditions (e.g. in patients with cerebrovascular or coronary artery disease). The usual dose for mild pain is 300–600 mg orally to a maximum daily dose of 4 g. In the treatment of rheumatic diseases larger doses, 5–8 g daily, are often required. Aspirin should be avoided in children less than 12 years of age and in breastfeeding mothers because of its association with Reye's syndrome, a rare disorder in children characterized by liver disorder and encephalopathy. The syndrome has a 20–40% mortality rate.

PARACETAMOL (ACETAMINOPHEN)

Paracetamol has similar analgesic and antipyretic effects to the other NSAIDs. However, since it lacks the antiinflammatory effects of the other NSAIDs, it is not a true NSAID. Paracetamol is the active metabolite of phenacetin and acetanilide, two previously used analgesic drugs which have been withdrawn from clinical use because of their toxicity. Proparacetamol is a prodrug that is converted rapidly to paracetamol following intravenous administration. Both paracetamol and proparacetamol are well absorbed in the duodenum and their rate of absorption can be used as a model for evaluating the speed of gastric emptying. The maximum daily dose of paracetamol is 4 g, and it is indicated for analgesia and temperature reduction in children as young as 3 months of age. The mechanism of action of paracetamol is similar to that of NSAIDs in preventing prostaglandin synthesis, but it appears to possess more central nervous system activity, explaining in part its lack of peripherally mediated antiinflammatory activity.

Paracetamol is associated with a much lower incidence of gastrointestinal mucosal irritation and damage than other NSAIDs. However, excessive doses can cause liver damage and, to a lesser extent, renal damage. Paracetamol is metabolized in the liver to aryl-containing metabolites that possess a strong affinity for sulphydryl groups. Normally these metabolites are inactivated by combining with glutathione or methionine. However, after an overdose they can accumulate and combine with molecules in liver cells to cause centrilobular hepatic necrosis. Treatment at an early stage includes gastric lavage, activated charcoal and intravenous fluid therapy. If the patient is assessed as at 'high risk' for hepatotoxicity as a result of high plasma paracetamol concentrations, the specific antidote is acetylcysteine, which is administered by intravenous infusion. Acetylcysteine preferentially binds the paracetamol metabolites, leading to a more rapid clearance of these potentially toxic breakdown products.

IBUPROFEN

Ibuprofen is a propionic acid derivative with analgesic properties similar to those of aspirin. It is rapidly absorbed after oral administration, with peak analgesia being reached within 1–2 h. The usual dose for mild to moderate pain is 400 mg every 4–6 h. It is better tolerated than aspirin, mainly due to less severe gastrointestinal disturbances, which occur in about 10–15% of patients. There have been a few reported cases of toxic amblyopia, and any patient developing ocular symptoms should discontinue ibuprofen treatment immediately.

Ibuprofen and other arylpropionic acids have an asymmetric carbon atom; each therefore exists as two distinct optical isomers or enantiomers. Only naproxen is marketed as the pure $S(-)$ enantiomer; the remainder of this group are available only as the racemic mixtures. The cyclooxygenase inhibitory activity resides in the $S(-)$ enantiomer. Interestingly, an oral dose of racemic ibuprofen results in higher blood concentrations of the $S(+)$ enantiomer, due to chiral inversion from the inactive $R(-)$ to the active $S(+)$ enantiomer. Approximately 60% of the inactive enantiomer of ibuprofen is converted to the active enantiomer.

INDOMETHACIN

Indomethacin, a methylated indole derivative, is a potent antiinflammatory drug but is less effective than aspirin as an analgesic for pain of noninflammatory origin. In addition to inhibition of prostaglandin synthesis, it is also an inhibitor of leucocyte motility. Indomethacin is rapidly and almost completely absorbed from the gastrointestinal tract after oral administration. Due to the high incidence of side-effects, indomethacin is reserved for the treatment of rheumatoid arthritis, osteoarthritis and ankylosing spondylitis. It is also useful in the management of acute attacks of gout, and can be of value in relieving the pain and inflammation of uveitis after ophthalmic surgery. Troublesome side-effects occur in approximately 30–35% of patients, and in 20% are severe enough to require reduction of dosage or complete withdrawal of the drug. The most common complaints are headache and gastrointestinal disturbances. Corneal deposits and retinal disturbances have been reported and patients on long-term indomethacin therapy should undergo routine ophthalmic examination.

Indomethacin has been used in neonates in the treatment of cardiac failure caused by a patent ductus arteriosus. Prostaglandin E causes dilatation of the ductus arteriosus, and inhibition by indomethacin may allow the ductus to close, thereby reducing the load on the heart. Successful closure can be expected in 70% of neonates.

PIROXICAM

Piroxicam is the most commonly used of the oxicam derivative, a class of enolic acid NSAIDs. It is approximately equivalent to aspirin and indomethacin for the treatment of rheumatoid arthritis, and is also recommended for the treatment of acute gout. It has occasionally been used for postoperative pain, but appears not to have any distinct advantage over other NSAIDs.

Piroxicam can be administered orally, rectally or intramuscularly. Like most NSAIDs it is well absorbed after oral administration and peak plasma concentrations are reached within 2–4 h. The elimination half-life varies between 30 and 70 h, and neither the age of the patient nor renal or hepatic dysfunction seems to have any major effect on the pharmacokinetics of piroxicam. The long half-life is a principal advantage for patients, permitting therapy with a single daily dose. The usual dose is 20 mg and is the same by all routes of administration. In addition to inhibition of cyclooxygenase, an additional mode of antiinflammatory activity of piroxicam and other oxicams is modulation of various cytokines, including IL-2, IL-6 and tumour necrosis factor α.

DICLOFENAC

Diclofenac is available for both oral and parenteral administration. It belongs to the phenylacetic acid class of NSAIDs and possesses the analgesic, antiinflammatory and antipyretic properties common to other NSAIDs. Diclofenac for parenteral use is dissolved in propylene glycol because it is poorly water soluble. It cannot be given intravenously in its undiluted form owing to an unacceptably high incidence of pain on injection and venous thrombosis. These adverse effects can be reduced following dilution with saline (or dextrose) and by injecting slowly or infusing as a dilute solution in 100 ml saline over 30 min.

After intravenous administration the elimination half-life of diclofenac is 1–2 h (Table 12.1). However, its pharmacodynamic effects follow a much longer time course, allowing for a dosing regimen of 75 mg every 12 h. Although rapidly and completely absorbed following oral administration, diclofenac undergoes significant presystemic hepatic metabolism to phenolic compounds which are conjugated with glucuronide or sulphate groups before renal excretion. Less than 1% of diclofenac is excreted unchanged in the urine. Diclofenac is bound extensively to plasma proteins. The high protein binding can result in clinically significant interactions with other highly protein-bound drugs (e.g. anticoagulants, digoxin and methotrexate). Diclofenac can cause displacement of competing drugs and thereby increase their potential toxicity.

KETOPROFEN

Ketoprofen is a propionic acid with similar analgesic, antipyretic and antiinflammatory effects to other NSAIDs. Although not widely licensed for intravenous use, administration of ketoprofen via this route has been reported without adverse effect. The pharmacokinetic properties of ketoprofen are similar to those of diclofenac (Table 12.1). It is well absorbed from the stomach, undergoes minimal presystemic absorption, and is highly plasma protein bound. Extensive metabolism of ketoprofen occurs in the liver, where it is conjugated to water-soluble metabolites. Less than 1% of the parent compound is excreted unchanged in the urine. Unlike diclofenac and ketorolac, significant amounts of ketoprofen (10–20%) are excreted in the bile.

KETOROLAC

Ketorolac, a carboxylic acid structurally related to tolmetin and zompirac, is the most potent NSAID available.[13] It is rapidly absorbed and undergoes negligible presystemic metabolism when administered orally, with peak levels in 30–45 min. Following intravenous injection, the time to onset of clinical effects is 15–20 min as a result of the hysteresis between peak plasma levels and its peak pharmacological effects.[14] Metabolism is less complete than with other NSAIDs and appears to take place primarily in the kidney rather than the liver. Metabolites account for 40% of the renally excreted breakdown products, primarily as conjugated or hydroxylated metabolites. However, 60% of the drug is excreted unchanged in the urine. The elimination half-life of ketorolac (5.4 h) is intermediate among the commonly used NSAIDs (Table 12.1).

The recommended intravenous dosing regimen of ketorolac has been changed because of concerns regarding adverse side-effects (e.g. bleeding, renal dysfunction). It is recommended that the first intravenous dose of 15–30 mg be followed by 10–30 mg every 4 h, with a maximum daily dose of 90 mg. Plasma protein binding is high (in common with other NSAIDs) and drug interactions can occur owing to displacement of other drugs that are extensively protein bound. Ketorolac is transferred from maternal to fetal circulations, but the resulting fetal–maternal plasma concentration gradient is much lower than that found with the more lipid-soluble opioid analgesics. Small amounts of ketorolac are excreted in breast milk, although it is unlikely that the newborn would receive more than 0.1–0.4% of the maternal dose.

TENOXICAM

Of the parenteral NSAIDs, tenoxicam is the most recent to be introduced into clinical practice and has gained widespread popularity for intravenous use. Its instability in solution has necessitated its preparation as a powder, which is reconstituted with water before use. Like other NSAIDs, tenoxicam possesses antipyretic, analgesic and antiinflammatory effects. Structurally, it is similar to piroxicam and belongs to the phenothiazine or oxicam group.

Tenoxicam has pharmacokinetic properties that are distinct from those of other NSAIDs. It has a rapid redistribution phase followed by a remarkably long elimination phase, with a terminal half-life of around 72 h (Table 12.1). Metabolism is extensive and takes place in the liver; less than 1% of the drug is excreted unchanged in the urine. Plasma protein binding is high, in common with the other NSAIDs, resulting in a small volume of distribution. There are as yet no data available regarding placental transfer or excretion into breast milk.

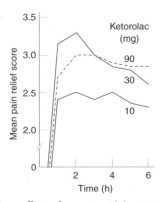

Fig. 12.4 Ceiling effect of nonsteroidal antiinflammatory drugs (NSAIDs) with respect to their analgesic efficacy in the early postoperative period. From Souter *et al.*[1]

PERIOPERATIVE USE OF NSAIDs

NSAIDs provide adequate postoperative analgesia following minor body surface procedures involving mild to moderate tissue damage (e.g. dental, nasal, arthroscopic and laparoscopic surgery).[15-17] The parenterally active NSAIDs are of particular benefit in the ambulatory surgery setting. Where surgery is more extensive and there is a visceral component to the pain (e.g. laparotomy or thoracotomy), NSAIDs do not provide adequate analgesia. The failure to control severe pain may be due in part to the ceiling effect exhibited by NSAIDs (Fig. 12.4). Above a threshold plasma concentration, additional analgesia cannot be achieved by increasing the drug concentration. The combination of an NSAID with an opioid is, however, effective in providing analgesia in patients who have undergone major, painful, surgical procedures. The addition of NSAID reduces the severity of pain as well as the opioid requirements. In the day-case setting this may have particular advantages in reducing unwanted opioid-related effects such as nausea, vomiting, inability to void, and sedation, and facilitating early discharge combined with good pain control.

REFERENCES

1. Souter AJ, Fredman B, White PF. Controversies in the perioperative use of nonsteroidal antiinflammatory drugs. *Anesth Analg* 1994; **79**: 1178–1190.

2. Dahl JB, Kehlet H. Non-steroidal anti-inflammatory drugs: rationale for use in severe postoperative pain. *Br J Anaesth* 1991; **66**: 703–712.

3. Brooks PM, Day RO. Nonsteroidal antiinflammatory drugs – differences and similarities. *N Engl J Med* 1991; **324**: 1716–1725.

4. Smalley WE, DuBois RN. Colorectal cancer and nonsteroidal anti-inflammatory drugs. *Adv Pharmacol* 1997; **39**: 1–20.

5. Furst DE. Meloxicam: selective COX-2 inhibition in clinical practice. *Semin Arthritis Rheum* 1997; **26**(Suppl. 1): 21–27.

6. McCormack K, Brune K. Dissociation between the antinociceptive and anti-inflammatory effects of the non-steroidal anti-inflammatory drugs. *Drugs* 1991; **41**: 533–547.

7. Jurna I, Brune K. Central effect of the nonsteroidal anti-inflammatory agents indomethacin, ibuprofen and diclofenac, determined in C fibre-evoked activity in single neurones of the rat thalamus. *Pain* 1990; **41**: 71–80.

8. Malmberg AB, Yaksh TL. Antinociceptor actions of spinal nonsteroidal anti-inflammatory agents on the formalin test in the rat. *J Pharmacol Exp Ther* 1992; **263**: 136–146.

9. Rice ASC, Lloyd J, Bullingham RES, O'Sullivan G. Ketorolac penetration into the cerebrospinal fluid of humans. *J Clin Anesth* 1993; **5**: 459–462.

10. Strom BL, Berlin JA, Kinman JL *et al*. Parenteral ketorolac and risk of gastrointestinal and operative site bleeding. *JAMA* 1996; **275**: 376–382.

11. Splinter WM, Rhine EJ, Roberts DW, Reid CW, MacNeill HB. Preoperative ketorolac increases bleeding after tonsillectomy in children. *Can J Anaesth* 1996; **43**: 560–563.

12. Camu F, Van LC, Lauwers MH. Cardiovascular risks and benefits of perioperative nonsteroidal anti-inflammatory drug treatment. *Drugs* 1992; **5**: 42–51.

13. Buckley MM, Brogden RN. Ketorolac. A review of its pharmacodynamic and pharmacokinetic properties, and therapeutic potential. *Drugs* 1990; **39**: 86–109.

14. Rice AS, Whitehead EM, O'Sullivan G, Lloyd J, Bullingham RE. Speed of onset of analgesic effect of intravenous ketorolac compared to morphine and placebo. *Eur J Anaesthesiol* 1995; **12**: 313–317.

15. Ding Y, White PF. Comparative effects of ketorolac, dezocine, and fentanyl during outpatient anesthesia. *Anesth Analg* 1992; **75**: 566–571.

16. Liu J, Ding Y, White PF *et al*. Effects of ketorolac on postoperative analgesia and ventilatory function after laparoscopic cholecystectomy. *Anesth Analg* 1993; **76**: 1061–1066.

17. Michaloliakou C, Chung F, Sharma S. Preoperative multimodal analgesia facilitates recovery after ambulatory laparoscopic cholecystectomy. *Anesth Analg* 1996; **82**: 44–51.

Section 4

CARDIOVASCULAR PHARMACOLOGY

13

DC Warltier, PS Pagel

INOTROPIC DRUGS

Heart failure occurs when the heart fails to provide adequate oxygen and metabolic substrates to peripheral tissues. The mechanism for development of heart failure is a reduction in overall pump performance resulting from decreases in intrinsic myocardial contractility, increases in afterload against which the heart ejects, or diastolic dysfunction. A reduction in inotropic state occurs in a variety of diverse pathological processes including myocardial ischaemia, stunning, hibernation or infarction, pressure or volume overload hypertrophy, idiopathic dilated cardiomyopathy and myocyte injury produced by drugs or infectious disease. Compensatory cardiovascular reflexes including sympathetic nervous system activation, parasympathetic nervous system withdrawal and stimulation of the renin–angiotensin–aldosterone (RAS) cascade may maintain adequate cardiac output at rest in the presence of decreased contractile function. During periods of haemodynamic stress, however, overall cardiac output may be inadequate. 'Cardiac reserve' is diminished with further reductions in contractility and, ultimately, cardiac output may even be inadequate under resting conditions. This progressive decrease in function characterizes the well-known stages of the New York Heart Association (NYHA) classification of patients with heart failure. Patients demonstrate significant cardiac reserve in stage I but suffer end-stage heart failure under resting conditions in stage IV.

Pooling of blood in the central venous or pulmonary circulation and concomitant increases in pressures occur as heart failure progresses. Homeostatic reflex increases in sympathetic nervous system tone and activation of the RAS cascade act to maintain arterial pressure by producing peripheral arteriolar vasoconstriction. However, undesirable increases in arterial forces opposing left ventricular ejection also occur, increasing myocardial oxygen consumption and further compromising pumping ability. Aldosterone secretion produces renal salt and water retention, increasing plasma volume and left ventricular preload, and exacerbating central venous or pulmonary arterial congestion. Enhanced sympathetic nervous system tone also reduces venous capacitance and increases venous return to the heart. These alterations in left ventricular afterload and preload increase end-systolic and end-diastolic left ventricular volumes and left ventricular end-diastolic pressures. When left ventricular end-diastolic pressures exceed approximately 25 mmHg, pulmonary vascular congestion, and subsequently pulmonary oedema, occur. The failing heart cannot adequately eject venous return, resulting in marked dilatation of the left ventricle. The usual increases in contractility, cardiac output and stroke work associated with an increase in end-diastolic volume (Frank–Starling relation) are not observed, and reductions in these indices of systolic function may occur as further ventricular dilatation develops (Fig. 13.1). Increased sympathetic and decreased parasympathetic nervous system activity produce compensatory

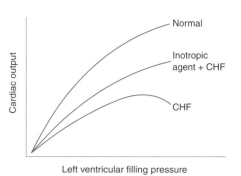

Fig. 13.1 Starling curves for normal and failing hearts (coronary heart failure; CHF) and the actions of an inotropic agent in the presence of CHF.

tachycardia, maintaining an adequate cardiac output. Unfortunately, such an increase in heart rate is an energy-inefficient means to increase cardiac output and may be especially detrimental in patients with coronary artery disease. Finally, end-organ hypoperfusion and death secondary to a reduction in cardiac output at rest occurs.

The search for new drugs that can increase contractility in failing myocardium has been remarkably unsuccessful.[1] The digitalis glycosides remain the only drugs available for the chronic oral management of heart failure, and their relative utility is controversial. The most successful way to treat heart failure is by allowing the left ventricle to eject against a reduced afterload. Diuretics help by reducing pulmonary and venous congestion. The lack of an efficacious, orally administered, inotropic drug has led to use of experimental procedures such as optimally timed atrioventricular (AV) sequential pacing, ventricular reduction surgery and skeletal muscle augmentation of pump performance. These are beneficial only in a small minority of patients with heart failure. In contrast, a variety of intravenous drugs have been used successfully in the treatment of acute heart failure.

Sympathomimetic amines, phosphodiesterase inhibitors and new drugs, including the myofilament calcium sensitizers, are presently used or will find future use for the treatment of reduced myocardial contractility in the perioperative period. Their use alone or in combination with vasodilators requires invasive monitoring to determine cardiac output at optimal left ventricular filling pressure and systemic vascular resistance. Intraoperative use of intravenous inotropes is especially common after cardiac surgery and cardiopulmonary bypass when decreased left ventricular systolic function may persist for several hours after separation from bypass. The mechanism for this reduction in contractility is multifactorial and may involve inadequate cardioprotection, postischaemic reperfusion injury (myocardial 'stunning') or interstitial myocardial oedema.[2] The use of intravenous inotropes enhances cardiac performance for short periods in the postoperative period until contractile dysfunction recedes.

CELLULAR MECHANISMS OF AUGMENTATION OF INOTROPIC STATE

Several processes affecting the interaction of actin and myosin in the sarcomere determine inotropic state. This interaction is both calcium (Ca^{2+}) and energy dependent. An increase in the concentration of intracellular Ca^{2+} causes the heart to contract during systole. A small amount of Ca^{2+} enters the myocyte through open voltage-gated Ca^{2+} channels of the sarcolemma upon membrane depolarization (Fig. 13.2). The amount of Ca^{2+}

> **Summary box 13.1 Cellular mechanisms of myocardial contractility**
>
> - Contractility controlled by intracellular Ca^{2+} concentration $[Ca^{2+}]_i$.
>
> - Increased $[Ca^{2+}]_i$ removes block by tropomyosin on the interaction between actin and myosin, allowing contraction to proceed.
>
> - Calcium crosses the cell membrane of myocytes via voltage-sensitive Ca^{2+} channels with each action potential and is also released from stores in the sarcoplasmic reticulum.
>
> - Calcium entry is balanced by removal, mainly by the Na^+–Ca^{2+} exchange pump, which extrudes Ca^{2+} in exchange for Na^+, which in turn are extruded in exchange for K^+ via the Na^+–K^+-ATPase pump.
>
> - The interconnection between Ca^{2+} and Na^+ means that an increase in $[Na^+]_i$ also increases contraction by a secondary increase in $[Ca^{2+}]_i$.

entering the cardiac myocyte depends on the number of channels and the duration that these channels remain in the open state. This small rise in Ca^{2+} concentration produces the release of a substantial amount of Ca^{2+} from the cisternae of the sarcoplasmic reticulum (SR) in the form of a 'Ca^{2+} transient'.

The initial influx of Ca^{2+} acts as a trigger for the release of stored Ca^{2+} from the SR. Release of Ca^{2+} from the SR is directly proportional to the amount and rate of trigger Ca^{2+} entering through sarcolemmal Ca^{2+} channels. Increased cytosolic Ca^{2+} concentrations act on the troponin–tropomyosin complex (proteins inhibitory to cardiac contraction), permitting an interaction between actin and myosin filaments to occur. Ca^{2+} binds to troponin C and produces a conformational change in the troponin–tropomyosin complex which allows the adenosine triphosphate (ATP)-dependent formation of cross-bridges between actin and myosin. The amount of Ca^{2+} present in the cytoplasm is directly related to the disinhibition of tropomyosin, the interaction of the actin and myosin filaments, and the force of contraction. The availability of intracellular Ca^{2+} for contractile activation is a primary factor involved in the modulation of contractility. Drugs that increase intracellular Ca^{2+} concentration produce a positive inotropic effect.[3] Sympathomimetic amines and phosphodiesterase inhibitors increase Ca^{2+} influx via receptor-linked sarcolemmal Ca^{2+} channels. Cardiac glycosides exert their positive inotropic activity indirectly by reversing the sodium Na^+–Ca^{2+} exchanger, thereby increasing intracellular Ca^{2+} concentration. In contrast, other new

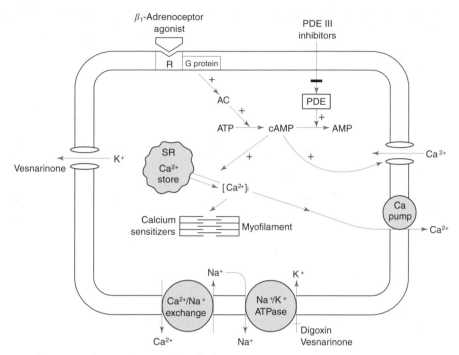

Fig. 13.2 Diagram illustrating the mechanisms by which various inotropic drugs can increase myocardial contractility. R, receptor; AC, adenylyl cyclase; ATP, adenosine triphosphate; cAMP, cyclic adenosine monophosphate; PDE, phosphodiesterase; SR, sarcoplasmic reticulum.

agents presently under clinical investigation increase inotropic state by enhancing the sensitivity of the contractile proteins to Ca^{2+} without altering the intracellular concentration of this ion.

Cytosolic Ca^{2+} is maintained at very low levels ($< 10^{-7}$ mol l^{-1}) during diastole by energy-dependent Ca^{2+} pumps in the sarcolemmal membrane and the SR. The Ca^{2+} uptake transporter in the SR is a primary determinant of the amount of Ca^{2+} retained by this organelle. Phosphorylation of the regulatory protein phospholamban by protein kinases causes increased Ca^{2+} uptake by the SR Ca^{2+}-ATPases. The Na^+–Ca^{2+} transporter also influences the amount of Ca^{2+} within the myocyte. This ion exchange system allows Ca^{2+} to be extruded from the cell in exchange for Na^+. Removal of intracellular Ca^{2+} allows relaxation of the sarcomere to occur when this ion dissociates from troponin C.

SYMPATHOMIMETIC AMINES

The sympathomimetic amines are drugs that mimic stimulation of the autonomic nervous system. The sympathomimetic amines can be divided into those that act directly on α- and β-adrenoceptors and those that act indirectly by promoting the release of noradrenaline from sympathetic adrenergic nerve endings. Noradrenaline, adrenaline and dopamine are endogenously pro-

duced catecholamines. In contrast, isoprenaline and dobutamine are manufactured synthetically (Fig. 13.3). These drugs are used clinically to enhance myocardial contractility. However, because of the widespread location of α- and β-adrenoceptors, sympathomimetic amines have a variety of pharmacological effects in other tissues. These actions are dependent on the specific drug and the distribution of adrenoceptors in each tissue.

Direct acting sympathomimetic amines have different selectivities for adrenoceptors because of differences in chemical structure. This selectivity may be highly dependent on the administered dose. For example, low doses of dopamine stimulate dopamine DA_1 receptors to produce vasodilatation, moderate doses activate β_1-adrenoceptors to enhance contractility and higher doses stimulate α_1-adrenoceptors to cause arterial vasoconstriction. In general, sympathomimetic amines may produce deleterious increases in myocardial oxygen consumption, and their use in patients with heart failure and concomitant coronary artery disease must be carefully weighed. Increasing cardiac output via a reduction in afterload should probably be the primary therapeutic approach in the pharmacological management of chronic, and even acute, heart failure.

Ephedrine and metaraminol are the most commonly used indirect sympathomimetic amines. They

---

Summary box 13.2 Inotropic drugs

- β_1-Adrenoceptor agonists:

    - increase intracellular cAMP concentration, which causes an increase in $[Ca^{2+}]_i$ and increased contractility.

- Phosphodiesterase III inhibitors:

    - inhibit the degradation of cAMP, thereby increasing $[Ca^{2+}]_i$. The effects can be synergistic with β_1-adrenoceptor agonists.

- Digitalis glycosides:

    - inhibit the Na^+–K^+-ATPase pump, increasing $[Na^+]_i$. This slows the removal of Ca^{2+} leading to increased contraction secondary to increase in $[Ca^{2+}]_i$.

- Myofilament calcium sensitizers:

    - enhance Ca^{2+} binding to the Ca^{2+}-specific regulatory site and stabilize the Ca^{2+}-bound conformation of troponin C. This allows prolonged interaction of actin and myosin filaments during contraction, resulting in a positive inotropic effect.

- Drugs with multiple mechanisms of action such as vesnarinone:

    - inhibit the delayed outward and inward rectified potassium currents

    - increase opening of sodium channels

    - are myofilament calcium sensitizers

    - produce mild inhibition of phosphodiesterase III.

---

increase arterial pressure by enhancing myocardial contractility and causing peripheral vasoconstriction. Ephedrine and metaraminol must gain access to the adrenergic nerve terminal in order to exert pharmacological activity.

CELLULAR MECHANISMS OF ADRENOCEPTOR STIMULATION

β-Adrenoceptors on the surface of the sarcolemma are coupled to adenylyl cyclase by a stimulatory guanine nucleotide-binding G (G_s) protein located in the cell membrane (Fig. 13.4). Adenylyl cyclase converts ATP to the second messenger, cyclic adenosine monophosphate (cAMP). cAMP binds to the regulatory subunit of protein kinase A, an enzyme that is responsible for the phosphorylation of sarcolemmal Ca^{2+} channels, troponin I and phospholamban. β-Adrenoceptor stimulation in the cardiac myocyte results in enhanced Ca^{2+} influx across the sarcolemma and accelerated Ca^{2+} uptake by the SR.

Stimulation of α_1-adrenoceptors located on vascular smooth muscle cell membranes causes an increase in intracellular Ca^{2+} concentration, resulting in contraction. The precise mechanism by which cytosolic Ca^{2+} concentrations are increased is under intense investigation. Binding of an agonist with the α_1-adrenoceptor ultimately causes an opening of receptor-operated Ca^{2+} channels within the vascular smooth muscle cell membrane. Stimulation of α_1-adrenoceptors increases activity of phospholipase C via activation of a coupled G protein (G_q). Cleavage of cell membrane phospholipids by phospholipase C causes a release of diacylglycerol and inositol 1,4,5-triphosphate (IP_3). IP_3 promotes release of Ca^{2+} from intracellular storage sites within the vascular smooth muscle cell, which produces contraction and causes activation of Ca^{2+}-dependent protein kinases and phosphorylation of respective substrates.

Cardiovascular adrenoceptors

The cardiovascular effects of sympathomimetic amines are dependent not only on the chemical structure of each drug but also on the number and location of adrenoceptors in each tissue. α_1-Adrenoceptors located in small arterioles and veins mediate increases in peripheral vascular resistance and decreases in venous capacitance, respectively. In contrast, β_2-adrenoceptors are responsible for vasodilatation. Cutaneous blood vessels have primarily α_1-adrenoceptors, whereas β_2-adrenoceptors play an important role in skeletal muscle perfusion via dilatation of arterioles. The cardiac actions of sympathomimetic amines are determined primarily by β_1-adrenoceptors. Thus, the effect of a sympathomimetic amine on arterial pressure is determined by the combined actions of the drug on heart rate, myocardial contractility, peripheral vascular resistance and venous return. A pure α_1-adrenoceptor agonist increases peripheral vascular resistance and decreases venous capacitance, the latter causing an increase in venous return to the heart. A pure β_1-adrenoceptor agonist increases heart rate, stroke volume and cardiac output, and decreases peripheral vascular resistance.

SPECIFIC SYMPATHOMIMETIC DRUGS

Adrenaline

Adrenaline (epinephrine), an endogenous catecholamine (Fig. 13.3), is an agonist of α_1-, α_2-, β_1- and β_2-adrenoceptors.[4] Intravenous infusion of adrenaline usually results in an increase in systolic arterial

(a) Endogenous

(b) Synthetic

Catechol

Adrenaline

Isoprenaline

Noradrenaline

Dobutamine

Dopamine

Dopexamine

Fig. 13.3 Chemical structures of (a) endogenous and (b) synthetic catecholamines.

pressure with little change in diastolic arterial pressure. Adrenaline produces positive inotropic and chronotropic effects by stimulation of β_1-adrenoceptors located on the cell membranes of cardiac myocytes and sinoatrial node cells, respectively. The duration of systole is modestly shortened concomitant with enhanced myocardial contractility. Adrenaline also has positive lusitropic properties, increasing the rate of myocardial relaxation and enhancing left ventricular filling. These combined effects result in a dramatic increase in cardiac output. Following bolus administration, an initial increase in heart rate may be followed by bradycardia secondary to increases in arterial pressure and baroreceptor reflex activation. Another catecholamine, noradrenaline, has even greater effects on baroreceptor activity, because it causes greater increases in peripheral vascular resistance and arterial pressure than adrenaline.

In addition to positive inotropic, chronotropic and lusitropic properties, adrenaline also has positive dromotropic effects, increasing conduction velocity and reducing the refractory period of the AV node, bundle of His, Purkinje fibres and cardiac muscle. The increase in AV nodal conduction may cause dangerous increases in ventricular rate in patients with atrial fibrillation. Increases in automaticity of latent pacemakers may occur because diastolic depolarization (phase 4) is also accelerated. These adrenaline-induced alterations in electrophysiology may contribute to the incidence of arrhythmias such as premature ventricular contractions, ventricular tachycardia and ventricular fibrillation. Cardiac arrhythmias occur more frequently in

the presence of the volatile anaesthetic halothane. Ventricular ectopy associated with adrenaline may be treated with lignocaine (lidocaine) or procainamide. However, these antiarrhythmics also produce direct negative inotropic effects that may offset the beneficial actions of adrenaline on contractility.

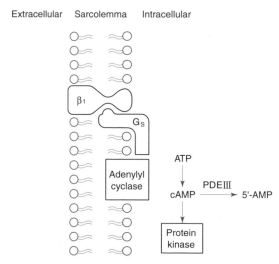

Fig. 13.4 β_1-Adrenoceptor stimulation activates adenylyl cyclase via a G protein. Adenylyl cyclase is responsible for the conversion of adenosine triphosphate (ATP) to adenosine monophosphate (cAMP), which acts as a second messenger via protein kinases. Phosphodiesterase (PDE) enzymes break down cAMP to 5'-AMP. Stimulation of β_1-adrenoceptors or inhibition of phosphodiesterase increases intracellular cAMP concentration.

a_1- and β_2-adrenoceptors are found on vascular smooth muscle cells. Stimulation of a_1 receptors by adrenaline constricts vascular smooth muscle primarily in small arterioles, especially those in the cutaneous, splanchnic and renal circulations. In contrast, activation of vascular β_2-adrenoceptors by adrenaline causes vasodilatation in skeletal muscle. The combined effect of adrenaline on blood flow to a specific tissue represents a balance of effects on a_1- and β_2-adrenoceptors located in the vascular supply of that organ. The effects of adrenaline on organ blood flow are also dose dependent. β_1-Adrenoceptors are more sensitive and are activated by lower doses of adrenaline. Vasodilatation and subsequent declines in arterial pressure occur primarily at lower doses of adrenaline. In contrast, the effects of adrenaline on a_1-adrenoceptors predominate at higher doses, resulting in increases in peripheral vascular resistance and arterial pressure. The use of high-dose adrenaline during cardiopulmonary resuscitation may be based on this intense a_1-adrenoceptor-mediated peripheral vasoconstriction and subsequent increases in coronary artery perfusion pressure. If so, other a_1-adrenergic agonists, including noradrenaline and phenylephrine, may also find a role in resuscitation.

The intense vasoconstriction produced by high doses of adrenaline after cardiopulmonary bypass may adversely impede left ventricular ejection by increasing afterload. The use of higher doses of adrenaline in combination with arterial vasodilators such as nitroprusside to enhance contractile performance and simultaneously decrease peripheral vascular resistance has become relatively commonplace. Veins also have a relatively high density of a_1-adrenoceptors. Adrenaline causes venoconstriction, resulting in enhanced venous return and increases in right and left ventricular filling pressures. a_1-Adrenoceptors also mediate direct vasoconstriction of the pulmonary vasculature produced by adrenaline. Thus, adrenaline increases pulmonary artery pressure by dual mechanisms.

a_1- and β_2-adrenoceptors are present in the coronary vessels, but the influence of adrenaline on coronary blood flow is usually indirect. An adrenaline-induced increase in myocardial oxygen consumption caused by tachycardia, increased left ventricular filling pressures, enhanced inotropic state and increased afterload produces increases in coronary blood flow by metabolic autoregulation. Direct stimulation of a_1-adrenoceptors by adrenaline may lead to a decrease in epicardial coronary artery diameter and a reduction in coronary blood flow in the presence of maximal coronary vasodilation (e.g. during intense myocardial ischaemia).

The actions of adrenaline and other sympathomimetic amines are confounded by prior administration of a- and β-adrenoceptor antagonists. For example, the expected decrease in vascular tone produced by β_2-adrenoceptor stimulation is blocked in patients receiving propranolol, a nonselective β antagonist. Adrenaline, in the presence of β-adrenergic blockade, would produce significantly greater peripheral vasoconstriction and considerably less pronounced positive inotropic and chronotropic effects. In fact, pharmacological blockade of β_1- and β_2-adrenoceptors could theoretically convert the haemodynamic effects of adrenaline to those of the pure a_1-adrenoceptor agonist, phenylephrine. β-Adrenoceptor antagonists competitively inhibit adrenoceptors. Higher doses of β-adrenoceptor agonists are able to overcome this competitive block and may be required in patients receiving β-adrenoceptor antagonists. Metabolic acidosis or hypothermia must also be corrected for maximal cardiovascular efficacy of adrenaline and other sympathomimetics to be achieved.[5]

Adrenaline has a wide variety of effects on other tissues. Activation of β_2-adrenoceptors by adrenaline causes relaxation of bronchial, gastrointestinal and uterine smooth muscle. Adrenaline activates a_1-adrenoceptors to contract gastrointestinal and urinary tract sphincters. Adrenaline-induced contraction of the splenic capsule may produce an increase in haematocrit. Stimulation of β_1-adrenoceptors located on juxtaglomerular cells of the afferent arteriolar wall causes the release of renin from the kidney and activation of the renin–angiotensin system. Lastly, adrenaline inhibits insulin secretion and stimulates glucagon release, producing an increase in blood glucose, lactate and free fatty acids.

Noradrenaline

Noradrenaline (norepinephrine) is the endogenous neurotransmitter released from adrenergic nerves during sympathetic nervous system stimulation. Noradrenaline stimulates a_1- and β_1-adrenoceptors but, in contrast to adrenaline, has little or no effect on β_2 receptors. These actions cause positive inotropic effects, vasoconstriction and increases in arterial pressure.[6] The hypertensive actions of noradrenaline may be especially useful for maintenance of coronary artery perfusion pressure in patients with severe coronary artery disease. Pronounced increases in arterial pressure produced by noradrenaline may be a desirable property during cardiopulmonary resuscitation and a potential advantage over adrenaline in this setting. Hepatic, skeletal muscle, splanchnic and renal blood flows are directly reduced by noradrenaline. When noradrenaline is used to treat severe hypotension, however, the increase in perfusion pressure may actually enhance blood flow to these tissues. Nevertheless, decreased perfusion of renal and splanchnic beds may represent a significant problem when high doses of noradrenaline are administered for prolonged periods of time.

Noradrenaline causes relatively greater increases in systemic vascular resistance and diastolic arterial pressure than adrenaline.[6] As a result of more profound peripheral vasoconstriction, baroreceptor reflex-mediated declines in heart rate are also greater during administration of noradrenaline compared with adrenaline. Direct positive inotropic effects and noradrenaline-induced increases in venous return resulting from reduced venous capacitance produce marked increases in ejection fraction and stroke volume. Two related non-catecholamines, phenylephrine and methoxamine, act only on α_1-adrenoceptors to produce peripheral vasoconstriction and do not enhance myocardial contractility under most conditions. Phenylephrine and methoxamine may produce α_1-adrenoceptor-mediated positive inotropic actions in certain states of heart failure. Like noradrenaline, selective α_1-adrenoceptor agonists increase arterial pressure but also may compromise tissue perfusion. In fact, use of pure α_1-adrenoceptor agonists to increase peripheral resistance and arterial pressure in the presence of a failing myocardium will cause a further reduction in cardiac output. Thus, peripheral hypoperfusion resulting from primary decreases in myocardial performance is treated most appropriately with a positive inotropic agent.

Noradrenaline is an ideal drug for treatment of the 'low cardiac output–low systemic vascular resistance' syndrome occasionally observed after cardiopulmonary bypass. However, it can induce internal mammary, gastroepiploic or radial artery graft spasm. Like adrenaline, noradrenaline may produce ventricular and supraventricular ectopy, although its arrhythmogenic potential is considerably lower. As a result, substitution of noradrenaline for adrenaline may be appropriate in the therapeutic management of cardiogenic shock when atrial and/or ventricular irritability is present. Increases in venous return and direct stimulation of pulmonary vascular α_1-adrenoceptors by noradrenaline may cause pulmonary hypertension and contribute to the development of right ventricular failure. The combined use of noradrenaline administered via the left atrium and the pulmonary vasodilator, prostaglandin E_1 (PGE_1), administered intravenously has been advocated to prevent right ventricular dysfunction in patients with reactive pulmonary vasculature after cardiopulmonary bypass.[4] PGE_1 exerts a relatively specific pulmonary vasodilating action and minimally affects systemic arterial tone, because the lungs rapidly metabolize this drug. In addition, lower doses of noradrenaline may be used when administered through the left atrium because it is also metabolized to a large degree by the lung. Lastly, metabolism in peripheral tissues limits the plasma concentrations of noradrenaline returning to the venous and pulmonary circulations.

Isoprenaline

Isoprenaline (isoproterenol) is a nonselective agonist of β_1- and β_2-adrenoceptors.[7] It is a synthetic catecholamine with low affinity for and devoid of activity at α-adrenoceptors. Isoprenaline produces marked cardiostimulatory effects, increasing heart rate, myocardial contractility and cardiac output, and simultaneously reducing peripheral vascular resistance via arteriolar vasodilatation. Isoprenaline-induced tachycardia results from β_1-adrenoceptor stimulation and baroreceptor reflex activation in response to decreases in arterial pressure. The increase in heart rate reduces and may interfere with left ventricular filling dynamics. Isoprenaline increases systolic and decreases diastolic arterial pressure. As a result, this drug produces marked increases in pulse pressure.

Isoprenaline is used clinically to increase heart rate during symptomatic bradyarrhythmias before insertion of a temporary or permanent pacemaker. It is also used after cardiac transplantation to increase cardiac output by increasing heart rate and myocardial contractility and reducing afterload. Isoprenaline also produces pulmonary artery vasodilatation and may be useful in the management of severe right ventricular failure. Isoprenaline increases automaticity and may cause supraventricular and ventricular arrhythmias. Large increases in myocardial oxygen consumption and simultaneous decreases in coronary artery perfusion pressure and diastolic filling time may lead to myocardial ischaemia or left ventricular subendocardial necrosis even in the presence of a normal coronary circulation. Isoprenaline may thus be especially deleterious in patients with coronary artery disease.

Dopamine

Dopamine is an endogenously produced catecholamine (see Fig. 13.3) and the immediate precursor of noradrenaline in adrenergic nerve terminals. The positive inotropic actions of dopamine are not related to dopamine receptors, but to its activity as an agonist of cardiac β_1-adrenoceptors. Dopamine is commonly used for inotropic support in the perioperative period.[7] Lower doses of dopamine selectively stimulate specific dopamine receptors (DA_1) in the renal and splanchnic vasculature, increasing blood flow to these organs. Dopamine-induced activation of DA_2 receptors in autonomic nervous system ganglia and adrenergic nerves also reduces noradrenaline release. The combined actions of dopamine on DA_1 and DA_2 receptors may produce a reduction in arterial pressure when low doses are administered. The renal vasodilating effects of lower doses of dopamine may be particularly useful in patients with impaired renal function or those at risk for decreases in renal perfusion. The increase in renal blood flow produced by dopamine enhances glomerular filtration rate, sodium excretion and urine output. It may also preserve renal function during simultaneous administration of other a_1-adrenoceptor agonists that directly reduce renal blood flow.[8] However, higher doses of dopamine stimulate a_1-adrenoceptors and produce arterial and venous vasoconstriction similar to that of noradrenaline. The stimulation of a_1- and β_1-adrenoceptors by higher doses of dopamine increases heart rate, preload and afterload. Thus, dopamine may not be the drug of choice for inotropic support of patients with raised pulmonary artery or left ventricular filling pressures.

Dobutamine

Dobutamine is a synthetic catecholamine (see Fig. 13.3) composed of two stereoisomers.[9] The (−) and (+) isomers of dobutamine are β_1-adrenoceptor agonists, but exert opposing a_1-adrenoceptor agonist and antagonist activity, respectively. Thus, dobutamine produces potent β-adrenoceptor stimulation with little or no effect on a_1-adrenoceptors.[10] Dobutamine causes peripheral vasodilatation by stimulation of β_2-adrenoceptors but has no activity at DA_1 receptors, in contrast to dopamine. Dobutamine causes less pronounced reductions in peripheral vascular resistance than isoprenaline. As a result, arterial pressure is maintained, and less pronounced baroreceptor reflex-mediated tachycardia occurs. However, dobutamine substantially increases heart rate in higher doses, presumably by activation of β_1-adrenoceptors. Doses of dobutamine that cause positive inotropic effects are frequently associated with increases in heart rate.[11] In contrast, dobutamine may cause indirect decreases in heart rate in patients with severe heart failure if increases in cardiac output and regional tissue perfusion produce a simultaneous reduction of endogenous sympathetic nervous system activity. Dobutamine-induced increases in heart rate and myocardial contractility cause a direct increase in myocardial oxygen consumption and may result in ischaemia in patients with coronary artery disease.

Dobutamine is often used to increase myocardial contractility, cardiac output and stroke volume in the perioperative period, especially in the presence of increased pulmonary vascular resistance after cardiopulmonary bypass.[12] In contrast to the effects of higher doses of dopamine, dobutamine reduces afterload and improves left ventricular–arterial coupling and mechanical efficiency in the presence of left ventricular dysfunction. The β_2-adrenoceptor stimulating actions of dobutamine also reduce pulmonary artery pressure and vascular resistance. In contrast, dopamine may increase pulmonary artery pressure because of a_1-adrenoceptor-mediated vasoconstriction of pulmonary vascular smooth muscle and increased venous return. Thus, dobutamine may be a better therapeutic option than

dopamine in patients with heart failure and raised pulmonary artery and left ventricular filling pressures.[13] Pulmonary vasodilatation by dobutamine may increase pulmonary shunt or ventilation–perfusion abnormalities.

Tolerance to the cardiac effects of sympathomimetic amines, including dobutamine, occurs during prolonged exposure to these drugs. Tolerance results from a reduction in the numbers or function of β-adrenoceptors or disabled coupling of the β receptor to the G_s protein via phosphorylation of the cytoplasmic portion of the receptor. Patients with chronic heart failure have a compensatory increase in sympathetic nervous system tone that is also associated with β-adrenoceptor desensitization. Interestingly, such desensitization may also occur acutely during cardiopulmonary bypass subsequent to release of endogenous catecholamines. Whether this interferes with separation from cardiopulmonary bypass has yet to be demonstrated. This process of β_1-adrenoceptor desensitization leading to tolerance to the actions of dobutamine and other related sympathomimetic amines represents a considerable problem in the treatment of left ventricular failure.[14] Substitution of other positive inotropes that do not stimulate β_1-adrenoceptors may allow recovery of responsiveness of these receptors to catecholamines over time. Recently, short-term intravenous infusion of dobutamine has been used to produce increases in cardiac performance long after drug administration is discontinued. The mechanism of this prolonged positive inotropic effect has not been established definitively but may have important clinical utility in end-stage cardiomyopathy.

Dopexamine

Dopexamine hydrochloride is a synthetic catecholamine structurally similar to dopamine and dobutamine (see Fig. 13.3). The pharmacological effects of dopexamine differ from those of dobutamine and dopamine in terms of the adrenergic receptor subtypes that are stimulated. Dopexamine is a potent β_2-adrenoceptor agonist with minimal β_1-receptor activity. It also has significant dopaminergic DA_1-receptor activity, with only minimal activity at DA_2 receptors and no a-adrenergic activity. In addition, dopexamine also has significant indirect sympathomimetic effects. It is a potent inhibitor of neuronal catecholamine reuptake (uptake 1), but unlike other indirect sympathomimetic agents, dopexamine does not displace noradrenaline from the sympathetic nerve terminals. These mechanisms, as well as the baroreceptor-mediated reflex increase in heart rate that results from dopexamine-induced reductions in systemic vascular resistance, are responsible for the positive inotropic and chronotropic effects of dopexamine. The decline in systemic vascular resistance is due mainly to arterial β_2-adrenoreceptor stimulation, with minor contributions from DA_1-receptor stimulation. Dopexamine may also produce a dose-related improvement in renal perfusion and a decline in renal vascular resistance.

Dopexamine has not proved to be particularly useful as an inotrope in cardiac anaesthesia. The inotropic effects are less with dopexamine than with dobutamine, whereas the effects on reducing systemic and pulmonary vascular resistance are greater. Infusion of doses greater than $6\,\mu g\ kg^{-1}\ min^{-1}$ are often required, and can produce unacceptable tachycardia. The main indication for this drug seems to be in improving splanchnic blood flow in patients with shock. The increase in mesenteric blood flow is secondary to β_2-adrenoceptor stimulation. Infusions of dopexamine up to $4\,\mu g\ kg^{-1}\ min^{-1}$ increase splanchnic and hepatic blood flow without altering limb perfusion and with only minimum decreases in arterial pressure.

Ephedrine

Ephedrine is a 'mixed' sympathomimetic amine that exerts direct and indirect actions on adrenoceptors. Ephedrine causes positive inotropic and vasopressor actions primarily by releasing noradrenaline from adrenergic nerves and indirectly activating α- and β_1-adrenoceptors. Ephedrine also produces direct stimulation of β_2-adrenoceptors, although the indirect actions are predominant. Ephedrine is often used in bolus doses to increase arterial blood pressure, especially in the presence of bradycardia, by increasing heart rate, stroke volume, cardiac output and peripheral vascular resistance. Thus, the haemodynamic effects of ephedrine are very similar to those of adrenaline.

Ephedrine is transported into the presynaptic terminals of adrenergic nerves and displaces noradrenaline from binding sites within and outside of the synaptic vesicles. Some of the displaced noradrenaline is released from the presynaptic nerve terminal and stimulates postsynaptic adrenergic receptors. Tachyphylaxis to the cardiovascular effects of ephedrine occurs as repetitive doses administered over a brief period of time acutely deplete stores of noradrenaline. Drugs that deplete noradrenaline from adrenergic nerves such as reserpine, or that inhibit the uptake of ephedrine into adrenergic nerves such as cocaine, will markedly diminish the effects of indirect sympathomimetics. Metaraminol has a similar mechanism but a longer duration of action than ephedrine.

PHOSPHODIESTERASE INHIBITORS

Phosphodiesterases are a group of structurally related enzymes that are responsible for a variety of physiological effects. The tissue distribution and subcellular isoforms of these enzymes have been studied intensively. Molecular investigations have identified seven subtypes responsible for cAMP or cyclic guanosine monophosphate (cGMP) hydrolysis. Phosphodiesterase inhibitors are a group of drugs that augment the intracellular actions of cAMP and cGMP by preventing their degradation.[9] Phosphodiesterase inhibitors may be 'selective' for a particular isoenzyme, but this selectivity is highly dose dependent. These drugs are not dependent on adrenoceptor activation for their positive inotropic effects.

The phosphodiesterase inhibitors include the bipyridine derivatives, amrinone and milrinone,[15] and newer imidazoline compounds, enoximone and piroximone. Several other drugs, including the methylxanthines theophylline and aminophylline, and the calcium sensitizers pimobendan and levosimendan, also have phosphodiesterase inhibiting activity. Vesnarinone, a drug with multiple modes of action including calcium sensitization and inhibition of Na^+–K^+-ATPase, is also a phosphodiesterase inhibitor. Unlike aminophylline and caffeine, which inhibit most isoforms of phosphodiesterase, drugs such as milrinone and enoximone are selective inhibitors of the cardiac phosphodiesterase III isoenzyme. This selective inhibition of phosphodiesterase III allows accumulation of cAMP in the cardiac myocyte by reducing metabolic breakdown (Fig. 13.4), while cGMP metabolism remains unaffected. The newer cardiac phosphodiesterase III inhibitors produce less pronounced positive chronotropic effects than catecholamines. These drugs are, however, arrhythmogenic because they increase intracellular cAMP and Ca^{2+} concentration.[16,17] The first clinically used drug in this class, amrinone, had a wide variety of side-effects including anorexia, abdominal pain, diarrhoea, headache, fever, liver function abnormalities and thrombocytopenia. In contrast, milrinone and enoximone are largely devoid of these adverse effects and have replaced amrinone for the acute management of heart failure in the perioperative period.

Phosphodiesterase III inhibitors not only increase myocardial contractility but also enhance left ventricular isovolumic relaxation and improve early ventricular filling. They also dose-dependently reduce peripheral and pulmonary vascular resistance by inhibiting phosphodiesterase and allowing the accumulation of cAMP in vascular smooth muscle. They are therefore often referred to as inodilators. The increase in cAMP concentration reduces intracellular Ca^{2+} levels and causes relaxation of the vascular smooth muscle cell. Decreases in peripheral and pulmonary vascular resistance enhance left and right ventricular ejection, respectively. This reduction in afterload contributes to the increases in cardiac output, left ventricular–arterial coupling and mechanical efficiency observed with these drugs. The relative importance of the positive inotropic effects versus the afterload-reducing properties in enhancing cardiac output has been debated intensely.[18] It is likely that both actions play important contributing roles in improving overall cardiovascular performance. Pulmonary artery vasodilatation may decrease hypoxic pulmonary vasoconstriction. Thus, phosphodiesterase inhibitors, like direct acting arterial vasodilators and dobutamine, may increase pulmonary shunt and, theoretically, cause arterial hypoxaemia. Phosphodiesterase inhibition also causes venodilatation, which reduces ventricular filling pressures and pulmonary congestion. This reduction in central venous, pulmonary capillary wedge and left ventricular end-diastolic pressures is not observed during administration of catecholamines. The decreases in preload and afterload produced by phosphodiesterase III inhibitors may contribute to reductions in myocardial oxygen consumption observed with these drugs in patients with heart failure despite simultaneous positive inotropic and chronotropic effects.

Phosphodiesterase III inhibitors are very useful in combination with other drugs in the treatment of acute left ventricular dysfunction. For example, the use of a phosphodiesterase III inhibitor in combination with a β_1-adrenoceptor agonist is pharmacologically rational. The β_1 agonist increases the concentration of cAMP in the cardiac myocyte via activation of adenylyl cyclase, whereas the phosphodiesterase III inhibitor prevents degradation of cAMP. The combined effects of these inotropic drugs are additive and may be synergistic in failing myocardium. Combination therapy also allows a reduction in dose of the β_1-agonist and attenuates the downregulation of the β_1-adrenoceptor associated with the use of high doses of sympathomimetic amines alone. As opposed to β_1-adrenoceptor agonists, phosphodiesterase III inhibitors require a loading dose before intravenous infusion. In patients undergoing cardiac surgery, a bolus loading dose is easily administered in the cardiopulmonary bypass reservoir before separation from bypass.

The phosphodiesterase III inhibitors enhance cardiac performance in patients with chronic NYHA class IV heart failure. Unfortunately, significant increases in mortality resulting from malignant ventricular arrhythmias have also been reported. Increases in intracellular concentrations of cAMP produced by either activation of adenylyl cyclase or inhibition of phosphodiesterase III are associated with arrhythmogenesis via an increase in intracellular Ca^{2+} concentration and development of afterpotentials. Thus, chronic oral therapy with phosphodiesterase III inhibitors in patients with congestive heart failure has largely been abandoned. Nevertheless, the phosphodiesterase inhibitors play an important role in the therapeutic management of acute heart failure requiring inotropic support. They

may be especially valuable in the treatment of right ventricular failure associated with pulmonary hypertension.[19]

DIGITALIS GLYCOSIDES

Digitalis glycosides are naturally occurring substances found in a variety of plants including foxglove. Their chemical structure contains a hydrophobic 23-carbon steroid nucleus and a hydrophilic unsaturated lactone ring (Fig. 13.5). Digitalis glycosides are the only positive inotropes currently available for the chronic oral treatment of congestive heart failure.[6] However, these drugs produce only modest increases in myocardial contractility compared with other drugs used intravenously for management of acute left ventricular dysfunction. The best known digitalis glycosides are digoxin and digitoxin, although a large number of related compounds have previously been used.

Digitalis glycosides selectively and reversibly bind to and inhibit the sarcolemmal Na^+–K^+-ATPase in the cardiac myocyte, by interacting with the K^+-binding site of the enzyme (see Fig. 13.2). Inhibition of this enzyme leads to an increase in the availability of intracellular Ca^{2+} during systole, thereby increasing myocardial contractility (Fig. 13.6). The Na^+–K^+-ATPase enzyme exchanges three intracellular Na^+ ions for two extracellular K^+ ions. This process is energy dependent because these ions must be moved across the sarcolemma against concentration gradients. Digitalis glycosides produce a slight increase in intracellular Na^+ concentration by inhibiting this pump. The increase in intracellular Na^+ causes a reduction in extrusion of Ca^{2+} from the cytoplasm by the sarcolemmal Na^+–Ca^{2+} exchanger. The SR stores the additional Ca^{2+} not extruded from the cytoplasm. This allows increased release of Ca^{2+} by the SR during the next myocyte contraction. A similar mechanism of action has been proposed for the Treppe phenomenon in cardiac muscle, during which sudden increases in heart rate are

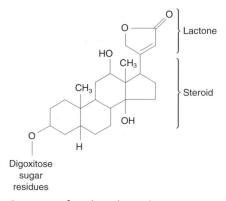

Fig. 13.5 Structure of cardiac glycosides.

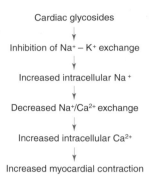

Cardiac glycosides

↓

Inhibition of Na⁺ – K⁺ exchange

↓

Increased intracellular Na⁺

↓

Decreased Na⁺/Ca²⁺ exchange

↓

Increased intracellular Ca²⁺

↓

Increased myocardial contraction

Fig. 13.6 Mechanism of the inotropic action of cardiac glycosides.

accompanied by an increase in contractile force. Under these conditions, a lag occurs in activity of the Na^+–K^+-ATPase concomitant with an abrupt increase in heart rate. As with digoxin, this causes a transient increase in intracellular Na^+ concentration.

An increase in the inotropic state produced by the digitalis glycosides is associated with decreases in left ventricular end-diastolic and end-systolic volumes. This reduction in left ventricular volume decreases wall tension and myocardial oxygen consumption in failing hearts despite concomitant increases in contractility. The compensatory increase in sympathetic nervous system tone that occurs in heart failure is reduced by the administration of digitalis glycosides, because these drugs improve cardiac output. Sympathetic nervous system withdrawal also decreases systemic vascular resistance and impedance to left ventricular ejection. The decrease in sympathetic tone may be partially related to direct actions of digitalis on the cardiac baroreceptors and may play an important role in reducing morbidity and mortality in patients with chronic congestive heart failure.[20]

Sarcolemmal Na^+–K^+-ATPase is responsible for maintaining a normal resting membrane potential. Inhibition of this enzyme by the digitalis glycosides produces dramatic alterations in cardiac electrophysiology and frequently leads to the development of a wide variety of arrhythmias, especially when large doses are administered. Potassium interacts with digitalis glycosides when binding to the Na^+–K^+-ATPase. As a result, there is a reduction in hyperkalaemia; hypokalaemia may profoundly increase digitalis toxicity. The side-effects of these drugs are toxic extensions of their beneficial pharmacological effects mediated by reduction in Na^+–K^+-ATPase activity. The digitalis glycosides have a low therapeutic ratio and a narrow margin of safety.

Digitalis glycosides are used for management of cardiac arrhythmias associated with a rapid ventricular response, since they decrease AV nodal conduction velocity. Digitalis glycosides are not commonly used acutely to increase myocardial contractility in the perioperative period because of the availability of far more efficacious agents with lower toxicity. However, they remain a mainstay in the oral treatment of chronic congestive heart failure.

MYOFILAMENT CALCIUM SENSITIZERS

Myofilament calcium sensitizers, including pimobendan, sulmazole and levosimendan, are a new group of drugs that may be beneficial in both the acute and chronic management of congestive heart failure.[21] These drugs are markedly different from the sympathomimetic amines, phosphodiesterase inhibitors and digitalis glycosides as they are not dependent on an increase in intracellular cAMP or Ca^{2+} concentration for their activity (Fig. 13.7). The myofilament Ca^{2+} sensitizers exert positive inotropic effects by modulating the response of the myofilament regulatory proteins or contractile elements to Ca^{2+} without specifically altering the availability of this ion. These drugs enhance Ca^{2+} binding to the Ca^{2+}-specific regulatory site of troponin C and stabilize the Ca^{2+}-bound conformation of this regulatory protein. This allows prolonged interaction of actin and myosin filaments during contraction, resulting in a positive inotropic effect. Myofilament Ca^{2+} desensitization occurs during myocardial hypoxia, ischaemia and stunning, and myofilament Ca^{2+} sensitizers may be particularly useful in these pathological conditions.

In addition to producing myofilament Ca^{2+} sensitization, many of the drugs in this class also partially inhibit vascular smooth muscle and cardiac phosphodiesterase. These actions cause arterial and venous vasodilatation and further augmentation of inotropic state. Myofilament Ca^{2+} sensitization may theoretically delay left ventricular relaxation and produce negative lusitropic effects. However, concomitant phosphodiesterase inhibition enhances relaxation and early ventricular filling during myofilament Ca^{2+} sensitization. The activity of one of these drugs, levosimendan, is dependent on

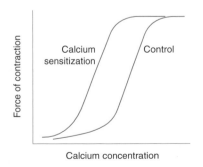

Fig. 13.7 Schematic calcium concentration–force of contraction relationships in cardiac muscle fibres in the presence and absence of calcium sensitization.

intracellular Ca^{2+} concentration, producing myofilament sensitization at relatively high intracellular Ca^{2+} concentrations in systole while having little effect at low intracellular Ca^{2+} concentrations in diastole.[22] As a result, the pharmacological activity of levosimendan may be selective for only a specific portion of the cardiac cycle.

Pimobendan and levosimendan decrease pulmonary capillary wedge pressure, mean arterial pressure and systemic vascular resistance, and dramatically increase cardiac output in patients with chronic left ventricular failure. Their hypotensive effects are similar to those of pure phosphodiesterase inhibitors and may be offset by increasing left ventricular preload with fluid administration. They augment myocardial contractility and improve left ventricular mechanical efficiency, while causing only minimal increases in heart rate and myocardial oxygen consumption.[23] Drugs that enhance myofilament Ca^{2+} sensitivity may also potentiate the positive inotropic effects of other agents that increase intracellular Ca^{2+} concentration. Most significantly, Ca^{2+} sensitizers may produce beneficial effects on left ventricular performance without the arrhythmogenicity associated with increased intracellular Ca^{2+} concentrations. This hypothesis remains to be tested, however.

THYROXINE

Thyroid hormone has profound effects on the cardiovascular system. Hyperthyroidism produces increases in heart rate, cardiac output, stroke volume and myocardial contractility whereas hypothyroidism produces the opposite haemodynamic changes. Circulating levels of the active hormone, triiodothyronine (T_3), may be significantly reduced in previously euthyroid patients after cardiopulmonary bypass.[24] The cardiovascular effects of T_3 are probably due to extranuclear effects at the cellular level. T_3 binds to receptors on both the plasma membrane and the SR of cardiac myocytes. This increases Ca^{2+}-ATPase and sodium channel activity, and activates adenylyl cyclase, resulting in an increase in intracellular Ca^{2+} and increased myocardial contractility.

In patients with poor myocardial function after cardiopulmonary bypass despite inotropic and intra-aortic balloon pump support, administration of T_3 produces substantial reductions in inotropic support and may allow successful weaning from cardiopulmonary bypass.[25] T_3 also has been used as an adjuvant agent in patients who are potential organ donors, to maintain adequate perfusion. Thus preliminary evidence suggests that the administration of T_3 to patients undergoing cardiac surgery may be of benefit; however, its routine use is not yet established.

SUMMARY

Development of drugs for improving cardiac performance in patients with acute and chronic heart failure continues to be an important goal. Unfortunately, drugs that effectively enhance myocardial function have been shown to be unreliable in the chronic oral therapy of heart failure because increased intracellular cAMP and Ca^{2+} concentrations produced by many of these drugs contribute to the development of malignant ventricular arrhythmias and sudden cardiac death.[26] New drugs presently under clinical investigation that act directly on contractile proteins may offer a unique mechanism of action by which inotropic state can be enhanced without adverse arrhythmogenesis. The sympathomimetic amines and the phosphodiesterase inhibitors are the most common drugs used to enhance contractility in patients with acute left ventricular dysfunction. Use of a specific drug is highly dependent on the haemodynamic status of the patient. A simple reduction in afterload with an arterial vasodilator should be strongly considered to increase cardiac output before an inotropic agent is selected.[11] Certain inotropic drugs might be more efficacious in specific pathological conditions. For example, β_1-adrenoceptor agonists may be less useful in diseases in which β_1-adrenoceptor desensitization occurs. Finally, the use of combinations of inotropic drugs acting by different mechanisms, or the use of inotropes in combination with arterial vasodilators, allows increases in pharmacological efficacy while simultaneously minimizing potentially adverse side-effects because smaller doses of individual drugs can be used.

REFERENCES

1. Armstrong PW, Moe GW. Medical advances in the treatment of congestive heart failure. *Circulation* 1993; **88**: 2941–2952.
2. Niroomand F, Kubler W. Hibernating, stunning and ischemic preconditioning of the myocardium: therapeutic implications. *Clin Investig* 1994; **72**: 731–736.
3. Feldman AM. Classification of positive inotropic agents. *J Am Coll Cardiol* 1993; **22**: 1223–1227.
4. DiSesa VJ. Pharmacologic support for postoperative low cardiac output. *Semin Thorac Cardiovasc Surg* 1991; **3**: 3–23.
5. Ford LE. Myocardial energetics. *Adv Exp Med Biol* 1993; **346**: 39–49.
6. Sanders MR, Kostis JB, Frishman WH. The use of inotropic agents in acute and chronic congestive heart failure. *Med Clin North Am* 1989; **73**: 283–314.
7. DiSesa VJ. The rational selection of inotropic drugs in cardiac surgery. *J Card Surg* 1987; **2**: 385–406.
8. Notterman DA. Inotropic agents. Catecholamines, digoxin, amrinone. *Crit Care Clin* 1991; **7**: 583–613.
9. Homoud MK, Chuttani K, Konstam MA. Positive inotropic agents in congestive heart failure. *Coron Artery Dis* 1993; **4**: 44–52.

10. Andersson KE. Some new positive inotropic agents. *Acta Med Scand Suppl* 1986; **707**: 65–73.

11. Butterworth J. Selecting an inotrope for the cardiac surgery patient. *J Cardiothorac Vasc Anesth* 1993; **7** (Suppl. 2): 26–32.

12. Vincent JL, Preiser JC. Inotropic agents. *New Horizons* 1993; **1**: 137–144.

13. Kikura M, Levy JH. New cardiac drugs. *Int Anesthesiol Clin* 1995; **33**: 21–37.

14. Zaloga GP, Prielipp RC, Buttenworth JF IV, Royster RL. Pharmacologic cardiovascular support. *Crit Care Clin* 1993; **9**: 335–362.

15. Colucci WS. Cardiovascular effects of milrinone. *Am Heart J* 1991; **121**: 1945–1947.

16. Tisdale JE, Patel R, Webb CR, Borzak S, Zarowitz BJ. Electrophysiologic and proarrhythmic effects of intravenous inotropic agents. *Prog Cardiovasc Dis* 1995; **38**: 167–180.

17. Lubbe WF, Podzuweit T, Opie LH. Potential arrhythmogenic role of cyclic adenosine monophosphate (AMP) and cytosolic calcium overload: implications for prophylactic effects of beta-blockers in myocardial infarction and proarrhythmic effects of phosphodiesterase inhibitors. *J Am Coll Cardiol* 1992; **19**: 1622–1633.

18. Packer M. The development of positive inotropic agents for chronic heart failure: how have we gone astray? *J Am Coll Cardiol* 1993; **22** (Suppl.): 119A–126A.

19. Doyle AR, Dhir AK, Moors AH, Latimer RD. Treatment of perioperative low cardiac output syndrome. *Ann Thorac Surg* 1995; **59** (Suppl.): S3–11.

20. van Zwieten PA. Pharmacotherapy of congestive heart failure. Currently used and experimental drugs. *Pharm World Sci* 1994; **16**: 234–242.

21. Hajjar RJ, Gwathmey JK. Calcium-sensitizing inotropic agents in the treatment of heart failure: a critical view. *Cardiovasc Drugs Ther* 1991; **5**: 961–965.

22. Pagel PS, Haikala H, Pentikainen PJ *et al.* Pharmacology of levosimendan: a new myofilament calcium sensitizer. *Cardiovasc Drug Rev* 1996; **14**: 286–316.

23. Just H, Drexler H, Hasenfuss G. Pathophysiology and treatment of congestive heart failure. *Cardiology* 1994; **84** (Suppl. 2): 99–107.

24. Holland FW II, Brown PS Jr, Weintraub BD, Clark RE. Cardiopulmonary bypass and thyroid function: a 'euthyroid sick syndrome'. *Ann Thorac Surg* 1991; **52**: 46–50.

25. Novitzky D, Cooper DK, Swanepoel A. Inotropic effect of triiodothyronine (T₃) in low cardiac output following cardioplegic arrest and cardiopulmonary bypass: an initial experience in patients undergoing open heart surgery. *Eur J Cardiothorac Surg* 1989; **3**: 140–145.

26. Teo KK, Ignaszewski AP, Gutierrez R *et al.* Contemporary medical management of left ventricular dysfunction and congestive heart failure. *Can J Cardiol* 1992; **8**: 611–619.

ANTIARRHYTHMIC DRUGS

Cardiac arrhythmia (synonym: dysrhythmia) is defined as an abnormality of rate, regularity or site of origin of the cardiac impulse, or a disturbance in conduction. This causes an alteration in the normal sequence of atrial and ventricular activation. Arrhythmias may be one, or even the only, sign of a pathological abnormality. They may cause adverse haemodynamic effects or induce dangerous tachyarrhythmias requiring immediate pharmacological intervention. The use of antiarrhythmic drugs should be based on knowledge of the physiology and pathophysiology of the arrhythmia itself, the pharmacology of the drugs and their specific indication range. Antiarrhythmic drugs have a variety of effects which on occasions may even be contradictory; they have the potential to terminate life-threatening arrhythmias but they can also generate arrhythmias (proarrhythmic effect).[1] Furthermore they are often associated with haemodynamic side-effects. This chapter tries to provide the necessary theoretical background for a rational use of antiarrhythmic drugs in the perioperative period.

BASIC CONCEPTS OF PHYSIOLOGICAL CARDIAC ELECTROPHYSIOLOGY

ANATOMY

A knowledge of the anatomy of the specialized conduction system responsible for the normal electrical activity of the heart is fundamental to the understanding of physiological and pathophysiological electrical signal transduction in the beating heart. The initial electrical impulse is generated by specialized cells which form the sinoatrial (SA) node, located at the junction of the right atrium with the superior vena (Fig. 14.1). The signal then travels to the left atrium via the Bachmann bundle and via anterior, middle or posterior internodal pathways to the atrioventricular (AV) node. The AV node, located in the right atrium close to the ostium of the coronary sinus, has a cell structure similar to that of the sinus node. In the caudal part of the AV node the composition of the conducting fibres changes and they form the common (His) bundle, which branches at the superior margin of the muscular interventricular septum and the central fibrous body into the left and right bundle branches. These continue subendocardially on both sides of the interventricular septum

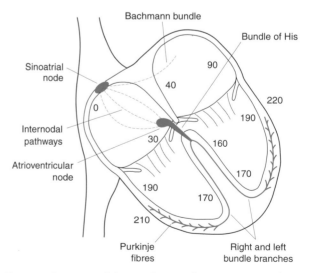

Fig. 14.1 Anatomy of the cardiac conduction system. The numbers show the time of appearance (in ms) of the impulse in different parts of the heart.

to the apex of the right and left ventricles. Terminal Purkinje fibres, connected with the ends of both bundle branches, form interweaving networks on the endocardial surface. This allows virtually simultaneous activation of both ventricular endocardial surfaces.

CELLULAR ELECTROPHYSIOLOGY

The regular beating of the heart is initiated by cyclical changes in the transmembrane potentials (action potentials) of cardiac cells. Three types of ion channels are involved in the cardiac action potential: fast sodium channels, slow calcium and sodium channels, and potassium channels. Cardiac fibres are mainly electrically quiescent, with a resting membrane potential (-50 to -95 mV) that is predominantly determined by the transmembrane K^+ concentration gradient. Depolarization is due to a net inward current of positive sodium and calcium ions, and repolarization to a net outward movement of positive potassium ions. The depolarizing currents carried by sodium and calcium channels have different roles in different regions of the heart. In the atria, ventricles and the His–Purkinje system, depolarization is characterized by a fast response with a large, rapidly rising phase 0, rapid propagation and a large safety factor for conduction. Phase 0 of the action potential is due to the rapid influx of Na^+, whereas Ca^{2+} currents contribute mainly to the plateau phase of the action potential. The depolarization in the sinoatrial and atrioventricular nodes depends on the slower opening of calcium channels, so that nodal conduction is slower than that in other cardiac cells. The differences between these two tissues lies in the lower negativity of the nodal resting potentials: only -55 mV, compared with -95 mV in the atria, ventricles and His–Purkinje system. At this level of negativity the fast sodium channels are inactivated and only the slow calcium–sodium channels can open to initiate the action potential. This slower nodal response prevents the cardiac impulse from travelling too rapidly from the atria to the ventricles, allowing the atria to eject into the ventricles before ventricular contraction occurs. This is an important safety feature of normal cardiac conduction.

The cardiac action potential and the underlying major ionic currents, lasting for several hundred milliseconds, can be divided into five distinct phases (Table 14.1; Fig. 14.2). Action potentials recorded in Purkinje fibres and in some ventricular muscle fibres show a brief, rapid phase of repolarization (phase 1) immediately after the initial action potential upstroke, which returns the membrane potential to near 0 mV. This is followed by the plateau phase of the action potential (phase 2). The main repolarization phase (phase 3) is caused by outward ion currents controlled largely by potassium channels.[2] At least eight major potassium channels have been identified in the heart[3] and they have assumed importance as pharmacological targets in cardiovascular medicine; K^+ channel blockers are antiarrhythmic drugs and also antidiabetic agents, whereas K^+ channel openers are used in the treatment of hypertension and coronary heart disease.[4]

Three potassium channels are important for the normal cardiac action potential. The transient outward potassium current (I_{to}) opens briefly after depolarization contributing to the early repolarization in phase 1, whereas the outward (delayed) rectifying current (I_k) opens at the end of the plateau phase, initiating repolarizing (phase 3). Another potassium current, the inward

Summary box 14.1 Cardiac electrophysiology

- Heart has two pacemakers, the sinoatrial (SA) and the atrioventricular (AV) nodes. The SA node has a much higher firing rate and thus is the controlling pacemaker.

- The impulses generated by the SA node pass to the left atrium via an intraatrial myocardial band (Bachmann bundle) and via the atria to the AV node. Conduction in the AV node is only 20–25% of that through the atria. This conduction delay allows completion of atrial contraction before ventricular activation.

- Activation of the myocardial cells involves three types of ion channels: fast Na^+ channels, slow Ca^{2+} and Na^+ channels, and K^+ channels. Depolarization is due to a net inward current of positive Na^+ and Ca^{2+} ions and repolarization to a net outward movement of positive K^+ ions.

- The cardiac action potential is divided into five distinct phases (0–4).

- Different classes of antiarrhythmic drugs act on different ion channels and thus on different phases of the action potential.

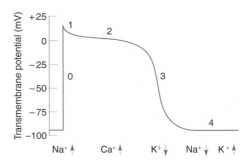

Fig. 14.2 Cardiac action potential showing the ion fluxes during the five phases.

Table 14.1 Phases and underlying ionic currents of a cardiac action potential

Cardiac action potential	Electrophysiology	Ionic currents
Phase 0	Rapid depolarization	Fast inward Na^+ currents (fast response fibres) Slow inward Ca^{2+} current (slow response fibres)
Phase 1	Initial rapid repolarization	Mainly via transient outward rectifying (I_{to}) K^+ channels
Phase 2	Plateau	Inward Ca^{2+} currents
Phase 3	Final rapid repolarization	Rapid outward K^+ currents (I_k)
Phase 4	Electrical diastole	High K^+ permeability, transport mechanisms (Na^+–Ca^{2+}–K^+)

rectifying (I_{ki}) current, is responsible for maintaining the resting diastolic phase of the action potential (phase 4). The I_{ki} channels close when the heart is depolarized, preventing them from initiating repolarization early in the action potential. The effectiveness of class III anti-arrhythmic drugs is based on their ability to block one or more of these potassium channels.

A normal action potential is followed by the effective refractory period (ERP), which is the minimum interval between two propagating responses. The ERP is closely linked to the absolute action potential duration, since the recovery of sodium channels (fast response) from inactivation closely parallels or even outlasts repolarization (slow response, slow inward Ca^{2+} recovery).

PATHOPHYSIOLOGY AND MECHANISMS OF ARRHYTHMIAS

Arrhythmias resulting from irregular generation of action potentials may arise due to alterations of impulse generation, impulse conduction or a combination of both at different levels of the conduction system. They may result from disruption of the normal electrophysiological processes by pathophysiological states such as hypoxia, ischaemia, pharmacological agents, electrolyte imbalance and/or pathological cardiac morphology.

CELLULAR MECHANISMS OF ARRHYTHMIAS

The underlying cellular mechanisms are complex and not completely understood. The electrophysiological mechanisms for abnormal impulse generation and propagation include depressed fast response, impaired automaticity, early and delayed afterdepolarizations and reentry of excitation.

Depressed fast response

The sodium channel responsible for the initial action potential depolarization exists in one of three functional states: open, closed inactive and closed resting. The closed states are potential dependent. The closed resting state is associated with a large (resting) negative (−90 mV) membrane potential, whereas the channel assumes the closed inactive state at membrane potentials of −60 mV. This is the normal resting potential in the SA and AV nodes. Fast conducting cardiac fibres have a high (negative) membrane potential. When in the closed resting state the channel readily opens in response to a depolarizing signal, whereas in the closed inactive state the channel is unable to open and is refractory, since even when the cell is stimulated the resulting inward sodium current is too small to generate an action potential. A partial loss of the membrane potential is associated with transition of the sodium channels to the closed inactivated state, and the overall conduction speed is slower. Thus, variability of the action potential response creates conditions of uneven conduction and refractoriness which ease excitation reentry or heart block.

Impaired automaticity

Both atrial and ventricular Purkinje fibres are capable of spontaneous diastolic depolarizations and repetitive automatic firing. This can accelerate spontaneous activity or induce abnormal activity in formerly quiescent fibres and is probably induced by ionic mechanisms (slow inward currents).

Early afterdepolarizations

Early afterdepolarizations (EADs) are oscillations in the transmembrane potential during the plateau and repolarization phases of the cardiac action potential; they cause secondary depolarizations before repolarization is complete. Possible ionic mechanisms include inward Na^+ and Ca^{2+} currents, slow inactivation of the fast inward Na^+ current or K^+ outward currents. EAD and EAD-triggered sustained rhythmic activity are more likely to occur at slow heart rates.

Delayed afterdepolarizations

Delayed afterdepolarizations (DADs) are oscillations in the transmembrane potential that occur after full repolarization of the action potential in early diastole. DAD is not self-initiating but depends on a previous action potential. Probably due to an excessive intracellular Ca^{2+} level, low K^+ levels and/or exposure to drugs such as catecholamines or digitalis, the resting membrane potential again transiently depolarizes. If the DADs reach threshold, a premature propagated response will occur. DADs have a potential to recur with an increased amplitude, and this can trigger activity that may induce coupled extrasystoles or runs of tachyarrhythmias.

Reentry of excitation

Reentrant arrhythmias occur by a recirculating activation following an initiating depolarization: the persisting action potential reexcites atrial or ventricular tissue at the end of their refractoriness. To initiate reentry, a one-way block of conduction due to a functional or anatomical barrier must be present to form a circuit (Fig. 14.3). A greatly slowed normal conduction and/or a markedly reduced refractoriness are other contributing factors. Reentry may occur in many sites; reentry at the AV node is the usual cause of paroxysmal supraventricular tachycardia, and at the level of the Purkinje fibres it is one of the causes of coupled ventricular premature beats and ventricular tachycardia.

PATHOPHYSIOLOGY OF SPECIFIC ARRHYTHMIAS

Sinus node dysfunction

Several underlying mechanisms and types of arrhythmias are associated with sinus node dysfunction (SND). SND is associated with a variety of disorders including: (1) neurogenic – inhibitory hypersensitive carotid sinus syndrome; (2) degenerative – fibrosis of pacemaker cells, autonomic nerves or ganglia; (3) metabolic – hypothermia, hypoxia and hypothyroidism; (4) increased vagal tone; and (5) drug mediated. The clinical correlates include sinus arrhythmias with or without wandering atrial pacemakers, type I or II SA block or sick sinus syndrome. SND can present as sinus bradycardia, pause or even sinus arrest.

AV junctional rhythm

A dysfunction of the sinus node pacemaker activity may allow pacemaker cells in the vicinity of the atrial AV node, or in the node itself, to assume generation of cardiac automaticity. This is most frequently induced by a slowing of the sinus rate (default), but an increased frequency of junctional depolarization (usurpation) of AV pacemaker activity can result in a junctional rhythm.

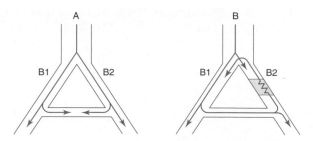

Fig. 14.3 Mechanism of reentry excitation. A: Normally an excitation impulse travelling down a Purkinje fibre passes down both branches to activate the myocardium. The impulses travelling along the connection between the branches cancel each other. When an area of unidirectional block develops in one of the branches (e.g. due to ischaemia), the anterograde impulse is blocked, but an impulse can be conducted in the retrograde direction via branch B2 and reenter branch B1. Transmission through the blocked area is slower than normal. If the delay in this retrograde impulse is sufficiently long that it reaches the myocardium after the refractory period, premature reexcitation occurs. This leads to arrhythmias, including ventricular tachycardia and fibrillation.

In addition to degenerative morphology, high (toxic) digitalis levels also give rise to this type of arrhythmia.

Atrial arrhythmias

A variety of arrhythmias is generated at the level of the atrial (supraventricular) conduction system, and these can result in severe haemodynamic disturbances, especially in patients with ventricular dysfunction. The term automatic atrial tachycardia is used to describe both automatic and triggered supraventricular tachycardias. The most common trigger for these arrhythmias is metabolic disturbances (e.g. hypokalaemia, alkalosis, digitalis toxicity), although it is a rare diagnosis in adults. Paroxysmal (reentrant) supraventricular tachycardia (PSVT) is initiated by a premature atrial or ventricular beat, has a sudden onset and termination, and is caused by either AV node reentry or reciprocation mechanisms. AV node reentry involves functional fast- and slow-conducting pathways within or in the vicinity of the AV node, whereas with reciprocation conduction to the ventricles is via the AV node, and the retrograde conduction is via a concealed accessory pathway. The resulting tachycardia is poorly tolerated and treatment should be directed at termination of reentry by increasing the refractoriness of the AV node or the accessory pathway.

Atrial flutter and fibrillation is a frequent cardiac disorder in elderly patients (5–10% in patients aged over 75 years, 12% of hospitalized patients)[5] with a high risk of systemic embolism due to mural thrombi. Degenerative disorders (chronic obstructive pulmonary and coronary artery disease, cardiomyopathies) but also acute events (heart surgery, rheumatic fever, myocarditis, hyperthyroidism) can all result in atrial flutter or fibrillation. The main therapeutic concern is control of ventricular rate with the prevention of fast atrial signal conduction to the ventricles.

A different, but rare (1–3 per 1000), form of paroxysmal supraventricular tachycardia is that resulting from accessory AV pathways (bundles of fast-conducting fibres connecting atria and ventricles). This fast and reentrant activation results in early activation and so-called tachyarrhythmias with ventricular pre-excitation (e.g. Wolff–Parkinson–White syndrome).

Ventricular arrhythmias

Ventricular arrhythmic beats are generated within the Purkinje system or the ventricular muscle, and occur because of increased automaticity. The idioventricular rhythm (40–60 beats per min), triggering a ventricular escape rhythm, occurs with AV heart block or sinus arrest, but is also seen in patients with acute myocardial infarction or after cardiopulmonary bypass.

Ventricular extrasystole (VES) occurs in about 50% of clinically normal adults and is not associated with cardiac pathology. However, VES can occur in patients with almost any significant cardiac disease. Excessive numbers of VESs are especially ominous in patients with myocardial ischaemia, especially after acute myocardial infarction, and may lead to haemodynamic instability and precipitate ventricular tachycardia, flutter and even fibrillation. The emphasis of VES risk evaluation is based on the circumstances of their occurrence. Circumstantial and transient VESs do not necessarily need to be treated, but identifiable imbalances should be corrected or removed. On the other hand, ventricular tachycardia needs immediate treatment for termination of the potentially fatal haemodynamic consequences.

INTRAOPERATIVE ARRHYTHMIA MONITORING

In the perioperative period the anaesthetist has to cope with a very different environment from that available to specialized electrophysiologists involved in the evaluation and diagnosis of cardiac arrhythmias. Operating rooms are a 'hostile' environment for physiological monitoring, with a high potential for monitoring artefacts. Standard perioperative arrhythmia monitoring should use five-lead surface electrocardiography (ECG) (standard limb leads plus one precordial lead). A combination of one of the inferior limb leads (II, III and aVF), an anterior precordial chest lead (modified V_1 or midclavicular lead) or even an intracavitary (oesophageal, transvenous) lead is best for P-wave detection and arrhythmia analysis.

INCIDENCE

Perioperative arrhythmia is relatively common during routine anaesthesia. The incidence depends on pre-existing disease, medication, dysrhythmia and the type of surgery. Large epidemiological studies in patients with American Society of Anesthesiologists class I or II have shown incidences varying from 3–5%[6] up to 11% in a retrospective study of 112 000 anaesthetics administered in a multicentre study of 17 201 anaesthetized patients.[7] However, only 0.9% of the patients required treatment for the arrhythmia, and a further 1.3% for a significant tachycardia or bradycardia.[7] These data suggest that perioperative arrhythmias are not a major cause of perioperative morbidity and mortality. For sub-populations with compromised physiological states, major disease and/or relevant drug therapy, a much higher incidence is likely.

CLASSIFICATION OF ANTIARRHYTHMIC DRUGS

Antiarrhythmic drugs form a rather heterogeneous group of compounds with a variety of effects, sites and mechanisms of action. The most widely used classification is that of Vaughan Williams, who grouped antiarrhythmic drugs into four classes (Table 14.2).[8] This was later modified by Harrison,[9] who subdivided group I into subclasses IA, IB and IC, incorporating effects on repolarization, determined by actions on K^+ channels.[9] Other classifications have also been described.[10]

Class I drugs, which are most effective against ventricular arrhythmias, alter the conductance of cations, mainly the fast inward Na^+ current, depressing phase 0 of the action potential – a local anaesthetic-like action. Their antiarrhythmic activity is due to slowing of conduction velocity, which terminates reentrant arrhythmias by blocking conduction in a limb of the circuit. Class I drugs also decrease contractility. There are major differences between the various class I agents with respect to their effects on cardiac conduction and ventricular repolarization or refractoriness (Fig. 14.4). These differences arise from different actions on the three distinct Na^+ channel states (closed resting, open, closed inactive) and on potassium channels. Class IA drugs have an intermediate intensity of action in blocking Na^+ channels, 1B are weakest and 1C the strongest. Class 1A drugs prolong the action potential, class 1B shorten it, and class 1C drugs have very little effect on repolarization and duration of the action potential. It is possible for a drug to belong to more than one of these subclasses. For example, moracizine has properties that place it in classes 1A, 1B and 1C.

Table 14.2 Classification of antiarrythmic drugs		
Classification	Mechanism of action	Antiarrhythmic agent
Class I	Sodium channel blockers (fast Na$^+$ influx)	
IA	Moderate to marked Na$^+$ channel block Phase 0 conduction depression (++), widens QRS Prolongs repolarization and lengthens APD and QT interval	Procainamide, disopyramide, moracizine, quinidine
IB	Mild to moderate Na$^+$ channel block Phase 0 conduction depression (+) Shortens repolarization and QT interval	Lignocaine, mexiletine, tocainide, phenytoin
IC	Marked Na$^+$ channel block Phase 0 conduction depression (+++) Little effect on repolarization	Propafenone, encainide, flecainide, indecainide
Class II	β-Adrenergic block	Propranolol, esmolol, acebutol, etc.
Class III	Prolongation of repolarization	Bretylium, amiodarone, sotalol
Class IV	Calcium channel block	Verapamil, diltiazem, etc.
Various	Muscarinic cholinergic block Increase of AV node ERP AV node conduction block	Atropine Digitalis Adenosine

APD, action potential duration; AV, atrioventricular; ERP, effective refractory period.

Class II antiarrhythmics are β-adrenoceptor antagonists. They have an indirect effect on the cardiac action potential, by inhibiting the actions of catecholamines, thereby decreasing sympathetic tone.

Pure class III drugs block one or more of the potassium channels involved in repolarization, but especially the delayed rectifying current (I_k) without significant effects on cardiac sodium channels. They delay membrane repolarization and increase refractoriness, with little effect on membrane depolarization (phase 0). In

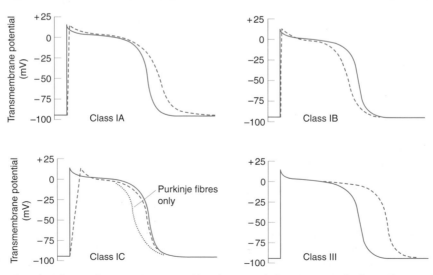

Fig. 14.4 Changes produced in the cardiac action potential by class I and class III antiarrhythmic drugs. Class IA drugs depress the maximum upstroke of phase 0 and prolong the action potential duration (APD); class IB drugs shorten the action potential, while class IC drugs markedly depress phase 0 upstroke but have little effect on the APD, except in Purkinje fibres where the duration is shortened. Class III drugs markedly prolong the APD (and the QT interval of the electrocardiogram).

general, block of potassium channels results in a prolongation of ventricular action potential duration, and its ECG surrogate, the QT interval. Pure class III drugs do not depress ventricular contractility. However, of the currently available class III drugs, amiodarone and sotalol have additional electrophysiological activities, and amiodarone has negative inotropic effects. Several pure class III drugs are under development. All other effects of the individual drugs may vary significantly, explaining their distinct actions on atrial and/or ventricular arrhythmias. One of the major drawbacks of the class III drugs is that their ability to prolong the action potential duration and refractoriness is diminished at high heart rates, so that they are the least effective when they are needed most. This phenomenon is referred to as 'reverse frequency-dependence'.

Class IV agents are predominantly L-type Ca^{2+} channel blockers. Various other drugs used for antiarrhythmic therapy do not fall easily into the Vaughan Williams classification (Table 14.2). For many drugs it is not clear which of their different effects, such as those on haemodynamics, microperfusion, metabolism or central/autonomic nervous system, are responsible for the main antiarrhythmic action.

INDIVIDUAL DRUGS, MECHANISMS AND INDICATIONS

CLASS 1A ANTIARRHYTHMIC DRUGS

These are used for the short- and long-term treatment of supraventricular and ventricular arrhythmias. They are especially useful for the treatment of recurrent PSVT, including that associated with Wolff–Parkinson–White syndrome. Other indications include atrial flutter or fibrillation, ventricular premature depolarizations and unsustained ventricular tachycardia. Doses and pharmacokinetic details are given in Table 14.3.

Quinidine

Quinidine is the *dextro* stereoisomer of quinine, a cinchona alkaloid. In addition to typical class IA electrophysiological actions, it has indirect anticholinergic properties. These actions lead to a decrease or even an increase of heart rate (vagolytic effect), prolonged conduction, prolonged atrial/ventricular ERPs and an increase in QRS and QT durations. Quinidine also has α-adrenergic blocking properties which may cause vasodilatation and a reduced preload, especially when given as a fast intravenous bolus. Many of these effects are more pronounced in conditions of ischaemia, hypoxia and tachycardia. In toxic concentrations or in combination with high digitalis concentrations, quinidine may induce sinus arrest, high grade AV block, 'torsades de pointes', polymorphic ventricular tachycardia and abnormal ventricular automaticity.

Summary box 14.2 Overview of main indications for different classes of antiarrhythmic drugs

- Class IA:
  ventricular ectopics, paroxysmal supraventricular tachycardia, atrial flutter or fibrillation, ventricular tachycardia.

- Class IB:
  ventricular tachycardia, digoxin-induced arrhythmias.

- Class IC:
  ventricular and supraventricular tachycardia (especially those due to reentry phenomena), atrial fibrillation and flutter (can convert recent-onset fibrillation or flutter to sinus rhythm).

- Class II:
  paroxysmal supraventricular tachycardia, atrial or ventricular premature beats, atrial fibrillation or flutter (slows ventricular rate).

- Class III:
  ventricular tachycardia, atrial fibrillation and flutter (can convert recent-onset fibrillation or flutter to sinus rhythm). Amiodarone is used in the management of patients with supraventricular and ventricular arrhythmias, and arrhythmias associated with the Wolff–Parkinson–White syndrome.

- Class IV:
  paroxysmal supraventricular tachycardia, atrial fibrillation and flutter. Not of benefit in treatment of ventricular arrhythmias.

- Atropine:
  sinus bradycardia.

- Digoxin:
  atrial fibrillation and flutter with rapid ventricular response.

- Adenosine:
  idiopathic and reentrant paroxysmal supraventricular tachycardia.

Quinidine still remains a useful antiarrhythmic for both supraventricular and ventricular arrhythmias. It can convert atrial fibrillation or flutter to sinus rhythm and maintain normal sinus rhythm. Quinidine is useful in managing reentry supraventricular tachycardia (e.g. in Wolff–Parkinson–White syndrome) and for the suppression of ventricular ectopy. Contraindications to its use include intraventricular conduction defects, AV block and aberrant impulses due to escape mechanisms.

		Effective plasma concentration ($\mu g\ ml^{-1}$)	Half-life (h)	Protein binding (%)	Metabolism[*]
Drug	**Dosage**				
Class IA					
Quinidine	0.2 g 4 hourly orally	2–6	6–7	80	Liver, hydroxylation
Procainamide	100 mg i.v. over 2–5 min then 30–90 $\mu g\ kg^{-1}\ min^{-1}$	3–10	4	20	Liver, acetylation
Disopyramide	0.2 g 4 hourly orally 0.2 mg kg^{-1} i.v. (for initial i.v. dose, see text)	2–4	5–7	30–40	Liver, n-dealkylation
Class IB					
Lidocaine	1 mg kg^{-1} i.v. 20–50 $\mu g\ kg^{-1}\ min^{-1}$	2–6	0.5–1	65	Liver, oxidation
Mexiletine	250–700 mg over 3 h i.v.	0.5–2	10–20	70	Liver
Phenytoin	0.5 g i.v.	10–20	16–24	80–90	Liver, hydroxylation
Class IC					
Propafenone	0.2–1 mg kg^{-1} i.v.	0.2–1	3.6	90	Liver
Flecainide	1 mg kg^{-1} i.v.	0.25–1	12	40	Liver, dealkylation
Encainide	0.5 g i.v.	10–20	3–11	80–90	Liver, hydroxylation

Table 14.3 Pharmacokinetics and dosage of class I antiarrhythmic drugs

[*] Organ and pathway. i.v., Intravenously.

Procainamide

Procainamide is the amide analogue of procaine hydrochloride. It has much less anticholinergic activity than quinidine and does not block α-adrenergic receptors. It is particularly effective in the treatment of life-threatening ventricular arrhythmias unresponsive to other therapies such as lignocaine (lidocaine). Procainamide is also used to maintain sinus rhythm following cardioversion. Myocardial contractility is minimally depressed in the normal heart but intravenous administration can cause hypotension, mainly due to peripheral vasodilatation, and it should not be given faster than 50 mg min^{-1}, especially in patients with left ventricular dysfunction.

Side-effects are comparable to those of quinidine, although in general less pronounced. Procainamide has an active metabolite with significant class III activity, which has to be taken into consideration especially during chronic treatment or in patients with impaired renal function. In some patients on long-term oral therapy a 'lupus-like syndrome' develops, with polyarthralgia or myalgia and other symptoms.

The indication range is comparable to that of quinidine, but with a special focus on the suppression of ventricular (tachy-) arrhythmias such as sustained ventricular tachycardia, ventricular couplets, multiform beats and the 'R on T' phenomenon.

Disopyramide

Disopyramide is chemically different from quinidine or procainamide. It is approved only for oral administration in some countries. Disopyramide is used as a racemate, and the enantiomers exhibit different properties. Both the racemate and (+)-disopyramide prolong action potential duration whereas (−)-disopyramide shortens the duration. In comparison with quinidine, disopyramide is comparable or even more effective for conversion of atrial flutter or fibrillation or ischaemia-induced ventricular arrhythmias.

Disopyramide has significant anticholinergic properties (10% the potency of atropine) which can offset its direct depressant effects on sinus and AV nodes. It has no α- or β-adrenergic antagonistic effects and has more pronounced negative inotropic effects than quinidine or procainamide, and should be administered with caution to patients with a history of congestive heart failure. Otherwise it is well suited and effective for the class IA indication profile: premature atrial/ventricular complexes, atrial flutter or fibrillation, paroxysmal AV nodal and reentrant tachycardia, and sustained ventricular tachycardia. For acute treatment of perioperative arrhythmias it is given intravenously: 0.2 mg kg^{-1} over 10–15 min, then 0.2 mg kg^{-1} over the next 45 min and a maintenance infusion of 0.4 mg kg^{-1} h^{-1}. The dose should be reduced in patients with diminished ventricular function.

CLASS IB ANTIARRHYTHMIC DRUGS

Drugs in this class produce only small changes in phase 0 depolarization and conduction velocity when resting membrane potentials are normal. When the membrane is depolarized or the frequency of excitation is increased, the depressant effects are significantly increased. In contrast to class IA agents, class IB drugs usually shorten repolarization and cause negligible changes in the ECG.

Lignocaine (lidocaine)

Lignocaine is used primarily for the emergency treatment of ventricular arrhythmias, particularly those due to acute ischaemia (e.g. myocardial infarction, heart surgery, etc.). It has a greater membrane-depressant effect on ischaemic and hypoxic myocardial cells than on normal tissues. Lignocaine has little effect on sinus node automaticity but it depresses normal and abnormal forms of automaticity in Purkinje fibres. It is generally ineffective against supraventricular and accessory pathway-induced (e.g. Wolff–Parkinson–White syndrome) arrhythmias. Sodium channels are blocked by lignocaine in the closed inactive state. In the atria, sodium channels spend only short periods in this state, which may explain the relative inefficiency of lignocaine against reentrant atrial arrhythmias.

Lignocaine is relatively safe and free from adverse cardiovascular side-effects. It causes minimal cardiodepression, although high doses can cause heart block. The most common side-effect is a dose-related central nervous system (CNS) toxicity. It is given intravenously because of extensive first-pass hepatic metabolism after oral dosing.

Mexiletine

Mexiletine is structurally similar to lignocaine and has comparable electrophysiological properties. It has minimal effects on atrial or ventricular refractory periods or sinus node function in the normal heart, but significant effects may occur in patients with conduction system abnormalities. The effect on myocardial contractility is minimal, even in patients with reduced ventricular function. Mexiletine is readily absorbed after oral administration with a bioavailability of 80–90% and is also available for intravenous administration. It is very effective for the treatment of chronic ventricular, but not supraventricular, arrhythmias and is often used in combination with another antiarrhythmic drug. Side-effects are similar to those of lignocaine.

Phenytoin (diphenylhydantoin)

Phenytoin is primarily an anticonvulsive agent with a narrow indication range as an antiarrhythmic agent. Because of a wide range of toxic side-effects, its use as an antiarrhythmic drug is limited to the treatment of arrhythmias caused by digitalis toxicity. The mechanism of action is similar to that of lignocaine, but some of its antiarrhythmic properties may be mediated by neural mechanisms (e.g. central modulation of vagal efferent activity, decreased sympathetic cardiac activity).

Even small doses of phenytoin are highly effective against multiform and/or complex ventricular premature beats, ventricular tachycardia and atrial tachycardia caused by digitalis. Side-effects are mainly CNS related, such as dizziness, fatigue, ataxia, nystagmus and stupor, but hyperglycaemia and hypocalcaemia occur with long-term treatment. Intravenous bolus injections can cause myocardial depression, hypotension, AV block and bradycardia. Phenytoin is poorly absorbed after oral and intramuscular administration. It has a long elimination half-life (± 22 h) and a potential for several drug–drug interactions owing to induction of hepatic cytochrome P450 enzymes. The hepatic metabolism of phenytoin is saturable within the therapeutic range of plasma concentrations (10–20 µg µl^{-1}) so that its pharmacokinetics are nonlinear (zero order).

CLASS IC ANTIARRHYTHMIC DRUGS

Class IC agents have a high affinity for sarcolemmal fast sodium channels and are the most potent agents in slowing conduction and suppressing inward sodium currents and spontaneous premature complexes. Their actions are mainly on the His–Purkinje systems, and the effects on repolarization, action potential duration and ERP are relatively small. The refractory period in both the AV node and accessory pathways is significantly increased. The effects on heart rate are small, although there is a substantial increase in the PR interval and QRS complex duration.

Propafenone

This agent is a class IC drug with a heterogeneous profile and some class IA and class II effects. While the primary mechanism of action is by blocking sodium channels, propafenone also has calcium and potassium channel and β-adrenergic blocking properties that contribute to its action. The action on potassium channels tends to counterbalance the prolongation of the action potential caused by block of the sodium and calcium channels. It is effective for the treatment of ventricular and supraventricular tachycardias (AV nodal and accessory pathway reentry, atrial flutter and fibrillation). It is useful in converting recent-onset atrial fibrillation or flutter to sinus rhythm, and for terminating paroxysmal supraventricular tachycardia. Its proarrhythmic and myocardial depressant effects limit its use, especially in patients with poor ventricular function.

Propafenone can be given orally or intravenously. After oral administration it is readily absorbed, but the bioavailability is low (5–12%), although it increases with increasing dose, suggesting enzyme saturability. The main metabolization is by cytochrome P450 enzymes. There is a risk of drug accumulation in patients with enzyme defects and/or hepatic dysfunction.

Flecainide

Flecainide is used mainly for the treatment of severe, life-threatening ventricular tachyarrhythmias and non-sustained ventricular tachycardia or high frequency premature ventricular beats. It may also be useful in treating severe supraventricular arrhythmias (AV nodal or AV accessory pathway reentrant tachycardias). The drug is almost completely absorbed after oral administration, and can also be given intravenously. With a long half-life (12–30 h) and high renal excretion (40%) there is a risk of accumulation in patients with renal insufficiency.

The main adverse effects are cardiovascular, including proarrhythmic actions and severe negative inotropic effects, especially in patients with impaired cardiac function. Both flecainide and encainide increase the risk of sudden death in patients with myocardial infarction and asymptomatic unsustained ventricular arrhythmias.[11] Their use is limited, therefore, to patients with severe and potentially life-threatening tachyarrhythmias.

Encainide

Encainide has a similar pharmacological profile to flecainide, with the same indication range and adverse effect potential. After oral administration encainide undergoes 30% hepatic first-pass metabolism by the cytochrome P450 enzyme system to two active metabolites. Some 10% of the population are poor metabolizers due to a genetic deficiency, and these individuals can have plasma concentrations 20 times those of extensive metabolizers.

CLASS II ANTIARRHYTHMIC DRUGS: β-ADRENERGIC ANTAGONISTS

The pharmacological effects of the β-adrenergic antagonists are complex and they are used whenever a block or modulation of sympathetic tone may be beneficial. For the treatment of arrhythmias no one drug offers distinct advantages, and the choice of drug in the individual patient is often based on pharmacodynamic or pharmacokinetic considerations. Representing the many substances, two drugs are discussed as representative of this class: propranolol as the 'prototype' β-adrenoceptor antagonist, and esmolol, which has an ultra-short action profile which makes it particularly suitable for perioperative use. Doses and pharmacokinetic details are given in Table 14.4.

> **Warning box 14.1** β-Adrenoceptor antagonists should be avoided in patients with
>
> - asthma or other bronchoconstrictive disorders
> - diabetes mellitus prone to hypoglycaemic reactions
> - peripheral vascular disease.

Propranolol

Propranolol is used for the management of ventricular and supraventricular arrhythmias and to prevent their recurrence. Its activity against supraventricular arrhythmias is by competitive inhibition of catecholamine binding to adrenergic receptors in the SA and AV nodes. A second effect includes an increase of background outward (potassium) currents. At concentrations higher

Drug	Dosage	Effective plasma concentration ($\mu g\ ml^{-1}$)	Half-life (h)	Protein binding (%)	Metabolism
Propranolol	0.025–0.05 mg kg^{-1} i.v. up to 3 mg	0.03–0.3	2–3	90	Liver, oxidation
Esmolol	0.5 mg kg^{-1} i.v.; 0.05–0.3 mg kg^{-1} min^{-1}	0.4–1.2	9 min	55	Plasma, esterases, hydrolysis

Table 14.4 Pharmacokinetics and dosage of class II antiarrhythmic drugs

i.v., Intravenously.

than those producing β-adrenoceptor antagonism it blocks sodium channels, producing a membrane-stabilizing (local anaesthetic) effect unrelated to β-adrenergic block. The role of this property in its antiarrhythmic action is uncertain. Automaticity in the SA node or Purkinje fibres is reduced in proportion to the degree of existing sympathetic tone. Propranolol slows the ventricular response to atrial flutter and fibrillation by prolonging the functional refractory period of the AV node. This effect is additive to the effects of digitalis and calcium-channel blockers. Propranolol can slow sinus tachycardia.

The oral bioavailability is low (around 10% after a single dose), but increases with multiple dosing. Adverse effects include hypotension, bradycardia and precipitation of congestive heart failure. Because it is nonselective, propranolol blocks β_2-adrenergic receptors responsible for bronchodilatation, and should not be used in patients with asthma or bronchospasm. It is also contraindicated in patients with diabetes receiving hypoglycaemic drugs.

Esmolol

Esmolol is an ultra-short-acting β-adrenergic antagonist, only used intravenously. The chemical structure of esmolol is similar to that of metoprolol but with a methyl ester group (Fig. 14.5), which makes it susceptible to rapid hydrolysis by erythrocyte esterases, giving it a unique pharmacokinetic profile with an elimination half-life of around 9 min. Esmolol is relatively β_1-receptor selective with no intrinsic (β-stimulating) activity. It is used for emergency treatment of rapid ventricular rates in patients with atrial flutter or fibrillation, as well as for sinus tachycardia.

Esmolol can be easily titrated by an initial bolus followed by an infusion adjusted to achieve the desired effect (Table 14.4). Untoward effects and mechanism of action are comparable to those of other β-adrenergic antagonists.

CLASS III ANTIARRHYTHMIC DRUGS

Substances in this class have a variety of pharmacological actions, but all prolong action potential duration and refractoriness in Purkinje and ventricular muscle fibres (see Fig. 14.4), by blocking one or more of the repolarizing K^+ channels (Table 14.5). These actions are less pronounced in atrial and AV nodal cells (exception bretylium). They all interact with the autonomic nervous system, but none alters vagal reflexes or the responsiveness of cardiac cholinergic receptors. Bretylium, like guanethidine, is taken up and stored in adrenergic nerve terminals, amiodarone causes some noncompetitive α- and β-adrenergic blockade, while sotalol is also a β-adrenergic antagonist. In addition to the three drugs described here, several class III drugs

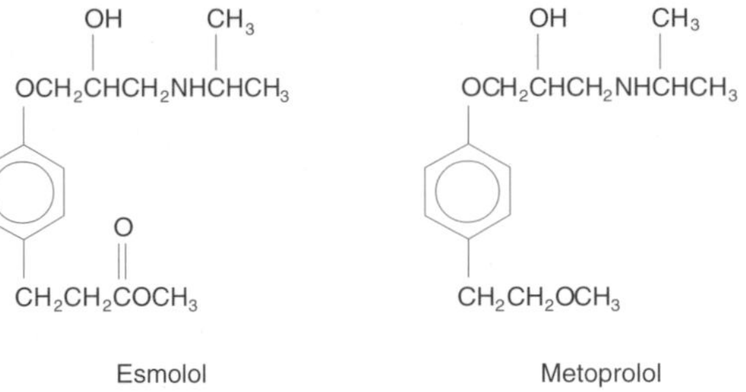

Fig. 14.5 Structure of esmolol and the related β-adrenoceptor antagonist, metoprolol.

are in different stages of development (see Table 14.5). Doses and pharmacokinetic details are given in Table 14.6.

Bretylium tosylate

Bretylium is an adrenergic neuron-blocking drug with antiarrhythmic activity. It has a complex pharmacology, including indirect effects through interactions with adrenergic neurons and direct effects on cardiac membranes. Bretylium is selectively concentrated in sympathetic ganglionic and postganglionic adrenergic neurons, where it releases stored noradrenaline and then inhibits further noradrenaline release by depressing neuronal excitability (chemical sympathectomy). It is indicated for the prophylaxis and treatment of ventricular fibrillation, especially after myocardial infarction, and other life-threatening ventricular arrhythmias (e.g. 'torsade de pointes' ventricular tachycardia). Its

Table 14.5 Effects of some class III antiarrhythmic drugs (potassium channel blockers) on the three important cardiac voltage-dependent potassium channels			
Drug	I_{to}	I_k	I_{ki}
Sotalol	+	+	+
Amiodarone	−	+	+
Clofilium	+	+	−
Tedisamil	+	+	−
Sematilide	−	+	−
Risotilide	−	+	−
Dofetilide	−	+	−

		Table 14.6 Pharmacokinetics and dosage of class III antiarrhythmic drugs			
Drug	Dosage	Effective plasma concentration ($\mu g\ ml^{-1}$)	Half-life	Protein binding (%)	Metabolism
Bretylium	5–10 mg kg^{-1} i.v.	1–10	9–13 h	> 5	No metabolism, renal elimination
Amiodarone	600 mg per 24 h orally 5 mg kg^{-1} bolus i.v. 1000 mg per 24 h i.v.	1–5	8–100 days	> 90	Liver, gut
Sotalol	80–320 mg every 12 h orally 20 mg bolus i.v. up to 1.5 mg kg^{-1}	0.1	10–15 h	< 10	Urinary excretion of unchanged drug

i.v., Intravenously.

antifibrillatory activity has given rise to the term 'pharmacological defibrillator'.

The major side-effect is hypotension, although initially there may be a rise in heart rate, blood pressure and myocardial inotropy as a result of catecholamine release. Within the therapeutic concentration range, bretylium causes few ECG effects. Because of poor oral absorption it is administered intravenously. It is not metabolized and is renally eliminated as the intact molecule.

Amiodarone

Amiodarone is potent antiarrhythmic agent with multiple cardiovascular actions. Its class III actions are due to reduction of the potassium outward current and consequent prolongation of the cardiac action potential and the QT interval in the ECG. Paradoxically this action may also result in a potential to induce polymorphic ventricular arrhythmias.[12] Amiodarone blocks cardiac sodium channels, a class I effect, with a selective affinity for inactivated channels, depressing the rate of rise of the action potential and conduction velocity in the ventricles, especially during fast heart rates. It is a noncompetitive inhibitor of α- and β-adrenoceptors, which results in vasodilatation, prolongation of the AV nodal refractory period and slowing of AV nodal conduction. Inhibition of β-adrenoceptors prolongs the ERP and slows SA rate (a class II effect). Amiodarone is used in the management of patients with supraventricular and ventricular arrhythmias, and arrhythmias associated with the Wolff–Parkinson–White syndrome. It also has a role in the management of atrial fibrillation. Amiodarone causes striking changes in cardiac metabolism, slowing oxidative metabolism and increasing energy (adenosine triphosphate ATP) reserve, which may explain its antianginal potency. Amiodarone blocks cal-

cium channels weakly and this, together with its actions on β-adrenoceptors, can result in myocardial depression following rapid intravenous administration. Myocardial depression is not a problem with chronic oral administration and congestive failure is rarely aggravated.

Amiodarone is poorly absorbed (bioavailability 45%) and peak concentrations occur 5–6 h after an oral dose. However, there is considerable latency between appearance in the blood and uptake in the myocardium, so that the maximum effect may not be reached for several weeks. It is extremely lipid soluble and concentrations in fat can reach up to 385 times the plasma concentration. The apparent volume of distribution is huge (5000 litres). With intravenous administration, therapeutic effects are seen within 1–30 min but the maximum effect may take 1–2 h. The elimination half-life after a single oral or intravenous dose is 4–6 h. However, with chronic oral therapy the half-life is extremely prolonged, up to 40 days. The indication range includes treatment of episodes of supraventricular tachycardia, atrial flutter and fibrillation, ectopic rhythm, and ventricular tachycardia or fibrillation after cardiac surgery or cardiac arrest.

Chronic oral therapy with amiodarone is associated with several side-effects, include pulmonary toxicity (fibrosis and probably immunologically mediated pneumonitis), hepatotoxicity, thyroid gland dysfunction, corneal microdeposits, blue-grey skin discoloration and neurological disturbances (tremor, sleep disturbances, peripheral neuropathy and extrapyramidal side-effects). Amiodarone potentiates the effect of warfarin, and the maintenance dose should be reduced by one-third to one-half in patients taking amiodarone. A poorly understood postoperative adult respiratory distress syndrome has been described after cardiac or pulmonary surgery in patients taking amiodarone.[12] Patients present 1–5

> **Warning box 14.2 Adverse effects of amiodarone**
>
> - Pulmonary toxicity, including pneumonitis and fibrosis, can occur with chronic use. A postoperative adult respiratory distress syndrome associated with a high mortality rate has been described.
>
> - Hepatotoxicity.
>
> - Thyroid gland dysfunction.
>
> - Corneal microdeposits.
>
> - Blue-grey skin pigmentation.
>
> - Neurological disturbances (tremor, sleep disturbances, peripheral neuropathy and extrapyramidal side-effects).
>
> - Interactions with the metabolism of warfarin and digoxin cause the plasma concentrations of these drugs to increase, potentiating their effects.

days after operation with diffuse pulmonary infiltrates and severe hypoxaemia. This syndrome, which has been described in patients given the drug intravenously for 3 days before pneumonectomy, is associated with a high mortality rate.

Sotalol

Originally synthesized as a nonselective β-adrenoceptor antagonist, sotalol has significant class III activity. Sotalol is available as a racemic mixture and the β-adrenergic effects reside with *l*-sotalol. D-Sotalol is a pure class III compound with only 2% of the β-adrenoceptor antagonism of the racemate. Sotalol delays cardiac repolarization by inhibiting the delayed rectifier potassium current, with a lesser effect on the inwardly rectifying and transient outward currents, and little or no effect on inward calcium or sodium currents. It has a potent antifibrillatory action modulated by its anti-adrenergic effects. It suppresses premature ventricular contractions and nonsustained ventricular tachycardia while preventing inducible ventricular tachycardia and fibrillation in patients with advanced structural heart disease.

Sotalol does not directly decrease myocardial contractility, although β-adrenergic blockade can reduce cardiac function in patients who are dependent on sympathetic activity to maintain cardiac output. Oral doses of sotalol are readily absorbed and the bioavailability is nearly 100%. Maximum plasma concentrations are reached within 2 h. Intravenous injection shortens significantly the onset of action. In patients with reduced renal function, dose and dosing intervals should be adjusted. Side-effects include a small prodysrhythmic potency (torsades de pointes, polymorphic ventricular tachycardia) and other side-effects comparable to those of other β-adrenoceptor antagonists.

CLASS IV ANTIARRHYTHMIC DRUGS

Class IV antiarrhythmics are all calcium channel blocking agents. Their main antiarrhythmic effects result from depression of calcium-dependent action potentials and slowing of AV nodal conduction. Doses and pharmacokinetic details are given in Table 14.7.

Verapamil and diltiazem

Both drugs depress the slow inward calcium current in all cardiac fibres, reduce the height of the action potential plateau, slightly shorten action potential duration in cardiac muscle fibres, and slightly prolong action potential duration in Purkinje fibres. They also depress SA node automaticity. Intravenously they are the preferred initial treatment for terminating sustained sinoatrial or AV nodal reentrant tachycardia or reciprocating (AV reentry, Wolf–Parkinson–White syndrome) tachycardias. About 60–80% of PSVTs are terminated within several minutes by intravenous verapamil. Both drugs increase the PR interval in sinus rhythm and slow

Table 14.7 Pharmacology and dosage of class IV antiarrhythmic drugs					
Drug	Dosage	Effective plasma concentration ($\mu g\ ml^{-1}$)	Half-life (h)	Protein binding (%)	Metabolism
Verapamil	5–10 mg i.v. bolus	0.01–0.03	3–7	90	Liver, *N*-/*O*-demethylation
Diltiazem	0.3 mg kg^{-1} i.v. bolus; 0.2–1.0 mg min^{-1} infusion	0.02	4–5	80–90	Liver
i.v., Intravenously.					

ventricular rate in patients with atrial fibrillation. Neither drug is of benefit in the treatment of ventricular arrhythmias.

Adverse effects are mainly cardiac. Caution should be exercised in patients with impaired myocardial function, those receiving β-adrenoceptor antagonists, in patients with hypotension or sick sinus syndrome. A diseased SA node is more sensitive to these drugs, and may be depressed to the point of sinus arrest. This may occur without overt evidence of 'sick sinus syndrome'. Extreme caution should be exercised in anaesthetized patients in whom there is a potential for additive or synergistic cardiovascular depressant effects.

OTHER ANTIARRHYTHMIC DRUGS (TABLE 14.8)

Atropine
Atropine is a competitive antagonist of actetylcholine at muscarinergic cholinergic receptors. It increases the heart rate and SA and AV node conduction time. The direct effect on the cardiac action potential, and therefore on ventricular arrhythmias, is minimal. Atropine is the drug of choice for bradycardia and hypotension due to vasovagal stimulation.

Cardiac glycosides
Digitalis glycosides are derived from the foxglove plants; digoxin from *Digitalis lanata* and digitoxin from *D. purpurea*. Digoxin is the one most widely used. Ouabain, which is available only in injectable form, is occasionally used when a rapid effect is desired. The onset of action after intravenous injection of ouabain 0.25–0.5 mg is 5–10 min.

The major therapeutic effect of digitalis is its inotropic effect on the failing heart, primarily by inhibiting the Na^+–K^+ adenosine triphosphatase (Na^+–K^+ pump), reducing intracellular potassium and increasing intracellular sodium and calcium concentrations. In addition it has direct and indirect actions on the autonomic nervous system which are mainly responsible for its antiarrhythmic activity. With therapeutic concentrations the predominant effect is parasympathetic activation, and increased sensitivity of the heart to acetylcholine; with toxic concentrations, sympathetic stimulation occurs. The vagal effects are predominantly on atrial and specialized conduction tissues. In addition there are interactions with the slow inward Ca^{2+} current during the cardiac action potential plateau (phase 2). Depending on the concentration and duration of exposure, these mechanisms reduce the action potential upstroke, conduction velocity and amplitude, increasing AV nodal refractoriness and conduction and slowing the ventricular rate in atrial fibrillation. Atrial fibrillation with a rapid ventricular response is one of the most common indications for digitalis.

Digitalis has a narrow therapeutic window and toxicity is a major concern. Extracardiac manifestations are often nonspecific and may be similar to those of congestive heart failure. Gastrointestinal symptoms (anorexia, nausea, vomiting and diarrhoea) are relatively common. However, cardiac arrhythmias are the most serious side-effects of digitalis toxicity. Digitalis-induced arrhythmias include atrial or ventricular premature beats, ventricular tachycardia, bigeminy, junctional rhythm and heart block. Hypokalaemia predisposes to toxicity, by enhancing the binding of digitalis to myocardial receptor sites and the development of spontaneous phase 4 depolarization and automatic rhythms. In patients with potentially life-threatening digitalis toxicity, digoxin-specific antibodies (Fab fragments) may be used to achieve rapid reversal. These bind digoxin with an affinity greater than that of digoxin for myocardial tissues.

The oral bioavailability of digitalis is 60–80%. Digoxin is not extensively metabolized and is eliminated

Table 14.8 Pharmacokinetics and dosage of other antiarrhythmic drugs

Drug	Dosage	Effective plasma concentration	Half-life	Protein binding (%)	Metabolism
Atropine	0.5–1.0 mg i.v.		2.5 h	50	Liver 50%, unchanged 50%
Digoxin	0.4–1.0 mg i.v.	1–1.8 ng ml^{-1}	1.5–2 h	20–25	Liver 40%, unchanged 60%
Adenosine	3 mg i.v. bolus, max. 12 mg i.v.	70–90 ng ml^{-1}	0.5 min		Liver

i.v., Intravenously.

by renal excretion, so that the dose needs to be adjusted in patients with renal failure. In contrast, digitoxin is almost completely metabolized to inactive metabolites. The elimination half-life of digoxin is 23–30 h, that of digitoxin considerably longer – 4–6 days.

Adenosine

Adenosine is an endogenous purine nucleoside with potent electrophysiological effects and major functions in vasomotor tone regulation. It binds with two different adenosine receptors (A_1 and A_2) and causes significant negative chronotropic effects on the SA node and negative dromotropic effects on the AV node, increasing AV node conduction time. These effects are due to a decreased action potential duration (increase of outward K^+ current) as well as partial Ca^{2+} channel blockade (in the presence of β-adrenergic stimulation). Adenosine has a narrow indication range: treatment of idiopathic paroxysmal and reentry supraventricular tachycardia, and PSVT associated with Wolff–Parkinson–White syndrome. In contrast to verapamil, adenosine has no effect on accessory pathway conduction and has no significant negative inotropic effect.

PERIOPERATIVE ARRHYTHMIAS: UNDERLYING CAUSES

The mechanisms responsible for the initiation of new, or the exacerbation of existing, cardiac dysrhythmias in the perioperative or immediate postoperative period are summarized in Table 14.9. Autonomic and physiological disturbances are the main causes of dysrhythmias.[13] Toxicity or side-effects associated with perioperatively administered drugs, airway or surgical stimulation, preexisting cardiac disease and technical problems are also important. Only limited data are available on the direct effect of anaesthesia-related drugs on dysrhythmia mechanisms, although local anaesthetics and halothane are known to affect the electrical properties of the heart. Halothane, thiopentone and propofol may facilitate ventricular arrhythmias due to catecholamines.

WHEN TO TREAT?

The decision when to treat arrhythmias in the perioperative period often differs from that in other situations. Indeed many perioperative arrhythmias do not require specific antiarrhythmic treatment. Drug therapy should be considered only when the arrhythmia cannot immediately be terminated by removing the precipitating or underlying cause, when circulatory function or myocardial oxygenation is severely compromised, or when the dysrhythmia predisposes the patient to life-threatening arrhythmias such as supraventricular tachyarrhythmias, ventricular tachycardia, flutter or fibrillation. Unnecessary treatment may potentially do more harm than good, owing to the untoward side-effects of antiarrhythmic drugs.[14]

The first step in the management of perioperative

Table 14.9 Underlying or contributing factors for perioperative and postoperative dysrhythmias			
Physiology	**Pharmacology**	**Technical**	**Perioperative**
Acid–base imbalance	Drug interactions	Equipment malfunction	Light anaesthesia
Electrolyte imbalance	Drug idiosyncrasy	Pulmonary artery or central venous catheter	Airway manipulation
Hypoxia	Catecholamines	Pacemaker malfunction	Surgical stress
Hypercarbia	Anaesthetic overdose	Electric shock	Autonomic imbalance
Cachexic states	Digitalis excess		Cardiac ischaemia
Obesity			Hypotension or hypertension
Endocrine dysfunction			CNS disorders
Stress			Temperature imbalance
Anxiety			

Drug	Dosage	Indications
Atropine	Bolus: 0.5–1.0 mg	Sinus bradycardia, AV block I, ventricular arrhythmias
Lignocaine	Bolus: 1 mg kg^{-1} Infusion: 10–50 μg kg^{-1} min^{-1}	
Propafenone	Bolus: 0.2–1.0 mg kg^{-1}	Supraventricular or ventricular tachyarrhythmias
Esmolol	Bolus: 0.5 mg kg^{-1} Infusion: 0.05–0.3 mg kg^{-1} min^{-1}	Non-compensatory sinus tachycardia, supraventricular tachycardia
Amiodarone	Bolus: 5 mg kg^{-1} Infusion: 10 μg kg^{-1} min^{-1}	Perioperative supraventricular or ventricular tachyarrhythmias
Verapamil	Bolus: 5–10 mg Infusion: 1.5 μg kg^{-1} min^{-1}	AV nodal reentrant paroxysmal tachycardia
Digoxin	Bolus: 0.4–1.0 mg	Slow ventricular rate in atrial flutter or fibrillation

Table 14.10 **Suitable antiarrhythmic drugs for emergency use in the perioperative period**

arrhythmias should be to ensure artefact-free ECG monitoring to allow the correct diagnosis of the dysrhythmia. Then potential causes of the dysrhythmia should be identified and corrected where possible. Only when this fails should drug therapy or electrical treatment be considered. Of course, immediate life-threatening arrhythmias such as ventricular tachycardia or fibrillation require immediate treatment before searching for underlying causes. For the specific indications within the perioperative setting, a limited number of drugs is suitable. The most important of these are summarized in Table 14.10.

REFERENCES

1. Kerin NZ, Somberg J. Proarrhythmia: definition, risk factors, causes treatment, and controversies. *Am Heart J* 1994; **128**: 575–585.
2. Merin RG. Cardiac cell membrane physiology: implications for the anaesthesiologist. *Curr Opin Anaesthesiol* 1995; **8**: 1–6.
3. Katz AM. Cardiac ion channels. *N Engl J Med* 1993; **328**: 1244–1251.
4. Escande D, Henry P. Potassium channels as pharmacological targets in cardiovascular medicine. *Eur Heart J* 1993; **14** (Suppl. B): 2–9.
5. Ganz L, Friedman P. Supraventricular tachycardia. *N Engl J Med* 1995; **332**: 126–173.
6. Cohen MM, Duncan PG, Pope WDB, Wolkenstein C. A survey of 112 000 anaesthetics at one teaching hospital (1975–1983). *Can Anaesth Soc J* 1986; **33**: 336–344.
7. Forrest JB, Cahalan MK, Rehder K *et al.* Multicenter study of general anesthesia. II. Results. *Anesthesiology* 1990; **72**: 262–268.
8. Vaughan Williams EM. A classification of antiarrhythmic actions reassessed after a decade of new drugs. *J Clin Pharmacol* 1984; **24**: 129–147.
9. Harrison DC. Antiarrhythmic drug classification: new science and practical applications. *Am J Cardiol* 1985; **56**: 185–187.
10. Task Force of the Working Group on Arrhythmias of the European Society of Cardiology. The Sicilian Gambit: a new approach to the classification of antiarrhythmic drugs based on their actions on arrhythmogenic mechanisms. *Circulation* 1991; **84**: 1831–1851.
11. Cardiac Arrhythmia Suppression Trial (CAST) Investigators. Preliminary report: effect of encainide and flecainide on mortality in a randomized trial of arrhythmia suppression after myocardial infarction. *N Engl J Med* 1989; **321**: 406–412.
12. Basler JR. The rational use of intravenous amiodarone in the perioperative period. *Anesthesiology* 1997; **86**: 974–987.
13. Atlee JL, Bosnjak ZJ. Mechanisms for cardiac dysrhythmias during anesthesia. *Anesthesiology* 1990; **72**: 347–374.
14. Dennis DM, Raatikainen MJP. Therapy of dysrhythmias. *Curr Opin Anaesthesiol* 1996; **9**: 90–97.

15

MFM James, LH Opie

DRUGS IN THE MANAGEMENT OF HYPERTENSION

Systemic hypertension is an extremely common 21condition which afflicts between 10% and 20% of the population; it is the most common cardiovascular disorder affecting patients presenting for anaesthesia. Although there are no absolute definitions of hypertension, it is generally accepted that a blood pressure lower than 140/90 mmHg is normal, a blood pressure between 140/90 and 160/95 mmHg represents borderline or labile hypertension, and either a systolic pressure greater than 160 mmHg or diastolic pressure of 95 mmHg is regarded as frankly hypertensive. Most of the hypertension with which anaesthetists are presented is so-called 'essential hypertension' in which there is no clearly defined underlying cause. Only 5% of all hypertensive patients present with secondary hypertension in which some other condition such as an endocrine abnormality, renal disease, preeclampsia, drug reactions or coarctation of the aorta can be demonstrated. Chronic hypertension significantly increases both morbidity and mortality, and the incidence of coronary artery disease, stroke and renal dysfunction are all increased in relation to the severity of hypertension. The impact of hypertension on anaesthetic outcome is the subject of considerable debate.

PHYSIOLOGY OF BLOOD PRESSURE CONTROL

Blood pressure is the product of cardiac output and peripheral resistance, each of which is regulated by several interacting processes. The control of blood pressure is mediated through complex, overlapping, mechanisms which interact to produce appropriate responses in a wide variety of circumstances. Only a brief overview of these mechanisms is provided here.

Neuronal control, through the autonomic nervous system, provides rapid response adaptations of the circulation to minute-by-minute variations, while hormonal and renal mechanism provide more prolonged and gradual regulation. These mechanisms are summarized in diagrammatic form in Fig. 15.1.

AUTONOMIC NERVOUS SYSTEM

Autonomic control of cardiovascular function is regulated by a feedback mechanism in which the stretch receptors on the high and low pressure sides of the circulation send inhibitory signals to central processing areas of the brain, altering the rate of traffic flow in parasympathetic and sympathetic nerves. Baroreceptors on the arterial side of the circulation are situated in the carotid sinus and aortic arch, and form the first line of defence against hypotension. A decrease in distending pressure decreases their discharge frequency, with a consequent rise in sympathetic outflow and reduction of vagal tone.[1] The responsiveness of these receptors is impaired by anaesthesia and declines with age and in severe hypertension, an effect that may be reversed by the use of antihypertensive drugs such as calcium antagonists.[2] Stretch receptors in the atria and pulmonary arteries sense alterations in the venous filling volumes and inhibit the output of antidiuretic hormone (ADH, vasopressin) from the posterior pituitary gland, and also sympathetic outflow. Abnormalities of sympathetic tone and blood volume may contribute to the hypertensive state.

ENDOCRINE FACTORS

Renin–angiotensin system
This coordinated hormonal cascade plays a central role in the control of renal function, fluid and electrolyte

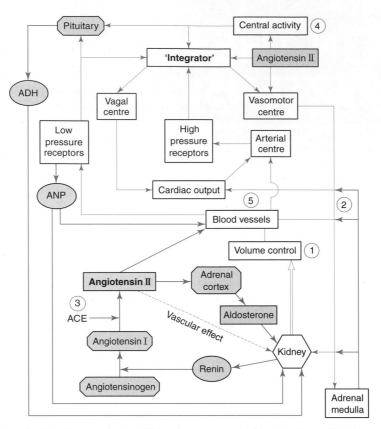

Fig. 15.1 Major pathways involved in the regulation of blood pressure and blood volume. The heavy lines indicate neural pathways and grey shading indicates hormonal regulation. The combination of blood vessel tone and blood volume will determine atrial stretch and the output of the low-pressure receptors; the same combination plus cardiac output determines arterial pressure. Atrial natriuretic peptide (ANP), antidiuretic hormone (ADH) and aldosterone all affect volume output from the kidney. Renin output is secondary to various interacting factors. See text for details. The numbers indicate sites of action of various agents used in the management of hypertension: 1, diuretics; 2, adrenergic antagonists; 3, angiotensin-converting enzyme (ACE) inhibitors; 4, centrally acting drugs; 5, direct vasodilators.

balance, and blood pressure regulation. Renin is produced by the juxtaglomerular apparatus in the kidney and cleaves angiotensinogen to produce angiotensin I. Angiotensin I is converted to angiotensin II by angiotensin-converting enzyme (ACE), a membrane-bound enzyme found on the plasma membranes of vascular endothelial cells. Renin release is increased by low sodium and chloride levels in the macula densa, decreased glomerular afferent arteriolar pressure, β_1-adrenoceptor stimulation, dopamine, prostaglandins and kinins. Release is inhibited by negative feedback from angiotensin II, vasopressin, atrial natriuretic peptide (ANP), nitric oxide and adenosine. Angiotensin II is one of the most powerful vasoconstrictor substances known, and it also stimulates the release of aldosterone from the adrenal cortex, resulting in sodium reabsorption in the kidney. Its major metabolite, angiotensin III is less powerful as a vasoconstrictor, but has a similar potency with regard to aldosterone release.

The renin–angiotensin system (RAS) also has important intrarenal effects, modulating renal vasoconstriction and increasing sodium and water reabsorption. In addition, angiotensin II stimulates the thirst centre in the hypothalamus, resulting in increased water intake. Angiotensin II also has direct effects on the brainstem, increasing sympathetic nervous system activity and peripherally stimulating sympathetic presynaptic receptors, thus enhancing the release of noradrenaline.[3]

The renin–angiotensin mechanism is also important at a local level, and all components of the system have been identified in tissues such as brain, heart and blood vessel walls.[4] Locally produced angiotensin II may be implicated in the development of cardiovascular pathology. Stimulation of local angiotensin II receptors leads to generation of inositol-1,4,5-triphosphate and diacylglycerol, which in turn will increase intracellular Ca^{2+} concentration (see Fig. 15.2). However, whether or not renin, angiotensinogen and angiotensin II are all actually synthesized at a vascular wall level remains the subject of dispute.[5]

Catecholamines

The endocrine function of the catecholamines is primarily related to acute responses such as the fight or flight response. Whether or not these agents are major factors affecting day-to-day or long-term blood pressure control, as postulated by the neurogenic theory of hypertension, is still open to dispute. Under normal circumstances, circulating noradrenaline does not exert significant endocrine effects as the noradrenaline concentration in plasma (< 400 pg/ml) is far below that required for vascular activity (> 2000 pg/ml), whereas adrenaline concentrations (< 80 pg/ml) are within the active range.[6] Noradrenaline released from sympathetic nerve terminals is locally active to promote a_1-mediated vasoconstriction and plasma noradrenaline concentration is mainly a reflection of this activity. Anti-adrenergic agents exert their effects primarily through actions on the sympathetic nervous system, rather than through actions on circulating catecholamines. Acute intra-operative events, such as the intubation response, may manifest increased catecholamine release and enhanced responses in hypertensive patients.

Atrial natriuretic peptide

ANP is produced from the atria in response to atrial distension. It increases renal blood flow, glomerular filtration rate (GFR) and sodium excretion, and decreases renin release, aldosterone production and release of vasopressin. It may have an integrated role in regulating the sympathetic nervous system, and may modulate the release of ADH. ANP inhibits vascular smooth muscle tone, but may also blunt baroreflex-mediated control of sympathetic activity in hypertension. ANP release is increased in patients with congestive cardiac failure.[7] It may be important in counteracting the undesirable effects of vasoconstrictor hormones during physical exercise and surgical stress.[8]

Antidiuretic hormone

The principal action of ADH is the reabsorption of water in the kidney. ADH is a potent vasoconstrictor, but under physiological conditions it has little direct effect on blood pressure as it exerts a central action which depresses cardiac output. Far more important is the renal effect, increasing water reabsorption and promoting sodium absorption and potassium excretion.[9] Thus ADH affects blood pressure primarily through effects on blood volume, rather than by alterations of vascular tone. Inhibition of ADH production is a feature of the postoperative period, and may contribute to fluid overload.

ENDOTHELIUM

Vascular endothelium plays a critical role in the regulation of vascular tone. The endothelium is a metabolically active site which extracts or metabolizes various substances including 5-hydroxytryptamine (5-HT) and angiotensin I. The endothelium also secretes a number of vasodilator substances including nitric oxide (NO), prostacyclin (prostaglandin I_2) and endothelium-derived hyperpolarizing factor. Several vasoconstrictors are also elaborated including the endothelins, angiotensin II and vasoconstrictor prostaglandins.[10] Endothelin-1 produces long-lasting vasoconstriction and is the most potent vasconstrictor yet identified. Vessel tone is dependent on the balance between these various factors, and the response of vascular smooth muscle to them, with the vasodilator factors normally predominant. The action of many vasoactive substances is mediated through endothelium-derived factors. These include acetylcholine, bradykinin, arachidonic acid, histamine, noradrenaline, 5-HT, substance P and vasopressin. Hypoxia, thrombin, stretch and a number of reducing substances inhibit the activity of vasodilator endothelial substances or increase the release of vasoconstrictors. Nitric oxide is extremely evanescent, as are many of the endothelial reactions, suggesting that these processes primarily mediate rapid vascular responses. This does not mean that the endothelium is inconsequential in hypertension, as inactivation of endothelium-derived nitric oxide can be shown in animal models of hypertension. Endothelial dysfunction may thus contribute to excessive vascular reactivity, and also contribute to the development of atherosclerosis and intravascular thrombus.[10] Current research into the development of antagonists of endothelium-derived substances (especially endothelin antagonists) may be of clinical significance in the future.

VASCULAR SMOOTH MUSCLE

Ionic balance across the cell membrane of vascular smooth muscle is critical in determining both the responsiveness of the cell to vasoconstrictor substances and also the concentration of calcium ions (Ca^{2+}) within the cytosol. The mechanisms controlling calcium flux across cell membranes are illustrated in Fig. 15.2. The sodium concentration gradient across the cell membrane is dependent on the sodium–potassium adenosine triphosphatase (ATPase) activity. Ca^{2+} is extruded from the cell in part by a Na^+–Ca^{2+} exchange mechanism which is driven by the inward Na^+ gradient. A rise in the cytosolic concentration of Na^+ diminishes this gradient and results in an increase in intracellular Ca^{2+} concentration, with a consequent increase in smooth muscle contraction. Altered ionic fluxes for sodium may thus result in increased intracellular Na^+ and raised cytosolic Ca^{2+} concentrations. Inhibition of the Na^+–K^+-ATPase

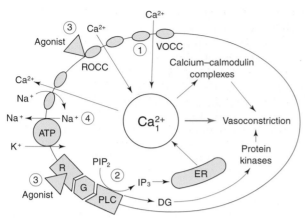

Fig. 15.2 Mechanisms regulating intracellular free cytosolic calcium concentrations. Ca^{2+} may enter the cell through voltage-operated calcium channels (VOCCs) in response to depolarization. Ca^{2+} influx may also follow binding of an appropriate agonist to a receptor-operated calcium channel (ROCC). Release of calcium from the endoplasmic reticulum (ER) is stimulated through the production of inositol triphosphate (IP_3) from phosphatidyl inositol biphosphate (PIP_2) by activated phospholipase C (PLC) in response to agonist binding to a receptor (R)–G protein (G) complex. The main extrusion mechanism for Ca^{2+} is the Na^+–Ca^{2+} antiporter, which is driven by the Na^+ gradient across the cell membrane. This gradient is maintained by the Na^+–K^+ adenosine triphosphatase (ATPase) pump. Calcium channel blockers affect vascular tone by inhibiting the influx of calcium through L-type VOCCs (1). Local angiotensin II receptors alter the production of IP_3 (2); this is a potential site for the action of angiotensin-converting enzyme inhibitors. Specific receptor antagonists alter agonist binding at receptor sites (3). Long-term diuretic use reduces the intracellular sodium content (4), thus increasing the efficiency of the Na^+–Ca^{2+} exchange pump and decreasing free cytosolic calcium concentration.

pump increases intracellular calcium by this mechanism. Enhanced cellular responsiveness to vasoconstrictors is a feature of hypertensive patients and of importance in their anaesthetic management.

PRINCIPLES OF PHARMACOLOGICAL CONTROL OF HYPERTENSION

Long-term treatment of hypertension results in significant reductions in the incidence of all cardiovascular and related complications. Current guidelines suggest that treatment should be instituted in patients with consistently raised arterial pressures of ≥ 90 mmHg diastolic or ≥ 140 mmHg systolic. Pharmacological interventions should be introduced on an individualized basis, with the aim of reducing the arterial pressure to below the above values. The heterogeneity of hyperten-

sion is such that it is impossible to predict the optimum form of management for any one patient; consequently the ideal regimen for an individual must be established by trial of various agents or combinations of agents.

A number of different groups of drugs may be used as first-line therapy. These include diuretics, adrenergic blocking agents (both α and β blockers), ACE inhibitors and calcium antagonists. Most of these agents are covered in detail in other chapters, and so this section will concentrate on their role in the management of hypertension and on the anaesthetic implications for patients receiving them.

The agents are grouped by their sites of action, and these are illustrated by the numbers in Fig. 15.1. The agents may be used as monotherapy or in combinations to achieve the best balance between control of blood pressure and side-effects.

DRUGS AFFECTING BLOOD VOLUME: DIURETICS

Many drugs used in the management of hypertension have some effect on blood volume, either directly or indirectly. Of these, the diuretics have the most obvious direct action. Although reduction in blood volume is an important component of the initial antihypertensive action of many drugs, prolonged diuretic therapy results in a gradual return of blood volume towards normal. The persistent antihypertensive effect of these drugs is more likely to be mediated through a reduction in the Na^+ content of vascular smooth muscle and consequently the cytosolic Ca^{2+} concentration (Fig. 15.2).

The diuretics used in hypertension can be divided into three groups: (1) the loop diuretics, which act mainly on the ascending limb of the loop of Henle; (2) the thiazides and related drugs acting at the proximal part of the distal convoluted tubule; and (3) potassium-sparing diuretics, which act at the terminal portion of the distal convoluted tuble and the collecting duct. The most potent natriuretics are the loop diuretics, which also have actions at the other sites, and which produce reabsorption of sodium in a dose-dependent fashion. The thiazides and related drugs (including indapamide) have a limited dose–response curve, and increasing dosage does not produce a proportionate increase in effect. The potassium-sparing diuretics act most distally in the nephron at the site of diminished Na^+–K^+ exchange.[3] The long-term use of diuretics has been shown to be associated with positive outcome benefit in several large studies. Despite their widespread use, the value of the diuretics has been questioned because of the side-effects. Besides the electrolyte disturbances, of which hypokalaemia and hypomagnesaemia are the most important, the thiazides may increase the risk of coronary artery disease through their effects on uric acid, glucose and lipid metabolism. The shorter-acting loop diuretics have not achieved the same popularity as the thiazides, but longer acting agents, such as torasemide, have been shown to be as efficacious and to have a similar side-effect profile.[11] The potassium-sparing agents are often combined with other diuretics to enhance natriuresis without excessive potassium loss. They should be avoided in renal failure where they may promote dangerous hyperkalaemia, and should generally not be used in combination with ACE inhibitors.

DRUGS AFFECTING ADRENERGIC RECEPTORS

The β-adrenergic blocking agents are competitive catecholamine antagonists at β-adrenergic receptors and have a well established place in the management of hypertension. Initial response to β blockade is brought about by a reduction in heart rate and cardiac output, and a more sustained response is the result of reductions in vascular tone, partly explicable by inhibition of renin release. Some agents (e.g. acebutolol, pindolol) have an intrinsic sympathomimetic effect, and the magnitude of the action on cardiac output is inversely proportional to this agonist activity. Blockade of peripheral presynaptic β_2 receptors at adrenergic nerve terminals causes a decreased release of noradrenaline and may contribute to a reduction in sympathetic vasoconstrictor tone. However, β blockers may merely shift the patient from a state of increased peripheral resistance and normal cardiac output to a state of low cardiac output with variable effects on peripheral vascular resistance.[12] Exceptions may include: (a) labetalol and carvedilol, which have both α- and β-blocking properties; (b) pindolol; and (c) bucindolol, which has nonspecific vasodilating properties. The adverse effects of the β blockers on airway resistance and blood glucose control can be mini-mized by the use of more selective β_1 antagonists such as atenolol.

Peripheral α-adrenergic blocking agents can be divided into nonselective α blockers and those that are more specific. The former are typified by phenoxybenzamine and phentolamine. Phenoxybenzamine is a long-acting agent which forms a covalent bond with α-adrenergic receptors, creating a noncompetitive block, which is particularly useful in the preoperative management of phaeochromocytoma (see below). Orthostatic hypotension is prominent and may contribute in intra-operative hypotension, and reflex tachycardia may result from its use. Phentolamine is a competitive, short-acting agent which also produces reflex tachycardia. Specific α_1-adrenergic blocking agents include prazosin, doxazosin and terazosin, and these lower blood pressure by a competitive inhibition of catecholamine-induced vasoconstriction.[13] Their selective postsynaptic α_1 action allows feedback inhibition by catecholamines at the presynaptic α_2 receptor, limiting further noradrenaline release at sympathetic nerve terminals. They cause dilatation of both arteries and veins, and the postural hypotension that they cause may limit their value. Prazosin is particularly likely to produce marked hypotension with the first dose. Sodium and water retention occur, but there is little change in renal function and these drugs are safe in renovascular hypertension. Ketanserin, the 5-HT receptor antagonist, has α_2 receptor blocking properties and may be of value in hypertensive crisis.[14] Urapidil, a postsynaptic α_1-adrenergic blocking agent, also exhibits some 5-HT antagonism, and both of these agents reduce peripheral vascular tone without an increase in heart rate or cardiac index.[15]

ANGIOTENSIN-CONVERTING ENZYME INHIBITORS

Initially, the ACE inhibitors were reserved for the treatment of severe unresponsive hypertension, but increasingly they are being used as first-line therapy. Interactions between the ACE inhibitors and other agents, notably the diuretics, can improve their efficacy significantly. Most of the ACE inhibitors are prodrugs which require conversion in the liver to the active compound after absorption. Impaired hepatic function can lead to slower onset of clinical action of these prodrugs.[4]

The mechanism of action of ACE inhibitors is complex, involving effects at the many sites at which angiotensin II is active (see Fig. 15.1). Plasma renin activity is usually increased due to the absence of inhibitory feedback from angiotensin II.[16] There is no consistent relationship between the level of systemic activation of the RAS and the efficacy of the ACE inhibitors, and the duration of hypotension exceeds the

Summary box 15.2 Angiotensin-converting enzyme (ACE) inhibitors

- Inhibit conversion of the inactive decapeptide angiotensin I to the active octapeptide angiotensin II by ACE.

- Two main mechanisms for reduction in blood pressure:

  - reduction in peripheral resistance with little effect on heart rate or cardiac output

  - reduces the renal retention of Na^+ secondary to reduction in aldosterone release.

- Effectiveness enhanced by concomitant administration of diuretics.

- With chronic use there is recovery of angiotensin II concentrations but blood pressure remains controlled.

- Few adverse effects; most common side-effect is persistent dry cough, possibly due to accumulation of bradykinin in the bronchial mucosa.

- Contraindicated in patients with bilateral renal stenosis (reduction in renal perfusion leads to renal failure).

duration of the ACE inhibition. Consequently, it has been suggested that tissue RAS activity is an important factor in the action of these drugs. ACE inhibitors generally increase renal blood flow and GFR, but in the presence of renal artery stenosis marked falls in GFR may occur with deterioration in renal function.

There is a wide range of ACE inhibitors available, and these drugs differ largely in terms of onset and duration of effect and, to a lesser extent, in terms of their route of elimination (Table 15.1). ACE inhibitors are contraindicated in patients with bilateral renal artery stenosis, and throughout pregnancy.

CENTRALLY ACTING AGENTS

A number of agents exert their antihypertensive effects primarily through actions on the central nervous system (CNS). These include methyldopa, reserpine and clonidine.

Methyldopa produces α-methylnoradrenaline, which is an intense stimulant of α_2-adrenergic receptors in the hypothalamus, and this is thought to be the predominant site of action, although a peripheral anti-adrenergic action cannot be excluded. Principal advantages of methyldopa include the preservation of renal, cerebral and myocardial blood flow, and minimal orthostatic hypotension. Its central parasympathetic action may produce bradycardia and it can cause significant sedation. Rebound hypertension on withdrawal of treatment occurs[17] and may be of relevance in the perioperative period. Reserpine depletes catecholamine stores, most notably in the CNS, and diminishes sympathetic outflow. Sedation is common and severe emotional depression may occur, although this is less relevant with the lower doses that are currently recommended. A reduction in anaesthetic requirements may be seen, but there is loss of responsiveness to indirect acting sympathomimetics, and an increased sensitivity to direct acting agents.

Table 15.1 Dosage and elimination of ACE inhibitors			
Drug	**Active substance**	**Elimination half-life (h)**	**Usual daily dose**
Class I: captopril-like			
Captopril	Captopril	4–6	25–50 mg twice daily
Class II: prodrugs			
Benazepril	Benazeprilat	21–22	5–80 mg in 1–2 doses
Cilazapril	Cilazaprilat	8–24	2.5–5 mg daily
Enalapril	Enalaprilat	11	5–20 mg in 1–2 doses
Fosinopril	Fosinoprilat	12	10–40 mg daily
Perindopril	Perindoprilat	27–60	4–8 mg daily
Quinapril	Quinaprilat	1.8	10–40 mg in 1–2 doses
Ramipril	Ramiprilat	34–113	2.5–10 mg daily
Trandolapril	Trandolaprilat	16–24	0.5–2 mg daily
Class III: water soluble			
Lisinopril	Lisinopril	7 or more	10–40 mg daily

Clonidine is a centrally acting α_2-adrenergic agonist which inhibits sympathetic outflow from the vasomotor centre, thus reducing blood pressure and cardiac output. It is particularly effective at reducing systolic blood pressure, with minimal orthostatic hypotension. Pretreatment with clonidine, in both normal and hypertensive patients, decreases anaesthetic requirements and enhances analgesia but may contribute to intraoperative hypotension and bradycardia.[18] An important consideration in anaesthesia is the severe rebound hypertension that may occur following withdrawal of the drug in patients receiving at least 0.2 mg per day for 1 week or longer. Rebound hypertension may occur as soon as 8 h and up to 36 h after the last dose.

A new generation of centrally acting agents, claimed to cause fewer central side-effects, acts on the imidazoline (I_1) receptors. These drugs, such as rilmenidine and moxonidine, have little effect on the central α_2 receptors that cause the central depressive side-effects.

DRUGS ACTING DIRECTLY ON BLOOD VESSELS

The calcium entry blockers are described in detail in Chapter 16. The short-acting direct vasodilators are considered later in the management of hypertensive crises, and also in Chapter 17.

Minoxidil is a potent arteriolar vasodilator, which may be effective in patients resistant to other medications. It may cause sodium retention and reflex tachycardia, and should only be given together with a β blocker and a diuretic. It may cause left ventricular hypertrophy as a side-effect, possibly due to sympathetic activation.

Calcium entry blockers

Calcium is rigorously excluded from the intracellular space, despite a 10 000-fold concentration gradient across the cell membrane. Ca^{2+} gains entry to the cytosol through either receptor- or voltage-operated channels (see Fig. 15.2). These latter can be divided into those permitting transient calcium currents (T channels), longer-acting channels passing larger quantities of calcium (L channels) and intermediate N channels. Most calcium entry blockers competitively inhibit the entry of calcium through the slow L channels in both the myocardium and peripheral vessels.[19] There are three main types of calcium antagonists, which have differing characteristics. Myocardial depression and vasodilatation may be potentiated by the combination of volatile anaesthetics and calcium antagonists. Long-acting calcium entry blockers are being used increasingly for the treatment of hypertension but the long-term safety of calcium antagonists as a group in hypertension has been questioned. Current evidence suggests that long-

term use of short-acting nifedipine may significantly worsen outcome in elderly hypertensive patients.[20]

HYPERTENSIVE CRISES

Hypertensive crisis is arbitrarily defined as a sudden, sustained increase of the diastolic pressure above 120 mmHg,[21] although the rate of increase in pressure is probably as important as the absolute level attained. The causes are summarized in Table 15.2. The urgency of the situation is determined more by symptomatology and end-organ dysfunction than by the specific value of the blood pressure. Thus patients with severe, but asymptomatic, hypertension should be regarded as urgent, and can be treated with oral drugs to reduce the pressure over 24 h. The presence of severe cerebral, renal or cardiac dysfunction may require intensive care unit (ICU) admission, invasive monitoring and intravenous therapy, and these cases should be regarded as true emergencies, even in the face of lower absolute arterial pressures. Maintenance of end-organ function is a more important objective than any predetermined target arterial pressure. Transient hypertensive episodes, such as those following endotracheal intubation, should not be regarded as hypertensive crises, unless they lead to sustained increases in arterial pressure.

The establishment of the definitive diagnosis is beyond the scope of this text, but it is critical that evidence of cerebral, cardiac and renal dysfunction is sought and that life-threatening surgical pathology is detected early, as the existence of such conditions will determine the selection of optimal therapy. In hypertensive crisis, the probability of secondary hypertension is markedly increased, and underlying pathology, particularly relating to the kidney, must be considered. In life-threatening situations, treatment may be required before a final diagnosis can be made but a good history (including drug history), a thorough clinical examination, electrocardiography, chest radiography and analysis of blood specimens should be performed to establish baselines.

URGENT HYPERTENSION

Where there is no immediate life-threatening complication, the aim should be a gradual reduction in blood pressure. Oral therapy with ACE inhibitors (such as captopril) or calcium entry blockers (such as nifedipine) are generally the first choice. Sublingual captopril is rapidly effective and has few side-effects, although it may be hazardous in the presence of renovascular disease. Short-acting nifedipine has little, if any, advantage given sublingually, as its absorption via this route is less efficient than when it is given as a bite-and-swallow capsule. Nifedipine capsules should be used with caution in patients with myocardial ischaemia

Table 15.2 Causes of hypertensive crisis	
Aggravated chronic hypertension (usually consequent on inadequate treatment and/or lack of compliance)	Essential Renovascular Parenchymal renal disease (e.g. glomerulonephritis)
Withdrawal of antihypertensive therapy	Notably with centrally acting agents (e.g. clonidine, α-methyldopa)
Drug ingestion or administration	β-agonists Cocaine, amphetamines, tricyclic antidepressants, monoamine oxidase inhibitor interactions
Central nervous system lesions	Head injury Spinal cord injury Guillain–Barré syndrome Tetanus
Collagen vascular diseases	
Surgical pathology	Ruptured cerebral aneurysm Thoracic aortic dissection
Surgical interventions	Carotid body manipulation Aortic cross-clamping Manipulations of secreting tumours
Preeclampsia or eclampsia	
Endocrine emergencies	Phaeochromocytoma Thyrotoxic crisis

as they may worsen the ischaemia or precipitate myocardial infarction. Prediction of the extent of blood pressure reduction is difficult and marked hypotension may follow the use of nifedipine; tachycardia is the major side-effect. The role of nifedipine in patients with raised intracranial pressure is debatable, as it may cause a reduction in cerebral perfusion pressure. Despite these disadvantages, the convenience of administration and relative infrequency of adverse effects make nifedipine a useful drug where there is little risk of myocardial ischaemia. Clonidine has a relatively slow onset of action and, like nifedipine, can cause steep reductions in perfusion pressure below critical levels. Diuretics have little place in the management of hypertensive emergencies unless there is accompanying pulmonary oedema.

HYPERTENSIVE EMERGENCIES

In the true emergency, the choice of drug therapy will depend on the underlying pathology, the severity of end-organ damage and the rate at which the blood pressure should be reduced. Intravenous agents are generally favoured, particularly those with short half-lives so that efficient titration of dosage to effect can be achieved with less risk of overshoot and hypotension (Table 15.3).

The aim should be to control arterial pressure whilst avoiding precipitous reductions which could impair end-organ perfusion. Where powerful intravenous agents are used, ICU management with invasive arterial pressure monitoring is advisable.

Sodium nitroprusside (SNP) is frequently the agent of choice owing to its rapid onset and offset of action, and generally good safety record. Current opinion favours the use of SNP as first-line therapy with replacement by longer-acting agents once the crisis is controlled.[22] Theoretically, SNP can cause cerebral vasodilatation, and its use in the presence of raised intracranial pressure is arguable, although it has been widely used in hypertensive encephalopathy. Nitroglycerin (glyceryl trinitrate) may be preferred in patients with significant myocardial ischaemia as it produces less tachycardia than SNP. However, it is slower in onset and its effect on arterial resistance is weak; about 15% of severe hypertensives are resistant to it and nitrate tolerance occurs with prolonged use.[23] Labetalol is a nonselective β-blocking drug with some α-adrenergic blocking properties (in a 7:1 ratio after intravenous injection) and may be useful in patients in whom tachycardia must be avoided. However, esmolol is more β_1 selective and its

Table 15.3 Drugs used for rapid blood pressure control				
Drug	**Administration**	**Onset**	**Duration**	**Comment**
Captopril	25 mg oral, sublingual	5–15 min Max 30–45 min	2–4 h	Hazardous in renal vascular disease; orally has slower onset
Nifedipine	Bite-and-swallow capsules 5–10 mg	10–30 min Max 30 min	3–6 h	Hypotension, hazardous in myocardial infarction; acute use only
Clonidine	0.1–0.2 mg oral	30–60 min	8–12 h	Sedation, heart block
Diazoxide	50–150 mg i.v. bolus	2–5 min	6–12 h	Hypotension, tachycardia, risk in myocardial infarction, hyperglycaemia
Enalapril	0.625–1.26 mg i.v. over 5 min	15 min	12–24 h	As for captopril
Hydralazine	5–10 mg i.v.	10–20 min	3–6 h	Hypotension, tachycardia
Esmolol	0.5–1.5 mg kg^{-1} i.v. then 50–100 μg kg^{-1} min^{-1} infusion	1–2 min	8–10 min	Depressed contractility, bronchospasm, heart block
Labetalol	20–80 mg i.v. every 10 min to max. 300 mg	5–10 min	3–6 h	As for esmolol; greater risk of bronchospasm
Magnesium sulphate	20–60 mg kg^{-1} i.v. Repeat boluses of 2 g as required to max. 20 g	1–3 min	10–15 min	Repeat doses hazardous in renal failure; potentiates nondepolarizing muscle relaxants
Phentolamine	5–10 mg i.v. every 15 min	2–4 min	3–10 min	Reflex tachycardia, angina
Trimethaphan	0.5–5 mg min^{-1} i.v.	1–5 min	10 min	Cycloplegia, paralytic ileus, hypotension, urinary retention
Nicardipine	5–15 mg h^{-1} i.v.	1–5 min	3–6 h	As for nifedipine but smoother blood pressure control
Nitroglycerin	5–100 μg min^{-1} i.v.	2–5 min	3–5 min	Headache, nausea, tolerance with prolonged use
Sodium nitroprusside	0.25–5 μg kg^{-1} min^{-1} i.v.	< 1 min	2–3 min	Cyanide toxicity with prolonged use; ICU monitoring required

Note: Onset times for oral agents indicate the commencement of action; 'max.' indicates the time at which the peak action of these agents may be expected to occur. With intravenous (i.v.) drugs, peak action is generally achieved within a few minutes of onset.

very much shorter duration of action may be preferable in the crisis situation. β blockers must be used with caution where peripheral vascular tone is elevated or where myocardial contractility is impaired. β blockers should be administered in small doses and titrated to effect. With esmolol the recommended loading dose of 1 mg/kg may be excessive in the crisis situation and 10 mg increments titrated to effect are to be preferred.

Intravenous verapamil will control blood pressure without producing tachycardia, but is also negatively inotropic. Nicardipine intravenously has been shown to be as efficacious as SNP and superior to nitroglycerin for control of mild to severe hypertension in the perioperative period. Although tachycardia and hypotension have been reported with this agent, comparative studies have shown nicardipine to produce less tachycardia than SNP. The onset of action is rapid, but it has a relatively long duration of action. Therapy may be commenced with 10 mg h^{-1} for 10 min, titrated against response in increments of 1–2.5 mg h^{-1} every 15 min thereafter. Hepatic dysfunction will delay clearance, and higher blood levels have been reported in the presence of renal failure.[24]

Preeclampsia and *eclampsia* are special circumstances where the blood pressure itself is a poor indicator of the level of risk, and considerations of fetal wellbeing alter drug selection. Hydralazine in doses of 5–10 mg is the most common first-line therapy but may cause reflex tachycardia. Magnesium sulphate is an effective vasodilator, but compensatory increases in cardiac output limit pressure reduction, and it is therefore mainly used to control convulsions rather than as an antihypertensive agent. If hydralazine is inadequate, consideration can be given to calcium entry blockers and labetalol. Intravenous nicardipine or nimodipine may prove particularly beneficial, but possible interactions between the calcium entry blockers and magnesium sulphate must be considered. SNP is generally avoided due to the risks of fetal toxicity. Diazoxide may cause precipitous falls in arterial pressure which may severely compromise uterine blood flow, and is no longer popular. Overaggressive reduction in blood pressure may compromise placental perfusion, and modest reductions in pressure rather than normalization should be the target.

PHAEOCHROMOCYTOMA

Pharmacological control of phaeochromocytoma commences with preoperative preparation. Although the benefit of preoperative a-adrenergic blockade has not been established conclusively, such preparation is now routine. Phenoxybenzamine is generally favoured because the competitive nature of the block produced by prazosin allows for breakthrough hypertension in the face of massive catecholamine release.[25] Phenoxybenzamine should be started with a dose of 20 mg daily in divided doses, but 250 mg daily may be required. Prazosin dosage should be increased in a stepped fashion from an initial daily dose of 2 mg to a maximum of 40 mg in divided doses. β blockers should be used only where there are clear indications of a predominance of β-mediated symptoms following the establishment of adequate a-adrenergic blockade. There have been a few recent reports on the use of calcium entry blockers, but there are insufficient data at present to assess their applicability and inadequate intraoperative control after diltiazem preparation has been reported.[26] Preoperative preparation is considered adequate when blood pressure is controlled to below 160/90 mmHg for 48 h and

orthostatic hypotension is present. Nasal congestion is also a useful indicator of adequate a blockade. The administration of an a blocker on the day of surgery is controversial, particularly phenoxybenzamine because of its prolonged duration of action. Where β blockade has been necessary, it is preferable not to have long-acting β blockade present at the time of surgery. A shorter-acting agent should be substituted on the day before operation, with the last dose given at least 12 h before induction. Drugs to be avoided include anticholinergics (particularly atropine), droperidol (which may inhibit catecholamine reuptake), substances that release histamine, and possibly halothane.

For intraoperative blood pressure control it is crucial to treat trends, rather than awaiting a specific level of pressure before changing treatment. Most authorities favour SNP, although adenosine infusions (at a rate of up to 200 μg kg^{-1} min^{-1}) have been used successfully. Phentolamine is no longer popular as both the onset and offset of action are rather slow. Calcium entry blockers, such as intravenous nicardipine, have been advocated on the rationale that they not only antagonize most of the peripheral actions of the catecholamines, but may also impede calcium-mediated hormone release. A similar rationale applies to the use of magnesium sulphate, which not only limits catecholamine release but is also an adrenergic antagonist and is highly effective against catecholamine-induced arrhythmias.[27] During the operation, β blockade is seldom necessary but, where needed, esmolol is the drug of choice; surprisingly low doses (10–20 mg) may be effective. Hypotension after tumour excision will generally respond to fluid therapy in a well prepared patient, but occasionally catecholamine support (usually with adrenaline) is needed for a few hours. Where magnesium sulphate has been used, calcium chloride (1 g) is an effective antagonist.

UNDIAGNOSED PHAEOCHROMOCYTOMA

This represents a considerable challenge as surgery in patients with undiagnosed phaeochromocytoma still carries a high mortality rate, although modern drugs and improved anaesthetic skills have reduced the risk considerably. The diagnosis should be suspected in patients in whom severe haemodynamic instability occurs during anaesthesia, without an obvious cause. Arrhythmias are frequently seen, and endtidal partial pressure of carbon dioxide may increase, but not as dramatically as may be seen with malignant hyperthermia or hyperthyroid crisis, which are the two major differential diagnoses. Other causes of hypertensive crises (see Table 15.2) should be considered. Once the condition is suspected, surgery should be halted immediately while pharmacological control is established. An infusion of SNP should be set up and titrated to effect;

nicardipine may be considered, but its use in this circumstance has not been reported. Alternatively, magnesium sulphate is rapidly effective in controlling both hypertension and arrhythmias, although doses of up to 12 g over a period of 15 min have been necessary. Where necessary, β blockade with esmolol should be instituted to control arrhythmias, but not before the establishment of adequate afterload reduction. Longer-acting β-blocking drugs should be avoided. Early establishment of large-bore central lines and central venous pressure monitoring is essential, as fluid requirements may be unpredictable.

MANAGEMENT OF HYPERTENSION DURING ANAESTHESIA

Preoperative hypertension predicts intraoperative haemodynamic instability and postoperative hypertension, but the influence of hypertension on perioperative mortality remains unresolved.[28] However, preoperative hypertension increases the risk of postoperative cardiovascular complications, overall morbidity and prolonged hospital stay.[29] The impact of antihypertensive therapy on perioperative morbidity is not clear-cut. A recent extensive review[30] concluded that none of the data currently available establishes definitively that the treatment of hypertension alters outcome following anaesthesia and surgery. Perioperative modulation of the sympathetic nervous system by β-adrenergic blockade, a_2-adrenergic stimulation with clonidine, deep anaesthesia or regional blockade may reduce the incidence of complications, but definitive outcome data are lacking.[30]

Delaying elective surgery on the grounds of hypertension is seldom justified unless the diastolic blood pressure is consistently above 115 mmHg or serious, treatable, end-organ dysfunction is present. Isolated systolic hypertension above 200 mmHg may also justify preoperative therapy, but the data are as yet unclear. Where end-organ dysfunction is less than optimally treated, operation should be delayed to allow institution of optimal therapy. Complications of drug treatment, such as marked electrolyte disturbances, may be grounds for delaying surgery.

The duration of time for which therapy should be introduced before subjecting the patient to surgery is also not established. For diuretic therapy to be useful, it should be instituted several weeks before operation. Agents such as the calcium entry blockers and the ACE inhibitors may be effective very rapidly and reduce the blood pressure within 24 h, but it is unlikely that such rapid reductions in blood pressure improve perioperative risks. If the objective is to reduce exaggerated cardiovascular responsiveness, treatment will take several weeks to be effective. It is of interest that the use of calcium entry blockers for at least 30 days will restore baroreceptor responsiveness, and thus should improve intraoperative haemodynamic stability.[31] The best plan for a patient with inadequately treated severe hypertension would appear to be to delay elective surgery for at least 1 month from the time of institution of appropriate antihypertensive therapy. Where surgery is urgent and cannot be delayed, attempts at short-term control of blood pressure before operation may do more harm than good. Careful anaesthetic management, with intraoperative control of cardiovascular function and fluid balance, is probably a better option.

PREOPERATIVE MANAGEMENT

Antihypertensive medication should not be withdrawn before surgery but should be continued for the entire perioperative period. Withdrawal of some drugs, including β blockers and particularly clonidine, can produce rebound hypertension or tachycardia, and consideration must be given to sustaining appropriate antihypertensive therapy throughout the perioperative period. All antihypertensive agents have implications for anaesthesia which are summarized in Table 15.4. Diuretics may produce electrolyte disturbances leading to increased arrhythmia risk. The β blockers may provoke bronchospasm and intraoperative bradycardia, and care must be taken in combining them with nonvagolytic anaesthetic combinations (for example, propofol, vecuronium and fentanyl). Calcium entry blockers may enhance the potential of the inhalational agents to cause vasodilatation, cardiac depression and conduction delays. There have been several studies that have suggested that marked hypotension and bradycardia may occur in patients taking ACE inhibitors, although the hypotension generally responded readily to fluid loading. A comparative study of the cardiovascular stability of untreated hypertensive patients or those taking one of ACE inhibitors, β blockers, calcium entry blockers or diuretics found no significant differences among any of the groups.[32]

The inclusion of a β blocker in the premedication may decrease the incidence of silent myocardial ischaemia but the impact of this on overall morbidity has not been established. Premedication with clonidine 5 μg kg^{-1} reduces intraoperative haemodynamic instability and may reduce the incidence of ST segment changes, but also increases the incidence of intraoperative bradycardia requiring intervention.[18]

INTRAOPERATIVE MANAGEMENT

Control of endotracheal intubation response

Hypertensive patients may show exaggerated haemodynamic responses at the time of tracheal intubation,

Table 15.4 Anaesthetic implications of antihypertensive medication		
Drug type	Action or side-effect	Comment
Diuretics Thiazides and loop diuretics	Hypokalaemia Hypomagnesaemia Hyperglycaemia Alkalosis	Relative hypovolaemia Arrhythmia risk Thiazides prolong muscle relaxant action
Potassium sparing	Hyperkalaemia Hyponatraemia	Risks in renal failure
Adrenergic antagonists β blockers	Decreased myocardial contractility Increased airway resistance	Bradycardia with vagotonic anaesthetic agents Rebound tachycardia Risk of myocardial infarction on withdrawal Risk in asthma and chronic obstructive airway disease
α blockers	Peripheral vasodilatation	Hypotension Poor response to blood loss
ACE inhibitors Captopril Enalapril Lisinopril and others	Inhibit conversion of angiotensin I to angiotensin II	Hypotension, bradycardia Relative hypovolaemia Airway angioedema (rare)
Centrally acting agents Methyldopa	Central α_2-adrenergic stimulation Orthostatic hypotension	Rebound hypertension Decreased anaesthetic requirements, sedation
Reserpine	Depletes catecholamine stores	Resistance to indirect-acting vasoconstrictors
Clonidine dexmedetomidine	Central α_2-adrenergic stimulation	Decreased anaesthetic and analgesic requirement Haemodynamic stability Bradycardia, hypotension Diuretic effect Severe rebound hypertension
Direct vasodilators Calcium entry blockers	Block calcium influx at L-type channels	Additive effects on contractility and vasodilatation with volatile agents and opiates Decreased anaesthetic requirement Potentiate neuromuscular blockade (especially with myopathies)

and it is essential that adequate depth of anaesthesia is attained before intubation is attempted. Induction agents alone are usually insufficient. In patients with ischaemic heart disease, esmolol (up to 2 mg kg^{-1}) is useful for controlling intubation-related tachycardia, and the opiates have a well established role in this regard; remifentanil may prove particularly useful. Numerous other drugs have been used with varying degrees of success for this problem, including lignocaine (1.5 mg kg^{-1}), the nitrates, magnesium sulphate (especially in preeclampsia, 40–60 mg kg^{-1}) and intravenous ACE inhibitors. Lignocaine is probably the least reliable and must be given at least 2–3 min before

intubation to be effective. Dexmedetomidine (0.6 μg kg^{-1} intravenously) reduces anaesthetic induction doses and may be useful for controlling intubation responses; however, it may produce postinduction hypotension in both the hypertensive and normotensive patient.

All these agents have their supporters and specific areas of application where they are particularly valuable. Overenthusiastic use of these techniques, however, may result in excessive hypotension in the interval between intubation and the commencement of surgery. If an exaggerated hypertensive response occurs, despite adequate depth of anaesthesia, aggressive treatment may result in severe hypotension. This response is usually short lived and, if no immediate risks are evident, the best plan is to observe the patient for a few minutes and treat the hypertension only if it is persistent.

Anaesthetic technique

There are no conclusive data to suggest that the anaesthetic technique itself affects outcome in hypertensive patients. However, tachycardia is most likely to occur where isoflurane or desflurane is used; arrhythmias are most common with halothane, and hypertension is more likely with an opioid-based technique. There are no significant differences in haemodynamic events in patients anaesthetized with sevoflurane or isoflurane, although there may be a trend towards a slower heart rate with sevoflurane.[33] Total intravenous anaesthesia with propofol–alfentanil mixtures may be associated with fewer cardiovascular emergence events than isoflurane.[34]

Intraoperative hypertensive crises are most commonly due to inadequate anaesthesia, although hypertensive crisis from other causes (see Table 15.2) may arise during anaesthesia. Phaeochromocytoma, thyroid crisis, carcinoid syndrome and malignant hyperpyrexia must all be considered and managed appropriately. Increasing depth of anaesthesia, correction of ventilatory abnormalities and provision of analgesia should be used before cardiovascular drugs. All of the agents used for hypertensive emergencies have been used for intraoperative hypertension. However, the possible interaction of cardiovascular drugs with anaesthetic agents must be born in mind. In particular, β blockers must be given cautiously and in smaller doses than is generally recommended for the non-anaesthetised patient.

Surgical interventions such as carotid artery or aortic clamping are associated with predictable episodes of hypertension, and plans should be made in advance to manage these episodes. A number of agents and techniques has been suggested, including preoperative clonidine, epidural anaesthesia, β blockers and vasodilators. During operation, nitroglycerin is generally the first choice if myocardial ischaemia is present, and is usually sufficient unless a suprarenal aortic cross-clamp is applied. SNP is valuable for resistant hypertension but its safety with regard to spinal cord ischaemia in thoracoabdominal aortic surgery has been questioned. A bolus of magnesium sulphate (2–4 g) has also proved valuable in controlling hypertension and arrhythmias at cross-clamp, and may offer some spinal cord protection.[35] Amrinone, an inodilator (loading dose, 1 mg kg^{-1}, infusion 5–20 $\mu g\,kg^{-1}\,min^{-1}$), has been compared successfully with SNP, and the use of adenosine has also been described. Too little information is currently available to recommend either of these drugs at the present time.

POSTOPERATIVE CARE

Postoperative hypertension is particularly likely after aortic surgery, carotid endarterectomy, coronary artery grafting and craniotomy. The extubation response may provoke a severe hypertensive and tachycardic response, and steps should be taken to protect the patient at this phase. Good postoperative analgesia should be established early – preferably *before* the patient recovers from anaesthesia. Immediate postanaesthesia hypertension and tachycardia are associated with a significant increase in risk of ICU admission and of death. The frequency of these events is associated with intraoperative hypertension, but unaffected by intercurrent medication.[36] Control of postoperative hypertension, once adequate analgesia is established, may be instituted with a wide variety of agents, as used for hypertensive crises. Of these, labetalol, hydralazine and nifedipine have been amongst the most widely used, with SNP and nitroglycerin being more popular for postcardiac surgical cases. Esmolol, given as a continuous infusion, may be particularly useful in patients after cardiac surgery.

The patient's normal antihypertensive drugs should be restarted as soon after anaesthesia as possible. Bed rest and opiate analgesia both tend to lower the blood pressure and may reduce the need for early reinstatement of normal oral therapy. However, if hypertension persists in the postoperative period, it would seem wise to reinstate an appropriate form of therapy, particularly in those at risk from ischaemic cardiac events.

SUMMARY

Hypertension represents a significant risk factor for perioperative morbidity. Good perioperative management of the hypertensive patient requires an understanding of the physiology of blood pressure control and a knowledge of the pharmacology of antihypertensive agents. Management of hypertensive crises may demand the use of powerful, intravenously administered, hypotensive agents. Preoperative preparation of the hypertensive patient includes good clinical evaluation of the extent of the disease processes and an appropriate decision, based on the adequacy of cardiovascular control, as to the advisability of proceeding with elective surgery. Intraoperative management is based on an understanding of the likely consequences of both the hypertensive disease and the medications that the patient may be taking. Good control of depth of anaesthesia, fluid balance and vascular tone is necessary. Establishment of good analgesia before recovery from anaesthesia, together with the use of appropriate cardiovascular drugs, forms the basis for the care in the postoperative period.

REFERENCES

1. Spyer KM. CNS organisation of reflex circulatory control. In: Loewy AD, Spyer KM (eds) *Central Regulation of Autonomic Functions*. New York: Oxford University Press, 1990: 3–16.

2. Kiowski W, Erne P, Bertel O, Bolli P, Bühler F. Acute and chronic sympathetic reflex activation and antihypertensive response to nifedipine. *J Am Coll Cardiol* 1986; **2**: 344–348.

3. Waeber B, Brunner HR. Antihypertensive agents: mechanisms of drug action. In: Hollenberg NK (ed.) *Hypertension: Mechanisms and Therapy*. Philadelphia: Current Medicine, 1994; 7.1–7.14.

4. Kellow NH. The renin–angiotensin system and angiotensin converting enzyme (ACE) inhibitors. *Anaesthesia* 1994; **49**: 613–622.

5. van Lutterotti N, Catanzaro DF, Sealy JE, Laragh JH. Renin is not synthesized by cardiac and extrarenal vascular tissues: a review of experimental evidence. *Circulation* 1994; **89**: 458–470.

6. Cryer PE. Physiology and pathophysiology of the human sympathoadrenal neuroendocrine system. *N Engl J Med* 1980; **303**: 436–444.

7. Zhu ST, Chen YF, Wyss JM et al. Atrial natriuretic peptide blunts arterial baroreflex in spontaneously hypertensive rats. *Hypertension* 1996; **27**: 297–302.

8. Blake DW, McGrath BP, Donnan GB et al. Influence of cardiac failure on atrial natriuretic peptide responses in patients undergoing vascular surgery. *Eur J Anaesthesiol* 1991; **8**: 365–371.

9. Breyer MD, Ando Y. Hormonal signalling and regulation of salt and water transport in the collecting duct. *Annu Rev Physiol* 1994; **56**: 711–739.

10. Daugherty MO, Rich GF, Johns RA. Vascular endothelium. *Curr Opin Anaesthesiol* 1995; **8**: 88–94.

11. Schmieder RE, Rockstroh JK. Efficacy and tolerance of low-dose loop diuretics in hypertension. *Cardiology* 1994; **84** (Suppl. 2): 36–42.

12. Messerli FH. Antihypertensive therapy – going to the heart of the matter. *Circulation* 1990; **81**: 1128–1135.

13. Grimm RH. a_1-Antagonists in the treatment of hypertension. *Hypertension* 1989; **13** (Suppl. 1): 131–136.

14. Vandenbroucke G, Floubert L, Evenpoel MC. Hemodynamic effects of ketanserin in the treatment of hypertension following CABG: a double-blind placebo-controlled study. *J Cardiovasc Thorac Anesth* 1990; **3** (Suppl. 1): 3.

15. Langtry HD, Mammen GJ, Sorkin EM. Urapidil: a review of its pharmacodynamic and pharmacokinetic properties, and therapeutic potential in the treatment of hypertension. *Drugs* 1989; **38**: 900–940.

16. Mirenda JV, Grissom TE. Anesthetic implications of the renin–angiotensin system and angiotensin-converting enzyme inhibitors. *Anesth Analg* 1991; **72**: 667–683.

17. Husserl FE, Messerli FH. Adverse effects of antihypertensive drugs. *Drugs* 1981; **22**: 188–210.

18. Hayashi Y, Maze M. Alpha 2 adrenoceptor agonists and anaesthesia. *Br J Anaesth* 1993; **71**: 108–118.

19. Foëx P. Drugs acting on the cardiovascular system. In: Healy TEJ, Cohen PJ (eds) *Wylie and Churchill-Davidson's A Practice of Anaesthesia*, 6th edn. London: Edward Arnold, 1995: 189–216.

20. Messerli FH. What happened to the calcium antagonist controversy? *J Am Coll Cardiol* 1996; **28**: 12–13.

21. Calhoun DA, Oparil S. Treatment of hypertensive crisis. *N Engl J Med* 1990; **323**: 1177–1183.

22. Friederich JA, Butterworth JF IVth. Sodium nitropusside: twenty years and counting. *Anesth Analg* 1995; **81**: 152–162.

23. Munzel T, Kurz S, Heitzer T, Harrison DG. New insights into echanisms underlying nitrate tolerance. *Am J Cardiol* 1996; **77**: 24C–30C.

24. Tran HT, Kluger J, Chow MSS. Focus on nicardipine HCl: iv formulation approved for the treatment of hypertension. *Hospital Formulary* 1994; **29**: 114–120.

25. Pullerits J, Ein S, Balfe JW. Anaesthesia for phaeochromocytoma. *Can J Anaesth* 1988; **35**: 526–534.

26. Munro J, Hurlbert BJ, Hill GE. Calcium channel blockade and uncontrolled blood pressure during phaeochromocytoma surgery. *Can J Anaesth* 1995; **42**: 228–230.

27. James MFM. Use of magnesium sulphate in the anaesthetic management of phaeochromocytoma: a review of 17 anaesthetics. *Br J Anaesth* 1989; **62**: 616–623.

28. Mangano DT. Perioperative cardiac morbidity. *Anesthesiology* 1990; **72**: 153–184.

29. Ferraris VA, Ferraris SP. Risk factors of postoperative morbidity. *J Thorac Cardiovasc Surg* 1996; **111**: 731–741.

30. Roizen MF. Anesthetic implications of intercurrent disease. In: Miller RD (ed.) *Anesthesia*, 4th edn. New York: Churchill-Livingstone, 1994: 903–1014.

31. Luna RL, Carrasco RM. Efficacy of verapamil in patients resistant to other hypertensive therapy. *Am J Cardiol* 1986; **57**: 64D–68D.

32. Sear JW, Jewkes C, Tellez JC, Foex P. Does the choice of antihypertensive therapy influence haemodynamic responses to induction, laryngoscopy and intubation? *Br J Anaesth* 1994; **73**: 303–308.

33. Rooke GA, Ebert T, Muzi M, Kharasch ED. The hemodynamic and renal effects of sevoflurane and isoflurane in patients with coronary artery disease and chronic hypertension. Sevoflurane Ischemia Study Group. *Anesth Analg* 1996; **82**: 1159–1165.

34. Mutch WA, White IW, Donen N et al. Haemodynamic instability and myocardial ischaemia during carotid endarterectomy: a comparison of propofol and isoflurane. *Can J Anaesth* 1995; **42**: 577–587.

35. Robertson CS, Foltz R, Grossman RG, Goodman JC. Protection against experimental ischemic spinal cord injury. *J Neurosurg* 1986; **64**: 633–642.

36. Rose DK, Cohen MM, DeBoer DP. Cardiovascular events in the postanesthesia care unit: contribution of risk factors. *Anesthesiology* 1996; **84**: 772–781.

16

HB van Wezel, JG van der Stroom, MB Vroom, M Pfaffendorf

CALCIUM ENTRY BLOCKERS

The concept of drug-mediated calcium antagonism was introduced by Albrecht Fleckenstein in the late 1960s, when he observed that verapamil mimicked in a reversible fashion the effect of calcium withdrawal on cardiac function and that the resulting loss of myocardial contractility could be overcome through increased calcium concentration.[1] Since their introduction in the early 1970s, the calcium entry blockers have been widely used in patients with coronary artery disease, hypertension and cardiac arrhythmias.

The family of calcium entry blockers consists of three major classes of pharmacological agents: phenylalkylamines (parent drug verapamil), dihydropyridines (parent drug nifedipine) and benzothiazepines (parent drug diltiazem). Their beneficial clinical effects are due to a wide range of pharmacological properties associated with the use of these agents.[2] These properties include coronary and peripheral vasodilatation, antispasmic effect, reduction in myocardial oxygen consumption and increase in supply, reduction in triggered electrical activity, prevention of intracellular calcium overload and antiplatelet effects. Furthermore, a large number of well documented clinical trials in patients with coronary disease has demonstrated that chronic oral use of calcium entry blockers leads to a reduction in angina and ischaemic episodes and to an increase in exercise tolerance.

For the management of hypertensive emergencies and acute hypertension developing in the perioperative period, the short-acting dihydropyridine nicardipine is being used increasingly.[3] Nicardipine is approved for this indication in most western European countries and the United States. For the prevention and therapy of supraventricular arrhythmias, verapamil and diltiazem are used. Nimodipine is being evaluated for the reduction of morbidity and mortality in patients with subarachnoid haemorrhage.

MECHANISM OF ACTION

At the end of the last century it was shown that calcium is essential for the excitation–contraction coupling process.[4] The intracellular concentration ($> 0.1 \mu$mol l^{-1}) of free calcium ions is more than four orders of magnitude lower than the extracellular concentration (1.3 mmol l^{-1}). An increase above 0.1μmol l^{-1} by a calcium ion influx and/or a release from intracellular stores results in an interaction of calcium with specific binding sites on regulatory proteins such as troponin C (in skeletal and cardiac myocytes) or calmodulin (in smooth muscle cells). These reactions trigger other processes, including the cross-bridging between actin and myosin, which finally result in muscle contraction. One major prerequisite of this system is the ability of the cell membrane to withstand the enormous concentration gradient of calcium ions, which means that under resting conditions the membranes must be virtually impermeable for Ca^{2+} (Fig. 16.1). Furthermore, active transport mechanisms such as the Ca^{2+} adenosine triphosphatase (ATPase) or the Na^{+}–Ca^{2+} exchanger eliminate free Ca^{2+} from the cytosol. On the other hand the huge concentration gradient allows a rapid increase of the intracellular free Ca^{2+} concentration simply by changing the membrane permeability for calcium ions.

CALCIUM ION CHANNELS

Calcium ion channels are specialized membrane-spanning proteins that selectively allow calcium ions to flow in the direction of their concentration gradient

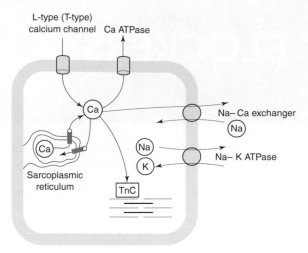

Fig. 16.1 Schematic representation of calcium handling in the myocytes: voltage-dependent Ca^{2+} influx via L-type calcium channels, Ca^{2+} release from the sarcoplasmic reticulum and the Na^+–Ca^{2+} exchanger. The Na^+ gradient is kept constant by the activity of Na^+–K^+ adenosine triphosphatase (ATPase). Contraction is initiated by interaction between Ca^{2+} and troponin C (TnC).

from the extracellular space to the cytosol. These calcium channels are glycoproteins which form a water-filled pore in the membrane. Specific binding sites for calcium in the interior of the pore form a selective filter for Ca^{2+}. The conformation of these channel proteins and thereby the calcium permeability of the whole membrane critically depends on the electrical potential

---

Summary box 16.1 Intracellular calcium and calcium channels

- Increases in intracellular Ca^{2+} concentration $[Ca^{2+}]_i$ are responsible for activation of widespread cellular processes, including muscle contraction, synaptic transmission, secretion and membrane excitability.

- Voltage-gated Ca^{2+}-selective ion channels are primarily responsible for the regulation of $[Ca^{2+}]_i$.

- Opening of these channels allows Ca^{2+} to enter the cell down a very large concentration from the extracellular fluid (1.3 mmol l^{-1}) to the cytosol (approximately 0.1 μmol l^{-1}).

- Calcium channel blockers prevent the opening of L-type Ca^{2+} channels, which are involved in excitation–contraction and excitation–secretion coupling, and impulse formation and propagation.

(voltage) over the membrane. This potential, which can range from -30 to -100 mV, dependent on the cell type, originates mainly from an unequal distribution of positive (Na^+, K^+) and negative charged (Cl^-) ions between the cytosol and extracellular space. The conformation of the calcium channel cycles in a voltage-dependent manner between an open state in which calcium can flow, an inactive state in which the channel is closed but refractory, and an impermeable but excitable resting state (Fig. 16.2). Depolarization increases the probability of the channel protein being in the open state, whereas after repolarization or at the resting potential the closed conformations are clearly favoured.

Several of these specialized voltage-operated channels have been characterized functionally by electrophysiological studies using specific blockers such as nifedipine, funnel web spider toxin ω-Aga-IVA or ω-conotoxin.[5] They are classified by their predominant location (e.g. the neuronal N-type or the Purkinje P-type calcium channel) or their functional characteristics (e.g. transiently activated T-type or long-lasting large-capacitance L-type calcium channel). The N-type channel, located almost exclusively on neuronal tissue, is activated by a strong depolarization and has a conductance of 12–20 pS (picoSiemens = $10^{-12} \times 1/\Omega$), and plays an important role in the regulation of neurotransmitter release. It is insensitive to organic calcium entry blockers, a property shared with the T-type channel. The T-type channel is more widely distributed and has been described in neurons, smooth muscle and skeletal muscle cells. In the heart it is found in pacemaker and conducting tissue. This type is activated by small depolarization and has only a small and transient conductance of 8 pS. These characteristics of the T-type channel suggest that it is more involved in the initiation of action potentials than in contributing to the cellular calcium homeostasis. L-type calcium channels are also widely distributed. They have large conductance (25 pS) and prolonged opening times that strongly influence the cellular calcium concentration. L-type channels are involved in excitation–contraction and excitation–secretion coupling, and in impulse formation and propagation. This channel is a complex with a molecular weight of about 400 kDa, composed from four subunits: the a_1 (212 kDa) which contains the binding sites for all calcium antagonists and the calcium conducting pore, the disulphide linked a_2/δ subunit (125 kDa), the intracellularly located β subunit (57 kDa) and the membrane-spanning γ subunit (25 kDa).

Although calcium channels are influenced primarily by the membrane potential, they can react to certain hormones, neurotransmitters and even mechanical stimuli such as stretch. Specific phosphorylation sites on the interior part of the channel protein allow their

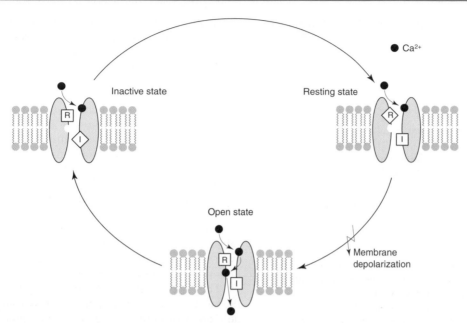

Fig. 16.2 Three conformational states of L-type calcium channels. Two specific binding sites form the selectivity filter for calcium ions (●). In the 'open state' Ca^{2+} can flow through, whereas in the refractory 'inactive state' and the excitable 'resting state' the channel is impermeable. The probability of changing from one state to the other is potential dependent. R, Resting state; I, Inactive state.

function to be modulated from inside the cell by protein kinases.[5] Many organic compounds interact with calcium channels but only those with a specific action on these structures will be discussed here.

CALCIUM ENTRY BLOCKERS

In 1964 Fleckenstein and coworkers[1] demonstrated that drugs are able to interfere with cellular calcium metabolism. They investigated a number of chemically heterogeneous compounds which induced an electromechanical uncoupling similar to a withdrawal of calcium. Resembling a classical pharmacological antagonism, this effect could be overcome in a concentration-dependent manner by increasing the extracellular calcium concentration. These experiments led to the term calcium antagonists. It is now recognized that this is not a true antagonism in the sense of competition for a similar binding site, but an interference of the compounds with the voltage-dependent calcium channels. Therefore a more appropriate terminology is calcium entry blockers. Alternative terms are calcium channel blockers, slow channel blockers, slow channel inhibitors, calcium channel inhibitors or calcium channel modulators.

The classical calcium entry blockers interact almost exclusively with L-type channels.[6] There are sites on the a_1 subunit of the L-type channel protein that selectively bind organic ligands and modulate the function of the whole structure. An inhibition (antagonism) and, although far less common, an activation (agonism) can be induced by this interaction. The main classes of therapeutic calcium entry blockers are 1,4-dihydropyridines (nifedipine), phenylalkylamines (verapamil) and benzothiazepines (diltiazem).

TYPES OF BINDING SITES

Since these three groups of calcium entry blockers represent very different chemical structures that are unlikely to interact with the same receptor, at least three distinct specific binding sites have been postulated. The affinity of these receptors is not constant but depends on the conformation of the channel protein. Since the latter is influenced by the membrane potential, the affinity of calcium entry blockers for their specific sites, and thereby their effect, is voltage dependent. Binding is highest in the 'inactive state' of the L-type channel. Once bound to the channel in this conformation, calcium entry blockers delay the recovery of the channel to the excitable 'resting state'. As a result the structure remains longer in the impermeable and refractory conformation and less Ca^{2+} can enter the cell. This 'modulated receptor model' is derived from the basic idea about the voltage-dependent mechanism of action of local anaesthetics on the fast Na^+ channel.

231

ALLOSTERIC INTERACTION OF CALCIUM ENTRY BLOCKERS

There is experimental evidence that all three receptors for calcium entry blockers are located on the a_1 subunit of the L-type channel and that they influence each other allosterically, i.e. the occupation of one receptor subtype influences the binding characteristics of the other two. For example, the benzothiazepine diltiazem inhibits the binding of the phenylalkylamine verapamil but promotes the binding of the 1,4-dihydropyridine nifedipine.

STEREOSELECTIVITY OF CALCIUM ANTAGONISTS

Calcium entry blockers bind stereoselectively to their specific binding site. If a compound is a mixture of two or more isomeric forms of the molecule, these will bind with different affinities and induce effects of different magnitude. Although the quality of the effect is generally the same for the isomers, in some cases, especially in the group of 1,4-dihydropyridines, the isomers can

produce opposite effects, one being an inhibitor of Ca^{2+} influx the other being an influx promoter.

Although L-type channels with their specific binding sites for calcium entry blockers are present in almost all excitable cells, there are remarkable tissue differences in the potency and efficacy of the compounds. Phenylalkylamines and benzothiazepines are nearly equipotent in vascular smooth muscle and cardiac myocytes. On the other hand, 1,4-dihydropyridines are more potent in dilating blood vessels than in depressing cardiac function. In therapeutic doses nifedipine and structurally related compounds have few or no cardiac depressing properties. Calcium entry blockers have little effect on venous smooth muscle, most probably because of a low density of L-type calcium channels. Therefore calcium entry blockers, in contrast to other vasodilators such as a_1-adrenoceptor antagonists or nitrates, have little influence on the cardiac preload.

This tissue selectivity might partly be explained by the fact that some tissues, such as veins, are less dependent on extracellular Ca^{2+} than others, such as the atrioventricular (AV) node. Since the affinity of the receptors for calcium entry blockers is voltage dependent, differences in the resting potential of different tissues (vascular smooth muscle −30 to −40 mV; cardiac myocyte −70 to −90 mV) might explain the vascular selectivity as it is seen for 1,4-dihydropyridines in arterial vascular smooth muscle compared with cardiac tissue.

FREQUENCY DEPENDENCY OF CALCIUM ENTRY BLOCKERS

The effect of calcium entry blockers is also dependent on the rate of conformation changes. Assuming that calcium entry blockers when bound to their specific receptor increase the time necessary for the channel to change its conformation from the refractory 'inactive' state to the excitable 'resting' state, an increase of stimulation frequency will result in an increasingly incomplete recovery. Thus, the efficacy of the calcium entry blockers increases with increasing stimulation frequency. This effect is most pronounced for the phenylalkylamines and weakest for the 1,4-dihydropyridines. Beside these functional differences there is a heterogeneity within the population of L-type calcium channels concerning the affinity for the ligands which are responsible for the diverse profiles of action seen with the different groups of calcium entry blockers but also among particular compounds within the same group.

CARDIOVASCULAR EFFECTS OF CALCIUM CHANNEL BLOCKERS

ARTERIAL BLOOD PRESSURE

All calcium entry blockers lower arterial blood pressure both when given acutely and with prolonged administration.[7] There appears to be little difference in blood pressure-lowering potency among the various agents, provided that adequate doses are given. There is evidence that calcium entry blockers are more potent in elderly patients and patients of African origin, presumably because of the lower activity of the renin–angiotensin system compared with young or white patients. Also, when pretreatment pressure is high, the pressure-lowering effect of calcium entry blockers will be more pronounced.

HEART RATE

Calcium entry blockers lower arterial pressure by decreasing peripheral resistance. This leads to baroreflex-mediated sympathetic activation, reflex tachycardia and increased cardiac output. An increase in plasma catecholamine and plasma renin activity usually accompanies the positive chronotropic effect.[7] Reflex tachycardia is particularly obvious following acute administration of calcium entry blockers, but may become less pronounced with chronic administration. Reflex tachycardia is especially common with the short-acting, water-soluble dihydropyridines nifedipine, nitrendipine and nicardipine. With verapamil, diltiazem and the longer-acting, lipid-soluble dihydropyridines usually no significant changes in heart rate occur. It has been suggested that the direct effect of these compounds on the sinus node prevents the reflex tachycardia that is so obvious with the old short-acting dihydropyridines.

CORONARY BLOOD FLOW

All calcium entry blockers are coronary vasodilators and therefore increase coronary blood flow (Table 16.1). It must, however, be emphasized that coronary blood flow is but one determinant of the myocardial oxygen supply–demand equilibrium. Other determinants, such as heart rate, contractility and arterial pressure, are also profoundly and variably affected by the different types of calcium entry blockers.[8] Thus, their overall effect on myocardial oxygenation will depend on an interplay of these mechanisms. Under certain conditions some calcium entry blockers may have a detrimental effect on the myocardial oxygen supply:demand ratio, leading to ischaemia, unstable angina pectoris and myocardial infarction.[9] The exact aetiology of these untoward effects is not clear, but most ischaemia-related adverse events have been associated with the short-acting nifedipine and not with its longer-acting formulation or any of the other calcium entry blockers. Generally, calcium entry blockers will improve oxygenation by unloading the heart, increasing coronary blood flow and reducing myocardial energy consumption.

CARDIAC CONDUCTION

The nondihydropyridine calcium entry blockers, in particular, decrease the automaticity of the sinus node, slow conduction in the AV node and have little or no effect on the automaticity of myocytes.[10] However, the electrophysiological properties vary considerably between drugs and may also depend on the route of administration. Intravenous administration of verapamil leads to significant reduction of AV conduction and even AV block. In contrast, after oral administration of verapamil, AV block is extremely rare. Both verapamil and diltiazem cause a slight prolongation of the PR interval in the electrocardiogram. The dihydropyridines in general have little effect on cardiac conduction.

MYOCARDIAL CONTRACTILITY

Although verapamil and diltiazem exert the most potent negative inotropic effect, all calcium entry blockers possess some degree of myocardial depressant activity.[11] This direct effect is partially offset by afterload reduction

Table 16.1 Pharmacodynamic profile of the parent compounds of the three major classes of calcium entry blockers			
	Phenylalkylamines (verapamil)	1,4-Dihydropyridines (nifedipine)	Benzothiazepines (diltiazem)
Peripheral vasodilatation	++	+++	+
Coronary vasodilatation	++	+++	+++
Conduction	– –	No effect	– –
Heart rate	–	(+)	–
Contractility	– –	(+)	–

and reflex sympathetic activation, especially with the dihydropyridines. Some of the newer agents such as isradipine, felodipine and amlodipine appear to have minimal negative inotropic activity even at supratherapeutic doses. Felodipine has been used successfully in patients with congestive heart failure.[12] As a general rule, however, most calcium entry blockers should be used with extreme care in patients with congestive heart failure. This applies to both chronic oral and acute intravenous applications.

DIASTOLIC RELAXATION
Calcium entry blockers appear to have a favourable effect on both early diastolic active relaxation and late diastolic passive distensibility. The effect on early relaxation may be heart rate dependent and seems to be most pronounced with verapamil, less so with diltiazem and almost absent with the dihydropyridines. The clinical importance of the reduction in left ventricular filling pressure in hypertensive patients is not fully understood.

CARDIOPROTECTION
Calcium entry blockers that lower heart rate should be reserved for patients following myocardial infarction, provided that they have normal left ventricular function. Verapamil especially appears to reduce the reinfarction rate significantly when therapy is started within 7 days after acute myocardial infarction.[13] Calcium entry blockers may exert a protective effect during global ischaemia associated with cardiopulmonary bypass by suppressing energy-dependent Ca^{2+}-mediated activity of the myocardium. Theoretically, the combination of blockade of slow channels with calcium entry blockers and of fast channels with cold cardioplegic hyperkalaemic solution may result in an even greater reduction in myocardial oxygen consumption than either intervention alone. However, although there are animal experimental studies showing that calcium entry blockers may protect against global ischaemic injury and reperfusion injury induced by extracorporeal circulation and aortic cross clamping,[14] there is no strong evidence demonstrating that they have a beneficial cardioprotective effect in cardiac surgical patients under clinical conditions.

CARDIOVASCULAR INDICATIONS OF CALCIUM CHANNEL BLOCKERS

ANGINA PECTORIS
The antianginal mechanisms of calcium entry blockers are complex and not yet fully understood. The drugs exert peripheral and coronary artery vasodilator activity and they have a depressant effect on myocardial

---

Summary box 16.3 Therapeutic indications for calcium channel blockers

- Angina pectoris (diltiazem and dihydropyridines); reduced myocardial oxygen consumption secondary to lowering of preload and coronary artery vasodilatation are the main mechanisms.

- Hypertension.

- Supraventricular tachydysrhythmias; verapamil and diltiazem are used for the treatment (intravenous) and prevention (oral) of supraventricular tachycardia, including atrial flutter.

- Cerebral artery vasospasm and cerebral protection; nimodipine reduces the risk of cerebral spasm after subarachnoid haemorrhage.

---

contractility and conduction. These actions may all mediate the beneficial effect of calcium entry blockers on the ratio between myocardial oxygen supply and demand.

Stable angina pectoris
Multiple double-blind placebo-controlled studies have clearly confirmed the efficacy of diltiazem, nicardipine, nifedipine, verapamil, felodipine and amlodipine in patients with stable angina pectoris, reducing attacks of pain and nitroglycerin consumption and improving exercise tolerance. Although monotherapy with calcium entry blockers appears to be safe and effective in patients with stable angina, these agents are usually combined with β-adrenoceptor antagonists and nitrates. This approach may be more efficacious than one drug used alone. Because adverse events may occur from this combination (heart block, bradycardia, congestive heart failure), the type and dosage of calcium entry blocker and β-adrenoceptor antagonist should be chosen carefully for each patient.

Surprisingly, there are no studies in patients with stable angina pectoris aimed at demonstrating a reduction in morbidity or mortality. This lack of information is partly due to the fact that the calcium entry blockers are relatively old drugs which were studied when relief from angina *per se* was considered a worthwhile therapeutic goal in symptomatic patients. An exception is the recent Angina Prognosis Study in Stockholm, which showed that verapamil administered to patients with stable angina pectoris offers the same prognostic benefits as metoprolol.[15]

Unstable angina pectoris
This is an ischaemic syndrome that covers a wide range of disorders, ranging from variant angina associated

with ST segment elevation and angiographically normal coronary arteries (Prinzmetal angina) to unstable angina pectoris with ST segment depression or elevation associated with severe multivessel coronary artery disease.

Calcium entry blockers are effective in the treatment of variant angina because of their ability to block spontaneous or drug-induced coronary vasospasm. Both verapamil and nifedipine appear to be more effective than propranolol at reducing symptomatic and asymptomatic episodes of myocardial ischaemia. This is in keeping with the concept that coronary vasospasm plays an important role in patients with angina at rest. Accordingly, in the management of patients with variant angina, the choice of calcium entry blocker (verapamil or nifedipine) is determined not so much by the effectiveness of the drug but by patient tolerance. In contrast, propranolol may exacerbate vasospastic phenomena rather than provide any benefit.

In 1989 the first metaanalysis of all clinical trials of calcium entry blockers in unstable angina and acute myocardial infarction was published.[16] Twenty-eight randomized trials involving 19 000 patients were included in the analysis, which suggested a slightly unfavourable effect of calcium entry blockers. No attempt was made to differentiate between the different classes of calcium entry blockers. Subsequently the Second Danish Verapamil Trial (DAVIT II) showed that there is an important difference among the different classes of calcium entry blockers, and reinfarction occurred significantly more frequently following acute myocardial infarction in patients treated with nifedipine but not with verapamil or diltiazem.[17] The chronic oral use of short-acting nifedipine in patients with coronary heart disease was reported to be associated with a dose-related increase in mortality rate.[18] At the same time the US National Heart, Lung and Blood Institute issued a statement warning that short-acting nifedipine should be used with 'great caution' if at all. This finding led to turmoil in the cardiological world and the major conclusion is that within the large family of calcium entry blockers there are important differences between and even within the classes.

The dihydropyridines act selectively on smooth muscle tissue and their therapeutic effect is obtained mainly by a reduction in afterload. Myocardial contractility and heart rate are either unchanged or increased. Under some conditions this may lead to increased myocardial oxygen consumption,[19] which of course is undesirable in patients with unstable angina or acute myocardial infarction. The short-acting form of nifedipine (used as monotherapy) in particular appears to possess these undesirable effects. The aetiology of these adverse effects is not yet fully understood, but it has been suggested that nifedipine may exert a direct proischaemic effect on the myocardium, especially during preexisting ischaemia.[18] The longer-acting slow-release formulation of nifedipine and its longer-acting derivatives felodipine, amlodipine and nicardipine appear to be safe, with or without concomitant β-adrenoceptor antagonist therapy.

In contrast to the dihydropyridines, the phenyl-alkylamines and benzothiazepines are less specific for vascular smooth muscle tissue. They exert a calcium antagonist effect at different levels, namely the myocardium, the conduction system and vascular smooth muscle tissue, resulting in negative inotropy and chronotropy, as well as afterload reduction.

SYSTEMIC HYPERTENSION

Calcium entry blockers are effective in the chronic treatment of systemic hypertension, but also for the acute management of hypertensive emergencies and perioperative hypertension. The mechanism of the antihypertensive properties of calcium entry blockers includes peripheral vasodilatation, antiadrenergic and natriuretic activities. They may be considered as a first-line therapy for initiating treatment in patients with essential hypertension. These include patients with preexisting disease (diabetes mellitus, asthma, gout, peripheral vascular disease) that limits or precludes the use of other antihypertensive agents. The calcium entry blockers reduce both systolic and diastolic pressure with a minimal number of side-effects (orthostasis). Left ventricular hypertrophy may regress in hypertensive patients treated with these agents.[20] Surprisingly, they do not appear to lower arterial blood pressure in normotensive patients.[20] For the management of acute hypertension and perioperative hypertension most calcium entry blockers are theoretically useful, but only the dihydropyridines, because their relative absence of negative inotropic effects, are commonly used. Nicardipine,[3] and in some countries also isradipine,[21] are approved for the prevention and therapy of hypertensive emergencies and perioperative hypertension. Both agents are available for intravenous administration.

SUPRAVENTRICULAR TACHYDYSRHYTHMIAS

Both verapamil and diltiazem are available for the oral or intravenous management of supraventricular arrhythmias associated with high ventricular rates. Except in rare situations, these agents are ineffective in converting acute or chronic atrial fibrillation to normal sinus rhythm. Virtually all cases of supraventricular tachycardia, including atrial flutter, respond promptly and predictably to intravenous verapamil or diltiazem, whereas only two-thirds of ectopic atrial tachycardias convert to sinus rhythm after adequate doses of these drugs.[22]

The recommended dose range of verapamil for terminating supraventricular tachycardia in adult patients with normal left ventricular function is 0.075–0.15 mg kg^{-1} infused over 1–3 min and repeated after 30 min. For diltiazem the recommended dose is a 0.25 mg kg^{-1} intravenous bolus, followed by a second bolus of 0.35 mg kg^{-1} if the response is inadequate, followed by a maintenance infusion of 10–15 mg h^{-1}.[23]

CORONARY ARTERY VASOSPASM AND PERIOPERATIVE MYOCARDIAL ISCHAEMIA

Coronary vasospasm or hyperdynamic coronary constriction is characterized by angina pectoris that occurs at rest in association with electrocardiographic ST changes, but not preceded by haemodynamic abnormalities. It has been suggested that coronary vasospasm plays an important role in the occurrence of perioperative myocardial ischaemia, since these ischaemic events are usually not associated with haemodynamic changes that may cause ischaemia.[24] Theoretically calcium entry blockers could be effective in the prevention and therapy of coronary artery spasm. However, it has been clearly demonstrated that the incidence of perioperative ischaemia is not altered by chronic treatment with these agents.[24]

CEREBRAL ARTERY VASOSPASM AND CEREBRAL PROTECTION

Cerebral arterial vasospasm leads to focal or diffuse constriction of one or more of the larger arteries at the base of the brain. Vasospasm occurs frequently between 4 and 14 days after subarachnoid haemorrhage and may cause irreversible neurological damage. The initial event in the development of vasospasm may be an intracellular influx of Ca^{2+} leading to contraction of large cerebral arteries.

Although verapamil and nifedipine have been shown to prevent cerebral arterial spasm in experimental studies, nimodipine has demonstrated a preferential cerebrovascular effect in patients with subarachnoid haemorrhage. Recently, Barker and Ogilvy[25] reported findings from a metaanalysis of all published randomized trials of prophylactic nimodipine used in patients with subarachnoid haemorrhage. Seven trials were included with a total of 1202 patients. They confirmed the significant efficacy of prophylactic nimodipine in improving outcome after subarachnoid haemorrhage. However, nimodipine does not appear to possess cerebral protective properties. Legault et al.[26] conducted a double-blind randomized clinical trial in patients undergoing cardiac valve replacement. They found a higher incidence of bleeding and an increased postoperative mortality rate in the patients given nimodipine. The effect on coagulation observed in this study does not appear to be a common property of all calcium entry blockers.

INDIVIDUAL DRUGS

DIHYDROPYRIDINES

The 1,4-dihydropyridines, such as nifedipine, are predominantly vasodilators at the level of peripheral resistance vessels and coronary arteries (Fig. 16.3). In concentrations that reduce blood pressure effectively, these compounds have little or no primary cardiac activity but, dependent on the time course of the onset of action, they can induce reflex activation of the sympathetic system which will, owing to the absence of a cardiodepressant action of the drug, result in a tachycardia.

The most common side-effects of 1,4-dihydropyridines are related to their vasodilator activity (headache, flush, palpitations). They induce a mild natriuretic effect which prevents the fluid retention often seen with other vasodilators. Since the introduction of nifedipine a large number of new 1,4-dihydropyridine derivatives has been developed. Although they generally display the

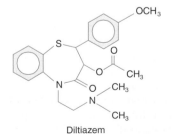

Fig. 16.3 Chemical structure of the three parent compounds of the major classes of calcium entry blockers. Highlighted are the characteristic, name-giving parts of the molecules: 1,4-dihydropyridines (nifedipine), phenylalkylamines (verapamil), benzothiazepines (diltiazem).

same pharmacodynamic behaviour as nifedipine, there are marked differences in their physicochemical characteristics (e.g. lipophilicity) which influences their pharmacokinetics. There are, however, some differences in clinical effects within the family of dihydropyridines that are of importance. To avoid reflex tachycardia and to allow a once-daily scheme of drug intake, more lipophilic compounds with a slow onset but long duration of action are preferred. For the same reasons, older drugs such as nifedipine or nisoldipine are available in slow-release formulations. Some drugs show selectivity towards particular vessel beds (e.g. nisoldipine – coronary arteries; nimodipine – cerebral arteries; manidipine – renal arteries) but this has been substantiated in clinical practice only for nimodipine.

Nifedipine

Nifedipine is the prototype of the dihydropyridines. It is used in the treatment of angina and hypertension, and in Raynaud phenomenon. In some countries an intravenous formulation is available. This is particularly useful in the management of acute and perioperative hypertension, because of the relative absence of a negative inotropic effect. The intravenous formulation is very light sensitive and must be administered in special black plastic syringes and infusion lines.

Nicardipine

Nicardipine is a newer dihydropyridine than nifedipine. It has a number of practical advantages over nifedipine, including the absence of light sensitivity and better solubility in water. After intravenous administration nicardipine produces arterial vasodilatation within 1–3 min. The duration of action after intravenous bolus administration is 10–15 min. It has been suggested that nicardipine has a higher degree of vasoselectivity and less negative inotropic activity than nifedipine. Equipotent doses (with respect to the effect on coronary blood flow) of intracoronary nifedipine and nicardipine resulted in a significant depression of left ventricular dP/dt (rate of rise in left ventricular pressure) in the patients given nifedipine only, and not in those given nicardipine.[27] In patients undergoing coronary artery bypass grafting surgery, nicardipine was equally effective as nitroprusside in controlling arterial blood pressure and maintaining stable haemodynamic conditions, especially in the control of hypertension following sternotomy.[3] In addition, patients treated with nicardipine showed a significantly lower incidence of ischaemic episodes than those treated with nitroprusside. These and other studies have led to the increasing use of nicardipine in the management of hypertension in peri-operative patients. To achieve rapid reduction of arterial blood pressure with nicardipine a bolus of 1–2 mg intravenously can be given, followed by a maintenance infusion at a rate of 10–15 mg h^{-1}. Once blood pressure is satisfactorily reduced, a maintenance infusion of 3 mg h^{-1} is usually effective.

First-generation calcium entry blockers such as nifedipine lack or have only a moderate degree of vascular selectivity and inhibit cardiac function at doses that cause arterial dilatation. This may lead to deterioration in patients with impaired left ventricular function and the combination of these drugs with β-adrenoceptor antagonists may adversely affect cardiac conduction and contractility. Development of newer agents has focused on obtaining a higher degree of vascular selectivity.

Felodipine

Felodipine has a higher degree of vascular selectivity than nifedipine, with a vascular : myocardial selectivity ratio greater than 100. Haemodynamic studies in patients with hypertension, coronary artery disease or congestive heart failure, or patients taking β-adrenoceptor antagonists, have shown that felodipine can produce profound arteriolar dilatation without signs of negative inotropic activity.[28]

Isradipine

Isradipine is a long-acting dihydropyridine derivative with potent arteriolar vasodilatation, negative chronotropic action and minimal effects on contractility and conduction.[20] Like nicardipine, isradipine has been approved for the intravenous prevention and therapy of perioperative hypertension in a number of European countries. However, due to its long duration of action (mean terminal half-life 8 h), this agent is not widely used.

Amlodipine

In contrast to agents whose duration of action is prolonged by the use of sustained-release gastrointestinal formulations, the metabolism of amlodipine allows a once-daily dosage. Amlodipine is inactivated by liver metabolism. It is bound extensively to plasma proteins. The haemodynamic effects and side-effects of amlodipine are similar to those of the other newer dihydropyridines. In particular, reflex tachycardia does not appear to occur and amlodipine can be used in patients with some reduction in myocardial contractility. However, the onset of action is much slower than that of, for example, nifedipine (3.5 h versus 30 min), possibly due to slow association with and dissociation from the receptor. It also has a very long half-life (35–50 h).

Lacidipine

Lacidipine is one of the newest dihydropyridines available for the treatment of hypertension.[29] Like amlodipine, it produces a sustained antihypertensive effect when given once daily. It is highly vascular-selective in all or most arterioles. Lacidipine has pronounced antiatherogenic properties in animal models of atherosclerosis, but whether this is also so in humans remains to be determined.

PHENYLALKYLAMINES

The first and main representative of this group is verapamil (Fig. 16.3), a vasodilator with additional cardiodepressant effects. Besides negative inotropy, these compounds also induce a negative chronotropic and dromotropic effect. For this reason no reflex tachycardia is seen with verapamil (given orally). In addition to the reduction of vascular tone and subsequent antihypertensive effect, verapamil can also be used for the treatment of supraventricular tachycardia. Although somewhat less common, the side-effects are comparable to those of 1,4-dihydropyridines. Verapamil should be used with caution in patients with heart failure or impaired atrioventricular conduction. In contrast to the 1,4-dihydropyridines, very few new phenylalkylamine derivatives have emerged. Gallopamil is a verapamil derivative discovered soon after verapamil. It has properties similar to those of verapamil.

BENZOTHIAZEPINES

This group is represented by diltiazem (Fig. 16.3), a compound with pharmacodynamic properties intermediate between those of 1,4-dihydropyridines and phenylalkylamines. For oral use immediate-release tablets and sustained-release preparations for both once-daily and twice-daily use are available. An intravenous preparation is also available. With long-term administration, saturation of hepatic first-pass metabolism is possible so that diltiazem pharmacokinetics become nonlinear. This can also result in a dose-related increase in absolute bioavailability. Diltiazem causes less negative inotropy than either verapamil or nifedipine, and evidence of adverse effects on cardiac function is unusual in patients with serious left ventricular dysfunction. Indeed, diltiazem may have beneficial effects in patients with congestive heart failure by decreasing afterload and improving cardiac output. Diltiazem also improves diastolic function in patients with hypertension, coronary disease and hypertrophic cardiomyopathy. The side-effect profile of diltiazem is superior to that of verapamil or nifedipine; this is a significant advantage in long-term treatment. Diltiazem, and probably also verapamil, are metabolized by the cytochrome

P450 enzyme, CYP 3A4. Both are potent inhibitors of this enzyme and interact with a variety of drugs including propranolol, carbamazepine, cyclosporine and benzodiazepines. They significantly increase the bioavailability of midazolam and triazolam, and prolong the elimination half-life.[30,31] These changes in pharmacokinetics are associated with profound and prolonged sedative effects.

Diltiazem is used mainly in the therapy of angina pectoris. Like all calcium entry blockers, it is a potent vasodilator with antihypertensive activity, but has never been used extensively for this indication.

FUTURE DEVELOPMENTS IN CALCIUM ENTRY BLOCKADE

A number of new calcium channel blocking agents are currently under development. At the present time clevidipine and mibefradil are undergoing clinical trials in patients.

CLEVIDIPINE

Clevidipine is an ultrashort-acting dihydropyridine, specially developed for intravenous use to control blood pressure during surgery.[32] Unlike most dihydropyridines, which are oxidized by the cytochrome P450 system, clevidipine is metabolized by ester hydrolysis by nonspecific tissue and blood esterases, resulting in rapid inactivation. The initial half-life of clevidipine in humans is 1.5 min, with a terminal half-life of about 10 min. Its hypotensive effect is rapid in onset and at the end of drug infusion blood pressure returns to baseline values within minutes.

Clevidipine reduces blood pressure by arteriolar dilatation without any detectable venodilatation or negative inotropic activity, even at higher infusion rates. The haemodynamic profile of clevidipine thus resembles that of the other longer-acting vasoselective calcium entry blockers (felodipine, amlodipine, isradipine), but because of its pharmacokinetic profile clevidipine allows for control of rapid changes in blood pressure such as may occur during and after (cardiac) surgery.

DRUG INTERACTIONS

Verapamil and β-adrenoceptor antagonists, when used in combination, can have additive negative inotropic effects. This may be worsened by concomitant use of cimetidine and possibly other H_2-receptor antagonists. Hyperkalaemia may develop in patients using verapamil who are given perioperative dantrolene.[32] Hypotension has been reported during fentanyl anaesthesia, when both esmolol and nicardipine were administered intravenously. This may be explained by the fact that dihydropyridines increase the bioavailability and plasma levels of some β-adrenoceptor antagonists.[33] Nicardipine can increase cyclosporin concentrations, making it necessary to monitor these levels carefully when both compounds are used together.

CONCLUSION

Calcium entry blockers have a variety of cardiovascular effects that make them extremely valuable for the chronic oral management of patients with hypertension, coronary artery disease and supraventricular arrhythmias. Their use in patients in the perioperative period is limited to the acute treatment of perioperative hypertension (nicardipine, isradipine) and some supraventricular arrhythmias (verapamil, diltiazem). It must be emphasized that acute myocardial ischaemia is not an indication for intravenous therapy with the currently available calcium entry blockers.

REFERENCES

1. Fleckenstein A. Specific inhibitors and promotors of calcium action in the excitation contraction coupling of heart muscle and their role in the prevention of myocardial lesions. In: Harris, P, Opie LH (eds). *Calcium and the Heart*. London: Academic Press, 1971: 135–188.
2. Braunwald E. Mechanism of action of calcium channel blocking agents. *N Engl J Med* 1983; **307**: 1618–1627.
3. van Wezel HB, Koolen JJ, Visser CA, Dijkhuis JP, Moulijn AC, Deen L. Antihypertensive and anti-ischemic effects of nicardipine and nitroprusside in patients undergoing coronary artery bypass grafting. *Am J Cardiol* 1989; **64**: 22H–27H.
4. Ringer S. A further contribution regarding the influence of the different constituents of the blood on the contraction of the heart. *J Physiol (Lond)* 1883; **4**: 29–42.
5. Hofmann F, Biel M, Flockerzi V. Molecular basis for Ca²⁺ channel diversity. *Annu Rev Neurosci* 1994; **17**: 399–418.
6. Triggle DJ. Calcium-channel drugs: structure–function relationships and selectivity of action. *J Cardiovasc Pharmacol* 1991; **18** (Suppl. 10): S1 S6.
7. Schmieder RE, Messerli FH, Garavaglia GE, Nunez BDI. Cardiovascular effects of verapamil in patients with essential hypertension. *Circulation* 1987; **75**: 1030–1036.
8. van Wezel HB, Bovill JG, Koolen JJ, Barendse G, Fiolet JWT, Dijkhuis JP. Myocardial metabolism and coronary sinus blood flow during coronary artery surgery: effects of nitroprusside and nifedipine. *Am Heart J* 1987; **113**: 266–273.
9. Brown BG, Bolson EL, Dodge HT. Dynamic mechanisms in human coronary stenosis. *Circulation* 1984; **70**: 917–922.
10. Singh BN, Nademanee K. Use of calcium antagonists for cardiac arrhythmias. *Am J Cardiol* 1987; **59**: 153B–162B.
11. de Buitleir M, Rowland E, Krikler DM. Hemodynamic effects of nifedipine given alone or in combination with atenolol in patients with impaired left ventricular function. *Am J Cardiol* 1985; **55**: 15E–20E.
12. Dunselman PH, Kuntze CE, van Bruggen A *et al.* Efficacy of felodipine in congestive heart failure. *Eur Heart J* 1989; **10**: 354–364.
13. Danish Study Group on Verapamil in Myocardial Infarction. Effect of verapamil on mortality and major events after acute myocardial infarction. *Am J Cardiol* 1990; **66**: 779–785.
14. Przyklenk K, Kloner RA. Effect of verapamil on post-ischemic 'stunned myocardium': importance of the timing of treatment. *J Am Coll Cardiol* 1988; **11**: 614–623.
15. Rehnquist N, Hjemdhal P, Billing E *et al.* Prevention of cardiac events in patients with angina pectoris: results of the APSIS study. *Eur Heart J* 1995; **16** (Suppl. H): 18.

16. Held P, Yusuf S, Furberg CD. Calcium channel blockers in acute myocardial infarction and unstable angina: an overview. *BMJ* 1989; **299**: 1187–1192.
17. Yusuf S, Held P, Furberg CD. Update on effects of calcium antagonists in myocardial infarction and angina in light of the Second Danish Verapamil Infarction Trial (Davitt-II). *Am J Cardiol* 1991; **67**: 1295–1297.
18. Furberg CD, Psaty BM, Meyer JV. Nifedipine. Dose-related increase in mortality in patients with coronary heart disease. *Circulation* 1995; **92**: 1326–1331.
19. van Wezel HB, Bovill JG, Koolen JJ, Barendse GAM, Fiolet JWT, Dijkhuis JP. Myocardial metabolism and coronary sinus blood flow during coronary artery surgery: effects of nitroprusside and nifedipine. *Am Heart J* 1987; **113**: 266–273.
20. Leslie J, Brister N, Levy JH *et al.* Treatment of postoperative hypertension after coronary artery surgery. Double blind comparison of intravenous isradipine and sodium nitroprusside. *Circulation* 1994; **90**: II-256–261.
21. Cummings DM, Amadio P, Nelson L, Fitzgerald JM. The role of calcium channel blockers in the treatment of systemic hypertension. *Arch Intern Med* 1991; **151**: 250–259.
22. Singh BN, Nademanee D, Baky S. Calcium antagonists: uses in the treatment of cardiac arrhythmias. *Drugs* 1983; **25**: 125–153.
23. Ellenbogen KA, Dias VC, Plumb VJ, Heywood JT, Mirvis DM. A placebo controlled trial of continuous intravenous diltiazem infusion for 24-hour heart rate control during atrial fibrillation and atrial flutter: a multicenter study. *J Am Coll Cardiol* 1991; **18**: 891–897.
24. Slogoff S, Keats AS. Does chronic treatment with calcium entry blocking drugs reduce perioperative myocardial ischemia? *Anesthesiology* 1988; **68**: 676–680.
25. Barker FG, Ogilvy CS. Efficacy of prophylactic nimodipine for delayed ischemia deficit after subarachnoid hemorrhage: a metaanalysis. *J Neurosurg* 1996; **84**: 405–414.
26. Legault C, Furberg CD, Wagenknecht LE *et al.* Nimodipine neuroprotection in cardiac valve replacement. *Stroke* 1996; **27**: 593–598.
27. Visser CA, Koolen JJ, van Wezel HB, Jonges R, Hoedemaker G, Dunning AJ. Effects of intracoronary nicardipine and nifedipine on left ventricular function and coronary sinus blood flow. *Br J Clin Pharmacol* 1986; **22**: 313S–318S.
28. Nordlander MIL, Messerli FH. Felodipine. In: Messerli FH (ed.) *Cardiovascular Drug Therapy*. Philadelphia: Saunders, 1996; 1040–1046.
29. Lee CR, Bryson HM. Lacidipine. A review of its pharmacodynamic and pharmacokinetic properties and therapeutic potential in the treatment of hypertension. *Drugs* 1994; **48**: 274–296.

30. Backman JT, Olkkola KT, Aranko K, Himberg JJ, Neuvonen PJ. Dose of midazolam should be reduced during diltiazem and verapamil treatments. *Br J Clin Pharmacol* 1994; **37**: 221–225.

31. Varhe A, Olkkola KT, Neuvonen PJ. Diltiazem enhances the effects of triazolam by inhibiting its metabolism. *Clin Pharmacol* Ther 1996; **59**: 369–375.

32. Rubin AS, Zablocki AD. Hyperkalemia, verapamil and dantrolene. *Anesthesiology* 1987; **66**: 246–249.

33. Rocha P, Guerret M, David D, Marchand X, Kahn JC. Kinetics and hemodynamic effects of intravenous nicardipine modified by previous propranolol oral treatment. *Cardiovasc Drugs Ther* 1990; **4**: 1525–1532.

17 QJW Milner, RD Latimer

VASODILATORS

The vasodilators are a disparate group of drugs acting either directly or indirectly on the mechanisms that maintain tone in vascular smooth muscle. These drugs have a number of uses:

- Control of systemic hypertension.
- Perioperative reduction in surgical bleeding.
- Treatment of heart failure and ischaemic heart disease.
- Treatment of hypertensive crises:
  — malignant hypertension
  — preeclampsia.

MAINTENANCE OF BLOOD PRESSURE

The maintenance of blood pressure depends on the complex interaction of a wide variety of factors that influence both the muscular tone of the veins and arteries and the cardiac output. The relationship between mean arterial blood pressure (MAP), cardiac output (CO) and systemic vascular resistance (SVR) is given by:

$$MAP = CO \times SVR$$

Mean arterial pressure is computed from the area under a pressure–time curve, and is approximately equal to:

$$MAP = \text{Diastolic Pressure} + \frac{\text{Systolic pressure} - \text{diastolic pressure}}{3}$$

Arterial blood pressure may be reduced by reducing any of the components of cardiac output and systemic vascular resistance. Cardiac output is the product of the stroke volume and heart rate, with both being influenced by the sympathetic and parasympathetic nervous systems. In addition, stroke volume is dependent on preload, afterload and myocardial contractility. Preload is the degree of stretch applied to a muscle and depends on venous return to the heart and thus the tone of the venous capacitance vessels. The afterload is the force against which the heart must contract to eject blood and depends on the vascular resistance in the arterial circulation. Arterial tone is determined by the activity of the autonomic nervous system, circulating vasoactive hormones, and locally acting agents and metabolites. Since the production of a specific arterial pressure is the product of such a wide range of determinants, changing just one aspect of the control mechanism will often cause a change in activity in another part of the system, in an attempt to maintain homeostasis, such as reflex tachycardia.

The drugs currently employed as vasodilators are not a homogenous group. However, the nitrovasodilators, sodium nitroprusside and the nitrates all work in a similar manner, by causing a local increase in the concentration of nitric oxide (NO).

NITRIC OXIDE

A series of remarkable discoveries in the past decade has revolutionized the way in which this simple compound is viewed.[1-3] Previously regarded as a toxic contaminant of nitrous oxide cylinders and an unwelcome constituent of cigarette smoke, nitric oxide is increasingly being recognized as a vitally important messenger in mammalian biology with central roles in cellular signalling, the regulation of vascular tone, peripheral neurotransmission and even cellular host defence mechanisms.

The intense scrutiny directed at this agent has shown it to have a pivotal role in the control of vascular smooth muscle tone and to be the pathway by which the nitrovasodilators work. The role of nitric oxide in the pathophysiology of sepsis and myocardial dysfunction suggests that future therapy of these conditions may be directed at influencing the production of this agent. An overview of its physiology is presented.

NITRIC OXIDE PHYSIOLOGY

The nitric oxide story began in 1980 with the observation by Furchgott and Zawadzki[1] that vascular smooth muscle relaxation in response to acetylcholine required the presence of an intact vascular endothelium. From this they proposed the existence of an endothelium-derived relaxing factor, which has subsequently been shown to be chemically and pharmacologically indistinguishable from nitric oxide.[4]

Nitric oxide is synthesized in vivo by the incorporation of molecular oxygen into the terminal guanidino nitrogen atom of the amino acid L-arginine, leaving a citrulline residue (Fig. 17.1). The reaction is catalysed by a family of enzymes, the nitric oxide synthetases (NOS) (Table 17.1), of which three have currently been described. They are large and complex haemoproteins similar to cytochrome P450 and require multiple cofactors for their activity. The isoforms of NOS are classified as endothelial (eNOS), neuronal (nNOS) and inducible (iNOS), and are encoded by genes on chromosomes 7, 12 and 17 respectively. The constitutive isoforms eNOS and nNOS synthesize nitric oxide continuously in small quantities in response to receptor stimulation or physical activation of the cells. In contrast, while iNOS is normally quiescent in a wide variety of healthy cells including endothelial cells, vascular smooth muscle cells, myocytes and immune cells such as macrophages and neutrophils, it can be produced in large quantities after exposure to stimuli such as endotoxin and certain cytokines (tumour necrosis factor, interleukin-1β and interferon-γ). The induced nitric oxide may be cytotoxic to some cells, invading pathogens and deoxyribonucleic acid. The regulation of iNOS expression in critical illness is currently the subject of considerable interest.

ROLE OF NITRIC OXIDE IN VASCULAR SMOOTH MUSCLE RELAXATION

Vascular smooth muscle relaxation is caused by a fall in intracellular calcium ion concentrations through the action of soluble guanylate cyclase. Activation of this enzyme by released nitric oxide is integral to the activity of sodium nitroprusside and the nitrates (Fig. 17.2). Guanylate cyclase increases the intracellular concentration of cyclic guanosine monophosphate (cGMP) and this in turn stimulates cGMP-dependent protein kinases, a subsequent reduction in intracellular calcium concentration and the dephosphorylation of myosin light chains in smooth muscle cells. The controlled release of nitric oxide from the vascular endothelium is a factor in determining resting peripheral vascular resistance, the regulation of coronary circulation, hypoxic pulmonary vasoconstriction and reperfusion-related ischaemic circulatory changes.

Nitric oxide is inactivated in blood by avid and extremely rapid binding to haemoglobin, forming nitrosylhaemoglobin which, in the presence of oxygen, is oxidized to methaemoglobin. Methaemoglobin is then converted back to haemoglobin in erythrocytes by methaemoglobin reductase, leaving nitrate as an end product.

OTHER PHYSIOLOGICAL ROLES FOR NITRIC OXIDE

Central nervous system

Neuronal NOS is found in all areas of the brain, suggesting that nitric oxide acts as a neurotransmitter. Nitric oxide may also have an influence in central pain modulation as β-endorphin analgesia is potentiated by L-arginine. Furthermore, there is some evidence to

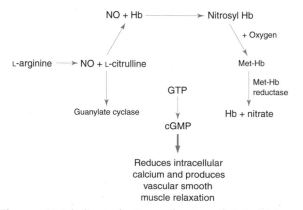

Fig. 17.1 Metabolic production and action of nitric oxide (NO). Hb, haemoglobin; Met-Hb, methaemoglobin; GTP, guanosine triphosphate; cGMP, cyclic guanosine monophosphate.

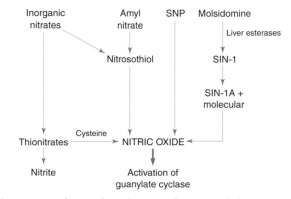

Fig. 17.2 Biochemical production of nitric oxide by nitrodilators. SNP, sodium nitroprusside; SIN, linsidomine.

Table 17.1 Characteristics of isoforms of nitric oxide synthetase

Isoform	Chromosome no.	Mol. wt.	Calmodulin dependent	Intracellular calcium dependent	Nitric oxide release	Cellular location
eNOS	7	133-kDa monomer	Yes	Yes	Picomolar 'puffs'	Endothelium, platelets, myocardium
nNOS	12	166-kDa dimer	Yes	Yes	Picomolar 'puffs'	Central and peripheral neurons
iNOS	17	131-kDa dimer	Yes	No	Nanomolar, sustained	Macrophages, fibroblasts, neutrophils, endothelium (vascular smooth muscle, cardiac myocytes), hepatocytes, Kupffer cells, certain tumour cells

eNOS, endothelial nitric oxide synthetase; nNOS, neuronal NOS; iNOS, inducible NOS.

implicate excessive nitric oxide production in the pathogenesis of conditions such as Huntington's disease and Alzheimer's disease, and that migraine sufferers may have an increased sensitivity to nitric oxide.

Platelets

Vascular endothelium secretes nitric oxide which diffuses into platelets, activating guanylate cyclase and reducing intracellular calcium levels, thereby reducing platelet adhesiveness to the endothelium. Platelets themselves also contain NOS, and the production of nitric oxide may be a self-regulatory function.

Respiratory system

Nitric oxide may play an important role in basal dilator tone in pulmonary and bronchial vessels, whilst the auto-inhalation of nitric oxide formed in the upper airways may lead to selective vasodilatation in pulmonary vessels supplying ventilated lung units and thus have a controlling influence in ventilation–perfusion matching.

PHARMACOLOGICAL ROLES OF NITRIC OXIDE

In addition to its role in the activity of the nitro-vasodilators (see below), nitric oxide is increasingly being used as a therapeutic agent. Inhaled nitric oxide is used selectively to reduce pulmonary vascular resistance in patients with chronic obstructive airway disease, adult respiratory distress syndrome (ARDS), persistent pulmonary hypertension of the newborn (PPHN), pulmonary hypertension in congenital heart disease and postoperative pulmonary hypertension after cardiac surgery.[5] Before this, pulmonary hypertension was usually treated with systemic vasodilators. Not only was systemic hypotension a significant problem, but

the resultant pulmonary vasodilatation was nonselective, increasing ventilation–perfusion (V-Q) mismatching and shunting. In contrast, inhalation of nitric oxide causes preferential vasodilatation in ventilated lung units, thus actively improving V-Q matching and decreasing the shunt fraction. In the treatment of PPHN, low concentrations of nitric oxide (5–80 p.p.m.) significantly improve oxygenation and in many patients obviate the need for extracorporeal membrane oxygenation.

The in vivo half-life of inhaled nitric oxide is only a few seconds and thus systemic hypotension is not a problem. It is a free radical and combines readily with other radicals such as superoxide to form peroxynitrite. The value of inhaled nitric oxide is limited by the production of methaemoglobin and rapid conversion of nitric oxide to nitrogen dioxide in the presence of oxygen. Nitrogen dioxide is a powerful oxidizing agent which initiates lipid peroxidation causing pulmonary oedema and pneumonitis. The rate of production of nitrogen dioxide is directly proportional to the oxygen concentration and the square of the nitric oxide concentration. Contact time between oxygen and nitric oxide should be kept to a minimum, with the gaseous nitric oxide being added to the ventilator fresh gas flow as close to the patient as possible. Methaemoglobin, nitric oxide and nitrogen dioxide levels must be monitored during therapy and an active scavenging unit attached to the ventilator.[6] Although nitric oxide up to 80 p.p.m. has been used successfully for periods of up to 80 days in patients, occupational health and safety standards suggest an upper limit of 25 p.p.m. exposure to nitric oxide and 5 p.p.m. to nitrogen dioxide. With the exception of PPHN, where nitric oxide concentrations of 80 p.p.m. may be needed initially to produce vasodilatation, in most patients clinical benefit may be achieved by concentrations of 5–15 p.p.m.

Nitric oxide and anaesthetic agents

Volatile anaesthetic agents are known to cause peripheral vasodilatation; however, evidence has emerged that rather than stimulating nitric oxide release, the halogenated anaesthetic agents, thiopentone and ketamine, actually inhibit its activity. Conversely propofol appears to stimulate the production and release of nitric oxide in endothelial cells.

THE NITROVASODILATORS

The increasing knowledge about nitric oxide has revolutionized our understanding of the pharmacological actions of the group of drugs known as the nitrovasodilators. The commonly used drugs in this group are sodium nitroprusside (SNP), glyceryl trinitrate and isorbide dinitrate or mononitrate.

SODIUM NITROPRUSSIDE

Chemical properties

SNP (Fig. 17.3) consists of a ferrous core surrounded by five cyanide groups and a nitrosyl group. The molecule is soluble in water and contains 44% cyanide by weight. In vivo, SNP reacts with oxyhaemoglobin, dissociating immediately and forming methaemoglobin with the

$$2Na^+ \left[\begin{array}{c} CN \quad CN \\ \diagdown \quad \diagup \\ CN-Fe-N=O \\ \diagup \quad \diagdown \\ CN \quad CN \end{array} \right]$$

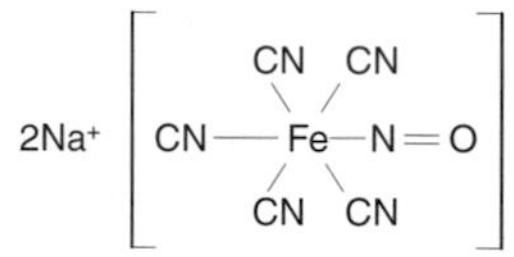

Fig. 17.3 Structure of sodium nitroprusside.

release of the five cyanide ions and nitric oxide. In contrast to the organic nitrates (see below), which require the presence of highly specific thiol compounds to generate nitric oxide, SNP generates nitric oxide spontaneously, functioning as a direct prodrug. SNP produces direct arterial and venous vasodilatation with the preservation of adequate blood flow to all organs, provided the mean arterial pressure is maintained above 55 mmHg and arterial occlusive disease is not present (Table 17.2). It is a potent pulmonary artery vasodilator and inhibits hypoxic pulmonary vasoconstriction. The effects on cardiac output are variable and depend on ventricular function and filling pressure. Where left ventricular end-diastolic pressure is raised, the reduction in afterload may increase cardiac output, whereas in normal subjects cardiac output may fall in line with a reduction in preload. Reflex tachycardia can be troublesome and may be treated with a short-acting β-adrenoceptor antagonist such as esmolol.

SNP is presented as a dry powder for reconstitution in 5% glucose or dextrose. SNP degrades spontaneously in light, yielding free cyanide ions, although it is still biologically active. The dry powder is contained in brown glass and the fresh solution should be wrapped in aluminium foil or other light-proof material. Although the powder can be reconstituted in saline, there are pharmaceutical reasons why this should not be done. The decomposition products of SNP react with minute quantities of organic substances forming highly coloured products; in the case of glucose or dextrose these are blue or dark red. Therefore any discoloured solution should be discarded. A solution of SNP should not be used more than 24 h after preparation.

Metabolism and toxicity (Fig. 17.4)

The five cyanide ions released by SNP react with methaemoglobin to produce cyanomethaemoglobin

	Heart rate	Contractility	Cardiac output	BP	SVR/PVR	Preload
GTN	Reflex ↑	Reflex ↑	↓↓	↓↓	↓↓	↓↓
Nitroprusside	Reflex ↑	↑	Variable	↓↓	↓↓/↓	↓↓
Hydralazine	Reflex ↑	↑	↓/↑	↓↓	↓	NC
Tolazoline	↑	NC	↑	↓↓	↓↓	
Trimetaphan	NC	NC	NC	↓↓	↓	↓

Table 17.2 **Summary of the effects of various vasodilators**

BP, blood pressure; SVR, systemic vascular resistance; PVR, pulmonary vascular resistance; GTN, glyceryl trinitrate; NC, no change.

which is nontoxic and remains in dynamic equilibrium with free cyanide. Normal adult methaemoglobin levels of about 0.5% are capable of binding the cyanide ions released from the dissociation of 18 mg SNP. The enzyme rhodanase uses thiosulphate to convert the remaining free cyanide ions to thiocyanate in the liver and most normal adults have a sufficient thiosulphate store to detoxify the cyanide released from 50 mg SNP. The risk of cyanide toxicity occurs only when SNP doses are high, or when thiosulphate and methaemoglobin are exhausted.

Cyanide binds to tissue cytochrome oxidase and inactivates oxidative phosphorylation causing acute cellular hypoxia and anaerobic metabolism with increasing metabolic acidosis. Blood cyanide concentrations exceeding 40μmol l^{-1} may be associated with clinical toxicity and fatalities have been reported at levels above 77μmol l^{-1}. Determining plasma cyanide levels is difficult and time consuming. However, in smoke inhalation injuries where cyanide toxicity also occurs, plasma lactate concentrations exceeding 10μmol l^{-1} correlate well with cyanide levels exceeding 40μmol l^{-1} and may provide a rapidly accessible guide to toxicity and need for treatment.

Whenever SNP is used, the possibility of cyanide toxicity should be borne in mind, although in practice if the recommended dosage regimens are followed it is extremely rare. The signs of toxicity include tachyphylaxis, with increasing dose requirements, evidence of confusion and central nervous system dysfunction, muscle twitching, vomiting and respiratory distress. Patients are not cyanosed since the cells cannot utilize oxygen and mixed venous oxygen concentration is high. Arterial blood gas analysis shows a marked metabolic acidosis with increasingly negative base excess and raised plasma lactate levels.

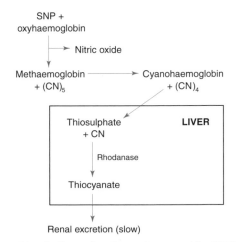

Fig. 17.4 Metabolism of sodium nitroprusside (SNP). CN, cyanide ion.

Summary box 17.1 Sodium nitroprusside toxicity and treatment

Signs of cyanide toxicity

- Cardiovascular signs: arrhythmias and hypertension.

- Central nervous system signs: confusion, loss of consciousness and convulsions.

- Metabolic acidosis: check plasma lactate level.

Treatment

- Stop SNP infusion.

- Ventilate with 100% oxygen.

- Sodium thiosulphate 150–200 mg kg^{-1} slowly intravenously.

- Sodium nitrite 6 mg kg^{-1} slowly intravenously.

- Correct metabolic acidosis with 8.4% sodium bicarbonate.

- Consider vitamin B_{12a} 25 mg h^{-1}.

As soon as toxicity is suspected the nitroprusside should be discontinued and 100% oxygen administered. Sodium thiosulphate 150–200 mg kg^{-1} intravenously is given, followed by an infusion at 6 mg kg^{-1} h^{-1} for each 1 mg kg^{-1} h^{-1} of SNP. Sodium thiosulphate is itself toxic in overdose. Additional methaemoglobin is created by giving sodium nitrite 6 mg kg^{-1} intravenously to create cyanomethaemoglobin. Sodium bicarbonate 8.4% (20 ml) is given to correct the metabolic acidosis. Hydroxycobalamin (vitamin B_{12a}) has been advocated as it binds cyanide, forming cyanocobalamin and acts as a temporary absorber of plasma cyanide. The dose is 22.5 mg hydroxycobalamin for each milligram of SNP administered. Unfortunately hydroxycobalamin has an extremely short half-life (5 min) and is also very expensive. Note that vitamin B_{12} (cyanocobalamin), which contains one hydryl group less than hydroxycobalamin, cannot trap significant quantities of free cyanide ions and therefore should not be used as a substitute.

Administration and dosage

SNP has an extremely rapid onset of action and is rapidly metabolized; it is administered only by continuous intravenous infusion. Its effects are seen within 30 s and a satisfactory degree of hypotension may be achieved in 2–3 min. An arterial catheter for continuous blood pressure monitoring is recommended. Initial infusion rates of $0.5–2\ \mu g\ kg^{-1}\ min^{-1}$ are adequate and a total maximum dose of $0.25\ mg\ kg^{-1}\ h^{-1}$ should not be exceeded ($1\ mg\ kg^{-1}\ h^{-1}$ for 5 h).

Side-effects

In addition to cyanide-related toxicity, SNP can cause reflex tachycardia. Arterial hypoxaemia may occur due to abolition of hypoxic vasoconstriction Rebound systemic and pulmonary hypertension can occur when administration is stopped. Despite causing renal vasodilitation the renin–angiotensin system is activated and this may lead to a pressure-related renal function decrease.

Contraindications

Few absolute contraindications to the use of SNP exist. The risk of cyanide toxicity may be increased in patients with abnormal thiocyanate metabolic pathways, or those with low levels of hepatic rhodanase. It has been stated that patients with Leber's optic atrophy or tobacco amblyopia should not receive SNP. However, this is based on one case report in 1975 and the validity of this has been questioned.[7] Patients with hepatic failure may be unable to produce adequate amounts of thiocyanate and those with renal failure may be unable to excrete this metabolite, which is itself toxic in high concentrations, and these should be considered relative contraindications. Thiocyanate, a metabolite of SNP, inhibits iodine binding and uptake, and SNP should be used with caution in patients with hypothyroidism.

Summary box 17.2 Side-effects of sodium nitroprusside

- Cyanide toxicity.

- Methaemoglobinaemia.

- Variable dose response.

- Reflex tachycardia.

- Photodegradation.

- Rebound systemic and pulmonary hypertension on its cessation, particularly if stopped abruptly.

- Because SNP causes pulmonary vasodilatation, the shunt fraction is increased and arterial hypoxaemia may occur.

- Despite renal vasodilatation the renin–angiotensin system is activated and a pressure-related fall in renal function is observed.

ORGANIC NITRATES

The organic nitrates glyceryl trinitrate (GTN, nitroglycerine), isosorbide dinitrate (ISDN), isosorbide mononitrate (ISMN) and amyl nitrate (Fig. 17.5) have long been the mainstay of treatment for angina, acute myocardial infarction and heart failure. Thomas Lauder Brunton recorded the first use of amyl nitrate in a patient with intractable angina in 1867, but until recently little progress was made in determining their exact mode of action. The revolution in our understanding of the actions of the vascular endothelium and the role of nitric oxide have shed great, but as yet incomplete, light on these agents.

Biotransformation of organic nitrates (see Fig. 17.2)
The organic nitrates are prodrugs which, although chemically heterogeneous, exert their pharmacodynamic action via a common pathway: the release of nitric oxide in vascular and nonvascular cells.[8] Nitric oxide stimulates the cytosolic enzyme guanylyl cyclase, leading to an increase in the concentration of intracellular cGMP. Their metabolism involves enzymatic and nonenzymatic pathways. Both glutathione-S-transferase and a cytochrome P450 enzyme are thought to compete for the nitrate. A specific thiol, N-acetylcysteine, present in cytosol is believed to be responsible for the nonenzymatic nitrate activation, and in both cases an unstable thionitrate may be the intermediary. In contrast, amyl nitrate is able to react with all available thiols forming S-nitrosothiols which rapidly decompose to release nitric oxide, producing smooth muscle relaxation.

Tolerance to nitrates
The rapid development of tolerance to organic nitrate therapy has long been recognized and the decrease in

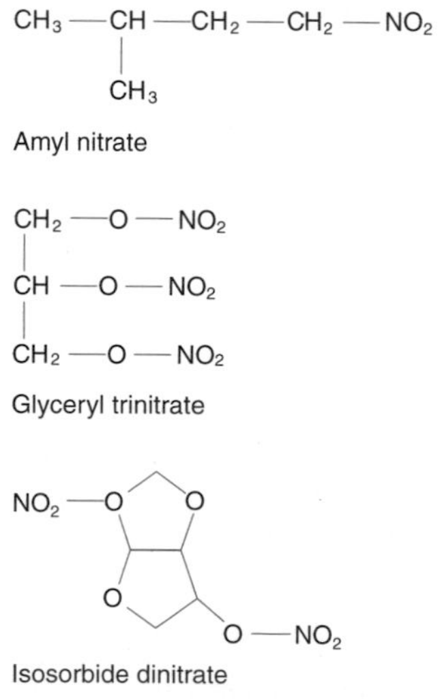

Fig. 17.5 Structure of commonly used organic nitrates.

vascular relaxation with repeated dosing appears to be matched by a reduction in the formation of nitric oxide.[9] This would suggest that tolerance is related to impaired biotransformation and not to desensitization or down-regulation of guanylate cyclase activity. It is not fully known whether this is a result of depletion of substrate (N-acetylcysteine) stores or downregulation of the enzyme systems that convert the organic nitrates into nitric oxide.

Haemodynamic effects

Low-dose nitrate therapy exerts its effects primarily on the venous capacitance system, causing venodilatation and decreased right and left ventricular filling pressures. As the dose is increased, the effect on arterial tone is more marked, decreasing vascular resistance and lowering arterial blood pressure (Table 17.2). The reduction in both preload and afterload decreases myocardial work. In addition, the nitrates have an effect on coronary arteries, increasing flow, reducing coronary artery spasm, dilating stenosed vessels and increasing collateral flow.

Through their action on platelet guanylate cyclase, the organic nitrates inhibit platelet aggregation. Indeed, it has been suggested that the value of nitrate therapy in unstable angina lies in its ability to inhibit platelet aggregation, and possibly a synergistic action with locally produced prostacyclin. Animal models have shown that prolonged nitrate therapy after myocardial injury may alter vascular and myocardial cell growth and proliferation, with reduction in ventricular dilatation and nonischaemic myocardial hypertrophy.

Presentation

Glyceryl trinitrate

GTN is available in a number of preparations although its effects are short lived (20–30 min); modified release preparations may prolong its action.
Dose: sublingually 0.3–0.6 mg as required; sublingual tablets should be supplied in brown bottles and discarded after 2 months; continuous intravenous infusion 0.01–0.4 mg min^{-1}. Both GTN and ISDN (below) are absorbed by polyvinyl chloride (PVC) infusion sets with a reduction in potency; glass or polyethylene is the preferred medium.

Topical GTN preparations are available, with patches releasing 5–10 mg per 24 h, and a 2% ointment can be applied transdermally under a sticking plaster (2–5 cm). The plasma half-life of GTN is approximately 5 min.

Isorbide Dinitrate

ISDN undergoes significant first-pass metabolism in the liver and the bioavailability is about 30–50%; it is rapidly converted to the mononitrate. The preparations are much more stable than GTN.
Dose: sublingually 5–10 mg; orally 30–120 mg daily; continuous intravenous infusion 2–12 mg h^{-1}. ISDN 1 mg may be given as a single intracoronary bolus before angioplasty.

Isosorbide Mononitrate

ISMN is the active metabolite of ISDN. It undergoes little first-pass metabolism and has virtually complete bioavailability.
Dose: orally 20 mg two or three times daily.

Summary box 17.3 Side-effects of organic nitrates

- Tolerance develops rapidly.

- Reflex tachycardia when given by intravenous infusion.

- Side-effects common to all nitrates include flushing, headaches, dizziness and weakness.

- Postural hypotension may occur.

- Absorbed by PVC giving sets.

- Increased intracranial pressure.

OTHER NITRIC OXIDE DONORS

Molsidomine

Molsidomine, a member of the sydnonimine group, is a potent preload reducing agent which also appears capable of dilating both stenosed and nonstenotic coronary arteries.

Mode of Action

Molsidomine, and its active metabolite linsidomine (SIN-1A), are a group of drugs with a terminal nitroso group which cause vascular relaxation after spontaneous hydrolysis and the release of nitric oxide. Unlike the nitrates, however, molsidomine does not require any cofactors for its action and tolerance appears to be less than with the nitrates; indeed molsidomine remained active in coronary artery strips that had previously been rendered unresponsive to GTN by prolonged exposure. Like other agents that activate guanylate cyclase, molsidomine inhibits platelet aggregation. Molsidomine is not currently used in the UK but is available in some other European countries and in Japan.

OTHER VASODILATORS

HYDRALAZINE

Mode of action

Hydralazine is a direct acting arterial vasodilator with little action on venous capacitance vessels, causing a fall in peripheral vascular resistance and a lowering of blood pressure (with particular effect on diastolic blood pressure). Baroreceptor activity is not affected and cardiovascular effects include increased heart rate (reflex), stroke volume and cardiac output. Postural hypotension is a less frequent problem than with other agents with greater venodilator activity. Pulmonary vascular resistance is reduced but at the expense of a decrease in arterial partial pressure of oxygen (Pao_2). The renin–angiotensin system is stimulated and sodium reabsorption increases with fluid retention and oedema. Hydralazine is a potent cerebrovasodilator and causes an increase in intracranial pressure in the closed skull. Although its exact mechanism of action is unclear, it does require an intact vascular endothelium for its effect and the generation of nitric oxide has been demonstrated in vitro. It is metabolized by acetylation in the liver. It has a relatively slow onset of action and plasma half-life is 2–3 h in normal subjects. It is 80% protein bound. The action is prolonged in 'slow acetylators' and the incidence of side-effects is increased.

Administration and dosage

Orally administered hydralazine is subject to considerable first-pass metabolism and bioavailability is 25–50%.

Dose: orally 25–50 mg twice daily; intravenous injection 5–10 mg slowly, repeated as desired; intravenous infusion, initially 0.2–0.3 mg min^{-1} reducing to maintenance rates of 0.05–0.15 mg min^{-1}.

Indications

Oral hydralazine is a useful agent when used in combination with other treatments for hypertension but when used alone causes tachycardia and fluid retention. Intravenously it is used in hypertensive emergencies such as preeclampsia. The use of hydralazine is limited by its toxicity, especially the occurrence of an immune disorder resembling systemic lupus erythematosus, with malaise, myalgia and arthritis in association with raised titres of antinuclear antibodies. This is particularly likely after prolonged use (6 months) and where the dose exceeds 100 mg daily. However, the majority of patients who develop positive antinuclear antibodies do not go on to develop the lupus syndrome and positive titres alone are not a contraindication to its continued use.

> **Summary box 17.4 Side-effects of hydralazine**
>
> - Development of an immune disorder resembling systemic lupus erythematosus (SLE). Hydralazine should not be used in patients with SLE.
>
> - Microscopic haematuria and/or proteinuria herald the onset of immune complex glomerulonephritis.
>
> - Tachycardia, palpitations, headache and flushing are common.
>
> - Tachyphalaxis is extremely common.
>
> - Peripheral neuropathy.

TRIMETAPHAN

Trimetaphan is a trimethyl sulphonium salt which reversibly blocks neurotransmission at autonomic ganglia (ganglion blockers). Ganglion blockers were amongst the first to be used clinically to achieve controlled perioperative hypotension. They cause interruption of impulse transmission from preganglionic to postganglionic fibres in both the sympathetic and parasympathetic nervous system by competitive inhibition of acetylcholine receptors. In addition they cause some direct arteriolar vasodilatation. Nerve conduction is not affected and they do not depolarize the ganglion. Trimetaphan has a rapid onset of action and hypotension lasts for 15–30 min.

Physiological effects

The physiological effects of trimetaphan are a consequence of its blockade of autonomic ganglia (Table 17.2). Changes in heart rate depend on the degree to which vagal tone is disturbed and a mild tachycardia is common. Stroke volume and cardiac output are reduced and this may be worsened by the use of inhalational anaesthetic agents, further depressing blood pressure. Trimetaphan causes a marked reduction in peripheral resistance, and cardiac work and myocardial oxygen consumption are decreased. Cerebral blood flow is decreased proportionally with intracranial pressure unchanged, although intraocular pressure is raised. Pronounced mydriasis occurs, which may confuse the unwary into altering the depth of anaesthesia; this also makes trimetaphan unsuitable during neurosurgery. Gastrointestinal stasis and urinary atony occur. Mild inhibition of plasma cholinesterase occurs and the duration of action of suxamethonium will be slightly extended. Trimetaphan has a mild direct neuromuscular blocking effect.

Dosage and administration

Trimetaphan is indicated only for the induction of hypotension during anaesthesia. Premedication with a β-adrenoceptor antagonist helps to attenuate the tachycardia.

Dose: 3–4 mg min^{-1} initially then adjusted according to response.

The combination of trimetaphan with SNP has been advocated to allow a reduction in the dose of both drugs and to reduce the toxicity of SNP. The effects appear to be synergistic rather than merely additive.

Side-effects

- The hypotension induced may persist for up to 1 h after cessation of the drug, particularly if high doses have been used.
- Histamine release occurs at high dosage.
- Tachycardia.
- Pupillary dilatation.
- Interaction with aminoglycoside antibiotics potentiating neuromuscular block.
- Inhibition of pseudocholinesterase may prolong the action of suxamethonium. Do not use in patients with abnormalities of plasma cholinesterases.

PROSTACYCLIN

Prostacyclin (prostaglandin (PG) I$_2$) is an ecoisanoid (derivatives of 20-carbon free fatty acids) synthesized from arachidonic acid in all vascular beds.

Actions

Like nitric oxide, prostacyclin is an endogenous substance with a wide variety of physiological actions, the significance of which are only beginning to be understood.

Physiological actions of prostacyclin include:

- Vasodilatation.
- Inhibition of platelet aggregation.
- Protective role against atheroma formation.
- Cytoprotective function.
- Decreased peripheral vascular resistance in sepsis.

Mode of action

Prostacyclin causes vasodilatation by increasing intracellular cyclic adenosine monophosphate (cAMP) levels through its action on specific PGI$_2$ receptors (probably a G protein) to stimulate adenylyl cyclase. cAMP in turn activates protein kinase A, which amongst other actions decreases free intracellular calcium levels and causes vascular smooth muscle relaxation. Prostacyclin also stimulates the release of nitric oxide from endothelial cells.

Prostacyclin is the most powerful inhibitor of platelet aggregation yet discovered. This effect is caused by stimulation of platelet cell-surface adenylyl cyclase receptors. Not only does it prevent platelet aggregation; it also disperses existing aggregates and inhibits thrombus formation. An important role for the intact vascular endothelium is the regulation of platelet activity, allowing platelets to adhere to damaged endothelium whilst at the same time controlling the formation of thrombus and maintaining luminal patency. The release of prostacyclin from vascular endothelial cells may be a controlling influence in this activity.

Prostacyclin also appears to be involved in a number of cytoprotective functions; in experimental models it reduces infarct size and enzyme release in myocardial infarction. In sheep, prostacyclin appears to protect the lungs against the effects of endotoxin, and in isolated cat livers it reduces the damage caused by hypoxia. The addition of prostacyclin to platelets increases their viability from 6–72 h.

Prostacyclin is used as an alternative anticoagulant to heparin during renal dialysis, particularly when heparin-induced thrombocytopenia occurs. The other areas where prostacyclin has shown most promise are in pulmonary hypertension, paediatric cardiac surgery and peripheral vascular occlusive disease. Studies in patients with peripheral vascular disease showed a significant increase in exercise tolerance and ulcer healing which persisted for up to 6 months after infusion of prostacyclin. Patients awaiting heart lung transplantation are frequently stabilized on prostacyclin until a donor organ becomes available.

Systemic infusion of prostacyclin in patients with ARDS has demonstrated a nonspecific fall in both systemic and pulmonary vascular resistance with a concomitant fall in P_{aO_2} due to intrapulmonary shunting. Extrapolating evidence from the use of inhaled nitric oxide in both ARDS and pulmonary hypertension,

---

Summary box 17.5 Clinical applications of prostacyclin

- ARDS.
- Peripheral vascular disease.
- Pulmonary hypertension.
- Heart failure.
- Cardiopulmonary bypass.
- Heart transplantation.
- Endotoxaemic sepsis.
- Alternative to heparin in renal dialysis.

investigators have successfully administered aerosolized prostacyclin to patients with these conditions. Delivery of drugs by this route achieves two goals. First, the vasodilator is targeted only at those vessels supplying ventilated lung units, avoiding the significant increase in intrapulmonary shunting that has characterized the use of vasodilators in these conditions. Second, the short half-life (2–3 min) of prostacyclin means that it has little systemic effect and treatment is not hampered by systemic hypotension. Both these criteria are also met by nitric oxide (see above); however, unlike nitric oxide, prostacyclin appears to have few side-effects, no toxic metabolites, and does not require a complicated delivery and monitoring system. Interestingly, the improvements in $P\text{ao}_2$ may not occur at the lowest pulmonary artery pressures, suggesting that at doses that maximally decrease the pulmonary artery pressure vasodilatation occurs in nonventilated areas and worsens shunt. Problems associated with aerosol administration include uncertainty of dosage and as yet unquantified effects on bronchial smooth muscle.

Presentation

Prostacyclin is presented in glass vials containing 500 µg of the freeze-dried agent. The initial dose is 5 ng kg^{-1} min^{-1}, slowly increased to a maximum of 20 ng kg^{-1} min^{-1}. Similar doses are used as a selective pulmonary artery vasodilator by direct infusion into the pulmonary artery just before harvesting donor lungs for allograft transplantation.

VASODILATORS ACTING ON POTASSIUM CHANNELS

NICORANDIL

Nicorandil (2-nicotinamidoethyl nitrate) is a new antianginal agent with potent vasodilator and antispasmodic properties which appear to be relatively specific to the coronary arteries.

Mode of action

Nicorandil has a dual mode of action. It is a nicotinamide nitrate ester and the nitrate group activates soluble guanylate cyclase in a manner similar to the organic nitrates. In addition it acts as an adenosine triphosphate (ATP)-sensitive potassium channel activator, causing vasodilatation by enhancing potassium transport across cell membranes[10] and may even promote the release of prostacyclin. It decreases both preload and afterload in a dose-dependent fashion and increases coronary blood flow. The drug has little effect on cardiac output, and has little negative inotropic effect. Initial studies indicate that tolerance is less of a problem than with organic nitrates.

Side-effects

The side-effect profile is similar to that of the organic nitrates with headache, flushing, nausea and the development of reflex tachycardia.

Dosage

Nicorandil has a long plasma half-life (6–8 h) and is suitable for the prevention of angina in patients who do not tolerate β-adrenoceptor antagonists.

Dose: 10–20 mg orally twice daily.

MINOXIDIL

The prodrug minoxidil is another vasodilator that acts predominantly on arterial resistance vessels, with little effect on venous tone.

Mode of action

Minoxidil undergoes extensive hepatic biotransformation by sulphotransferases to its active metabolite, minoxidil-N-O-sulphate. The latter stimulates ATP-sensitive K^+ channels in arterial smooth muscle, causing an increase in polarization of the cell membrane and preventing Ca^{2+} influx.

Minoxidil causes a reflex increase in sympathetic stimulation to the heart, increasing contractility and cardiac output. Although minoxidil is a renal vasodilator, the fall in arterial blood produced by the drug can often decrease renal perfusion pressure and urine output. It is a potent stimulator of renin secretion. It is

---

Summary box 17.6 Side-effects of minoxidil

- Reduced renal perfusion causes salt and water retention due to increased renal tubular reabsorption, rather than as a result of renin secretion.

- Reflex sympathetic activity causes tachycardia and increased myocardial work.

- Electrocardiographic changes, including inverted T waves and ST elevation, often appear with the start of treatment; they regress with time and are not associated with ischaemia or changes in cardiac enzymes.

- Pericardial and pleural effusions are rare complications.

- Hypertrichosis occurs in all patients who receive minoxidil for extended periods, and may be related to increased cutaneous blood flow. It reverses on cessation of treatment, but may make the use of minoxidil unacceptable to women.

well absorbed from the gut and only 20% is excreted unchanged in urine, the remainder being metabolized in the liver. Plasma half-life is 3–4 h but its duration of action may be up to 24 h following a single dose. Because of reflex sympathetic activity minoxidil is reserved for patients with refractory hypertension, and should then be combined with a β-adrenoceptor antagonist.

Dosage

Minoxidil is available as an oral preparation in 2.5- and 10-mg tablets. Usual dose is 5–40 mg daily.

DIAZOXIDE

Diazoxide is a powerful vasodilator acting directly on vascular smooth muscle by opening specific K^+ channels in the cell membrane. Although structurally similar to the thiazide diuretics, it has no diuretic action and instead causes renal sodium and water retention with oedema formation. Diazoxide causes significant hyperglycaemia by inhibiting the release of insulin from pancreatic β cells. Owing to its highly alkaline nature (the solution has a pH of 11), it cannot be given intramuscularly. A single intravenous bolus of 300 mg is usually given to control blood pressure, but up to 1200 mg may be required. The drug works within 5 min with a duration of action of 2–6 h. It is metabolized in the liver and 50% is excreted unchanged by the kidney. Protein binding is greater than 90%.

Because of its side-effects the use of diazoxide is limited to hypertensive emergencies such as preeclampsia and hypertensive encephalopathies, and to severe hypertension that is resistant to other agents.

Summary box 17.7 Side-effects of diazoxide

- Sodium and water retention.

- Hyperglycaemia.

- Leucopenia and thrombocytopenia.

- Reflex tachycardia.

The two sulphonylureas glibenclamide and tolbutamide both block K^+ channels and will competitively inhibit the action of nicorandil, minoxidil and diazoxide at these receptors.

ADENOSINE

The purine nucleotide adenosine is present in virtually all mammalian cells and, although its actions were first described in 1929 by Drury and Szent-Grygori, it has only recently been used as a therapeutic agent.[11] At least two specific adenosine receptor types have been identified in the cardiovascular system, A_1, a high-affinity receptor inhibiting adenylyl cyclase, and A_2 receptors that mediate vasodilatation throughout the vasculature. A_1 receptors also activate K^+ channels by an action that is independent of cAMP. Adenosine acts within 30 s and has a plasma half-life of 10 s, being cleared from the plasma by facilitated transport into erythrocytes and vascular endothelial cells and then degraded by deaminases.

Clinical uses of adenosine

- Diagnosis and treatment of tachyarrhythmias.
- Vasodilator (particularly pulmonary).
- Myocardial protection against ischaemia–reperfusion injury.

The opening of specific ATP-gated K^+ channels by specific membrane A_1 receptors in the atria and sinoatrial node causes:

- Shortening of the atrial action potential.
- Hyperpolarization of the sinoatrial node.
- Decrease in atrioventricular (AV) node action potential amplitude.

Adenosine is therefore extremely effective at terminating supraventricular tachycardias, especially where the AV node is involved in reentrant circuits such as in Wolff–Parkinson–White syndrome.[12] The transient effects of adenosine allow rapid differentiation of supraventricular and ventricular tachycardias where electrocardiographic diagnosis is difficult, and the use of verapamil may cause severe hypotension. Adenosine is ineffective in most ventricular tachycardias except those caused by catecholamines where it attenuates the catecholamine-induced calcium influx.

Adenosine is an effective pulmonary artery vasodilator causing minimal effects on blood pressure and an increase in cardiac output when infused at $50\,\mu g$ $kg^{-1}\,min^{-1}$ in patients with pulmonary hypertension following cardiac surgery.[13] It has a protective effect on myocardial cells exposed to ischaemia-related reperfusion injury, reducing oxygen free radical formation, lipolysis and superoxide anion production, and inhibiting noradrenaline release from sympathetic nerve terminals. The endogenous release of adenosine following myocardial ischaemia is postulated as an autoprotective mechanism to maintain cellular integrity following injury. Adenosine attenuates reperfusion injury following regional myocardial ischaemia, and infusing adenosine into the coronary circulation may be a valuable tool in augmenting both surgical and pharmacological coronary revascularization.[14]

Dosage: Diagnosis and treatment of tachyarrhythmias

– 3 mg intravenous bolus (ideally via a central vein) followed by 6 and 12 mg if unsuccessful.

Summary box 17.8 Side-effects of adenosine

- Bradycardia and sinus arrest (usually of short duration).

- Other arrhythmias.

- Sensation of dyspnoea.

- Bronchospasm.

- Facial flushing.

Contraindications

In atrial fibrillation adenosine shortens the atrial action potential and therefore decreases the refractory period and worsens the arrhythmia. Patients with sick sinus syndrome and second- and third-degree heart block should not receive adenosine. Asthma is a relative contraindication because of the development of bronchospasm.

URAPIDIL

The use of many of the vasodilators described above is hampered by the inevitable development of sympathetically mediated reflex tachycardias caused by decreases in arterial baroreceptor stimulation. There is considerable interest in the production of vasodilators that do not induce this increase in heart rate.

Mode of action

Urapidil is a short-acting selective α_1-adrenoreceptor antagonist causing a reduction in peripheral vascular resistance and a fall in blood pressure. In addition it has agonist activity at central serotonin (5-hydroxytryptamine $(5\text{-HT})_{1A}$) receptors in the central medullary region of the brain. These receptors have been shown to inhibit serotonergic neurons that are excitatory to preganglionic sympathetic neurons of the spinal cord. Antagonism at central α_1 receptors may also help to attenuate the reflex tachycardia accompanying a fall in systemic blood pressure. Unlike clonidine, urapidil has no action at central α_2 receptors.

Most of the action of urapidil is on arterial tone, but there is some effect on venous tone, causing a fall in right ventricular end-diastolic volume and a decrease in circulating atrial natriuretic factor (ANF) concentrations (see below). Little change in cardiac output or ejection fraction occurs.

Urapidil has 75% oral bioavailability and a half-life of 4–5 h. Plasma protein binding is 80% and the volume of distribution $0.77\,l\,kg^{-1}$. The drug is mainly metabolized in the liver and only 15% appears unchanged in urine.

Dosage: oral 50–100 mg twice daily; intravenous bolus 25 mg or $0.4\,mg\,kg^{-1}$ and infusion of $0.002\,mg\,kg^{-1}\,min^{-1}$.

Indications

Urapidil is indicated for the long-term treatment of hypertension and the perioperative control of blood pressure. It is particularly suited to use in cardiovascular surgery because it causes little increase in myocardial work.[15]

ENDOTHELIN ANTAGONISTS

Mounting evidence supports the local regulation of vascular tone by agents released from endothelial cells themselves. Not only does the endothelium produce prostacyclin (see above), the most potent vasodilator yet discovered, it also produces a 21-amino-acid peptide endothelin,[16] the most potent vasoconstrictor to be discovered. Endothelin synthesis is induced by a number of independent vasoactive substances such as thrombin, adrenaline, angiotensin II and vasopressin. It is formed from an intermediate preprohormone (preproendothelin) by proteolytic cleavage under the influence of endothelin-converting enzyme. Three isoforms of endothelin (ET) have been identified and sequenced, ET-1, ET-2 and ET-3, and these have been shown to be active at two distinct receptor types, ET_A and ET_B. Both receptors mediate endothelin-dependent vasoconstriction. In addition ET_B stimulation also causes vasodilatation via the release of nitric oxide and prostacyclin, thus modulating the vasoconstrictive response to endothelin. Disordered production of endothelin has been implicated in the pathophysiology of a number of cardiovascular diseases such as myocardial infarction, atherosclerosis, congestive heart failure and pulmonary hypertension.

Two endothelin receptor antagonists are being developed, BQ 123 and Bosentan (RO-47-0203). Bosentan is a mixed antagonist at both endothelin receptor types and is currently undergoing clinical trials.

ATRIAL NATRIURETIC FACTOR

ANF is an endogenous peptide hormone released by atrial myocytes that acts as a regulator of fluid homeostasis. It is a potent and selective relaxant of vascular smooth muscle. The relaxation mediated by ANF is due to a direct action on the vascular smooth muscle itself and is independent of the endothelium. In contrast to nitric oxide, which activates soluble guanylate cyclase, ANF activates particulate guanylate cyclase, causing a concentration- and time-dependent increase in cGMP. ANF acts via specific receptors, the density of which vary widely throughout the vascular bed, explaining the heterogenicity of its action in different vascular beds. From observations that atrial distension leads to natriuresis, there would seem to be a direct humoral connection between the heart and renal function.[17]

Summary box 17.9 Effects of atrial natiuretic factor

- Activation of particulate guanylate cyclase.

- Alteration of regional blood flow.

- Inhibition of the release of other vasoactive hormones.

- Natriuresis with effects on renal tubular function.

INFLUENCE OF ANF IN DISEASE

In rats rendered hypertensive and anuric by angiotensin II and vasopressin, ANF lowers blood pressure and promotes diuresis. Furthermore raised levels of circulating ANF have been found in patients with essential hypertension.

Congestive heart failure is associated with humoral imbalance including raised concentrations of plasma noradrenaline, increased activity in the renin–angiotensin–aldosterone system, raised circulating vasopressin levels and raised ANF concentration. In addition there appears to be a direct link between the degree of heart failure and the increase in circulating ANF concentration. Indeed patients with raised right atrial pressure and high circulating ANF levels demonstrate predictable decreases in ANF levels as their clinical condition improves.

CLINICAL IMPLICATIONS

ANF is degraded by the enzyme neutral endopeptidase. Candoxatril is a neutral endopeptidase inhibitor and is being investigated as monotherapy in essential hypertension, and as a vasodilator in heart failure. Treatment with candoxatril in congestive cardiac failure produces natriuresis and a reduction in both left and right filling pressures.

REFERENCES

1. Furchgott RF, Zawadzki JV. The obligatory role of endothelial cells in the relaxation of arterial smooth muscle by acetylcholine. *Nature* 1980; **288**: 373–376.

2. Moncada S, Palmer RM, Higgs EA. Nitric oxide: physiology, pathophysiology and pharmacology. *Pharmacol Rev* 1991; **43**: 109–142.

3. Quinn AC, Petros AJ, Vallance P. Nitric oxide: an endogenous gas. *Br J Anaesth* 1995; **74**: 443–451.

4. Luscher TF. Endothelium derived nitric oxide: the endogenous nitrovasodilator in the human cardiovascular system. *Eur Heart J* 1991; **12** (Suppl. E): 2–11.

5. Hurford WE. Inhaled nitric oxide therapy. *Curr Opin Anaesthesiol* 1996; **9**: 117–126.

6. Wessel DL, Adatia I, Thompson JE, Hickey PR. Delivery and monitoring of inhaled nitric oxide in patients with pulmonary hypertension. *Crit Care Med* 1994; **22**: 930–938.

7. Freidrich JA, Butterworth JF. Sodium nitroprusside: twenty years and counting. *Anesth Analg* 1995; **81**: 152–162.

8. Feelisch M. Biotransformation to nitric oxide of organic nitrates in comparison to other nitrodilators. *Eur Heart J* 1993; **14** (Suppl. 1): 123–132.

9. Zhang LM, Castresana MR, Newman WH. Tolerance to nitroglycerin in vascular smooth muscle cells: recovery and cross-tolerance to sodium nitroprusside. *Anesth Analg* 1994; **78**: 1053–1059.

10. Quast U, Guillon JM, Cavero I. Cellular pharmacology of potassium channel openers in vascular smooth muscle. *Cardiovasc Res* 1994; **28**: 805–810.

11. Aggarwal A, Warltier DC. Adenosine: present uses, future indications. *Curr Opin Anaesthesiol* 1994; **7**: 109–122.

12. Rankin AC, Brooks R, Ruskin JN, McGovern BA. Adenosine and the treatment of supraventricular tachycardia. *Am J Med* 1992; **92**: 655–664.

13. Fullerton DA, Jones SD, Grover FL, McIntyre RC Jr. Adenosine effectively controls pulmonary hypertension after cardiac operations. *Ann Thorac Surg* 1996; **61**: 1118–1124.

14. Forman MB, Velasco CE, Jackson EK. Adenosine attenuates reperfusion injury following regional myocardial ischemia. *Cardiovasc Res* 1993; **27**: 9–17.

15. Van der Stroom JG, van Wezel HB, Vergroesen I *et al.* Comparison of the effects of urapidil and sodium nitroprusside on haemodynamic state, myocardial metabolism and function in patients during coronary artery surgery. *Br J Anaesth* 1996; **76**: 645–651.

16. Yanagisawa M, Kurihara H, Kimura S *et al.* A novel potent vasoconstrictor peptide produced by endothelial cells. *Nature* 1988; **332**: 411–415.

17. de Bold AJ, Kuroski-de Bold ML, Boer PH *et al.* A decade of atrial natriuretic factor research. *Can J Physiol Pharmacol* 1991; **69**: 1480–1485.

Section 5

OTHER SYSTEMS AND SPECIAL TOPICS

18

AW Schuster, P Dorinsky

DRUGS ACTING ON THE RESPIRATORY SYSTEM

The lung diseases most often requiring pharmacological intervention are those involving lung obstruction and/or bronchospasm. The most common of these disorders are asthma, chronic bronchitis and emphysema. Asthma is characterized by reversible airflow obstruction, predominantly in the third to seventh generations of the bronchi. Bronchoconstriction occurs in response to specific and/or nonspecific stimuli and reverses either spontaneously or in response to therapy. Subjects with asthma have intermittent attacks of bronchospasm with tightness of the chest, expiratory wheezing and dyspnoea. Acute attacks of asthma can progress to status asthmaticus, a medical emergency requiring urgent pharmacological intervention. Asthma is increasing in prevalence and severity, particularly in the young, and has a rising mortality rate in most industrial countries. The characteristic pathological features of asthma in adults are bronchial hyperreactivity and inflammation. Inflammatory changes result in damage to the bronchial epithelium and eosinophil infiltration, mucosal oedema and mucus plugging. Some degree of inflammatory changes are present even in patients with mild asthma. Bronchial hyperreactivity occurs to a wide variety of stimuli such as cold air, atmospheric pollutants and, in sensitive individuals, allergens such as pollen and domestic dust mites. These stimuli can trigger bronchospasm.

In many individuals an asthmatic attack consists of two phases. The immediate phase occurs abruptly and is due mainly to bronchospasm triggered by the release of mediators such as leukotrienes and histamine from mast cells and other cells including eosinophils, platelets and macrophages. The late phase or delayed response is a progressive inflammatory reaction initi-

ated during the first phase by the release of chemotaxins that attract leucocytes into the bronchial mucosa. The late phase develops at a variable time after exposure to the initiating stimulus.

The pathological features of chronic bronchitis include enlargement of the mucus-secreting glands and inflammation of the small airways. Although features of chronic bronchitis may coexist with emphysema, the latter is characterized primarily by enlargement and/or destruction of alveoli. Patients with chronic bronchitis also have clinical features that include sputum production and expiratory wheezing, whereas these are generally lacking in patients with emphysema. Individuals with emphysema respond poorly to bronchodilator and antiinflammatory therapy, while patients with asthma respond quite well to these agents and those with chronic bronchitis have an intermediate response.[1,2]

PHYSIOLOGY OF AIRWAY CONTROL

A rational approach to the pharmacological therapy of bronchoconstrictive disorders requires an understanding of airways regulation. The tone of the bronchial muscles is regulated by parasympathetic innervation, by circulating adrenaline and noradrenaline, and by other neurohumoral mediators referred to as nonadrenergic noncholinergic (NANC) mediators. The parasympathetic cholinergic pathway which originates in the vagus nerve has an important regulatory role in the human airway. Cholinergic efferent nerves synapse in ganglia within the airway and postganglionic nerve fibres then innervate the airway smooth muscle and mucous glands. These fibres release acetylcholine which can result in bronchoconstriction, increased mucous secretion and vasodilatation. Cholinergic pathways play an important role in the pathogenesis of airway obstruction in asthma, chronic bronchitis and emphysema.

There are three distinct subtypes of muscarinic receptors in the airways. The M_1 subtype is present in the parasympathetic ganglia and mucus-secreting glands. The M_2 subtype is found in parasympathetic nerve terminals and is autoinhibitory in nature. It is believed that abnormal functioning and/or absence of M_2 receptors is important in the pathogenesis of bronchospasm induced by β-adrenoceptor antagonists. The M_3 subtype is located in the smooth muscle and mucous glands of the airway. When acetylcholine binds to airway M_3 muscarinic receptors, it causes the release of cyclic guanosine monophosphate (cGMP) which in turn stimulates the release of intracellular calcium ions (Ca^{2+}), causing smooth muscle contraction. Anticholinergics inhibit acetylcholine from binding to muscarinic receptors located in the respiratory epithelium, submucosal glands, mast cells and airway smooth muscle, thus preventing release of cGMP and inhibiting bronchoconstriction.

While the bronchi have a rich parasympathetic innervation, there is no sympathetic innervation of bronchial smooth muscle and all sympathetic effects are due to circulating adrenaline and noradrenaline acting on β_2-adrenoceptors. Stimulation of these receptors results in bronchodilatation. The main physiological relaxant in the bronchi, however, is thought to be the NANC inhibitory mediator, which is a potent bronchodilator. Neither the source nor the identity of this mediator is known, although there is some evidence that it may be either vasoactive intestinal peptide or nitric oxide. A second class of NANC mediators are the excitatory neuropeptides such as substance P and neurokinin A, which are thought to have a role in the delayed phase of asthma. Substance P, which is also involved in nociception, increases mucus secretion in bronchial glands while neurokinin A is a potent vasoconstrictor.

BRONCHODILATORS

β-ADRENOCEPTOR AGONISTS

The β-adrenoceptor agonists used in asthma and other obstructive lung disorders are selective for the β_2-receptors; nonselective β_2-adrenoceptor agonists such as adrenaline and isoprenaline are no longer used in the routine management of asthma. The drugs currently used include the resorcinols (orciprenaline (metaproterenol), isoetharine and terbutaline) and saligenins (salbutamol and salmeterol). The resorcinols and saligenins are noncatecholamines because they lack hydroxyl groups at positions 3 and 4 of the benzene ring. They have a modified central catecholamine nucleus (Fig. 18.1), which results in β_2-receptor selectivity and a longer duration of action. Orciprenaline was the first noncatecholamine used as a bronchodilator, but is not as β_2 selective as, for example, salbutamol. Resorcinols and saligenins also have bulky substituents on the N atom, which increases potency and makes them less susceptible to metabolism by monoamine oxidase and to neuronal uptake (uptake 1). Because of the resorcinol ring structure, drugs such as orciprenaline are not degraded by catechol-*O*-methyltransferase (COMT).

The main effect of these agents is to dilate the bronchi by activating β_2-adrenoceptors on the bronchial smooth muscle. This stimulates adenylyl cyclase, increasing cyclic adenosine monophosphate (cAMP) concentration. cAMP, acting via protein kinases, provides the energy for compartmental shifts in calcium, which results in smooth muscle relaxation. There is also evidence indicating that β_2-adrenoceptor agonists may open activated potassium channels by direct linkage to a G protein. This process may occur at very low concentrations and influence airway relaxation independent of cAMP.[3] β-Adrenoceptor agonists also have limited anti-inflammatory actions. They inhibit mediator release from mast cells and may stimulate release of relaxant factors from bronchial epithelial cells. They may also inhibit vagal tone, increase mucus clearance by an action on the cilia, and reduce microvascular leakage thereby reducing oedema.

Although β_2-adrenoceptor antagonists have no effect on airway tone in normal individuals, in patients with hyperreactive airways they can precipitate serious acute bronchospasm, which of course does not respond to the usual doses of β_2-adrenoceptor agonists. Thus nonselective antagonists such as propranolol should be avoided in these patients, and even selective antagonists should be used with caution since none is so selective that this danger can be ignored.

The β_2-adrenoceptor agonists can be classified according to their duration of action into short and long acting. In general, the short-acting agonists have an onset of action that occurs within minutes and the peak effect is reached within 30–60 min. The longer-acting agents generally have a slower onset, usually 10–20 min, and reach their peak effectiveness in 2–4 h. The short-acting agents provide bronchodilatation for 4–6 h (up to 8 h with fenoterol) and protection from provocation for 2–4 h, whereas the longer-acting agents provide bronchodilatation and bronchoprotection for up

---

Summary box 18.1 Actions of β_2-adrenoceptors agonists that are potentially of benefit in obstructive lung disease

- Bronchial smooth muscle relaxation.

- Enhanced mucociliary clearance.

- Inhibition of mediator release from mast cells and basophils.

- Reduced vascular permeability.

- May reduce the release of acetylcholine by an action on prejunctional receptors on cholinergic nerves.

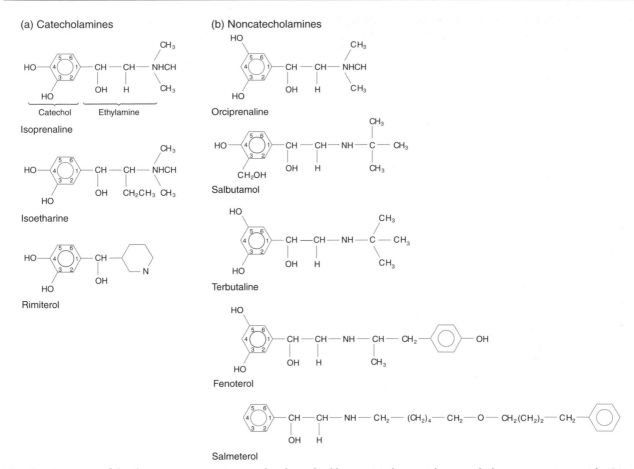

Fig. 18.1 Structure of β_2-adrenoceptor agonists used as bronchodilators: (a) drugs with a catecholamine structure, with -OH groups at positions 3 and 4 of the benzene ring; (b) noncatecholamines.

to 12 h (Table 18.1). The short-acting drugs include salbutamol, fenoterol, rimiterol and terbutaline. Bambuterol, a prodrug of terbutaline, is also available. The maximum effect of these drugs is reached within 20–30 min when given by inhalation, with a duration of 4–6 h. Rimiterol has an even faster onset, the effect appearing within 20 s of inhalation, and a short duration, the bronchodilatation declining after 30 min. Salbutamol (albuterol) has a hydroxymethyl group on the catechol ring. Since the hydroxymethyl group is not a substrate for COMT, it is resistant to methylation by COMT, a property that contributes to its duration of action. The short-acting β_2-adrenoceptor agonists are useful in the treatment of incidental bronchospasm and are the agents of choice in the treatment of acute asthma as well as in treating bronchospasm in other chronic obstructive lung disorders.

Formoterol and salmeterol xinafoate are long-acting drugs. The effects of formoterol appear within 1–3 min after inhalation, while with salmeterol effects are apparent only after 10–20 min. For both drugs broncho-

dilatation lasts for up to 12 h. The part of the salmeterol molecule that is responsible for binding to the β_2 receptor is identical to salbutamol (Fig. 18.1). The extended therapeutic effect of salmeterol is believed to be due to the binding of its long lipophilic side-chain to an exoreceptor adjacent to the active portion of the β_2 receptor. The exoreceptor anchors the agonist and permits nearly continuous stimulation of the β_2 receptor. The long-acting drugs are indicated for the management of asthma that reacts inadequately to treatment with steroids, and for chronic bronchitis and emphysema. They may be useful in the treatment of exercise-induced asthma. Long-acting β_2-adrenoceptor agonists should not be used in the treatment of acute asthma. Salmeterol may have contributed to approximately 20 deaths that occurred in the first 8 months after its release in the United States. Although the drug itself is not intrinsically harmful, its use in acute asthma may delay access to more rapid acting β_2 agonists, thus allowing potentially life-threatening bronchospasm to develop.

Because of the high incidence of side-effects (see

Table 18.1 Pharmacokinetic properties of inhaled β-adrenoceptor agonists			
Agent	Onset (min)	Duration (h)	Peak effect (min)
Salbutamol	5–15	4	60
Bitolterol	3–5	5	60
Adrenaline	1–5	1–2	–
Isoetharine	1–5	2–3	30
Orciprenaline	1	3–4	45
Rimiterol	20 s	1–2	–
Pirbuterol	5	4–6	30–60
Terbutaline	5–30	4	60
Salmeterol	20	8–12	180
Formoterol	1–3	12	–

undergo substantial first-pass metabolism in the liver. It is also possible to administer some of these agents intravenously. Although this approach may be useful in patients with refractory, life-threatening, respiratory symptoms, its utility is limited by an unacceptably high incidence of significant side-effects.

Side-effects

The side-effects of inhaled drugs are minor relative to the orally administered agents and are due largely to β_1-receptor stimulation, since even selective β_2 agonists stimulate β_1 receptors at high doses (Table 18.2). Muscle tremor, caused by direct stimulation of the β_2-adrenoceptors in the skeletal muscles, is the limiting side-effect of orally administered β_2-adrenoreceptor agonists. Cardiovascular side-effects with oral administration are also common and include tachycardia, palpitations, hypertension and a prolongation of the QTc interval on the electrocardiogram. Prolongation of the QTc interval may lead to ventricular arrhythmias including torsades de pointes. Because of these side-effects, oral administration should be used with caution in patients who are taking other sympathomimetic agents and in those with congestive heart failure, arrhythmias, coronary artery disease, hypertension, hyperthyroidism or epilepsy.

below) oral adrenergic agents β_2-adrenoceptor agonists are seldom used for bronchodilatation. This route can, however, be useful in young children who cannot manipulate inhalers. Another indication is in adults in whom inhalation triggers bronchospasm. Oral delivery is significantly confounded by the variability in gastrointestinal absorption and by the first-pass effect of hepatic metabolism. To compensate for the first-pass effect, larger doses must be given orally, with the result that side-effects are also increased.

Inhalation of aerosol, powder or nebulized solution is by far the most common and effective means of delivering these drugs. Aerosol delivery is highly effective and is characterized by a rapid onset of action and a significant decrease in the incidence of side-effects.[4] A critical determinant of the delivery of inhaled drugs is the particle size. The ideal size is 1–5 μm; these particles are deposited in the small airways, where they are most effective. Particles larger than 10 μm are deposited mainly in the mouth, while those smaller than 0.5 μm are inhaled into the alveoli and then exhaled without being deposited. Even under ideal circumstances, however, only about 2–10% of the inhaled drug is deposited in the small bronchi. Most of the remainder is swallowed. Fortunately the β_2-adrenoceptor agonists used for this purpose are either poorly absorbed from the gastrointestinal tract and/or

Table 18.2 Receptor selectivity of β-adrenoceptor agonists			
	Receptor stimulation		
Agent	α	β_1	β_2
Salbutomol	o	±	+3
Bitolerol	o	±	+3
Adrenaline	+1	+1	+1
Isoetharine	o	+1	+2
Isoprenaline	o	+1	+1
Orciprenaline	o	+1	+2
Pirbuterol	o	±	+3
Salmeterol	o	±	+3
Terbutaline	o	±	+3

Paradoxical bronchoconstriction has been reported after nebulized salbutamol, but not terbutaline, suggesting that this reaction could be specific to the drug preparation rather than a class effect.[5]

METHYLXANTHINES

The naturally occurring methylated xanthines (methylxanthines) caffeine, theophylline and theobromine, present in coffee beans, tea leaves, cocoa seeds and cola nuts, have been used for hundreds of years in the treatment of bronchospasm. The methylxanthines most frequently used today are theophylline and aminophylline, the ethylenediamine salt of theophylline (Fig. 18.2). The methylxanthines have low water solubility but the formation of salts, such as in aminophylline, markedly increases this. In plasma, aminophylline dissociates to yield the parent theophylline. The most important pharmacological property of these drugs is their ability to relax smooth muscle, especially bronchial muscle. In addition they stimulate the central nervous system (CNS) and cardiac muscle, and have a diuretic action on the kidneys. Theophylline is the most effective of the methylxanthines as a bronchodilator. However, it is less effective than β_2-adrenoceptor agonists, has a very narrow therapeutic window and has declined in importance for the treatment of asthma. A plasma theophylline concentration of 20 μg ml^{-1} (the upper limit of the therapeutic range) produces 45–60% of maximum bronchodilatation compared with the 80–90% that can be achieved with β_2-adrenoceptor agonists. Theophylline also causes myocardial stimulation, resulting in an increase in cardiac output and a decrease in central

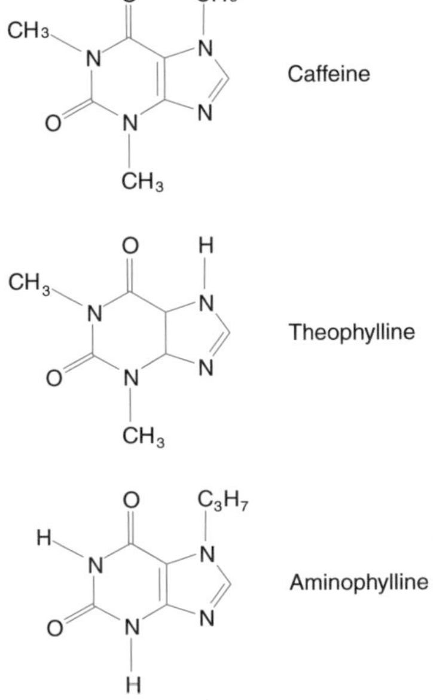

Fig. 18.2 Structure of the methylxanthine bronchodilators.

> **Summary box 18.2 Methylxanthines**
>
> - Caffeine, theophylline and theobromine are ingredients in coffee, tea, coca and cola beverages.
>
> - Theophylline and aminophylline (the ethylenediamine salt of theophylline) are the drugs in this class most commonly used in obstructive lung diseases.
>
> - Most important pharmacological property of the methylxanthines is smooth muscle relaxation, especially of the bronchial muscles.
>
> - Stimulation of the CNS and cardiovascular system is responsible for most of the side-effects.
>
> - Theophylline is the most effective bronchodilator in this class, but is less effective than β_2-adrenoceptor agonists. This, together with a narrow therapeutic window, limits its usefulness.
>
> - The mechanisms of smooth muscle relaxation are not fully understood. The most likely candidate seems to be adenosine receptor antagonism. Inhibition of phosphodiesterase is relevant only at concentrations above those producing a therapeutic effect.

venous pressures. It may also improve diaphragm function, especially when this muscle is fatigued, as is often the case in patients with chronic bronchitis and emphysema. These effects can contribute to the improvement in ventilatory function and to the decreased sensation of dyspnoea produced by theophylline in many patients with obstructive lung diseases. Lastly, theophylline is an immunomodulator, increasing suppressor T-cell counts in the peripheral blood of antigen-challenged asthmatics and inhibiting the late phase response to allergens.[6]

The best-characterized cellular actions of the methylxanthines are inhibition of phosphodiesterase, the enzyme that inactivates cAMP, and antagonism of the receptor-mediated actions of adenosine. However, the exact mechanism of action remains unknown. Until recently it was believed that relaxation of the bronchial smooth muscle occurred via the inhibition of phosphodiesterase. However, phosphodiesterase is only minimally inhibited at therapeutic concentrations of theophylline. Nevertheless there is a strong correlation between the rank order of methylxanthines for inhibiting phosphodiesterase and their effectiveness in asthma. This may reflect their ability to selectively inhibit a particular isoform of this enzyme, phosphodiesterase-4.[7] A large body of evidence now suggests that adenosine receptor antagonism is the most important mechanism responsible for the pharmacological actions of these drugs in doses that are used clinically. Theophylline is relatively nonselective for the different subtypes of adenosine receptors. Enprofylline, a new methylxanthine which is more potent than theophylline as a bronchodilator in asthmatic patients but is without obvious CNS effects, is a poor antagonist of most but not all adenosine receptors. This has been used as an argument that adenosine does not play a role in asthma. However, recent work has demonstrated that both theophylline and enprofylline are antagonists at the adenosine A_{2B} receptor, whereas enprofylline is a poor antagonist at the A_{2A} receptor.[8] Other mechanisms relevant to the use of these drugs in obstructive lung disorders are inhibition of mediator release, increased sympathomimetic activity, altered cellular function and reduced respiratory muscle fatigue.

Pharmacokinetics

The methylxanthines are well absorbed after oral administration. Food can slow the rate, but not the extent, of absorption. Theophylline is metabolized primarily in the liver (90%) by several cytochrome P450 enzymes, and is eliminated in the urine as 1,3-dimethylxanthine. Less than 10% of the drug is excreted unchanged in the urine. The major metabolic pathways are N-demethylation and hydroxylation. In infants less than 1 year of age, however, nearly half of the drug is excreted as unchanged theophylline in the urine. Theophylline, or its salt aminophylline, has its onset of action within 3–4 min after intravenous administration and within 30 min after oral administration. Its peak effect when given intravenously is at about 60 min, while after an oral dose the peak effect occurs at 2 h. The average half-life of the drug is 5.2 (range 3–9.5) h in adults and 3.6 h in children aged 5–15 years. The average half-life is shorter in smokers (4.3 h) than in nonsmokers (7 h), possibly due to enzyme induction in smokers.

Factors leading to increased levels of theophylline (i.e. decreased theophylline clearance) include heart failure, liver disease, respiratory failure, prolonged fever, hypothyroidism, extremes of age or any acute life-threatening illness. Clinically significant drug interactions are also common and a host of drugs can decrease theophylline clearance (Table 18.3). Drugs that are enzyme inducers increase the clearance of theophylline (see Chapter 28 for details of enzyme inhibitors and inducers).

The rate at which individuals metabolize theophylline is quite heterogeneous. As a result, a given dose of theophylline may produce widely varying plasma concentrations. Therefore drug levels should be monitored frequently. The therapeutic range for theophylline is $10–20\ \mu g\ ml^{-1}$. Generally, the loading dose for intravenous aminophylline is $5–6\ mg\ kg^{-1}$ over 30 min followed by a continuous infusion at a rate of $0.5–1\ mg\ kg^{-1}\ h^{-1}$. As a general guideline, each $0.6\ mg\ kg^{-1}$ increment in the aminophylline infusion rate ($0.5\ mg\ kg^{-1}$ for theophylline) will change the aminophylline concentration by approximately $1\ \mu g\ ml^{-1}$. In obese children and adults weighing more than 120% of their ideal body weight, the initial dose should be based on ideal body weight to avoid overdosing.[9]

Side-effects

Since theophylline has such a narrow therapeutic window, side-effects and toxicity are sometimes seen at blood concentrations considered to be therapeutic. Minor side-effects such as nausea, vomiting, tachycardia, tachypnoea and tremor become more prominent with increasing blood levels. However, they may also occur at therapeutic or subtherapeutic levels and necessitate discontinuing treatment. The major life-

Table 18.3 Factors that affect theophylline pharmacokinetics	
Factors that increase clearance	**Factors that decrease clearance**
Smoking Alcohol Low carbohydrate, high protein diet Cystic fibrosis	Heart failure Liver cirrhosis Viral infections Pneumonia
Enzyme-inducing drugs	**Enzyme-inhibiting drugs**
Phenytoin Carbamazine Barbiturates Rifampicin	Cimetidine Macrolide antibiotics, e.g. erythromycin Azole antifungal agents Oral contraceptives

threatening side-effects of the methylxanthines are seizures and ventricular arrhythmias. These usually occur when the plasma theophylline concentration exceeds 35 μg ml^{-1} and they can occur without warning signs. Theophylline-induced convulsions are relatively refractory to therapy and have a reported mortality rate of 50%.[10] Serious ventricular arrhythmias are uncommon at therapeutic levels of theophylline but life-threatening ventricular arrhythmias may occur at toxic concentrations. They are usually responsive to lignocaine (lidocaine). Aminophylline or theophylline should be injected slowly over 20–30 min to avoid severe toxic symptoms. Rapid intravenous injection of 500 mg aminophylline has resulted in sudden death that is probably due to cardiac arrhythmias. Volatile anaesthetics, especially halothane, increase the risk of ventricular arrhythmias when used concomitantly with theophylline. Halothane sensitizes the myocardium to endogenous catecholamines, whereas theophylline increases the release of endogenous catecholamines.

MUSCARINIC RECEPTOR ANTAGONISTS

The main agent used specifically as a bronchodilator is ipratropium bromide. Ipratropium is a quaternary ammonium compound formed by the addition of an isopropyl group to the N atom of atropine (Fig. 18.3). Oxitropium is a quaternary ammonium derivative of hyoscine (scopolamine). The newest drug in this class is tiotropium, also with a quaternary ammonium structure, which has a prolonged and persistent bronchodilator activity due to extremely slow dissociation from the muscarinic receptor. These drugs are administered by inhalation and the effects are almost exclusively confined to the airways, since less than 1% of an inhaled dose is absorbed systemically. Because of their quaternary structure, little of the dose that is swallowed is absorbed from the gastrointestinal tract.

Ipratropium is considered the drug of choice in the treatment of chronic obstructive lung disease but it is less effective than β_2-adrenoceptor agonists in the treatment of asthma. Combined treatment with a β_2-adrenoceptor agonist is, however, more effective than either agent alone. In Europe inhalers containing a mixture of ipratropium and fenoterol are available, but are recommended for use in chronic bronchitis or emphysema rather than asthma. Ipratropium protects incompletely against bronchoconstriction induced by stimuli that have effects only partially mediated through vagal reflex mechanisms such as cold air, histamine and allergens. In contrast to atropine, it does not reduce mucociliary clearance in normal subjects and thus does not contribute to the accumulation of secretions in the lower airway. After inhalation the onset of action is 15–30 min with a peak effect at 1–2 h and duration of action of 3–6 h.

Because of the low systemic uptake from the lungs or gastrointestinal tract, ipratropium has few side-effects. Unlike atropine it does not cross the blood–brain barrier and therefore has almost no CNS side-effects. The most common systemic side-effects are headache, dry mouth, nausea, cough, nervousness and dizziness. Cardiovascular or ocular side-effects are uncommon, even when doses in excess of those recommended are administered. Ipratropium is contraindicated in patients with atropine hypersensitivity.

ANTIINFLAMMATORY AGENTS

The main antiinflammatory agents used in the treatment of obstructive lung disorders are the bischromones (sodium cromoglycate and nedocromil) and the glucocorticosteroids.

The chromones (Fig. 18.4) are used in the treatment of mild to moderate asthma to prevent asthama attacks, but are ineffective in treating acute bronchospasm since they are not bronchodilators. They inhibit both phases of asthma caused by allergens or exercise, probably by inhibiting the release of histamine and other autacoids from sensitized pulmonary mast cells.[11] Long-term treatment with these drugs can reduce bronchial hyperreactivity and airway inflammation.

Summary box 18.3 Anticholinergic drugs

- Ipratropium is the main drug used as a bronchodilator. Others in this class are oxitropium and tiotropium.

- All are quaternary ammonium compounds, so systemic uptake and passage of the blood–brain barrier is minimal.

- Ipratropium is an isopropyl derivative of atropine; oxitropium is a derivative of hyoscine (scopolamine).

- Act on muscarinic M$_3$ receptors on bronchial smooth muscle.

- Less effective in asthma than β_2-adrenoceptor agonists, but combinations are more effective than either drug given alone.

- Anticholinergic drugs are considered the bronchodilators of choice in patients with chronic bronchitis or emphysema.

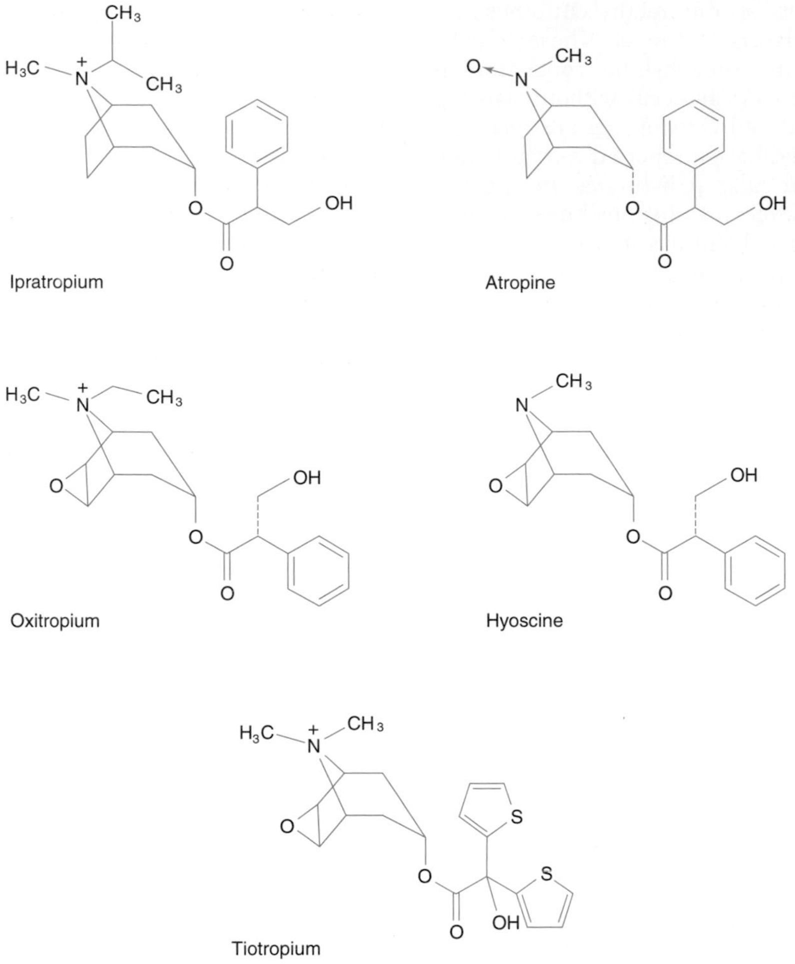

Fig. 18.3 Muscarinic receptor antagonists.

SODIUM CROMOGLYCATE (CROMOLYN SODIUM)

Sodium cromoglycate attenuates bronchospasm induced by various provocative stimuli such as inhaled allergens, cold air, fog, pollutants and exercise. It inhibits the activation and recruitment of cells (e.g. eosinophils and mast cells) that play an important role in the inflammatory processes that characterize asthma. Cromoglycate works best when given before a potentially provocative agent and should not be used during an acute asthmatic attack. It may be necessary to administer cromoglycate for 4–6 weeks before a therapeutic response is noted in patients with asthma. Cromoglycate is effective only when administered by inhalation, using either a solution delivered by aerosol spray or nebulizer, or powered drug mixed with lactose delivered by a special turboinhaler. Peak plasma concentrations occur within 15 min and cromoglycate has a half-life of approximately 80 min. Nearly 10% of

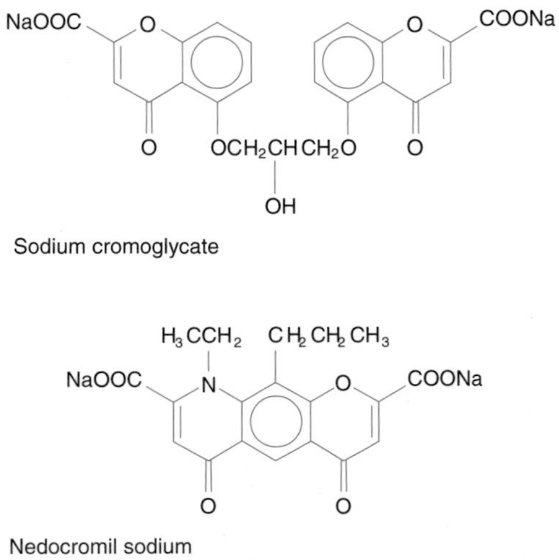

Fig. 18.4 Sodium cromoglycate and nedocromil.

Summary box 18.4 Chromones

- Available drugs are sodium cromoglycate and nedocromil.

- Effective only when administered by inhalation.

- Are not bronchodilators but inhibit the activation and recruitment of cells (e.g. eosinophils and mast cells) that play an important role in the inflammatory processes that characterize asthma. Mast cell stabilization is not an important mechanism.

- Other mechanisms include antagonism of inhibition of cytokinin release, inhibition of platelet-activating factor interaction with platelets, suppression of nonmyelinated vagal sensory nerve endings, inhibition of phosphodiesterase and reduction of airway permeability.

- Corticosteroid-sparing effects may be particularly useful in patients with corticosteroid-dependent asthma.

- Nedocromil may be slightly more effective than cromoglycate, especially in younger patients.

- Few side-effects; those that do occur are usually minor.

the drug is absorbed systemically after inhalation. Cromoglycate is not metabolized after absorption but is excreted unchanged in the bile and urine. Drug that is swallowed is absorbed minimally from the gastrointestinal tract.

Although the exact mechanism of action remains unknown, cromoglycate is thought to inhibit calcium influx by phosphorylating a membrane protein with the result that mediator release from mast cells is inhibited. It also inhibits C-fibre sensory nerve activation in animals and may inhibit reflex-induced bronchospasm. Other mechanisms include suppression of nonmyelinated vagal sensory nerve endings, inhibition of phosphodiesterase and reduction of airway permeability.

Side-effects

Cromoglycate sodium causes few side-effects; those that do occur are usually minor and include cough, wheezing, dry throat, joint swelling, nausea, headache, nasal congestion, rash and urticaria. Transient bronchospasm that can be reversed with inhaled β_2 agonists may also occur. More serious side-effects have been reported and are most often attributable to allergic reactions (i.e.

laryngeal oedema, angioedema, urticaria and anaphylaxis). Patients who are lactose deficient should use the lactose-free preparation to avoid gastrointestinal discomfort.

NEDOCROMIL SODIUM

Nedocromil sodium is a pyranoquinolone (Fig. 18.4) that is structurally different from cromoglycate, but with similar pharmacological properties. Like cromoglycate, nedocromil has corticosteroid-sparing effects and may be particularly useful in patients with corticosteroid-dependent asthma. Nedocromil may be slightly more effective than cromoglycate, especially in younger patients.[9] Systemic absorption of nedocromil after inhalation is low (less than 10% with 2.5% due to absorption from the gastrointestinal tract). Once absorbed, it is not metabolized and is excreted unchanged via the urinary and gastrointestinal tracts. The side-effects from nedocromil are usually mild and transient. The most commonly reported side-effects are headache, nausea, vomiting, dizziness and altered taste.

GLUCOCORTICOSTEROIDS

Systemic steroids have long been used to treat severe asthma, but the more recent development of formulations for inhalation, which significantly reduce the risk of side-effects, has allowed them to be used also for moderate asthma. Individuals who require inhaled β_2-adrenoceptor agonists four or more times weekly

Summary box 18.5 Glucocorticosteroids

- Very effective in the management of chronic asthma and of benefit in patients with other chronic obstructive lung diseases with a predominantly inflammatory component.

- Main antiinflammatory actions include inhibition of leucocyte chemotaxins, reduced recruitment and activation of eosinophils and other inflammatory cells. Also decrease generation of leukotrienes and platelet-activating factor.

- Usually given by inhalation. Full effect may be achieved only after several days or weeks of treatment.

- Use of high-dose inhaled steroids is as effective as oral therapy in many patients.

- In status asthmaticus, intravenous hydrocortisone is used in the acute phase followed by oral therapy.

- Adverse effects with inhaled steroids are uncommon.

benefit from the addition of steroids.[12,13] The main compounds used by inhalation are beclomethasone, budesonide, triamcinolone, flunisolide and fluticasone. Oral steroids, prednisone, prednisolone and hydrocortisone, are used for chronic asthma or acute, severe or rapidly deteriorating attacks. The use of high-dose inhaled steroids is, however, probably as effective as oral therapy in many patients. In status asthmaticus intravenous hydrocortisone is used in the acute phase, followed by oral therapy.

Inhaled glucocorticoids are considered to be first-line agents in the treatment of asthma. They are also beneficial to patients with other chronic obstructive lung diseases. Although the effects of these drugs on airway function seem to be dose dependent, 2–4 weeks of continuous use may be necessary before maximum benefit is obtained.

For an acute exacerbation of asthma or chronic obstructive lung disease, intravenous hydrocortisone or methylprednisolone in doses of 60–120 mg every 6 h may be required. Intravenous therapy is continued until there is sustained clinical improvement, at which time the intravenous corticosteroids may be tapered. Oral therapy with prednisone or an equivalent oral agent is then begun at a daily dose of 0.5–1.0 mg kg^{-1} and reduced by 10 mg every 3–4 days. Inhaled corticosteroids can be resumed when the daily dose falls to 20 mg.

Mechanism of action

In general, the corticosteroids pass through cell membranes and bind to specific cytoplasmic receptors. There is a single glucocorticoid receptor population present in the cytoplasm of bronchial endothelial and epithelial cells. Once bound to these receptors, the steroid–receptor complex translocates to the cell nucleus, attaches to nuclear binding sites and initiates messenger RNA synthesis. This stimulates the production of proteins that produce the characteristic actions of steroids (Fig. 18.5). The beneficial effects of corticosteroids in asthma are probably due to their ability to inhibit the inflammatory processes that occur. Corticosteroids affect numerous aspects of inflammation including leucocyte traffic and function, regulator protein synthesis, catecholamine receptor binding affinity and density, eicosanoid synthesis and vascular endothelial integrity.

Corticosteroids have many actions that may be important in the treatment of asthma and other chronic obstructive lung disorders. Specifically, corticosteroids inhibit the transcription of various proinflammatory cytokines. In addition, corticosteroids inhibit airway mucous secretion and upregulate β adrenoceptors at the gene transcriptional level. They also inhibit immunoglobulin E synthesis. However, this effect takes hours or

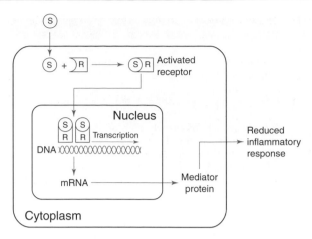

Fig. 18.5 Cellular mechanism of action of steroids used in obstructive lung disorders. The glucocorticoid receptor (R) is present in the cytoplasm predominantly in an inactive form but becomes activated by binding to a steroid molecule (S) and translocates to the nucleus. Two receptor–steroid complexes (dimers) interact with DNA to produce messenger RNA (mRNA) for specific mediator proteins that are responsible for the antiinflammatory and other cellular actions of the steroids.

days to develop. Finally, inhaled corticosteroids improve lung function, decrease the need for inhaled β_2 agonists, decrease airway responsiveness to allergens, and decrease circulating levels of eosinophils, basophils and neutrophils.

It is important to note that narrowing of the airway lumen in asthma and other chronic obstructive lung disorders is the result both of bronchial smooth muscle hyperactivity and of mucosal oedema and inflammation. Patients may have only partial relief from bronchodilators since the events that mediate bronchoconstriction are often inflammatory and do not respond to bronchodilators. Corticosteroids can block inflammation and the late-phase response of asthma.

Pharmacokinetics

Corticosteroids are available in oral, inhalational and intravenous forms. The various corticosteroids differ in their relative potencies and duration of action owing to the structural modifications that influence pharmacokinetic properties of these drugs. Corticosteroids can be placed into one of three categories: (1) short-acting drugs (e.g. hydrocortisone); (2) intermediate-acting drugs (e.g. prednisone, prednisolone, methylprednisolone); and (3) long-acting drugs (e.g. dexamethasone, triamcinolone, betamethasone).

Although antacids can inhibit absorption, the corticosteroids are generally well absorbed orally and drugs such as prednisone and prednisolone reach peak plasma concentrations 1–2 h after ingestion. By contrast, inhaled glucocorticoids differ in their rates of absorption. For example, betamethasone and dexamethasone are well absorbed and often produce systemic side-effects, whereas triamcinolone acetonide, beclomethasone dipropionate and flunisolide are poorly absorbed, rapidly metabolized and associated with fewer systemic side-effects. Budesonide and flunisolide undergo extensive hepatic first-pass metabolism, which reduces their bioavailability. Budesonide and beclomethasone, the main compounds given by inhalation, are the most potent of the steroids used in asthma.

Once absorbed, these compounds bind avidly to corticosteroid-binding globulin and can readily cross the placenta. Elimination is primarily hepatic and 70% is conjugated in the liver to inactive or poorly active compounds, while only a small amount is excreted unchanged in the urine. Drugs that can impair elimination of glucocorticoids include ketoconazole, oral contraceptives, erythromycin and troleandomycin. Liver disease can also potentially reduce glucocorticoid clearance. However, since corticosteroids can be metabolized by other mechanisms (e.g. lung esterases), the impact of liver disease on glucocorticoid clearance is usually not clinically significant. Finally, numerous drugs can accelerate glucocorticoid elimination, and these include aminoglutethimide, carbamazepine, ephedrine, phenobarbitone, phenytoin and rifampicin.

Side-effects

Side-effects are common with all orally administered steroids and with the inhaled agents that have significant systemic absorption (e.g. betamethasone, dexamethasone). Changes in appetite, insomnia and personality changes are the most common short-term side-effects, while cataracts, glucose intolerance, osteoporosis, hypertension and peptic ulcers are more common long-term complications of the corticosteroids. Although inhaled corticosteroids are generally well tolerated, there is concern for the their possible adrenal inhibitory effects. However, the relationship between a measurable change in adrenal function and the risk of clinically important systemic side-effects has not been established.[14] In addition, a review of the risk of systemic toxicity from inhaled steroids suggests that regular treatment with up to 800 μg beclomethasone daily in adults or up to 400 μg daily in children is unlikely to have clinically important effects on adrenal function, bone metabolism or growth.[14]

Oral candidiasis and dysphonia caused by steroid myopathy of the laryngeal muscles are also common side-effects of inhaled glucocorticoids. These side-effects can be diminished with regular rinsing of the mouth following each administration, or by using a spacer device that aids in drug delivery such that a higher proportion of a given dose reaches the distal airways rather than being trapped in the oropharynx. Rare side-effects include the immediate and delayed hypersensitivity reactions such as rash, angioedema, urticaria and bronchospasm.

HISTAMINE H$_1$-RECEPTOR ANTAGONISTS

Although release of histamine from mast cells by allergens is a trigger for bronchospasm in patients with allergic asthma and some types of exercise-induced asthma, antihistamines are relatively ineffective in the treatment of asthma. This is because histamine is only one of several mediators released from mast cells and other cells, such as leukotrienes, neurokinin A and platelet-activating factor that are more important as bronchoconstrictors. Some of the nonsedating antihistamines such as cetirizine and azelastine, which may also inhibit the release of leukotrienes, are reasonably effective in mild atopic asthma, decreasing the number of attacks and allowing a reducion of concomitant therapy. Ketotifen, a 5-hydroxytryptamine antagonist with some H$_1$-receptor antagonism, may be useful in childhood asthma.

FUTURE THERAPY

LEUKOTRIENE ANTAGONISTS

Leukotrienes are arachidonic acid metabolites produced by inflammatory cells such as mast cells, macrophages, eosinophils and basophils. The cysteinyl leukotrienes are believed to play a role in regulating airway tone and inflammation in patients with asthma. Specifically, the leukotrienes increase vascular permeability, increase mucous production, increase oedema, induce bronchoconstriction and promote inflammatory cell inflammation. Leukotriene inhibitors such as the leukotriene (LT) D$_4$-receptor antagonists, accolate and pranlukast, exert their effects either by blocking arachidonate 5-lipoxygenase synthesis or by preventing mediators from binding to their receptors, thus blocking bronchoconstriction. The exact role of leukotriene inhibitors in the treatment of asthma is still being defined. However, cysteinyl leukotriene inhibitors such as accolate and pranlukast have been described as the first new treatment for asthma in 25 years.[15] Accolate, which is given orally, prevents antigen and exercise-induced bronchospasm. It has bronchodilator activity about 30% that of salbutamol and its effects are additive with β_2-adrenoceptor agonists.

ANTIINFLAMMATORY DRUGS

Several potentially useful antiinflammatory drugs are currently undergoing clinical trials. Zileutin is a 5-lipoxygenase inhibitor which prevents the production not only of the bronchoconstrictor leucotrines, LTC$_4$

and LTD_4, but also of LTB_4, one of the major chemotaxins that recruits leucocytes into the bronchial mucosa and then activates them. Inhibitors of cyclic nucleotide phosphodiesterase selective for inflammatory cells are also being developed and may be an improvement on the methylxanthines.[16] Deoxyribonuclease, which acts to hydrolyse excess DNA produced by inflammatory cells, has proven useful in the treatment of the pulmonary symptoms in cystic fibrosis.[17,18] In this condition DNA from the nuclei of lysed cells makes a substantial contribution to the viscosity of the inflammatory infiltrate. It is currently being assessed in chronic bronchitis, where purulent secretions also contribute to airway obstruction.

REFERENCES

1. Corbridge TC, Hall JB. The assessment and management of adults with status asthmaticus. *Am J Respir Crit Care Med* 1995; **151**: 1296–1316.

2. Petty TL. Diagnosis and treatment of chronic obstructive pulmonary disease. *Chest* 1990; **97**: 1S–33S.

3. Kume H, Graziano MP, Kotlikoff MI. Stimulatory and inhibitory regulation of calcium-activated potassium channels by guanine nucleotide binding proteins. *Proc Natl Acad Sci USA* 1992; **89**: 11051–11055.

4. American Thoracic Society. Standards for the diagnosis and care of patients with chronic obstructive pulmonary disease (COPD) and asthma. *Am Rev Respir Dis* 1987; **136**: 225–244.

5. Finnerty JP, Howarth PH. Paradoxical bronchoconstriction with nebulized albuterol but not with terbutaline. *Am Rev Respir Dis* 1993; **148**: 512–513.

6. Ward AJ, McKenniff M, Evans JM. Theophylline: an immunomodulatory role in asthma? *Am Rev Respir Dis* 1993; **147**: 518–523.

7. Barnette MS, Christensen SB, Underwood DC, Torphy TJ. Phosphodiesterase-4: biological underpinnings for the design of improved inhibitors. *Pharmacol Commun* 1996; **8**: 65–73.

8. Feoktistov I, Polosa R, Steven T, Biaggoni I. Adenosine A_{2B} receptors: a novel therapeutic target in asthma? *Trends Pharmacol Sci* 1998; **19**: 148–153.

9. Guidelines for the diagnosis and management of asthma. National Heart, Lung and Blood Institute. National Asthma Education Program. Expert panel report. *J Allergy Clin Immunol* 1991; **88**: 425–534.

10. Zwillich CW, Sutton FD, Neff TA. Theophylline-induced seizures in adults: correlation with serum concentrations. *Ann Intern Med* 1975; **82**: 784–787.

11. Brogden RN, Sorkin EM. Nedocromil sodium: an updated review of its pharmacological properties and therapeutic efficacy in asthma. *Drugs* 1993; **45**: 693–715.

12. Israel E, Drazen JM. Treating mild asthma – when are inhaled steroids indicated? *N Engl J Med* 1994; **331**: 737–739.

13. Barnes PJ. Inhaled glucocorticoids for asthma. *N Engl J Med* 1995; **332**: 868–875.

14. Fahy JV, Boushey HA. Controversies involving inhaled beta-agonist and inhaled corticosteroids in the treatment of asthma. *Clin Chest Med* 1995; **16**: 715–733.

15. Rogers DF, Giembycz MA. Asthma therapy for the 21st century. *Trends Pharmacol Sci* 1998; **19**: 160–163.

16. Nicholoson CD, Shabid M. Inhibitors of cyclic nucleotide phosphodiesterase isoenzymes – their potential utility in the therapy of asthma. *Pulmonary Pharmacol* 1994; **7**: 1–17.

17. Harris CE, Wilmott RW. Inhalation-based therapies in the treatment of cystic fibrosis. *Curr Opin Pediatr* 1994; **6**: 234–238.

18. Wilmott RW, Fiedler MA. Recent advances in the treatment of cystic fibrosis. *Pediatr Clin North Am* 1994; **41**: 431–451.

19 JG Bovill

HISTAMINE AND HISTAMINE ANTAGONISTS

HISTAMINE

Histamine is a basic amine formed by the decarboxylation of the amino acid L-histidine (Fig. 19.1). It has important functions as a neurotransmitter, as a regulator of inflammatory and immunological reactions, and in gastric acid secretion as well as in the pathophysiology of allergy and anaphylaxis. Histamine is widely distributed throughout the animal kingdom and is present in many venoms, bacteria and plants. In mammals most histamine is synthesized and stored in secretory cytoplasmic granules of mast cells in the tissues and the basophils in the blood. Within these granules it is posi-

Summary box 19.1 Histamine

- Basic amine formed from L-histidine.

- Found mainly in mast cells (tissues) and basophils (blood).

- Highest concentrations in the lungs, skin, gastrointestinal tract and vascular endothelium.

- Widespread biological activity:

  - neurotransmitter

  - regulator of inflammatory and immunological processes

  - regulates gastric acid secretion.

- Intimately involved in allergy and anaphylaxis.

- Actions mediated via three specific receptors, H_1, H_2 and H_3.

tively charged and held as an ionic complex with negatively charged granule constituents such as heparin and proteases. The turnover rate of histamine in mast cells and basophils is low and, when depleted, it may take several weeks for the concentration to be restored. The release of histamine, and many other mediators, from mast cells and basophils is common during allergic disorders. Histamine synthesis and release is inhibited by glucocorticoids. A fully differentiated mast cell contains up to 1000 granules which, in addition to histamine, also contain heparin, proteases and hydrolytic enzymes. The human body contains sufficient histamine in its tissues, neatly packaged in the granules of its mast cells and basophils, to destroy itself if released all at one time.[1]

Histamine is present in all human tissues in concentrations from 0.1 to 20 μg g^{-1}. The concentration is higher in the lungs, skin, the gastrointestinal tract and blood vessel endothelium, sites corresponding to the highest density of mast cells. The name histamine is derived from the Greek word for tissue, *histos*. The concentration of histamine in the plasma is normally low ($<$ 1 ng ml^{-1}) but may reach 40 ng ml^{-1} or higher during anaphylactic or anaphylactoid reactions. Concentrations above 12 ng ml^{-1} are associated with severe hypotension, bronchospasm and ventricular arrhythmias.[2]

Histamine is rapidly cleared from the blood by two metabolic pathways (Fig. 19.1). The metabolites have little or no activity. The steroid-derived muscle relaxants, pancuronium and vecuronium, although not stimulating the release of histamine, are potent inhibitors of histamine-N-methyltransferase in humans.[3] However, this is not associated with an increase in plasma histamine concentrations and appears not to be of any clinical significance.[4] It may be that other enzyme pathways (e.g. diamine oxidase) compensate for the inhibition of histamine-N-methyltransferase by these drugs.

HISTAMINE RECEPTORS

The biological effects of histamine are mediated via three receptor subtypes, H_1, H_2 and H_3, which are linked to G protein but activate different cell-signalling systems. The three types of histamine receptors can be activated preferentially by analogues of histamine.

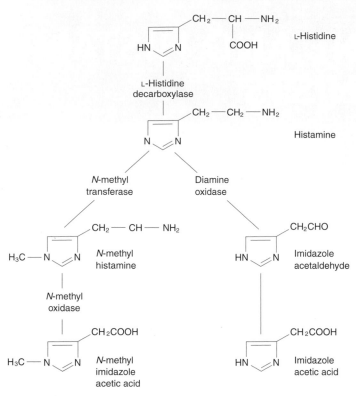

Fig. 19.1 Formation and metabolism of histamine.

The prototypal agonist at the H_1 receptor is 2-methyl-histamine, whereas 4(5) methylhistamine is selective for the H_2 receptor. (R)-a-methylhistamine, a chiral analogue of histamine, is a highly selective agonist at the H_3 receptor.

H_1 receptors are widely distributed throughout the body. They are present throughout the central nervous system (CNS), with high densities found in the hypothalamus. They appear to have a role in maintaining wakefulness, and this may explain the sedating properties of some H_1 antagonists. Most of the important effects of histamine in allergic diseases, including bronchoconstriction and contraction of the gut, are mediated through H_1 receptors. Other effects, including the cardiovascular responses, involve both H_1 and H_2 receptors. In humans the predominant cardiovascular effect is vasodilatation and a lowering of blood pressure. This response is also responsible for the cutaneous flushing commonly observed with histamine release. The vasodilator effects of histamine are mediated by H_1 receptors on the vascular endothelial cells and H_2 receptors on vascular smooth muscle. Activation of H_1 receptors results in the local production of nitric oxide. The mechanism by which activation of H_2 receptors leads to vasodilatation is not well understood. Histamine, acting via H_2 receptors, has positive inotropic and chrono-

tropic effects on the heart. In the pulmonary circulation H_1 receptors mediate vasodilatation while H_2 agonists cause vasoconstriction. The hypotension and shock associated with anaphylaxis are secondary to increased vascular permeability and vasodilatation, while changes in atrioventricular conduction may be partly responsible for the tachycardia.

Injection of histamine intradermally causes a combination of effects known as the 'triple response', described by Sir Thomas Lewis in 1927. This consists of a reddening of the skin and a wheal with a surrounding flare. The reddening is due to dilatation of the small arterioles and precapillary sphincters, and the wheal is caused by local oedema due to leakage of fluid from postcapillary venules made more permeable by histamine.

Histamine typically induces a contraction in non-vascular smooth muscle in the bronchi, gut and the uterus, mediated via H_1 receptors. There are marked species differences in the response of smooth muscle to histamine. While the uterus of some species responds to histamine with contraction, in the human uterus, gravid or not, the response is negligible. Guinea-pigs are exquisitely sensitive to histamine, and they die from asphyxia due to severe bronchospasm after even small doses of histamine. The contraction of the guinea-pig

Summary box 19.2 Pharmacological activity associated with individual histamine receptors

H_1
- Vasodilatation.

- Increased vascular permeability and oedema.

- Pulmonary artery vasoconstriction.

- Coronary artery vasoconstriction.

- Activation of vagal afferent nerves in airways.

- Bronchospasm.

- Gut contraction.

- Adrenaline release from adrenal medulla.

- Stimulation of cutaneous nerve endings, pain and itching.

H_2
- Control gastric acid secretion.

- Increased lower airway mucus secretion.

- Relaxation of vascular smooth muscle.

- Positive inotropy.

- Slow atrioventricular conduction.

- Increased atrial and ventricular automaticity.

- Bronchodilatation.

- Suppression of lymphocyte proliferation.

- Suppression of antibody production by β-lymphocytes.

- Relax stomach and gallbladder smooth muscle.

H_3
- Modulation of histamine synthesis and release.

- Inhibit vagally mediated bronchoconstriction.

- Vasodilatation.

- Tonic inhibition of gastric acid secretion.

- Inhibit gut contraction by inhibition of acetylcholine at nicotinic synapses in autonomic nerve terminals.

- Presynaptic regulation of neurotransmission processes in the CNS.

terminal ileum formed the basis of the original bioassay for histamine. The mouse, in contrast, is relatively insensitive to the effects of histamine, whereas humans lie somewhere in between.

Although H_1 receptors are dominant in human bronchial smooth muscle, H_2 receptors are also present, where they have a dilatatory function. However, H_2-mediated bronchodilatation is probably minimal and of little clinical consequence. Patients with asthma tolerate H_2 antagonists well. In humans other mediators such as leucotrines are probably more important in producing bronchospasm than histamine. Histamine H_2 receptors play an essential role in the regulation of acid secretion by gastric parietal cells. Histamine interacts with acetylcholine and gastrin via H_2 receptors to control acid production. H_2-receptor antagonists are potent inhibitors of gastric acid secretion.

The H_3 receptor was first discovered in the CNS,[5] but has now been identified in many peripheral tissues, including the cardiovascular system. Knowledge as to the physiological significance of H_3 receptors is growing rapidly. H_3 receptors are highly sensitive to histamine. They are activated at histamine concentrations two orders of magnitude lower than those required to activate H_1 or H_2 receptors, and appear to act as autoreceptors, through which histamine inhibits its own release and synthesis.[6] The release of the monoamine neurotransmitters noradrenaline, dopamine and serotonin in the central and peripheral nervous systems is also inhibited by histamine through H_3 receptors.

The discovery of the H_3 receptor has led to the realization that, in addition to its generally unfavourable effects, histamine also has beneficial effects through interacting with the H_3 receptor. H_3 agonists antagonize gut contractions caused by H_1-receptor stimulation. In the gastric mucosa H_3 receptors have a tonic inhibitory role in the regulation of basal acid secretion. H_3-receptor activation may inhibit M_3-mediated cholinergic stimulation of acid secretion through mechanisms operating downstream to the receptor sites. In the lungs, H_3-receptor activation inhibits cholinergic neurotransmission and vagally mediated bronchoconstriction. Cholinergic mechanisms are important in airway diseases such as asthma, and H_3 agonists offer potential therapeutic benefit. In the cardiovascular system H_3 receptors are found on postganglionic sympathetic neurons supplying blood vessels and the heart. They are also present in the endothelium where they mediate vasodilatation by releasing nitric oxide (NO) and prostacyclin. The coronary vasodilatation caused by histamine is mediated by both H_2 and H_3 receptors, and this is dependent on nitric oxide.[7]

Specific H_3-receptor agonists thus might be of potential value in asthma and in some cardiovascular and gastrointestinal diseases. A number of potent

H_3-receptor agonists have been synthesized in recent years, and some are undergoing the early phases of clinical trials. One difficulty in developing suitable drugs has been finding compounds that are free of H_1- or H_2-agonist activity.

HISTAMINE AND ALLERGY

Hypersensitivity is a special type of reaction in which tissue damage occurs as a result of an immune response to a foreign substance. The term allergy is often used synonymously with this reaction. Histamine is one of the major mediators of allergy, although the clinical expression of allergic diseases such as allergic rhinitis and urticaria depends on the actions of multiple mediators, many of which, like histamine, are also derived from mast cells. In addition to involvement in immediate hypersensitivity reactions, histamine also acts as a regulator of immune responses.

Anaphylaxis is a form of immediate hypersensitivity in which there is an explosive response to antigen challenge, usually within minutes, with release of active mediators. Multiple organ systems are involved, the most prominent being cardiovascular, cutaneous, respiratory and gastrointestinal. Anaphylaxis is immunologically mediated, via immunoglobulin (Ig) E, and occurs upon exposure to an antigen to which the subject has previously been sensitized. The usual causative antigen is a drug, insect venom or food. The reaction can be evoked by a minute quantity of an antigen and is potentially fatal (for details see Chapter 27). There is a rapid release of histamine and other mediators that collectively cause increased permeability of the postcapillary venules, leading to oedema formation, vasodilatation, bronchial and visceral smooth muscle contraction, and an increase in secretion, particularly of the respiratory tract (Fig. 19.2).

Although histamine has a prominent role in anaphylaxis, measurement of plasma histamine concentration is of little value in establishing the diagnosis of an anaphylactic reaction. Blood sampling needs to be done within 10 min of a reaction, at which time resuscitation is the priority. Meticulous and complicated handling of samples is also necessary. A more useful alternative is to measure methylhistamine since it is more stable and its concentration remains raised for longer.[8] A highly sensitive and specific test for anaphylaxis is the mast cell tryptase assay. The concentration of this enzyme, released from immunologically activated mast cells but not basophils, is raised for between 1 and 6 h after a reaction.[9] Mast cell tryptase should be measured in all patients suspected of an allergic reaction during anaesthesia.

An anaphylactoid reaction is clinically and pathologically identical to anaphylaxis but without involvement of an IgE antibody and corresponding antigen

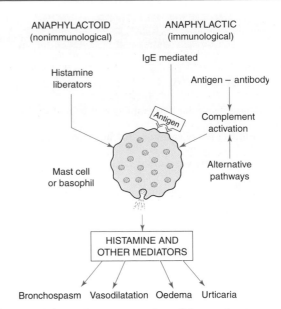

Fig. 19.2 Schematic representation of the mechanisms involved in the release of histamine and other mediators during anaphylactic and anaphylactoid reactions. IgE, immunoglobulin E.

(Fig. 19.2).[2] Many inflammatory products, such as the complement fragments C3a, C4a and C5a (anaphylatoxins), and interleukins 1, 3 and 5, bring about or enhance the release of histamine. A large number of drugs and therapeutic and diagnostic substances stimulate the release of histamine from mast cells directly without previous sensitization, especially when given intravenously. Among these are thiopentone, morphine, pethidine, suxamethonium, tubocurarine and atracurium, iodinated radiographic contrast media and plasma expanders based on cross-linked gelatins.[10] In most cases the reaction is mild and short lived, with cutaneous flushing, mild to moderate hypotension, tachycardia and moderate bronchospasm. In the occasional patient, however, a full-blown anaphylactic-like reaction is triggered, which may be fatal.

It is probable that adverse events related to histamine release are more common than is realized. These adverse effects can be prevented or attenuated by pretreatment with H_1 and H_2 antagonists, but not by either drug alone.[11-13] Histamine stimulates the release of endogenous catecholamines. This may give protection from some of the adverse reactions, especially bronchospasm. Intravenous histamine usually produces bronchospasm only in patients taking β-blockers.

HISTAMINE H₁ ANTAGONISTS

The main therapeutic role of these drugs is in the treatment of allergic diseases involving IgE-mediated hypersensitivity, such as allergic rhinitis, hay fever and urticaria. Although histamine is not a major mediator in asthma, it contributes to the pathogenesis of the disease and antihistamines, particularly the newer nonsedating drugs, have a role in its therapy. H_1 antagonists, in combination with an H_2 antagonist, are also used in the prophylaxis and treatment of anaphylactic and anaphylactoid reactions.

Numerous compounds capable of antagonizing the effects of histamine are available. They have little structural resemblance to histamine but a feature common to many is a substituted ethylamine containing a nitrogen atom in an alkyl chain or a ring (Fig. 19.3). H_1 antagonists are often classified according to the chemical group containing the substituted ethylamine (Table 19.1). They are competitive antagonists of histamine at the H_1 receptor, except for terfenadine and astemizole,

which are unsurmountable (noncompetitive) antagonists. Many of the older first-generation drugs (e.g. chlorpheniramine) are small water-soluble compounds that cross the blood–brain barrier relatively easily. This accounts for many of their side-effects, which are not directly related to antagonism of the H_1 receptor, but may be caused by antagonism at other receptors such as the muscarinic cholinergic, 5-hydroxytryptamine (5-$HT)_3$ or a_1-adrenergic receptors. Some, particularly the phenothiazines, produce a high incidence of sedation, which limits their clinical usefulness. Several have marked antimuscarinic effects causing dry mouth, blurred vision and constipation. Because of these properties the first-generation H_1 antagonists are seldom used specifically for their antihistamine effects, but are used for their actions at nonhistamine sites. Some of the phenothiazines (e.g. promethazine and

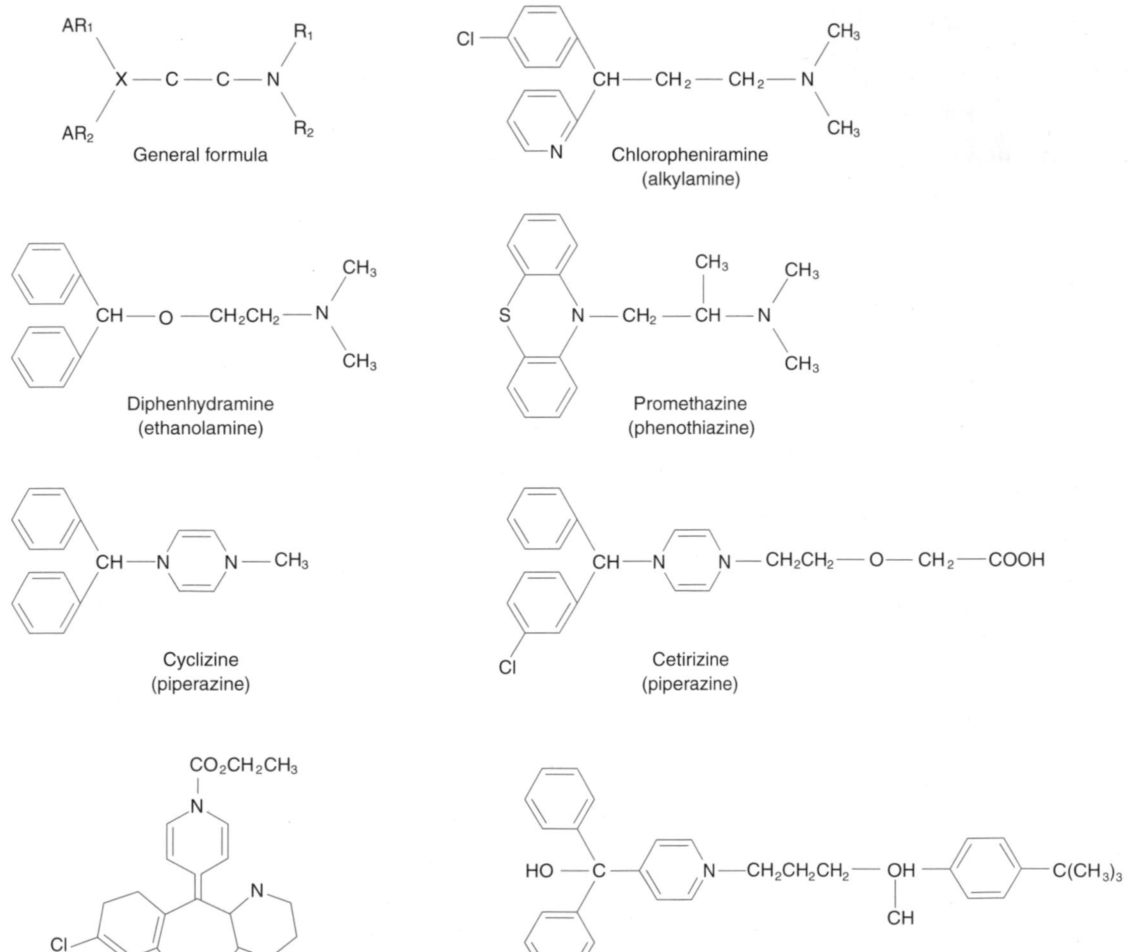

Fig. 19.3 Chemical structures of some commonly used H₁ antagonists.

Table 19.1 Pharmcological characteristics of some commonly used H₁ antagonists

Drug	Sedation	Antimuscarinic effects	Oral absorption	Presystemic metabolism	Active metabolites	Dose (mg)	$t_{1/2}$ (h)
Ethanolamines							
Diphenhydramine	+++	+++	>90%	70%	No	25–50	3–8
Alkylamines							
Chlorpheniramine	+	++	>80%	<20%	No	4–8 (oral), 5–20 (i.v. or i.m.)	30
Dexchlorpheniramine	+	++	Extensive	NA	No	2	20–24
Acrivastine	0	0	Extensive	Minimal	Yes	8	1.5 (2–3)
Piperazines							
Hydroxyzine	+++	+++	Extensive	NA	Yes	25–100	20
Cetrizine	0/+	0	Approx. 100%	<10%	No	10	7–10
Cyclizine hydrochloride	+	+++	Extensive	NA	No	50	NA
Cinnarizine	+	+	Extensive	NA	No	25	3
Phenothiazines							
Promethazine	+++	+++	>80%	75%	No	25–50 (oral)	7–14
Mequitazine	0/+	0/+	70%	Approx. 99%	No	5	40
Piperidines							
Terfenadine	0	0	Aprox. 100%	Approx. 100%	Yes	60	1–3 (4–5)
Loratadine	0	0	>90%	>90%	Yes	10	12
Azelastine	+	0	82%	Negligible	Yes	2	16 (48)
Miscellaneous							
Clemastine	++	+	Extensive	NA	No	2	4–6
Astemizole	0	0	90%	>90%	Yes	10–30	1–5 (10–14) days
Ketotifen	0/+	0	>90%	Low	Yes	1–2	22

Drugs in italics are second-generation nonsedating antihistamines. NA, data not available; i.v., intravenous; i.m., intramuscular.

trimeprazine) are used for premedication. Those with antimuscarinic effects, such as promethazine, diphenhydramine and cyclizine, are useful as antiemetics. Where a specific antihistamine effect is wanted, the second-generation nonsedating H_1 antagonists are preferred.

'SEDATING' H₁ ANTAGONISTS

The first-generation H_1 antagonists form a heterogeneous group of chemical compounds with two aromatic rings connected by a two- or three-atom chain to a tertiary amino group (Fig. 19.3). The aromatic rings confer lipophilicity so that they can readily enter the CNS. Sedation or drowsiness is a common adverse effect of the classical antihistamines. The incidence is dose related and varies among the chemical classes. Ethanolamines and phenothiazines generally have marked sedative effects, whereas the alkylamines cause only mild sedation (Table 19.1).

Ethanolamines

The prototype antihistamine of this group is diphenhydramine. It has antimuscarinic and pronounced central sedative properties and also an antitussive effect. The mechanism of the latter is unclear, but diphenhy-

---

> **Summary box 19.3 Clinical uses of H₁ antagonists**
>
> - Prophylaxis and treatment of allergic disorders (drugs that lack sedative and antimuscarine actions preferred):
>
>   - allergic rhinitis
>
>   - hay fever
>
>   - urticaria
>
>   - asthma
>
>   - anaphylactic and anaphylactoid reactions (in combination with an H_2 antagonist).
>
> - As antiemetics:
>
>   - motion sickness
>
>   - labyrinthine disorders (e.g. vertigo, Menière's disease)
>
>   - drug-induced, including postoperative emesis.
>
> - Mild forms of Parkinson's disease.
>
> - For sedation.

---

dramine is a common ingredient of propriety preparations for the treatment of coughs and colds. It is an effective antiemetic, especially useful for prevention and treatment of motion sickness. Because of its anticholinergic properties, it is occasionally used in the treatment of patients with mild forms of Parkinson's disease. It is also of use in the treatment of drug-induced extrapyramidal effects.

Piperazine derivatives

Cinnarizine is an H_1-receptor antagonist and a calcium channel blocker used for the treatment of vertigo and emetic symptoms due to Menière's disease and related labyrinth disorders. It is also effective in motion sickness. It is used for peripheral and cerebral vascular disorders, because of its calcium channel-blocking properties.

Cyclizine has antimuscarinic properties and is a potent antiemetic, effective for the control of postoperative and drug-induced nausea and vomiting. It has been used to prevent motion sickness, although diphenhydramine and promethazine are more effective. It is available in oral and parenteral formulations. In contrast to many other first-generation antihistamines, sedation is not marked. Cyclizine is available in tablet form as the hydrochloride and in injectable form as the lactate. Because of its anticholinergic action, blurred vision and dry mouth are associated with clinical doses. When given by rapid intravenous injection, tachycardia may be a problem. Meclozine is a related drug which, like cyclizine, is used primarily for motion sickness.

Alkylamines

The prototype drug in this class is chlorpheniramine maleate, which is a very potent H_1 antagonist with only weak antimuscarinic and moderate antiserotonin actions. It also produces less sedation than some other antihistamines. Transient CNS stimulant effects may be seen when injected intravenously. Chlorpheniramine is a racemic mixture, with the antihistamine action residing mainly in the (+)-*laevo*-isomer (dexchlorpheniramine). This isomer is also available commercially.

Phenothiazines

Promethazine has prominent sedative effects as well as antimuscarinic and dopamine D_2-blocking effects. These make it useful as an antiemetic, and it is especially useful for the prevention and treatment of motion sickness. Like other phenothiazines, it has weak a_1-adrenergic blocking effects and can lower blood pressure if injected rapidly intravenously. Intramuscular injection can be painful.

Trimeprazine tartrate is a phenothiazine with H_1-antagonist activity which produces marked sedation. It is used mainly for its marked effect in the relief of pruritus, and is also popular for the premedication of children (dose 2 mg kg^{-1}).

Mequitazine is a phenothiazine with a greater affinity for peripheral than for central H_1 receptors. Although it crosses the blood–brain barrier, its transport into the CNS is complex and animal studies suggest that a threshold concentratient gradient exists, below which little passage occurs. This may partly explain the reduced sedative effects compared with other phenothiazines. Mequitazine has only weak anticholinergic activity. It is available only in oral form. The half-life is long, approximately 40 h, and the apparent volume of distribution is very high, 4000 litres, as a result of extensive protein and tissue binding. Mequitazine may also undergo extensive enterohepatic recirculation and because of this, and its extensive protein binding, its pharmacokinetics may be altered in patients with hepatic disease.

Miscellaneous

Clemastine fumarate is a first-generation H_1-receptor antagonist with a long duration of action. It has high H_1-receptor specificity and only weak antimuscarinic effects. The incidence of CNS side-effects is generally low. Sedation is less than with most other first-generation drugs but more than with second-generation antihistamines such as loratadine. It is available in parenteral form, and is useful for the prophylaxis and treatment of acute anaphylaxis. It can be given intravenously in a dose of 2 mg, together with an H_2 antagonist such as ranitidine, to patients at risk of an allergic reaction, for example before giving protamine to a patient undergoing a repeat cardiac operation. The onset is rapid after intravenous administration.

'NONSEDATING' H_1 ANTAGONISTS

The newer second generation of H_1-receptor antagonists such as terfenadine and astemizole are large, lipophilic molecules with a charged side-chain, and are extensively bound to albumin. These drugs have difficulty in crossing the blood–brain barrier and produce little or no sedation or central anticholinergic symptoms when given in the recommended doses, although higher doses may be associated with some CNS depression, especially if taken in combination with other CNS-depressing drugs. Cetirizine, for example, is the carboxylic acid metabolite of the first-generation H_1 antagonist, hydroxyzine. Cetirizine is a highly potent H_1-receptor antagonist which is considerably more polar than hydroxyzine and therefore less likely to cross the blood–brain barrier. It causes significantly less sedation and mental impairment than the parent compound.

All of the second-generation H_1-receptor antagonists are extensively absorbed after oral administration. None

is available for parenteral use, but azelastine is available as a nasal spray. Loratadine, astemizole and terfenadine undergo greater than 90% presystemic metabolism in the liver with the formation of metabolites with significant antihistamine activity. In the case of terfenadine, first-pass metabolism is virtually complete and most of the clinical effects with the recommended doses are due to the pharmacologically active metabolite, terfenadine carboxylate. Terfenadine is potentially cardiotoxic whereas the metabolite is not. Ketotifen undergoes demethylation to form nor-ketotifen, which has similar potency as the parent drug. Cetirizine is eliminated mainly by renal excretion of the unchanged drug. The main indication for these drugs is the treatment of allergic disorders such as allergic rhinitis and skin allergies including urticaria. Azelastine is of benefit in the management of asthma, producing a significant and long-lasting bronchodilatation. The use of azelastine by nasal spray by patients with rhinitis is superior to oral use, giving protection for at least 12 h. Ketotifen, in addition to H_1 antagonism, also has a membrane-stabilizing action similar to that of sodium cromoglycate, inhibiting the release of chemical mediators from mast cells and basophils. This makes it useful in the prophylaxis of bronchial asthma.

The incidence of side-effects of these drugs, when given in the recommended doses, is very low. There have, however, been a number of reports of patients treated with terfenadine who developed prolongation of the QT interval of the electroencephalogram associated with the life-threatening ventricular arrhythmia, torsades de pointes. This was associated with unusually high plasma concentrations of terfenadine resulting either from portacaval shunting due to cirrhosis of the liver or interactions with drugs inhibiting cytochrome P450 hepatic enzymes, such as ketoconazole or erythromycin. Similar cardiac dysrhythmias have been reported with overdosage of astemizole. These drugs should, therefore, not be used in patients with severe liver disease, nor should they be coadministered with hepatic enzyme inhibitors such as ketoconazole or erythromycin. Ketotifen should not be administered concomitantly with oral antidiabetic agents since the combination can lead to a reversible fall in the platelet count in some patients. The mechanism of this interaction is not known.

H_2-RECEPTOR ANTAGONISTS

Currently four H_2-receptor antagonists are available: cimetidine, ranitidine, famotidine and nizatidine. They competitively inhibit the actions of histamine at all H_2 receptors. A combination of H_1 and H_2 antagonists is more effective than an H_1 antagonist alone in the prevention of reaction to drug-induced histamine release.[11–13] The value of combined therapy in the prevention and treatment of anaphylactic and anaphylactoid reactions is less well established. In some studies a beneficial effect was reported, but not in others. Since H_2 antagonists block some of the desirable effects of histamine, such as positive inotropy and coronary artery dilatation, they should be used with caution. In addition, H_2 receptors exert a negative feedback on histamine release, and antagonism of this might lead to an increase in histamine release.

The main clinical use of H_2-receptor antagonists is as inhibitors of gastric acid secretion. Their introduction in the mid-1970s was a major breakthrough in the treatment of peptic ulceration. They inhibit both basal and stimulated gastric secretion of acid and pepsin, with a reduction in the volume of gastric juice. Acid secretion may be inhibited by 90% or more. All are given orally and are well absorbed, but undergo varying presystemic metabolism, from 25–50% in the case of cimetidine and ranitidine to less than 10% with famotidine and nizatidine.[14] Cimetidine was the first clinically available H_2 antagonist. The newer drugs are more potent than cimetidine (ranitidine five times, famotidine 40 times, nizatidine 10 times). Famotidine and nizatidine have a duration of action considerably longer than that of cimetidine, so that a single daily oral dose is sufficient. Adverse reactions to cimetidine are rare with the doses used to treat patients with peptic ulcers. Cimetidine binds to androgen receptors, displacing dihydrotestosterone, and may cause gynaecomastia and impotence in men. A decrease in oestradiol metabolism induced by cimetidine may also be a factor in these symptoms. The frequency of gynaecomastia is about 1 in 1000 but is dose related. The incidence is higher in patients given high doses, for instance for the treatment of the Zollinger–Ellison syndrome.[15] None of the other three H_2 antagonists has antiandrogenic effects.

Cimetidine is a potent inhibitor of hepatic cytochrome P450 enzymes, responsible for the phase I metabolism of many drugs, including opioids, benzodiazepines, lignocaine and warfarin. P450 inhibition will cause a greater than expected drug plasma concentration and thus more pronounced clinical effect, which also may be prolonged. The P450 inhibition by cimetidine comes about because of an interaction directly with the P450 haem iron through one of the nitrogen atoms of the imidazole nucleus. Ranitidine, which contains a furan ring in place of imidazole, does not inhibit P450, although it does form a complex with hepatic cytochrome P450, but more weakly than cimetidine. As far as is known, neither famotidine nor nizatidine inhibits P450 enzymes.

There have been case reports of cardiac arrhythmias (bradycardia and atrioventricular dissociation) in patients given bolus intravenous injections of cimetidine. Intravenous doses of cimetidine should therefore be given slowly (over 10 min) to patients with cardiovascular disease. Cardiac arrhythmias may be related to antagonism of cardiac H_2 receptors. However, cimetidine also increases plasma prolactin levels, an effect mediated by antagonism of dopamine receptors. Increased prolactin concentrations can precipitate arrhythmias.

These drugs are effective in reducing the volume of gastric secretions and raising the pH in surgical and obstetrical patients requiring urgent operations, and so protect against aspiration damage to the lungs. Of the four available drugs, ranitidine is most widely used for this purpose. An oral dose of ranitidine (150 mg given 60–90 min before surgery) will produce a peak effect at the time of induction of anaesthesia, and the effect will last for 5–8 h. Alternatively, ranitidine may be given intravenously (dose 50 mg). For reduction of gastric acidity during prolonged surgery or in intensive care patients, ranitidine can be given as a continuous infusion of 200–400 mg per 24 h.

REFERENCES

1. Settipane GA. *Histamine H, and H, Receptors*. Providence, Rhode Island: OceanSide Publications, 1988–1989.
2. McKinnon RP, Wildsmith JAW. Histaminoid reactions in anaesthesia. *Br J Anaesth* 1995; **74**: 217–228.
3. Futo J, Kupferberg JP, Moss J et al. Vecuronium inhibits histamine N-methyltransferase. *Anesthesiology* 1988; **69**: 92–96.
4. Levy JH, Adelson D. Effects of vecuronium-induced histamine N-methyltransferase inhibition on cutaneous responses to histamine. *Agents Actions* 1992; (Special Conference Issue): C211–C212.
5. Arrang JM, Garbarg M, Schwartz JC. Auto-inhibition of brain histamine release mediated by a novel class (H_3) of histamine receptor. *Nature* 1983; **302**: 832–837.
6. Schwartz JC, Arrang JM, Garbarg M, Pollard H. A third histamine receptor subtype: characterisation, localisation and functions of the H_3-receptor. *Agents Actions* 1990; **30**: 13–23.
7. Kostic MM, Jakovljevic VLJ. Role of histamine in the regulation of coronary circulation. *Physiol Res* 1996; **45**: 297–303.
8. Fisher M, Baldo BA. Anaphylaxis during anaesthesia: current aspects of diagnosis and prevention. *Eur J Anaesthesiol* 1994; **11**: 263–284.
9. Laroche D, Vergnaud M, Sillard B et al. Biochemical markers of anaphylactoid reactions to drugs. Comparison of plasma histamine and tryptase. *Anesthesiology* 1991; **75**: 945–949.
10. Marone G, Stellato C, Mastronardi P, Mazzarella B. Nonspecific histamine-releasing properties of general anesthetic drugs. *Clin Rev Allergy* 1991; **9**: 269–279.
11. Hosking MP, Lennon RL, Gronert GA. Combined H_1 and H_2 receptor blockade attenuates the cardiovascular effects of high-dose atracurium for rapid sequence endotracheal intubation. *Anesth Analg* 1988; **67**: 1089–1092.
12. Philbin DM, Moss J, Akins CW et al. The use of H_1 and H_2 histamine

antagonists with morphine anesthesia: a double-blind study. *Anesthesiology* 1981; **55**: 292–296.

13. Lieberman P. The use of antihistamines in the prevention and treatment of anaphylaxis and anaphylactoid reactions. *J Allergy Clin Immunol* 1990; **86**: 684–686.

14. Desager J-P, Horsmans Y. Pharmacokinetic–pharmacodynamic relationships of H₁-antihistamines. *Clin Pharmacokinet* 1995; **28**: 419–432.

15. Jensen RT, Collen MJ, Pandol SJ *et al*. Cimetidine-induced impotence and breast changes in patients with gastric hypersecretory states. *N Engl J Med* 1983; **308**: 883–887.

20 RN Sladen

DIURETICS

Diuretics are drugs that increase water and electrolyte excretion. However, they are as often misused, with important consequences for haemodynamic stability and renal function. In this chapter the emphasis will be on diuretic therapy in the perioperative period, and not on long-term diuretic usage, for example in chronic hypertension. Each class of diuretic is described with respect to its clinical pharmacology, indications and adverse effects. The causes of diuretic resistance are summarized and strategies for dealing with it are presented. The final section deals with the use of diuretics for specific clinical indications such as renal protection, oliguria and renal insufficiency, and acute renal failure.

CLINICAL PHARMACOLOGY OF DIURETICS

CLASSIFICATION AND SITE OF ACTION

Diuretics have three broad mechanisms of action: osmotic or water diuresis (e.g. mannitol), inhibition of sodium and chloride reabsorption or natriuresis (e.g. loop diuretics, thiazides and potassium-sparing diuretics) and inhibition of sodium bicarbonate reabsorption (e.g. the carbonic anhydrase inhibitors). The oldest of the currently used diuretic agents, acetazolamide, has an unsubstituted sulphonamide group ($-SO_2NH_2-$) which confers carbonic anhydrase inhibition. Most diuretics subsequently developed, including frusemide, bumetanide, chlorothiazide and metolazone, are sulphonamide derivatives, although their sodium transport inhibitory activity is far greater than carbonic anhydrase inhibition. Ethacrynic acid is a phenoxyacetic acid derivative.

Diuretics may be classified according to their chemical structure, site of action within the nephron (Fig. 20.1) or natriuretic potency (Table 20.1). Diuretics

Summary box 20.1 Diuretics

- Drugs that increase the excretion of sodium and water by an action on the kidneys.

- *Osmotic diuretics* are inert substances that are filtered but not reabsorbed from the filtrate. The primary effect is to increase the amount of water excreted.

- *Carbonic anhydrase inhibitors* increase the excretion of sodium bicarbonate in the proximal tubule. Not used as diuretics but used for treatment of glaucoma.

- *Loop diuretics* inhibit $Na^+–K^+–2Cl^-$ cotransporter in the thick ascending loop of Henle, resulting in the excretion of 15–20% of filtered Na^+ (normally less than 1% excreted). Main adverse effects are hypokalaemia, metabolic alkalosis, hyponatraemia, hypovolaemia and hyperuricamia. Ototoxicity can occur with high doses, especially with ethacrynic acid.

- *Thiazide diuretics* inhibit $Na^+–K^+–2Cl^-$ cotransporter in the distal convoluted tubule. Less potent than loop diuretics; about 5% of filtered Na^+ excreted. Side-effects similar to those of the loop diuretics.

- *Potassium-sparing diuretics* are weak diuretics acting in the collecting tubules. Can cause hyperkalaemia and metabolic acidosis. Two main groups:

  - Na^+ channel blockers (e.g. triamterene and amiloride)

  - aldosterone antagonists (e.g. spironolactone).

acting on the loop of Henle are the most powerful agents, causing the excretion of 20–25% of a filtered sodium load and thus the greatest tubular sodium loss (i.e. fractional excretion of sodium) (Table 20.1). The thiazide group and metolazone are moderately potent, resulting in the excretion of 5–8% of filtered sodium, and the potassium-sparing diuretics are mildly potent, causing the excretion of only 2–3% of filtered sodium.

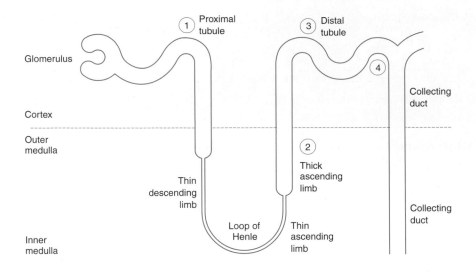

Site	Segment	Sodium reabsorption (%)	Diuretic effects of blockade
1	Proximal tubule	60–70	Relatively weak – sodium can be reabsorbed distally
2	Medullary thick ascending loop of Henle	15–25	Potent – important site for sodium reabsorption with relatively few distal sites
3	Early distal tubule	5–8	Less potent – less important site for sodium reabsorption
4	Late distal tubule, collecting ducts	<3	Relatively weak – little sodium reabsorption

Fig. 20.1 Tubular transport systems and the primary sites of sodium reabsorption and diuretic action. Modified from Warnock DG. Diuretic agents. In: Katzung BG (ed.) *Basic and Clinical Pharmacology*, 5th edn. East Norwalk: Appleton and Lange, 1992: p. 212, Fig. 15-2, with permission.

LOOP DIURETICS

Examples: frusemide, bumetanide, piretanide, torasemide, ethacrynic acid.

Mechanisms of action

Loop diuretics are initially secreted into the proximal tubular fluid and thence gain access to the cells of the medullary thick ascending loop of Henle (mTAL). Their primary action is inhibition of sodium chloride reabsorption in the mTAL, where up to 25% of all sodium reabsorption occurs. There is limited capability for reabsorption of sodium ions beyond this level.

The primary inhibitory site of action of loop diuretics appears to be at the sodium–potassium–2chloride symporter situated at the luminal membrane (Fig. 20.2). An energy-dependent sodium–potassium adenosine triphosphatase (ATPase) pump is situated in the basolateral cell membrane and pumps Na^+ out into the interstitium against its concentration gradient and maintains a low intracellular concentration. This favours the inward movement of Na^+ from the tubular lumen, facilitated by the luminal symporter system, creating sufficient energy to draw K^+ in against its concentration gradient. Inhibition of these active transport pumps at the luminal and basolateral membranes by loop diuretics may provide renal protection during ischaemia, by decreasing mTAL oxygen requirement. Loop diuretics have modest carbonic anhydrase inhibitory activity in the proximal tubule, but this appears to be unimportant clinically.

Loop diuretics also inhibit mTAL uptake and increase urinary excretion of magnesium, calcium and uric acid. In addition, they have specific vasodilator effects. In the kidney, frusemide dilates cortical vessels, which may protect against ischaemic insults and tubuloglomerular feedback that results in cortical vasoconstriction. Intravenous injection, especially of larger doses, is followed by prompt venodilatation, which may be helpful in acute pulmonary oedema or congestive cardiac failure, by lowering raised left ventricular filling pressures.

Table 20.1 Classification of diuretic agents based on electrolyte handling

Class	Examples	Site of action	Mechanism	FENa (%)	K	HCO$_3^-$
Loop diuretics	Frusemide, ethacrynic acid, bumetanide	mTAL	Inhibits Na–K–2Cl symporter	20–25	+	−
Thiazides	Chlorothiazide, hydrochlorthiazide, metolazone	Early distal tubule	Inhibit sodium chloride uptake	5–8	++	±
Potassium sparing	Triamterene, amiloride	Late distal tubule, collecting ducts	Inhibit Na$^+$ uptake	< 5	−	−
	Spironolactone	Late distal tubule, collecting ducts	Aldosterone antagonism	< 5	−	−
Carbonic anhydrase inhibitors	Acetazolamide	Proximal tubule	Decreased intracellular H$^+$ formation (bicarbonate loss)	< 5	+	+++
Osmotic diuretics	Mannitol	Throughout tubule	Osmotic pressure: prevention of water absorption by permeable segments of the nephron	< 5	+	±

FENa, fractional excretion of sodium (sodium clearance/creatinine clearance × 100%); mTAL, medullary thick ascending loop of Henle; Na, sodium; K, potassium; Cl, chloride; H$^+$, hydrogen ion; HCO$_3^-$, bicarbonate; +, increased urinary loss; −, decreased or no urinary loss.

Indications

Diuresis

The most common perioperative indications for loop diuretics are fluid overload, pulmonary congestion and pulmonary oedema. The initial benefit may be through venodilatation, but ultimately the goal is to decrease intravascular volume, venous return and ventricular pressures. Loop diuretics may be very helpful in the therapy of hyperkalaemia, hypercalcaemia and hypermagnesaemia. In all cases, saline infusion should be provided to preserve the intravascular volume. This approach is also effective for halide intoxication (bromide, fluoride or iodine), but not for the elimination of lithium, which may be worsened.

Renal Protection

In animal models, prior administration of frusemide provides protection against ischaemic or nephrotoxic insults, but in clinical practice loop diuretics are usually given to treat oliguria, that is, they are given *after* a renal insult, rather than before. The most appropriate prophylactic use of loop diuretics is to maintain high urine flow rates in the pigment nephropathies: intravascular haemolysis or rhabdomyolysis. Increased tubular flow 'washes out' nephrotoxic pigments and cellular debris, and prevents tubular obstruction and damage. Small doses of frusemide may be added to mannitol if there is an inadequate response to osmotic diuresis, but aggressive fluid replacement remains the essential and most effective means of renal protection in these situations.

Dosage

Frusemide is the 'first-line' loop diuretic used in anaesthesia and critical care. After intravenous injection its onset of action is rapid, within 5 min. The duration of effect is variable, depending on intravascular volume. In hypovolaemia, the effect may be quite short lived. In hypervolaemic patients or in the presence of other diuretics (mannitol, dopamine, etc.), very small doses of frusemide can elicit a brisk diuresis lasting 2–3 h.

During operation it is best to start with 5–10 mg intravenous frusemide and repeat as indicated based on the amount and duration of subsequent diuresis. In patients with resistant oedematous states (e.g. congestive cardiac failure) who have been on chronic diuretic therapy or who have a low glomerular filtration rate (GFR), the required intravenous dose is usually of the order of 20–40 mg or greater. Bolus doses of 80 mg or

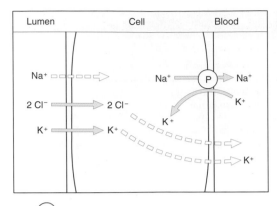

| Lumen | Cell | Blood |

P — Na⁺, K⁺–ATPase (Na pump)

□□□□ Passive movement

▬▬▬ Primary active or secondary active transport

Net result: reabsorption Na⁺, K⁺, 2 Cl⁻ ions

Fig. 20.2 Transport mechanisms in the medullary thick ascending loop of Henle. At the apical (luminal) membrane of the tubular cell, sodium is reabsorbed passively together with active transport of potassium and two chloride ions (Na^+–K^+–$2Cl^-$ symporter). This is the primary site of action of loop diuretics. At the basolateral membrane an energy-dependent active transport system (Na^+–K^+-ATPase) pumps out Na^+ in exchange for K^+ and enhances the gradient for Na^+ absorption at the luminal membrane. From Wingard LB, Brody TM, Larner J, Schwartz A. Diuretics: drugs that increase excretion of water and electrolytes. In: Wingard LB, Brody TM, Larner J, Schwartz A (eds) *Human Pharmacology: Molecular-to-clinical.* London: Wolfe Publishing, 1991: p. 249, Fig. 19-3, with permission.

more should be given slowly because of the potential for hypotension induced by venodilatation; bolus doses greater than 240 mg should be avoided because of the risk of ototoxicity and because of the greater effectiveness of concomitant therapy (see below).

Ethacrynic acid (25–50 mg intravenously) or bumetanide (1 mg intravenously) are reserved for situations of frusemide resistance or given concomitantly when GFR is impaired.

Adverse effects

Acute Hypovolaemia
Acute hypovolaemia and hypotension may be caused by the initial venodilation; inappropriate administration to 'make urine' when oliguria is secondary to preexisting hypovolaemia; and/or subsequent loss of urinary concentrating ability by the 'washing out' of the hypertonic medullary countercurrent mechanism. The latter effects are common to all diuretic agents, whether by inhibition of active sodium chloride transport or osmotic activity. The resultant diuresis is usually short lived, but may be sufficient to cause hypotension and further exacerbate

renal ischaemia. Acute tolerance to diuretics develops commonly because the initial volume depletion activates sodium-conserving mechanisms, which reduces GFR and stimulates renal tubular reabsorption of sodium and water.

Hypokalaemic Metabolic Alkalosis and Tachyarrhythmias
Loop diuretics induce potassium (K^+) wasting, and hydrogen ion (H^+) is excreted in exchange to conserve this vital ion, resulting in extracellular alkalosis. The increased delivery of sodium to the distal tubule and collecting duct, as well as the contraction of the extracellular fluid, induces aldosterone secretion, which further enhances urinary loss of potassium.

The most important consequence of hypokalaemic metabolic alkalosis is an increased potential for both ventricular and supraventricular arrhythmias, especially in patients on digoxin therapy. Digoxin toxicity may be unmasked or exacerbated. Diuretic-induced hypomagnesaemia frequently accompanies hypokalaemia, and significantly increases myocardial irritability.[1] This situation occurs most commonly in the postoperative period, when a large sustained diuresis is induced to mobilize sequestered fluid.

Particular care should be used with diuretic therapy in patients with right ventricular failure (e.g. right ventricular infarction, cor pulmonale, severe pulmonary hypertension), because these patients are very dependent on the maintenance of a high right ventricular preload.

Ototoxicity
The nephrotoxic and ototoxic effects of aminoglycoside antibiotics may be worsened by the concomitant administration of loop diuretics. If hypovolaemia is induced, the nephrotoxins are concentrated in the tubules. Sustained high doses of loop diuretics (e.g. more than 250 mg intravenous frusemide in an attempt to 'convert' oliguric to nonoliguric acute renal failure) may cause ototoxicity and temporary or permanent hearing loss.[2]

Chronic Diuretic Therapy
The adverse effects of chronic therapy of all diuretic classes and their potential impact on anaesthetic management are summarized in Table 20.2. Patients who present for surgery on chronic diuretic therapy (e.g. for hypertension or congestive heart failure) almost inevitably have a decreased plasma volume. This may predispose to hypotension during induction and maintenance of either general or regional anaesthesia, and preparation for anaesthesia should include adequate fluid loading. These patients also may have decreased total body potassium (and/or magnesium) levels. Extracellular hypokalaemia and arrhythmias, particularly in

Table 20.2 Preoperative evaluation of patients on chronic diuretic therapy			
Diuretic class	**Chronic conditions**	**Adverse effects**	**Anaesthetic implications**
Loop diuretics	CHF, hypertension, cirrhosis, nephrotic syndrome, chronic renal insufficiency, hypercalcaemia	Decreased plasma volume Hypokalaemia Hypomagnesaemia Metabolic alkalosis Hyperuricaemia	Haemodynamic instability Arrhythmias Acute alkalosis (hyperventilation)
Thiazide diuretics	CHF, hypertension	Decreased plasma volume Hypokalaemia Hypomagnesaemia Metabolic alkalosis Hyperuricaemia Glucose intolerance	Haemodynamic instability Arrhythmias Acute alkalosis (hyperventilation) Hyperglycaemia
Potassium-sparing diuretics	Combination therapy for cirrhosis, CHF, hypertension	Hyperkalaemia	Hyperkalaemia (decreased GFR), arrhythmias
Carbonic anhydrase inhibitors	Glaucoma	Metabolic acidosis	Acute acidosis (hypovolaemia), hyperkalaemia (decreased GFR)

CHF, congestive heart failure; GFR, glomerular filtration rate.

patients on digoxin therapy, will be exacerbated by acute respiratory alkalosis caused by excessive mechanical ventilation during anaesthesia. Patients with chronic obstructive lung disease compensate for chronic respiratory acidosis with a metabolic alkalosis, which may be exacerbated by diuretic-induced hypokalaemia and aldosterone activation.

Hyperuricaemia is a recognized complication of loop diuretic therapy, especially when extracellular volume depletion results in enhanced proximal tubular reabsorption of uric acid. However, it appears that acute gout is very rarely precipitated, even in susceptible patients.

High doses of frusemide have been reported to interfere with colorimetric methods of serum creatinine assay to the extent that it becomes unmeasurable. Enzymatic methods of measuring serum creatinine concentration are not affected.

THIAZIDE DIURETICS
Examples: hydrochlorthiazide, chlorothiazide, metolazone.

Mechanisms of action
The thiazides inhibit sodium chloride reabsorption in the early distal tubule. Only about 15% of the glomerular filtrate reaches this segment and only 5–8% of sodium reabsorption occurs here, so that thiazides are less potent diuretic agents than the loop diuretics.

Summary box 20.2 Clinical uses of thiazide diuretics

- Heart failure.

- Hypertension; may have action unrelated to their diuretic action but exact mechanism poorly understood.

- In severe resistant oedema the combination of loop and thiazide diuretics is often effective.

- Reduce urinary calcium excretion in patients with hypercalcuria and renal stone formation.

Indications
The only true indication for thiazide diuretic therapy in the immediate perioperative period or intensive care unit is as concomitant therapy with loop diuretics in states of resistant oedema or low GFR.

Adverse effects
The adverse effects of thiazide diuretics occur as a consequence of chronic administration and should be evaluated when patients present for surgery (Table 20.2). They include hypokalaemic metabolic alkalosis, muscle weakness, impaired glucose tolerance and hyponatraemia. Thiazides compete for uric acid secretion, which may result in hyperuricaemia, and calcium excretion is also impaired.

POTASSIUM-SPARING DIURETICS

Examples: spironolactone, triamterene, amiloride.

Mechanisms of action

These drugs act on the remote distal tubule and collecting duct, and have weak diuretic activity, because less than 5% of filtered sodium is reabsorbed in these segments. They are usually used in combination with loop diuretics or thiazides to augment diuresis and restrict potassium loss induced by these agents. Potassium-sparing diuretics can be divided into two groups: aldosterone antagonists (e.g. spironolactone) and sodium transport inhibitors (e.g. triamterene, amiloride). They are not available for parenteral injection and are seldom used in the perioperative period; indeed, because of their propensity to induce hyperkalaemia, they should be discontinued in critically ill patients at risk for renal insufficiency or acute renal failure.

Aldosterone is a steroid hormone produced by the zona glomerulosa of the adrenal cortex, and is released under the influence of adrenocorticotrophic hormone, angiotensin II and intravascular hyponatraemia and/or hypovolaemia. Its release and actions are opposed by atrial natriuretic peptide (ANP). Aldosterone enters the distal tubular cytoplasm and attaches to a receptor, then migrates to the nucleus where it induces the formation of messenger RNA, which induces the synthesis of a protein which enhances the permeability of the apical (luminal) membrane to Na^+ and K^+. The reabsorption of Na^+ stimulates the basolateral membrane Na^+–K^+-ATPase pump, the intracellular concentration of potassium rises, and it follows its concentration gradient out into the lumen. The net effect of aldosterone's action is Na^+ reabsorption and K^+ loss.

Spironolactone is a competitive aldosterone antagonist and therefore inhibits sodium retention and potassium excretion. It is a synthetic steroid analogue which binds to cytoplasmic mineralocorticoid receptors, preventing the receptor complex from translocating to the collecting duct cell nucleus (Fig. 20.3). Because aldosterone's effects are mediated via protein synthesis, the onset and offset of action of spironolactone is slow. Its onset of action takes 2–4 days for full potency. Although the drug itself is rapidly metabolized, its effects last for 48–72 h after it is discontinued, so that hyperkalaemia is a potential danger if a patient develops acute renal insufficiency or failure.

Spironolactone is most useful in the long-term treatment of refractory oedematous states such as chronic liver failure, which are characterized by intravascular hypovolaemia, sodium retention and secondary hyperaldosteronism. In these situations, loop diuretics or thiazides merely exacerbate intravascular hypovolaemia and hypokalaemic metabolic alkalosis, and may induce hepatic encephalopathy by increasing ammonia transport into the brain. In the presence of alkalosis, the lipophobic ammonium moiety (NH_4^+) is converted to lipophilic ammonia (NH_3), which easily crosses lipid cell membranes, so-called nonionic diffusion trapping.

Adverse effects

The most important adverse effects are related to potassium and chloride retention: hyperkalaemia and hyperchloraemic metabolic acidosis. Hyperkalaemia may be life threatening in patients with acute renal insufficiency or acute renal failure. To some degree, these effects may be balanced when spironolactone is used in combination with thiazide diuretics. Spironolactone can cause gynaecomastia.

Normokalaemic, hypochloraemic, metabolic alkalosis can occur in patients on a combination of spironolactone and frusemide, and is associated with diuretic resistance.[3] Correction of the metabolic alkalosis by substituting acetazolamide for frusemide enhances the response to frusemide when it is subsequently restarted.

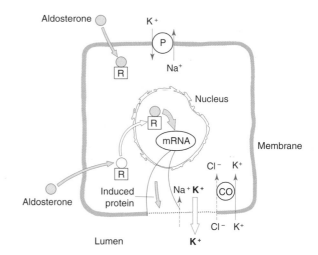

Fig. 20.3 Mode of action of aldosterone. Aldosterone enters the distal tubular cytoplasm and attaches to a receptor, then migrates to the nucleus where it enhances the production of a protein that increases the permeability of the luminal membrane to sodium and potassium ions. The net effect of aldosterone's action is sodium reabsorption and potassium loss. Spironolactone acts by preventing the attachment of aldosterone to the cytosolic receptor. R, receptor; mRNA, messenger ribonucleic acid; CO, cotransporter (= symporter); P, sodium–potassium adenosine triphosphatase pump. From Wingard LB, Brody TM, Larner J, Schwartz A. Diuretics: drugs that increase excretion of water and electrolytes. In: Wingard LB, Brody TM, Larner J, Schwartz A (eds) *Human Pharmacology: Molecular-to-clinical*. London: Wolfe Publishing, 1991: p. 249, Fig. 19-4, with permission.

OSMOTIC DIURETICS

Examples: mannitol, urea, isosorbide, glycerol.

Mechanisms of action

Osmotic diuretics are small molecules that draw water into the renal tubule. Mannitol is the archetypal osmotic water diuretic, i.e. it is not a natriuretic agent. It is an 'inert' sugar that is not metabolized by the body, remains largely confined to the blood, and is directly excreted by the kidneys. It prevents water reabsorption in all segments of the tubule that are freely permeable to water: the proximal tubule, descending loop of Henle and the collecting duct.

Mannitol also induces diuresis by a number of other mechanisms, many of which also confer protection against renal cortical ischaemia. It expands the intravascular volume by increasing osmotic pressure and drawing fluid in from the extracellular space. This increases ventricular preload, cardiac output, renal blood flow (RBF), transglomerular pressure gradient and GFR. Its osmotic effect increases tubular flow rate by preventing water reabsorption; this in turn prevents or diminishes tubular obstruction by cellular debris in the ischaemic proximal tubule.

Volume expansion of the atria by the osmotic effect of mannitol stimulates the release of ANP; this may be one of its most important benefits. Osmotic haemodilution may protect against the 'no-reflow' phenomenon, that is, hypoperfusion caused by red cell aggregation and endothelial swelling in the vessels of the inner medulla as a consequence of renal ischaemia. Mannitol is a free-radical scavenger and may attenuate reperfusion injury after ischaemia. Finally, mannitol may increase the activity of vasodilator intrarenal prostaglandins, notably prostacyclin (prostaglandin I_2), which may further protect against ischaemic injury.

Indications

Diuresis

Mannitol is used for its osmotic effect to decrease intracellular and interstitial fluid, and to provide renal protection. It is administered to prevent or decrease raised intracranial pressure during and after neurosurgical procedures, head injury and in the presence of brain tumours, or to decrease intraocular pressure. Its inclusion in cardioplegia solutions during cardiopulmonary bypass (CPB) helps to attenuate ischaemia-induced myocardial oedema.

Renal Protection

There is considerable laboratory evidence that mannitol protects against ischaemic and nephrotoxic acute renal injury, but there are few controlled, prospective clinical studies.

Prophylactic administration of mannitol before aortic cross-clamping has been used widely for nearly 30 years, although in a saline-loaded canine model of thoracic aortic cross-clamping, neither mannitol, dopamine nor a mannitol–dopamine combination prevented a 25–50% decrease in GFR and RBF.[4] Even with the use of a continuous infusion of 20% mannitol at 100 ml h^{-1}, infrarenal aortic cross-clamping results in a 38% decrease in RBF although urine flow is well maintained.

Mannitol is routinely added to the pump prime before instituting CPB to protect renal function. Despite its use, subclinical markers of glomerular and tubular injury (e.g. microalbuminuria, urinary *N*-acetyl-*β*-D-glucosaminidase) are consistently raised.[5] None the less, the incidence of acute renal failure after uncomplicated CPB in patients with previously normal renal function is less than 3%. Mannitol washes out the hypertonic renal medulla and impairs the renal concentrating ability for several hours after CPB, resulting in an osmotic diuresis of 200–400 ml h^{-1}. This can exacerbate postoperative hypovolaemia and hypokalaemia.

Osmotic diuresis with mannitol is advocated for many situations where there is a high risk of nephrotoxic injury. These include use of radiocontrast dyes, intravascular haemolysis (transfusion reactions), myoglobinaemia (rhabdomyolysis) and conjugated hyperbilirubinaemia (obstructive jaundice).

Dosage

Bolus dosing of mannitol is provided by 6.25–12.5 g (25–50 ml of a 25% solution), given 10–20 min before a defined insult (e.g. aortic cross-clamping) and repeated if necessary every 4–6 h. In the aggressive management of closed head injury or postsurgical oedema, as much as 25–50 g mannitol may be administered every 3 h. Alternatively, a continuous infusion of 5–10% mannitol may be given at 50 ml h^{-1}. The solution must be warmed if crystallization has occurred.

Adverse effects

Rapid administration of mannitol can precipitate pulmonary oedema by excessive expansion of the intravascular space. If it is not excreted promptly, mannitol may generate a hyperosmolar syndrome (serum osmolality greater than 320 mOsm kg^{-1}). Water intoxication may result with a normal or decreased serum sodium concentration. Serial testing of serum osmolality is used as a guide to the limits of mannitol dosing during aggressive therapy in closed head injury: the mannitol dose is decreased if the serum osmolality exceeds 310 mOsm kg^{-1}. Note that, in the presence of mannitol, serum osmolality cannot be calculated from serum sodium concentration[*] and must be measured directly. The

---

[*]Serum osmolality = (Na/2 + K + BUN/3 + glucose/18) mOsm kg^{-1}, where Na = serum sodium concentration, K = serum potassium concentration, BUN = blood urea nitrogen.

maximum cumulative dose in a 24-h period should be no greater than 1.5 g kg^{-1}. Excessive mannitol-induced diuresis may lead to acute hypovolaemia and actually worsen renal function.

CARBONIC ANHYDRASE INHIBITORS
Example: acetazolamide.

Mechanisms of action
Carbonic anhydrase, a metalloenzyme containing zinc, is a family of five isoenzymes which catalyses the reversible combination of water and carbon dioxide to form carbonic acid in the luminal brush border of the proximal tubular cell. Carbonic acid in turn serves as a source of H$^+$ which is exchanged for filtered bicarbonate, which is thus preserved. Acetazolamide results in diuresis together with an obligatory loss of bicarbonate. However, although the proximal tubule is the major site for sodium reabsorption in the nephron, the fractional excretion of sodium induced by carbonic anhydrase inhibition is relatively low, around 3–5%. There are several reasons for this. Only a portion of the proximal tubule is affected by carbonic anhydrase inhibition. Acetazolamide decreases the GFR. Finally, and most importantly, most of the Na$^+$ that escapes is reabsorbed more distally, especially at the mTAL.

Indications
The indications for intravenous acetazolamide in the perioperative period are as an adjunct to reverse iatrogenic metabolic alkalosis, or to alkalinize the urine in rhabdomyolysis and myoglobinuria. In neither situation is acetazolamide first-line therapy.

Metabolic Alkalosis
The major adverse affects of metabolic alkalosis are hypokalaemia (as a result of movement into cells in exchange for H$^+$) which predisposes to arrhythmias, and hypoventilation (i.e. carbon dioxide is retained to normalize pH). It is important to distinguish metabolic alkalosis due to excess administration of bicarbonate (e.g. via the citrate in transfused blood, which is converted to bicarbonate on a mol : mol basis), from that which has resulted from excessive diuresis (contraction alkalosis and hypokalaemia). In the former, judicious administration of acetazolamide may be helpful in restoring ventilatory drive; in the latter, it may simply exacerbate hypovolaemia. Bicarbonate excretion is usually limited in the presence of hypokalaemia, because the renal tubules preferentially eliminate H$^+$ in exchange for K$^+$. Therefore, the initial step in the treatment of metabolic alkalosis is the careful restoration of normal intravascular volume and aggressive replacement of chloride and potassium. Only if alkalosis persists should acetazolamide be considered.

Renal Protection
The primary management of rhabdomyolysis and myoglobinuria includes aggressive maintenance of intravascular volume and high tubular flow with fluid and mannitol administration. Urinary alkalization (i.e. keeping the urinary pH > 6.0) retards the conversion of myoglobin to toxic ferrihaematin and decreases the risk of tubular injury. Usually this is accomplished by the addition of sodium bicarbonate (25 mmol l^{-1}) to the intravenous fluid. Addition of acetazolamide may be considered if metabolic alkalosis develops and myoglobinuria persists.

Dosage
The standard dose of acetazolamide is 250–500 mg intravenously. Doses may be repeated every 6–12 h, but it is seldom required to continue a course for longer than 24 h. The electrolyte and acid–base status should be carefully reassessed and acetazolamide discontinued once the pH starts to return to near normal values. Excess or protracted administration of acetazolamide may result in metabolic acidosis and hypovolaemia.

DOPAMINERGIC AGENTS
Examples: dopamine, dopexamine, fenoldopam.

Mechanisms of action
Dopamine receptors in the renal and splanchnic vasculature mediate vasodilatation and increase RBF and GFR, whereas those in the luminal and basolateral membranes of the proximal tubule inhibit sodium reabsorption and promote diuresis. There are two subtypes of dopamine, DA$_1$ and DA$_2$. DA$_2$ receptors are sited on the presynaptic terminal of postganglionic sympathetic nerves, and inhibit the release of noradrenaline from presynaptic vesicles in a similar fashion to the presynaptic a_2 receptor.

Based on the receptor subtypes, dopamine agonists and antagonists may be categorized as selective or nonselective agents. Dopamine is a mixed DA$_1$ and DA$_2$ agonist; however, DA$_2$ stimulation may further facilitate renal vasodilatation by decreasing intrarenal noradrenaline release. The advantages of a selective DA$_1$ agonist such as fenoldopam therefore become apparent. Haloperidol, chlorpromazine and metoclopramide are nonselective dopaminergic antagonists, but there are few clinical data on their ability to inhibit dopamine-induced diuresis.

Dopamine
In the low dose range (1–3 μg kg^{-1} min^{-1}) dopamine acts as a nonselective dopaminergic agonist. Dopamine may enhance renal function by several mechanisms. Its renal vasodilator action increases RBF and blocks the renal

vasoconstrictor effects of noradrenaline. Its β_1-mediated inotropic effect increases cardiac output and thereby RBF and renal perfusion pressure. Stimulation of tubular DA$_1$ receptors evokes saliuresis.

Clinically and experimentally, the diuretic effect of dopamine is consistently demonstrable, whereas its dopaminergic effect on RBF and GFR is difficult to separate from its inotropic effect on cardiac output. Even if it acts primarily as a saliuretic, dopamine could protect the renal tubules by suppressing the sodium pump, decreasing oxygen consumption and by increasing tubular flow. However, there are relatively few data suggesting that prophylactic administration of low-dose dopamine protects the kidney from injury. In established chronic renal insufficiency (GFR $<$ 50 ml per min per 1.73 m^{-2}) dopamine may induce natriuresis but does not significantly increase GFR or RBF.

In a study comparing equi-inotropic doses of dopamine and dobutamine after cardiac surgery, the two agents had similar effects on GFR and RBF. However, dopamine induced a threefold greater urine flow rate and sodium excretion than dobutamine, suggesting that it primarily affected tubular dopaminergic receptors.[6] In another study on haemodynamically stable patients with normal renal function, low-dose dopamine (200 μg min^{-1}) appeared to have only a diuretic effect, with no improvement in creatinine clearance.[7] In contrast, low-dose dobutamine (175 μg min^{-1}) consistently improved creatinine clearance, without a diuretic effect, presumably through its inotropic effect on cardiac output and blood pressure.

Dopexamine

Dopexamine is a synthetic analogue of dopamine which has a predominantly β_2-receptor effect, and about one-third the effect of dopamine on the renal vasculature. As such it is more an inodilator than a diuretic, although it may promote diuresis in patients with congestive heart failure by both its cardiac and renal actions.[8]

Fenoldopam

Fenoldopam is a benzazepine dopamine analogue which is a selective DA$_1$-receptor agonist, i.e. it is devoid of β- or α-adrenergic activity. It antagonizes noradrenaline-induced vasoconstriction, and thus has the potential to be a potent vasodilator–diuretic. It has a rapid onset and offset of effect, with an elimination half-life of 10 min. When administered by intravenous infusion at 0.1–0.5 μg kg^{-1} min^{-1} to hypertensive patients, it provides a dose-dependent reduction in blood pressure, mild reflex tachycardia, and marked increases in RBF, urine flow and sodium excretion, although there is little change in GFR.[9]

Indications

Diuresis

Dopamine is indicated as a diuretic if urine output remains low ($<$ 0.5 ml kg^{-1} h^{-1}) after reasonable attempts have been made to restore adequate intravascular volume and cardiac output. The saliuretic and diuretic response to low-dose dopamine are impaired by intravascular hypovolaemia (e.g. preoperative fluid restriction), which activates tubular salt and water conservation.[10]

Renal Protection

Despite its widespread clinical use as a 'renal protective' agent, there are few data that actually support a beneficial effect of low-dose dopamine on renal outcome.

Aortic and cardiac surgery. Dopamine induces a significant saliuresis and improves creatinine clearance during infrarenal aortic cross-clamping.[11] However, extravascular fluid volume expansion to maintain a pulmonary artery occlusion pressure between 12 and 15 mmHg is just as effective as mannitol or dopamine in maintaining GFR in this situation.[12] Prophylactic administration of dopamine during CPB has not been demonstrated to prevent tubular enzymuria or to benefit renal function in patients with normal or moderately abnormal ($<$ 50 ml min^{-1}) creatinine clearance.[13,14]

Transplantation. Although in healthy volunteers low-dose dopamine reverses the marked decrease in RBF caused by oral cyclosporin A, it has not consistently prevented renal dysfunction after transplantation. The use of prophylactic dopamine during renal transplantation has not decreased posttransplant renal insufficiency or acute renal failure, and may actually cause more problems with tachycardia and arrhythmias.

Sepsis. In septic shock, low-dose dopamine is frequently coadministered with dobutamine, adrenaline or noradrenaline in the belief that this confers renal protection. In patients with sepsis without vasopressor support, short-term low-dose dopamine administration doubled urine flow and increased creatinine clearance by 60% without affecting systemic haemodynamics.[15] However, after 48 h the renal response had decreased significantly, suggesting the possibility of downregulation of the dopaminergic receptors. Moreover, patients in septic shock who required vasopressor support did not respond to low-dose dopamine.

Nephrotoxic insults. Low-dose dopamine increases the renal clearance of aminoglycosides, but it has not yet been shown to protect against nephrotoxicity. In patients with obstructive jaundice about to undergo surgery, low-dose dopamine does not appear to confer additional renal protection to good hydration and a bolus of frusemide at induction of anaesthesia.[16] However, dopamine did reverse the impairment of urine flow and serum creatinine induced by recombinant interleukin-2 in patients undergoing therapy for metastatic urological cancer.[17]

Adverse effects

Dopamine's β_1-adrenergic activity may cause unwanted tachycardia or tachyarrhythmias in susceptible patients even at low doses. At doses above 10 μg kg^{-1} min^{-1} dopamine causes increasing renal vasoconstriction through its α_1-adrenergic action and biotransformation to noradrenaline, which diminishes urine flow rate. Even low-dose dopamine may contribute during haemorrhagic shock.[18] Inadvertent subcutaneous extravasation of a dopamine infusion may cause intense vasoconstriction and even tissue necrosis; for this reason it is always preferable to infuse dopamine via a central venous catheter.

ATRIAL NATRIURETIC PEPTIDE

Examples: atrial natriuretic peptide, urodilatin.

Mechanisms of action

For many years it had been postulated that a natriuretic hormone existed to account for diuresis observed with volume loading. Finally in 1981 de Bold *et al.*[19] demonstrated that injection of an extract of atrial tissue in rats caused natriuresis. Subsequently a family of natriuretic peptides was identified, including atrial natriuretic peptide (ANP, produced in atrial myocytes), brain natriuretic peptide, C-type natriuretic peptide and urodilatin (produced in the kidney itself).

The major trigger for ANP release is increased atrial volume. The renal effect of ANP is a prompt, sustained increase in GFR and natriuresis even when arterial pressure is decreased. The vasodilator effects of ANP are mediated through guanylate cyclase activation and increased cyclic guanosine monophosphate levels. As such, ANP antagonizes the vasoconstrictor effects of noradrenaline, angiotensin II and endothelin.

Hypotension or hypovolaemia triggers the release of renin from the afferent arteriole, which causes the formation of angiotensin II, which in turn stimulates the release of aldosterone from the adrenal cortex. Angiotensin II and aldosterone cause vasoconstriction and sodium retention, which ultimately results in the reexpansion of the intravascular volume. This causes atrial distension which triggers the release of ANP. ANP inhibits the release of renin, its action on angiotensinogen to form angiotensin II, angiotensin-induced vasoconstriction, the stimulation of aldosterone secretion by angiotensin II, and the actions of aldosterone on

the collecting duct. Thus, the actions of ANP promote vasodilatation and sodium excretion. The therapeutic administration of fluids that distend the atrium and release ANP is an important intervention to curtail renal vasoconstriction and sodium retention. Release of ANP appears to be a reflex response to counteract the cascade of vasoconstriction and salt retention induced by angiotensin, aldosterone and antidiuretic hormone (ADH) (Fig. 20.4). ANP inhibits renin secretion and aldosterone release and blocks the salt-retaining action of aldosterone. It also inhibits ADH secretion from the posterior pituitary and antagonizes its effect on the V_2 receptor in the collecting duct. All these actions promote natriuresis.

An example of the protective role of endogenous ANP is illustrated by the observation that, in patients undergoing mitral valve replacement, the acute reduction in left atrial pressure following surgery results in a significant reduction in urine output and sodium excretion, the magnitude of which are related to the degree of reduction in left atrial pressure.[20] In other words, patients with mitral valve disease and high left atrial pressure have a constant stimulus to ANP release. When the valvular gradient is removed and atrial stretch diminishes, ANP levels decrease, with the observed effect on salt excretion and urine flow rate.

Indications, limitations and adverse effects

Diuresis

When ANP is administered exogenously it acts as a potent venodilator, and decreased cardiac preload results in decreased systemic blood pressure. Urodilatin lacks the systemic vasodilator effects of ANP, and is a more potent diuretic agent. In certain oedematous

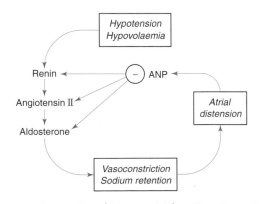

Fig. 20.4 Interactions between atrial natriuretic peptide (ANP) and the renin–angiotensin–aldosterone system. From Sladen RN. Renal Physiology. In: Miller RD (ed.) *Anesthesia*, 4th edn. New York: Churchill Livingstone, 1994: 663–688, with permission.

disease states, notably congestive heart failure, cirrhosis and the nephrotic syndrome, there is a markedly blunted response to the natriuretic effect of ANP. In the first two situations, enhanced proximal tubular reabsorption of sodium decreases distal sodium delivery to the major site of ANP action.

In patients with severe chronic renal insufficiency, infusion of a synthetic atrial peptide (atriopeptin III) induces natriuresis and increases GFR.[21] However, the individual response is quite variable, and high doses are associated with a significant decrease in systolic blood pressure. Anaritide, a synthetic analogue of ANP, has a natriuretic and diuretic effect in patients with cirrhotic ascites and/or oedema, but high doses also produce hypotension.[22]

DIURETIC RESISTANCE

ACUTE TOLERANCE ('BRAKING PHENOMENON')

Shortly after diuretic administration is commenced, acute tolerance develops with a decreased saliuretic response to repeated doses, thought to be secondary to the contraction in extracellular fluid induced by diuresis. In response to acute hypovolaemia, sympathetic and renin–angiotensin activation increases sodium reabsorption in the proximal tubule, mTAL and distal tubule ('braking phenomenon' or 'postdiuretic sodium retention'). This can be counteracted by fluid repletion.[23]

CHRONIC TOLERANCE

Long-term administration of loop diuretics is associated with a gradually increasing dose requirement. An important mechanism for chronic tolerance to loop diuretic therapy is hypertrophy of the tubular epithelium of the distal tubule, presumably because mTAL blockade allows increased concentrations of sodium to reach this segment. This results in increased capacity of the electroneutral Na^+–Cl^- transport system and an increased number of Na^+–K^+-ATPase pumps on the surface of the basolateral membrane. The result is that an increased amount of the Na^+ is reabsorbed downstream from the mTAL. This site is blocked by thiazide diuretics, which may in part account for the synergistic effect of combining a loop and thiazide diuretic in resistant states. In addition, administration of thiazides may actually prevent distal tubule hypertrophy.

DISEASE STATES

Diuretic resistance ('refractory oedema') is encountered in disease states such as renal insufficiency, congestive heart failure, hepatic cirrhosis and the nephrotic syndrome. The abnormal response to diuretic therapy can be explained by altered pharmacokinetics and/or pharmacodynamics.

Normal diuretic pharmacokinetics and pharmacodynamics

The dose–response curve for diuretic action has a typical sigmoidal shape (Fig. 20.5), based on the relationship between urinary diuretic concentration and sodium excretion rate.[3] Once a threshold concentration is reached, sodium excretion increases with progressive increase in urinary diuretic concentration until a maximal response is achieved. Pharmacokinetic factors such as dose, bioavailability, tubular secretory capacity and time course of delivery affect the urinary diuretic concentration, whereas the pharmacodynamic response of the tubules to a given concentration of diuretic affects sodium excretion. In normal individuals loop diuretics cause a maximum fractional sodium excretion of 20–25%, suggesting that they can completely inhibit sodium reabsorption at the mTAL.

Diuretics block sodium absorption at the luminal border of the mTAL, so it is the concentration of diuretic in the urine that determines diuretic activity. Loop diuretics are highly protein bound, and GFR itself plays little role in drug delivery into the urine. Instead, they are actively secreted into the tubular fluid by the organic acid secretory pump in the straight segment of the proximal tubule.

Altered diuretic pharmacokinetics and pharmacodynamics

Diuretic resistance may occur because of decreased diuretic delivery to the luminal border of the tubule (pharmacokinetic effect), or because of decreased sodium excretory response to a given concentration of drug in the urine (pharmacodynamic effect). In the

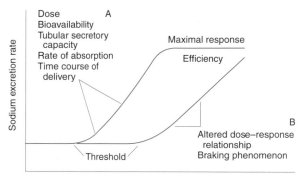

Fig. 20.5 Dose–response curves of loop diuretic action, illustrating both the pharmacokinetic (A) and pharmacodynamic (B) determinants of the response. In diuretic-resistant states (dotted line), the dose–response curve is shifted to the right. From Sica DA, Gehr TW. Diuretic combinations in refractory oedema states: pharmacokinetic–pharmacodynamic relationships. *Clin Pharmacokinet* 1996; **30**: 232, Fig. 2.

latter case, the threshold concentration for response will be raised and/or the dose–response curve will be flattened and shifted to the right (Fig. 20.5).

Renal insufficiency is considered the archetype for pharmacokinetic resistance. In uraemia, secretion of accumulated endogenous organic acids competes with loop diuretics at the proximal tubule, so that decreased diuretic reaches the luminal border of the mTAL. The renal clearance of frusemide correlates directly to blood urea nitrogen (BUN) and creatinine clearance.

Hepatic failure is the archetype for pharmacodynamic resistance; diuretics reach the luminal border of the tubule but, for reasons not completely understood, there is resistance to their action at the mTAL site.[23] However, pharmacokinetic factors also play a role. In hepatic cirrhosis, congestive heart failure and nephrotic syndrome, the effective intravascular volume is markedly decreased leading to increased absorption of Na^+ in the proximal tubule. Thus less Na^+ is available for diuretic action at the mTAL and distal tubule.

STRATEGIES FOR OVERCOMING DIURETIC RESISTANCE

Strategies for overcoming diuretic resistance are summarized in Table 20.3, and include correction of abnormal haemodynamic parameters, use of higher doses of diuretic agents, administration of human albumin, continuous infusions and combination therapy.[3]

Correction of abnormal haemodynamic parameters

Depleted intravascular volume or lowered blood pressure decreases the filtered load of Na^+ and tubular diuretic delivery. Therefore the most important initial step in improving diuretic response is the restoration of normal haemodynamic parameters. If diuretic response remains impaired, enhancement of RBF by low-dose dopamine, or of cardiac output by inotropic agents, should be attempted.

Table 20.3 Strategies for overcoming diuretic resistance

- Correction of abnormal haemodynamic parameters:
  - restoration of depleted intravascular volume
  - increased renal blood flow – inotropic support or low-dose dopamine.
- Increased dosage of diuretic agents.
- Albumin infusion to increase drug delivery.
- Continuous diuretic infusion.
- Combination therapy:
  - same class (loop + loop)
  - sequential nephron blockade (loop + thiazide).

Utilization of higher doses of diuretic

In severe renal insufficiency only about one-fifth of the dose of frusemide reaches the urine, and only about one-tenth of the dose of bumetanide or torasemide.[23] The reason for this disparity is that frusemide is almost entirely dependent on renal elimination for its clearance, and its serum levels remain persistently high, whereas bumetanide and torasemide undergo considerable hepatic biotransformation. In normal patients the intravenous dose of frusemide that achieves maximal diuretic response is 40 mg. Therefore, in severe renal insufficiency this would have to be increased fivefold (i.e. to 200 mg), whereas the dosage of bumetanide and torasemide would have to be increased tenfold, from 1 to 10 mg and from 20 to 200 mg respectively. The risk of ototoxicity limits the dose of frusemide to 250 mg, especially when administered concomitantly with aminoglycoside antibiotics. Because loop diuretics are highly protein bound, administration of human albumin to hypoalbuminaemic patients markedly increases the diuretic efficacy of frusemide.

Continuous diuretic infusion

The duration of time over which a diuretic is delivered into the urine is a critical determinant of diuretic response. Thus, it is logical that administration of a diuretic by continuous infusion may provide a greater and more sustained response than bolus injection (Fig. 20.6). It may also decrease the potential for rebound sodium retention or angiotensin activation triggered by high plasma concentrations of the loop diuretic, as well as making titration to effect easier and complications related to high peak doses less likely.[3,24] The potential advantage of continuous infusion therapy has been demonstrated in normal individuals, after cardiac surgery, in liver disease and in severe renal insufficiency. Because of the increased magnitude of saliuresis and diuresis achievable by continuous diuretic infusion, there is potentially an increased risk of all the usual adverse diuretic effects, particularly hypovolaemia, hypokalaemia and hypomagnesaemia.

Combination of loop diuretics with thiazide diuretics

The combination of loop diuretics with thiazides appears to induce a synergistic diuretic response. Segmental nephron blockade of sodium absorption with low doses of a loop diuretic at the mTAL and a thiazide at the distal tubule is more effective than high doses of either agent used alone. This may be very helpful in fluid and solute elimination in situations of low GFR (as long as the low GFR is not due to volume depletion) or in other situations of diuretic tolerance or resistance. It can also avoid the potential for ototoxicity from high doses of loop diuretics.

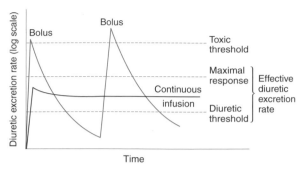

Fig. 20.6 Bolus versus continuous infusion of a loop diuretic. Following an intravenous bolus there is a rapid increase and decrease in diuretic excretion rate. However, most of this is 'wasted' because the maximum sodium excretion rate is quickly achieved, and the diuretic effect is short lived. The high peak level of diuretic may simply serve to induce drug toxicity. In contrast, when administered by continuous intravenous infusion, lower (i.e. subtoxic but effective) levels are sustained for the duration of infusion. This results in a sustained, titratable diuresis even in diuretic-resistant states.

Choice of Thiazide Diuretic

Metolazone, a thiazide-like diuretic, is the agent most commonly used in combination with frusemide in diuretic-resistant states. It blocks sodium absorption both proximally and distally to the mTAL (Fig. 20.7). Like frusemide, metolazone undergoes extensive tubular secretion and is active at the luminal surface of the tubular cells. Metolazone is available only as an oral formulation with very unpredictable gastrointestinal absorption. Therefore the onset of synergistic diuretic effect may vary between 12 and 48 h. The combination of frusemide and metolazone is capable of generating a large diuresis even in states of very low GFR; once diuresis commences, the doses of frusemide and metolazone should be reduced sharply. About 80% of metolazone is excreted unchanged by the kidney. Therefore, when it is used in renal insufficiency, it will accumulate and have a very long duration of action.

An alternative approach in acute situations is to combine intravenous frusemide with intravenous chlorothiazide 0.5–1.0 g twice daily. Even the addition of an intravenous diuretic of the same class, such as bumetanide 1 mg or ethacrynic acid 25–50 mg, appears to enhance the diuretic effect of frusemide markedly. Combination diuresis can cause an impressive and exaggerated diuresis which may result in profound hypovolaemia, hypokalaemia, hypomagnesaemia, metabolic alkalosis and potential for arrhythmias.

DIURETIC AGENTS IN OLIGURIA AND ACUTE RENAL FAILURE

The first step in the management of perioperative oliguria is to assume that it is due to hypovolaemia until otherwise proven. The finding of a prerenal pattern on urine analysis (urine : plasma osmolar ratio > 1.4 : 1, urine : plasma creatinine ratio > 50 : 1, urinary sodium < 20 mEq l^{-1}, fractional excretion of sodium (FENa) < 1%) supports this assumption. Diuretic therapy should be considered for oliguria under the following conditions: (a) there are unequivocal signs of fluid overload; (b) oliguria persists despite fluid challenges and restoration of stable haemodynamics; and (c) there is evidence of pigment nephropathy (haemolysis, rhabdomyolysis), although even here intravascular volume expansion remains the primary intervention.

LOOP DIURETICS

Urinary sodium and water excretion can be increased by loop diuretics even in the presence of marked renal impairment, although there is only anecdotal and uncontrolled evidence that they prevent or ameliorate the course of acute renal failure. For any effect to be obtained they must be given within 18 h of the ischaemic or toxic event, and at high doses or by continuous infusion because of the impaired diuretic delivery to the tubule.

Rapid administration of high-dose frusemide can cause abrupt hypotension from systemic venodilatation, and repeated dosing, particularly in combination with aminoglycosides, may cause ototoxicity. Single boluses should be limited to no more than 250 mg intravenously, with a daily limit of < 1 g per day. As discussed above, the use of continuous frusemide infusion or combined therapy with thiazide diuretics is a safer and more effective alternative.

LOW-DOSE DOPAMINE

The successful use of low-dose dopamine as a replacement or adjunct to high-dose frusemide therapy in resistant oliguria has been reported frequently, but almost all studies have been uncontrolled. Low-dose dopamine can increase urine flow, but to be effective must be started within 17 h of the onset of low urine output. Although the relative roles of dopaminergic and inotropic stimulation in this response remain unclear, a true dopaminergic effect is suggested by a study on surgical intensive cave unit patients who had remained oliguric despite fluid resuscitation to stable haemodynamics.[25] Low-dose dopamine increased mean urine output from 0.29 to 1.04 ml kg^{-1} h^{-1} without a change in haemodynamics; urine flow decreased when dopamine was stopped and increased when it was restarted.

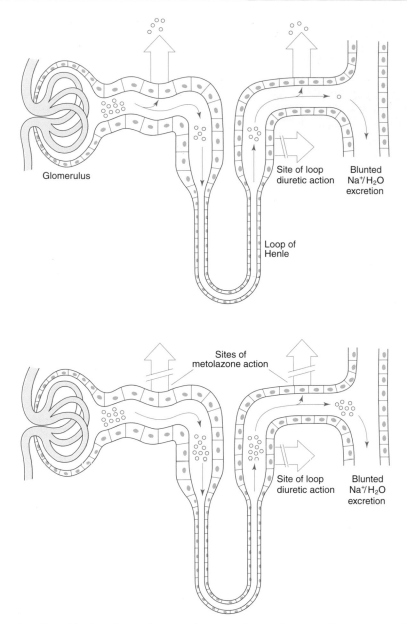

Fig. 20.7 Segmental nephron block with metolazone. The upper figure illustrates the exaggerated sodium reabsorption that occurs at the proximal and distal tubules in diuretic-resistant states. This blunts the responsiveness to loop diuretics at the medullary thick ascending loop of Henle. The lower figure illustrates the application of segmental nephron block by the addition of metolazone, which blocks sodium reabsorption at the proximal and distal tubule, to a loop diuretic, which blocks sodium reabsorption at the ascending loop of Henle. From Sica DA, Gehr TW. Diuretic combinations in refractory oedema states: pharmacokinetic–pharmacodynamic relationships. *Clin Pharmacokinet* 1996; **30**: 231, Fig. 1.

ATRIAL NATRIURETIC PEPTIDE

Of all the diuretic agents, ANP has been studied most carefully and has shown the most encouraging results in the reversal of functional impairment in ischaemic and nephrotoxic acute renal failure. In animal models of ischaemic acute renal failure, postinjury infusion of ANP or its analogues with or without dopamine consistently improves RBF and GFR, induces natriuresis, and limits the extent of histological injury and subsequent azotaemia. This has been confirmed in a number of clinical studies involving patients with acute renal failure of differing aetiologies, in whom the use of either ANP or one of its analogues, urodilatin or anaritide, resulted in improvement of renal function and avoided the need for haemodialysis in a significant number of patients. However, the initial promise shown by ANP in reversing the effects of ischaemic and/or nephrotoxic injury to the kidney after the insult appears to be confined to oliguric acute tubular necrosis. In a large placebo-controlled study involving 504 critically ill patients with acute tubular necrosis, anaritide improved the dialysis-free survival rate from 8% to 27% in patients who were oliguric (urine flow < 400 ml daily), but dialysis-free survival worsened in patients without oliguria. The authors postulated that this disparity may be due to a fundamental difference in the underlying pathology of oliguric and nonoliguric acute tubular necrosis, with the latter having a much more benign outcome.

REFERENCES

1. Casthely PA, Yoganathan T, Komer C, Kelly M. Magnesium and arrhythmias after coronary artery bypass surgery. *J Cardiothorac Vasc Anesth* 1994; **8**: 188–191.
2. Rybak LP. Ototoxicity of loop diuretics. *Otolaryngol Clin North Am* 1993; **26**: 829–844.
3. Sica DA, Gehr TW. Diuretic combinations in refractory oedema states: pharmacokinetic–pharmacodynamic relationships. *Clin Pharmacokinet* 1996; **30**: 229–249.
4. Pass L, Eberhart R, Brown J et al. The effect of mannitol and dopamine on the renal response to thoracic aortic cross-clamping. *J Thor Cardiovasc Surg* 1988; **95**: 608–612.
5. Ip-Yam PC, Murphy S, Baines M et al. Renal function and proteinuria after cardiopulmonary bypass: the effects of temperature and mannitol. *Anesth Analg* 1994; **78**: 842–847.
6. Hilberman M, Maseda J, Stinson E et al. The diuretic properties of dopamine in patients after open-heart operation. *Anesthesiology* 1984; **61**: 489–494.
7. Duke GJ, Briedes JH, Weaver RA. Renal support in critically ill patients: low-dose dopamine or low-dose dobutamine? *Crit Care Med* 1994; **22**: 1919–1925.
8. Ghosh S, Gray B, Oduro A, Latimer R. Dopexamine hydrochloride: pharmacology and use in low cardiac output states. *J Cardiothorac Vasc Anesth* 1991; **5**: 382–389.
9. Murphy MB, McCoy CE, Weber RR et al. Augmentation of renal blood flow and sodium excretion in hypertensive patients during blood pressure reduction by intravenous administration of the dopamine-1 agonist fenoldopam. *Circulation* 1987; **76**: 1312–1318.
10. Bryan AG, Bolsin SN, Vianna PTG, Haloush H. Modification of the diuretic and natriuretic effects of a dopamine infusion by fluid loading in preoperative cardiac surgical patients. *J Cardiothorac Vasc Anesth* 1995; **9**: 158–163.
11. Salem MG, Crooke JW, McLoughlin GA et al. The effect of dopamine on renal function during aortic cross-clamping. *Ann R Coll Surg Engl* 1988; **70**: 9–12.
12. Baldwin L, Henderson A, Hickman P. Effect of postoperative low-dose dopamine on renal function after elective major vascular surgery. *Ann Intern Med* 1994; **120**: 744–747.
13. Myles PS, Buckland MR, Schenk NJ et al. Effect of 'renal-dose' dopamine on renal function following cardiac surgery. *Anaesth Intensive Care* 1993; **21**: 56–61.
14. Costa P, Ottino GM, Matani A et al. Low-dose dopamine during cardiopulmonary bypass in patients with renal dysfunction. *J Cardiothorac Anesth* 1990; **4**: 469–473.
15. Lherm T, Troche G, Rossignol M. Renal effects of low-dose dopamine in patients with sepsis syndrome or septic shock treated with catecholamines. *Intensive Care Med* 1996; **22**: 213–219.
16. Parks RW, Diamond T, McCrory DC et al. Prospective study of postoperative renal function in obstructive jaundice and the effect of perioperative dopamine. *Br J Surg* 1994; **81**: 437–439.
17. Memoli B, Libetta C, Conte G, Andreucci VE. Loop diuretics and renal vasodilators in acute renal failure. *Nephrol Dial Transplant* 1994; **4**: 168–171.
18. Segal JM, Phang T, Walley KR. Low-dose dopamine hastens onset of gut ischemia in a porcine model of hemorrhagic shock. *J Appl Physiol* 1992; **73**: 1159–1164.
19. de Bold AJ, Borenstein HB, Veress AT, Sonnenberg H. A rapid and potent natriuretic response to intravenous injection of atrial myocardial extract in rats. *Life Sci* 1981; **28**: 89–94.
20. Shannon RP, Libby E, Elahi D et al. Impact of acute reduction in chronically elevated left atrial pressure on sodium and water excretion. *Ann Thorac Surg* 1988; **46**: 430–437.
21. Windus DW, Stokes TJ, Morgan JR, Klahr S. The effects of atrial peptide in humans with chronic renal failure. *Am J Kidney Dis* 1989; **13**: 477–484.
22. Fried T, Aronoff GR, Benabe JE et al. Renal and hemodynamic effects of atrial natriuretic peptide in patients with cirrhosis. *Am J Med Sci* 1990; **299**: 2–9.
23. Brater DC. Diuretic resistance: mechanisms and therapeutic strategies. *Cardiology* 1994; **84** (Suppl. 2): 57–67.
24. Rudy DW, Voelker JR, Greene PK et al. Loop diuretics for chronic renal insufficiency: a continuous infusion is more efficacious than bolus therapy. *Ann Intern Med* 1991; **115**: 360–366.
25. Flancbaum L, Choban PS, Dasta JF. Quantitative effects of low-dose dopamine on urine output in oliguric surgical intensive care unit patients. *Crit Care Med* 1994; **22**: 61–68.
26. Cedidi C, Kusz ER, Meyer M et al. Treatment of acute postoperative renal failure after liver and heart transplantation by urodilatin. *Clin Invest* 1993; **71**: 435–436.
27. Allgren RL, Marbury TC, Rahman SN et al. Anaritide in acute tubular necrosis. *N Engl J Med* 1997; **336**: 828–834.

21 MA Gerhardt, MB Howie

ENDOCRINE SYSTEMS AND METABOLIC DISORDERS

DIABETES MELLITUS

Diabetes mellitus is the most common endocrine disease, affecting 2% of the general population. The prevalence is greater in the surgical population. Although the pathognomonic feature of diabetes mellitus is an increased blood glucose concentration (> 6.6 mmol l^{-1} (120 mg dl^{-1}): 1 mmol l^{-1} = 18.2 mg dl^{-1}), the systemic nature of the disease can have a great impact on anaesthetic and perioperative management.[1]

Presenting symptoms of diabetes mellitus are typically polyuria and polydipsia secondary to hyperglycaemia. The capacity of the proximal renal tubules to reabsorb glucose is approximately 10 mmol l^{-1}, and when exceeded results in glycosuria and an osmotic diuresis. As with any diuresis, electrolyte disturbances are common (hypokalaemia and hypomagnesaemia), and can present perioperatively when poor glycaemic control results in hypovolaemia, electrolyte abnormalities and a metabolic acidosis. Blood analysis of glycosylated haemoglobin (haemoglobin A_{1c}; $HgbA_{1c}$) can document the stability of glucose control. $HgbA_{1c}$ is a nonenzymatically produced haemoglobin. Frequent hyperglycaemia promotes glycosylation and is reflected by a markedly raised level of $HgbA_{1c}$. As an integral component of red blood cells, $HgbA_{1c}$ provides insight into blood glucose control over the prior three months (life span of red blood cells is $\sim$ 120 days).

Type 1 diabetes mellitus (insulin-deficient diabetes; juvenile-onset diabetes) is an autoimmune disease resulting from destruction of the insulin-producing β-islet cells of the pancreas.[2] Patients with type 1 diabetes are unable to produce insulin and are thus dependent on exogenously administered insulin for blood glucose control and survival. Type 1 diabetes is associated with a thin body habitus and additional endocrine abnormalities, e.g. thyroid disorders. When control of blood glucose is lost, patients develop diabetic ketoacidosis.

Type 2 diabetes mellitus (insulin-resistant diabetes; adult-onset diabetes mellitus) results from either impaired insulin production and/or insulin receptor desensitization.[3] Type 2 diabetics are usually obese. Dietary control, weight loss and oral hypoglycaemic agents may control blood glucose levels without insulin therapy. Failure of conservative treatment requires institution of insulin therapy to avoid diabetes mellitus complications. Type 2 diabetes mellitus predisposes patients to nonketotic hyperosmolar coma rather than ketoacidosis.

Hyperglycaemia may occur as a consequence of another condition, and is termed secondary diabetes mellitus. Secondary diabetes mellitus may be reversible with resolution of the underlying process. Pregnancy, pancreatic disease and surgery, glucocorticoid excess (Crushing's syndrome or pharmacological therapy), pheochromocytoma and acromegaly are some of the causes of secondary diabetes mellitus. Gestational diabetes mellitus increases the risk of morbidity and mortality of both mother and fetus.[4] Polyhydramnios and a large-for-gestational age fetus complicate delivery. Postpartum, the infant may develop severe hypoglycaemia and requires close monitoring.

MOLECULAR PHARMACOLOGY AND PHYSIOLOGY

The protein structure of insulin was determined in 1953 by Frederick Sanger at the University of Toronto, for which he earned the Nobel prize. Insulin is a 51–amino–acid polypeptide consisting of an α and a β chain linked by two disulphide bonds. It is stored in the β-islet cells of the pancreas as a precursor molecule, proinsulin. When secreted from the pancreas, proinsulin is cleaved enzymatically to insulin and C peptide. Insulin exerts its effects via interaction with the insulin receptor, found on cellular membranes.[5] Binding of insulin to the receptor promotes cellular uptake and phosphorylation of glucose. In the liver, glycogen synthesis and inhibition of protein catabolism is promoted. The brain, heart and kidney rely on insulin to preserve cellular energy and oxidative metabolism. Insulin is both metabolized by hepatic mechanisms and excreted by the kidney.

A variety of hormones modulate insulin secretion, including those produced by the sympathetic nervous system. Rudimentary control occurs through blood glucose concentrations. When blood glucose rises, insulin secretion is increased to bring levels back to normal. When blood glucose levels fall, glucagon secretion increases with opposing effects; insulin secretion declines and blood glucose levels rise secondary to hepatic glycogenolysis. Augmentation of insulin secretion occurs with β-adrenergic receptor stimulation. Parasympathetic activation also results in increased insulin secretion. However, a_2-adrenergic receptor activation results in inhibition of insulin release.

In addition to glucose homeostasis, insulin exerts physiological effects on adipose, liver and muscle tissue. Activation of lipoprotein lipase and intracellular lipase increases fatty acid deposition in adipose tissue. Insulin inhibits hepatic glycogenolysis and catabolism of amino acids while promoting glycogen synthesis. Anabolic effects occur in muscle tissue, where amino acids are actively transported into cells and incorporated into proteins. Small glycogen stores in muscle are also replenished by insulin.

COMPLICATIONS OF DIABETES

When blood glucose is poorly controlled the diabetic patient is prone to develop both acute and chronic complications. Peripheral vascular disease is a serious cause of diabetes mellitus morbidity, contributing to dysfunction of the cardiac, vascular, renal and neural systems in addition to poor circulation leading to infectious disease (especially of the lower extremities). Microvascular disease afflicts virtually every organ system. Poor circulation predisposes the diabetic patient to ulceration and infection of the foot and lower extremities ('diabetic foot ulcers'). Diabetic retinopathy secondary to microvascular disease leads to blindness. Following surgery, microvascular disease is responsible for poor wound healing. Involvement of large and medium-sized arterial conduits leads to cerebrovascular disease, coronary artery disease and disease of the aorta and its major branches.

Diabetes mellitus predisposes patients to peripheral neuropathies and autonomic nervous system dysfunction. Classic diabetic neuropathy is a symmetric, bilateral loss of sensation with or without neuropathic pain/paraesthesias in the distal extremities, the so-called glove-stocking neuropathy. Autonomic dysfunction has several consequences.[6] Diabetic patients frequently have hypertension, yet are prone to orthostatic hypotension despite adequate intravascular volume. Not only does cerebrovascular disease result in increased risk of stroke, but hyperglycaemia (>11 mmol l^{-1}) during cerebral ischaemia results in a more severe neurological deficit. Autonomic neuropathy predisposes patients to gastroparesis, with delayed emptying of gastric contents, and an increased risk of aspiration during induction of anaesthesia.

Cardiac disease is common in patients with diabetes mellitus. Autonomic neuropathy results in asymptomatic angina and painless (silent) myocardial infarction, and classic signs and symptoms of coronary artery disease are absent or not reliable. Obligate loss of potassium and magnesium due to osmotic diuresis increases the risk of cardiac dysrhythmias.

Renal dysfunction and urological infectious disease are associated with diabetes mellitus, and renal failure is a serious complication of advanced diabetes and may necessitate haemodialysis or organ transplantation. Atherosclerosis of renal arterioles contributes to the development of hypertension and renal ischaemia. Hypertension accelerates renal failure.

Acute complications of diabetes mellitus, ketoacidosis, nonketotic hyperosmolar coma and hypoglycaemia, are life threatening and demand immediate attention. All three produce mental status changes which may range from confusion to unconsciousness. Frequent monitoring of blood glucose during anaesthesia is required since assessment of mental status is not available. Furthermore, sudden loss of glycaemic control is commonly associated with a physiological stress and requires investigation, particularly in the preoperative and late postoperative periods.

Diabetic ketoacidosis occurs in type 1 diabetes mellitus when insulin therapy is inadequate. Elevations of blood glucose in diabetic ketoacidosis are typically into the 25–50 mmol l^{-1} range. Insulin deficiency

Table 21.1 Insulin preparations and pharmacokinetics				
Preparation	Onset (h)	Peak (h)	Duration (h)	Human preparation
Fast				
Soluble	0.5–1	2–4	4–8	Yes
Semilente	2	6	14–16	No
Intermediate				
Isophane	2–4	4–12	12–24	Yes
Lente	2–4	6–12	18–24	Yes
Long				
Protamine zinc	6–8	12–18	24–36	No
Ultralente	4–8	10–20	24–36	No

results in increased utilization of free fatty acids by the liver, where they are preferentially converted to aceto-acetate and β-hydroxybutyrate. These are responsible for the ketosis and anion gap acidosis. Lactic acidosis may be superimposed from inadequate tissue perfusion. Initial serum potassium measurements may be normal due to acidosis despite significant depletion of total body stores due to urinary potassium loss. Concomitant hypomagnesaemia and hypophosphataemia also require correction. Patients with type 2 diabetes mellitus are prone to develop nonketotic hyperosmolar coma when glycaemic control is lost. Unlike diabetic ketoacidosis, acidosis and the production of ketones is usually absent.

Hypoglycaemia is a life-threatening acute complication that demands immediate intervention. Heightened sympathetic outflow can produce signs and symptoms of both anxiety and hypoglycaemia. An anxious diabetic patient should never be sedated preoperatively prior to ruling out hypoglycaemia. Postoperatively, hypoglycaemia is one of three immediately life-threatening causes of delayed emergence from anaesthesia (along with hypoxia and hypotension). Hypoglycaemia results in catecholamine secretion; β-adrenergic receptor antagonist therapy may abolish the signs and symptoms of hypoglycaemia.

TREATMENT OF DIABETES MELLITUS

Insulin

Insulin preparations are of bovine, porcine or human origin. Bovine and porcine insulin differ from human insulin by three and one amino acid residues, respectively. Human insulin, produced by recombinant DNA technology, is used by most patients. Insulin potency is determined by bioassay against an international standard and expressed as units of activity per volume. The most common preparation has 100 units ml^{-1}. All insulin preparations require refrigeration for storage. Prior to use, the bottle should be gently rolled to insure even resuspension.

Insulin is available in short, intermediate and long-acting preparations (Table 21.1). Soluble (regular) human insulin is a rapidly acting solution that can be administered by subcutaneous or intravenous routes. When given subcutaneously, onset of action occurs in 20–30 minutes with a peak at 2–3 h and 4–6-h duration. When given intravenously the onset is within a few minutes and the duration is approximately 30 min; therefore a continuous infusion is frequently utilized to provide appropriate therapy. Soluble insulin is usually mixed in normal saline as a 1 unit ml^{-1} solution. Insulin has variable absorption to glass and plastic intravenous lines. Priming the tubing may help eliminate initial delivery variance.[7]

When soluble insulin is injected subcutaneously absorption is slow because it must dissociate into monomers in the tissue before absorption. This often results in hyperglycaemia occurring 1–3 h after a meal due to inadequate insulin levels, and possibly excessive insulin levels a few hours later with the risk of hypoglycaemia. Recombinant DNA technology has allowed the development of insulin analogues that are monomeric and are therefore rapidly absorbed. When injected at mealtimes they result in earlier bioavailability of insulin and thus more effective control of blood glucose. Currently one of these analogues (Lys(B28), Pro(B29), referred to as Lispro insulin)) is available for clinical use.[8]

The intermediate- and long-acting forms are depot preparations that make use of protamine or zinc to prolong their action. Isophane insulin (NPH: *N*eutral solution, *P*rotamine, *H*agedorn's laboratory insulin) is an intermediate-acting preparation prepared with protamine. Patients using these preparations who

---

Summary box 21.1 Diabetes mellitus

- Two types:

  - Type 1: insulin-deficient diabetes. An autoimmune disease with destruction of the insulin producing β-islet cells of the pancreas. Patients are dependent on exogenously administered insulin.

  - Type 2: insulin-resistant diabetes. Due to impaired insulin production and/or insulin receptor desensitization.

- Drug treatment:

  - Insulin – nowadays usually human. Available in short, intermediate and long-acting preparations

  - Oral hypoglycaemic drugs:

    - Sulphonylureas, e.g. tolbutamide. Act mainly by stimulating insulin release from β-islet cells

    - Biguanides, e.g. metformin. No action on insulin production or release, lower blood glucose by decreased hepatic glucose output, increased peripheral glucose utilization. Have little potential for hypoglycaemia

    - Thiazolidinediones (troglitazone). Decrease insulin resistance without directly stimulating insulin secretion

    - α-Glucosidase inhibitors (acarbose). Inhibit uptake of carbohydrates from intestine.

present for cardiac surgery are at increased risk for reaction to protamine. Ultralente insulin is a long-acting preparation formed with zinc rather than protamine. Zinc retards the release of insulin and these preparations have a duration of 12–24 h. Protamine zinc insulin, which contains both protamine and zinc, has a duration of 24–40 h. Within the last decade, many patients have been converted to 70/30 insulin for added therapeutic convenience and simplification. This is a mixture containing 70% isophane insulin and 30% soluble insulin. It is important to note that all intermediate-and long-acting insulin preparations are suspensions, not solutions. Thus they cannot be given intravenously as drug microembolization would result.

Oral hypoglycaemic drugs

The main groups of oral hypoglycaemic drugs are the biguanides and sulphonylureas. Newer drugs include thiazolidinedione derivatives and α-glucosidase inhibitors. The oral hypoglycaemic drugs are only effective in patients with some endogenous insulin secretion, i.e. type 2 diabetes mellitus.

Sulphonylureas

These drugs, which are structurally related to sulphona-mides, act mainly by stimulating insulin release from β-islet cells of the pancreas by inhibiting ATP-sensitive potassium channels. The decrease in K^+ flux partially depolarizes the β-cell membrane, leading to an increased influx of Ca^{2+} through voltage-sensitive calcium channels and release of insulin (Fig. 21.1). Insulin sensitivity is also increased, possibly due to upregulation of insulin receptors. They enhance the effect of insulin to stimulate glucose uptake into muscle and fat cells.

The first-generation sulphonylureas were tolbuta-mide, chlorpropamide, tolazamide and acetohexamide. Second- and third-generation drugs include gliben-clamide, glipizide, gliclazide and glyburide. The second-generation agents are 10–100 times more potent than the first-generation drugs, but their maximum hypogly-caemic effects are similar. The sulphonylureas are rapidly and completely absorbed after oral administration, with peak effects within 2–4 h. They are pre-dominantly (90–95%) metabolized by the liver to inactive or only weakly active metabolites that are excreted in the urine. Chlorpropamide has an active metabolite. All are highly protein bound (> 90%), mainly to albumin. For the first-generation drugs this binding is ionic and thus they can be readily displaced from protein binding sites by other binding drugs such as NSAIDs, coumarins and some uricosuric drugs, e.g. sulphinpyrazone. This interaction can result in severe hypoglycaemia. Because the protein binding of the second-generation drugs is nonionic they are less read-ily displaced. Hypoglycaemia can also occur when

sulphonylureas are given with hepatic enzyme inhibi-tors such as monoamine oxidase inhibitors, some anti-biotics (including sulphonamides, trimethoprim and macrolides) and azole antifungal drugs.

Tolbutamide is a short-acting drug, with a half-life of 5 h, and is given in divided daily doses. It is the least likely of the sulphonylureas to cause hypoglycaemia. Chlorpropamide has a long duration of action, with a half-life of 35 h, so that a single morning oral dose is suf-ficient. It is much more likely to cause hypoglycaemia than tolbutamide, and hypoglycaemia can be prolonged. For this reason it should be avoided in the elderly and in patients with impaired renal function.

The sulphonylureas are generally well tolerated. The most common side-effect is hypoglycaemia, due either to overdosage, increased insulin sensitivity, or change in diet or energy expenditure. Mild hypoglycaemia can usually be managed by adjusting the dose, but severe cases can persist for several days, especially with the longer acting drugs. Allergic skin rashes, and rarely blood dyscrasias and transient leucopaenia, have been reported. The latter may be related to the sulphonamide structure. Chlorpropamide causes flushing when taken with alcohol. This is due to inhibition of aldehyde dehydrogenase leading to high concentrations of acetaldehyde (a disulfiram-like action). Chlorpropamide can cause fluid retention due to stimulation of ADH release. The sulphonylureas are contraindicated in preg-nancy since they cross the placenta and stimulate release of insulin in the fetus.

Biguanides

The only drug currently available in this class is metformin. Metformin has no action on insulin release and is effective in patients with nonfunctioning β-islet cells. It stimulates the tyrosine kinase activity of the

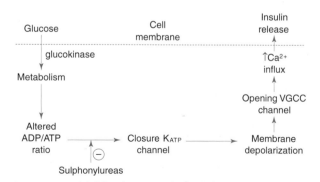

Fig. 21.1 A model for the control of insulin secretion by glucose in the pancreatic β-cell. Following transport of glucose into the cell there is a change in the ADP/ATP ratio which leads to closure of a K_{ATP} channel and membrane depolarization. Depolarization opens voltage-gated calcium channels (VGCC) and the resulting influx of Ca^{2+} causes exocytosis of insulin.

intracellular portion of the β-subunit of human insulin.[9] The blood glucose-lowering effect of metformin is the net result of decreased hepatic glucose output, increased peripheral glucose utilization, decreased fatty acid oxidation and increased splanchic glucose turnover.[10] As it does not increase insulin production it has little potential for hypoglycaemia. Metformin suppresses appetite, an additional benefit in the obese diabetic. It raises high density lipoprotein cholesterol and reduces triglycerides, thus improving the adverse plasma lipid profile common in diabetics. Metformin is well absorbed from the gastrointestinal tract and is excreted unchanged by the kidneys. The half-life is about 3 h. With chronic use metformin can interfere with the absorption of vitamin B_{12}.

Accumulation of metformin can occur in patients with renal insufficiency, and interference with pyruvate metabolism can lead to severe lactic acidosis. This has a mortality rate of about 50%.[11] Buformin and phenformin, which have a risk factor for lactic acidosis 20 times greater than metformin, were removed from the market in the seventies. Lactic acidosis is more likely in situations associated with anaerobic metabolism, and metformin should not be given to patients with renal disease, liver disease or severe pulmonary or cardiac disease predisposing to hypoxia. It is recommended to switch patients taking metformin to another oral hypoglycaemic prior to cardiac or other major surgery.

Thiazolidinediones

Type 2 diabetes mellitus is characterized by both resistance to insulin and reduced insulin secretion in response to glucose. A major breakthrough in the therapy of this form of diabetes has been the development of a number of thiazolidinedione derivatives that decrease insulin resistance without directly stimulating insulin secretion.[12] Of these compounds, troglitazone has recently become available for clinical use and several others (ciglitazone, pioglitazone and englitazone) are undergoing clinical development. In addition to beneficial effects on glucose metabolism, they also have profound effects on circulating lipids. The exact mechanism by which these drugs improve insulin sensitivity is uncertain, but may involve regulation of gene expression mediated by the interactions of thiazolidinediones with a family of nuclear receptors known as the peroxisome proliferator-activated receptors (PPARs).

Troglitazone is given orally in a daily dose of 200–600 mg and may be combined with other diabetic therapy. It is well absorbed with peak plasma concentrations at 2–3 h. There is a very low incidence of side-effects. One to 2% of patients develops mild, reversible changes in aminotransferase activity. However, a small number of patients have developed more severe idiosyncratic hepatocellular injury.[13]

α-Glucosidase Inhibitors

Dietary carbohydrates must be digested into monosaccharides before they can be absorbed. This process involves α-glucosidases, enzymes located on the surface of the small intestinal microvilli. Acarbose, miglitol and voglibose are reversible inhibitors of α-glucosidases. Acarbose was the first of these drugs to be used in the management of patients with type 2 diabetes who are inadequately controlled by diet with or without other oral hypoglycaemic drugs. Acarbose competes with dietary oligosaccharides for α-glucosidases, and has a higher affinity for the enzymes. Because binding is reversible, digestion and absorption of complex carbohydrates after a meal is slower than usual but not prevented. There is, therefore, a reduced rise in blood glucose after a carbohydrate meal. Postprandial insulin levels are also reduced but fasting insulin is generally unchanged. Acarbose can also be used in insulin-dependent diabetic patients to improve glycaemic control. The delayed digestion and absorption of carbohydrates allows better synchronization of insulin pharmacokinetics with changes in glucose levels after a meal.

Less than 2% of the ingested acarbose is absorbed, so that systemic adverse effects are uncommon. The most common side-effects are flatulence, abdominal distension and diarrhoea due to fermentation of unabsorbed carbohydrates in the colon.

ANAESTHETIC MANAGEMENT OF THE DIABETIC PATIENT

There are two preoperative goals for the anaesthetist caring for the diabetic patient: avoidance of hypoglycaemia in the perioperative period and assessment of end-organ dysfunction resulting from diabetes mellitus. Noninsulin-dependent type 2 diabetics should forego oral hypoglycaemic therapy on the morning of surgery. Patients on insulin therapy should receive one-half of their usual morning dose of insulin, and the blood glucose concentration should be measured 1 h before surgery. Patients treated with insulin should be instructed to observe for hypoglycaemic symptoms (tremor, nervousness, tachycardia) and to drink clear fruit juice (i.e. apple or grape juice) should any suspicion of low blood sugar levels arise. Anxiety and hypoglycaemia produce similar signs and symptoms. Do not sedate an 'anxious' diabetic patient until hypoglycaemia has been ruled out. Patients with diabetes mellitus are at increased risk of aspiration due to gastroparesis. Preoperative treatment with metoclopramide and an H_2-histamine receptor antagonist may decrease aspiration risk.

During the operation blood glucose determinations should be made at least hourly, and should be

Table 21.2 Insulin sliding scale	
Blood glucose (mmol l^{-1})	Dose of soluble insulin
> 4.5 to < 11	No additional treatment
11–14	2 units
14–16.5	4 units
16.5–19	8 units
19–22	12 units
> 22	Initiate insulin infusion

maintained between 5 and 10 mmol l^{-1}. Hypoglycaemia should be treated by glucose (or dextrose) infusion. Severe hypoglycaemia (blood glucose $\leq$ 3.5 mmol l^{-1}) should be treated with an intravenous bolus of 50 ml of 50% glucose followed by a glucose infusion. If blood glucose concentrations exceed 15 mmol l^{-1}, insulin therapy is indicated. For brief procedures subcutaneous doses may be sufficient; an insulin sliding scale is presented in Table 21.2. In cases anticipated to last more than 2 h insulin infusion is indicated. The authors routinely give a small bolus dose (5–10 units) intravenously and commence an infusion (1–5 units h^{-1}). Serial glucose determinations are made every 30 minutes until stable glucose concentrations are achieved at < 12 mmol l^{-1}, whereupon hourly measurements may suffice. Additional bolus doses and adjustment of the infusion rate may be required, particularly when catecholamine infusions are required for inotropic support of the heart. Potassium and magnesium therapy is usually required.

PHAEOCHROMOCYTOMA

Phaeochromocytoma is a neuroendocrine-derived tumour which secretes the catecholamines noradrenaline and adrenaline. These are responsible for the signs and symptoms of phaeochromocytoma. A phaeochromocytoma is usually found on the adrenal medulla, although bilateral adrenal medulla (about 10%) or extramedullary sites are possible. It is frequently associated with other endocrine abnormalities. Phaeochromocytoma is a secondary cause of hypertension, with tumour excision resulting in a cure. Intraoperative activation of an undiagnosed phaeochromocytoma is a medical emergency, with a mortality rate approaching 50%. Parturition can also precipitate exacerbation of catecholamine secretion. Extreme hypertension (e.g. 300/150 mmHg) and tachycardia appear acutely, and require immediate treatment and cessation of the surgical procedure.

Blockade of a_1-adrenergic response is the primary therapeutic goal in the management of phaeochromocytoma. A variety of a_1-adrenoceptor antagonists have been used (Table 21.3). Phenoxybenzamine, phentolamine and labetalol are the most commonly used. Unlike virtually all other clinically useful antagonists, phenoxybenzamine binding to the a_1-adrenoceptor is

Table 21.3 a_1-Adrenergic receptor antagonists			
Antagonist	Specificity	Dose	Route
Phenoxybenzamine	a_1	0.5–1.0 mg kg^{-1}	po
Phentolamine	$a_1 = a_2$	0.5–1.0 mg 50 μg kg^{-1} (–titrate)	iv CI
Labetalol	a_1; $\beta_1 = \beta_2$	5–50 mg 0.5 mg min^{-1} (–titrate) 15–300 mg BID	iv CI po
Prazosin	a_1	2–20 mg per day	po
Terazosin	a_1	1–5 mg QID	po

Specificity refers to adrenergic receptor subtype. Abbreviations for routes of administration; po, oral; iv, intravenous bolus; CI, continuous infusion intravenously; BID, twice daily; QID, 4 times daily. Titrate, starting dose is given and must be adjusted to desired response. Note, for labetalol, loading dose to effect must be given intravenously immediately before CI.

not competitive. Rather, it covalently attaches to the receptor and effectively eliminates that receptor from any further response. Labetalol also possesses unique pharmacological properties, antagonizing both a_1- and β-(β_1 and β_2)adrenergic receptors.

ANAESTHETIC MANAGEMENT

Two primary goals must be satisfied prior to surgery, haemodynamic stability and restoration of intravascular fluid volume. This usually requires 1–2 weeks to achieve. Phenoxybenzamine therapy is utilized to prevent hypertensive episodes. Development of orthostatic hypotension and nasal congestion suggests adequate a_1-adrenoceptor blockade. The patient should be free of cardiac arrhythmias and electrocardiographic changes. Labetalol is a good choice to manage tachycardia. If a β-adrenoceptor antagonist is administered prior to sufficient a_1-adrenergic receptor blockade, a hypertensive episode may be precipitated. This is thought to occur when peripheral vascular β_2-adrenergic receptors (vasodilatory) are blocked leaving unopposed vasoconstriction via a_1 receptors. Phenoxybenzamine therapy is continued up to the day of surgery.

Intraoperative management

Prior to tumour removal, the chief concern is a hypertensive crisis, and management should be tailored to decrease the likelihood of catecholamine secretion, either from the tumour or due to anxiety. Following ligation and tumour excision hypotension is the primary problem. Aggressive volume administration will be required to maintain haemodynamic stability.

Preoperative sedation is required to decrease anxiety. Benzodiazepines provide excellent anxiolysis. Theoretically, the a_2-adrenergic agonist clonidine may have particular benefit. In addition to anxiolysis and sedation, clonidine decreases sympathetic outflow. Glucocorticoid therapy may be required if bilateral adrenalectomy is anticipated. Hyperglycaemia is common in the preoperative period, and may require treatment.

Most intravenous induction agents have been used safely, but ketamine is contraindicated. Rapid, aggressive treatment of hypotension or hypertension is indicated as this promotes catecholamine secretion. Phenylephrine is the drug of choice to treat hypotension, although higher than usual doses may be required due to preoperative a_1-adrenergic receptor blockade. Ephedrine promotes catecholamine release, which may result in uncontrolled hypertension and is best avoided. Prior to tumour excision, therapy to decrease blood pressure may be required. However, agents with a long duration of action may complicate management following tumour removal when hypotension prevails. Nitroprusside is commonly used in this situation. Phentolamine, labetalol, and calcium channel blockers have also been

used. Tachycardia is problematic as administration of β-adrenergic receptor antagonists (e.g. esmolol, metoprolol) may result in hypertension from unopposed a_1-adrenergic receptor blockade.[14] Rapid volume administration is required after tumour removal. Occasionally, a phenylephrine or noradrenaline infusion may be required to support blood pressure.

ADRENAL CORTEX

The adrenal cortex synthesizes many steroid hormones derived from cholesterol, of which the most important are the corticosteroids (glucocorticoids and mineralocorticoids). Synthesis of corticosteroids (glucocorticoids and mineralocorticoids) occurs in the adrenal cortex under the influence of the anterior pituitary adrenocorticotrophic hormone (ACTH). The primary glucocorticoid is cortisol (hydrocortisone) whereas aldosterone is the primary mineralocorticoid. Release of cortisol is controlled by a negative-feedback mechanism involving the hypothalamus and the anterior pituitary. Low blood cortisol levels result in the release of ACTH, which stimulates cortisol synthesis and release by activating adenylyl cyclase. This increases cyclic AMP activity, which acting via protein kinase A increases the activity of cholesterylester hydrolase. This enzyme, which converts cholesterol to pregnenolone (Fig. 21.2), is the rate-limiting step in steroid synthesis. This conversion also involves the cytochrome P450 enzymes. Inhibitors of cytochrome P450 such as ketoconazole and aminoglutethimide are used to suppress excessive steroid production in Cushing's syndrome when surgical removal of the hormone-secreting tumour is not successful.

MOLECULAR PHARMACOLOGY

Glucocorticoid receptors (GR) are cytoplasmic metalloproteins which regulate gene expression.[15] Corticosteroids are transported into the intracellular matrix, where they bind with the GR. The hormone-receptor complex then interacts with additional intracellular proteins known as heat shock proteins prior to binding to the DNA.[16] Heat shock proteins facilitate the biochemical response. The GR is then transported into the nucleus where specific regions of DNA, known as glucocorticoid response elements, provide recognition and binding sites for the activated GR. Corticosteroid-responsive genes are then activated, resulting in synthesis of new proteins. These are responsible for the physiological effects.

The glucocorticoids have profound effects on carbohydrate and protein metabolism, as well as influencing immune and inflammatory responses. The name glucocorticoids derives from their role in glucose metabolism. They mobilize glucose from stores and increase

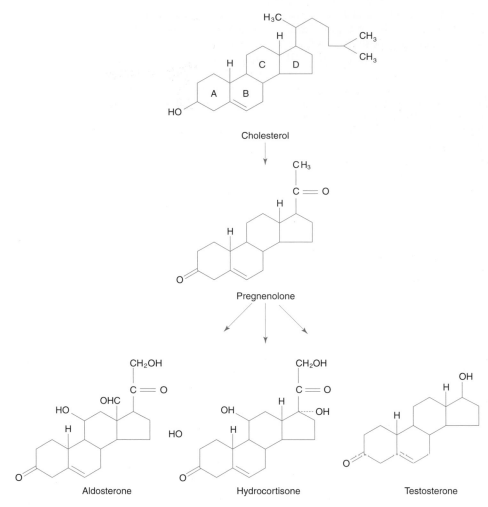

Fig. 21.2 Formation of adrenal steroids from cholesterol.

Summary box 21.2 Glucocorticosteroids

- Cortisol synthesized from cholesterol in the adrenal cortex under a negative-feedback control by ACTH.

- The glucocorticoids have profound effects on carbohydrate and protein metabolism, as well as influencing immune and inflammatory responses.

- Endogenous and synthetic glucocorticosteroids are used in the management of diseases with an inflammatory or autoimmune component, to prevent rejection after organ transplantation, and for patients with adrenal insufficiency.

- Chronic use associated with several adverse effects. Also results in suppression of endogenous cortisol production.

glyconeogenesis and glucose secretion by the liver. Glucose uptake and utilization in the peripheral tissues is suppressed. Lipolysis is increased. Glucocorticoids inhibit protein synthesis and stimulate the catabolism of proteins, particularly in the muscles, to amino acids. The amino acids are then available for conversion to glucose. Calcium absorption from the gastrointestinal tract is decreased and its excretion by the kidneys is increased. This can result in osteoporosis. The glucocorticoids have profound antiinflammatory effects. The accumulation of neutrophils and monocytes at the site of inflammation is suppressed and their phagocytic and antigen-processing activity is inhibited. While useful in treating inflammatory diseases these actions compromise the immune system and predispose patients to an increased risk of infection. The endogenous glucocorticosteroids all have some mineralocorticoid activity.

THERAPEUTIC USES OF GLUCOCORTICOSTEROIDS

Particularly synthetic glucocorticosteroids are used in the management of diseases with an inflammatory or autoimmune component, such as asthma and rheumatoid arthritis, and in the prevention of rejection after organ transplantation. A variety of endogenous and synthetic glucocorticosteroids are used therapeutically. A major goal in the development of synthetic drugs is to produce steroids without mineralocorticoid activity.

Hydrocortisone is available as either succinate or phosphate salts for oral and intravenous administration. It is the drug of choice when a rapid effect is required, e.g. acute adrenal insufficiency or as perioperative replacement therapy. Prednisolone can also be given intravenously. It has about 0.8 of the mineralocorticoid activity of hydrocortisone. Prednisone is a prodrug that is converted to prednisolone in the body. For chronic therapy synthetic steroids without mineralocorticoid activity are preferred, such as dexmethasone, betamethasone or triamcinalone.

Adverse effects

Long-term use of glucotricosteroids is associated with several adverse effects, especially when high doses are given for antiinflammatory activity. These effects are similar to the clinical manifestation of Cushing's syndrome (see below). Fluid retention and oedema result in the characteristic moon face. Disturbances of glucose metabolism leads to hyperglycaemia and occasionally diabetes.

ADRENAL INSUFFICIENCY

Adrenal insufficiency (Addison's disease) can result from hypopituitary or adrenal dysfunction; however the most common presentation for the anaesthetist is adrenal insufficiency secondary to glucocorticoid therapy. Chronic corticosteroid therapy results in negative feedback on the pituitary and adrenal glands. Both absolute and relative deficiency can result in adrenal crisis. Pharmacological doses of glucocorticoids result in adrenal suppression for weeks to months following steroid therapy. Failure to adequately replenish adrenal steroids results in cardiovascular collapse. Although a single dose of steroids does not place a patient at risk, any patient treated for more than 48 h requires supplementation.

Anaesthetic management consists of appropriate pharmacological therapy to avert adrenal crisis. Therapeutic replacement can be accomplished with any of the commonly available glucocorticoids. Typically the adrenal cortex produces about 20–30 mg of cortisol daily. Increased amounts are required to prevent an adrenal crisis when the stress of surgery and illness are superimposed. Many clinical regimens have been successfully employed. Administration of hydrocorti-

sone 100 mg intravenously 8 h prior to induction of anaesthesia, at induction and 8 h following surgery is adequate for most surgical procedures. The patient should resume their preoperative therapy on the first postoperative day. Although glucocorticoids may produce hyperglycaemia and impair wound healing, failure to replenish these hormones can be life-threatening. Thus, corticosteroids should always be administered when they are indicated.

ADRENAL HYPERFUNCTION (CUSHING'S SYNDROME)

Corticosteroid excess (Cushing's syndrome) can result from pituitary tumours, ectopic ACTH secretion from a peripheral malignancy, adrenal tumours or glucocorticoid therapy. Elevated ACTH results from pituitary or ectopic tumours. Lung cancer is the most frequent malignancy associated with ectopic ACTH production. A dexamethasone suppression test is used to diagnose a suspected Cushing's syndrome. Failure of a small dose of dexamethasone to reduce plasma cortisol levels confirms the diagnosis. Chronic Cushing's syndrome is a secondary cause of diabetes mellitus with its attendant complications. Hypokalaemia may predispose the patient to dysrhythmias. In patients in whom Cushing's syndrome develops from corticosteroid therapy, the adrenal function is completely suppressed. Despite their Cushinoid appearance, these patients require continued therapy with corticosteroids.

THYROID DYSFUNCTION

The thyroid hormones are responsible for regulating cellular metabolic activity and oxygen consumption. Thyroid hormone deficiency or excess results in disease, which may progress to a life-threatening disorder. Only emergency surgery should be performed in patients with uncontrolled thyroid dysfunction. Thyroid storm is a hypermetabolic state whose differential diagnosis includes malignant hyperthermia, neuroleptic malignant syndrome, phaeochromocytoma and awareness under anaesthesia.

The anterior pituitary gland secretes thyroid stimulating hormone (TSH). TSH promotes thyroid uptake of iodine and its incorporation into thyroxine (T_4; levothyroxine). T_4 is bound to thyroglobulin, a carrier protein. T_3 and T_4 are inactive when bound to thyroglobulin. In peripheral tissues, thyroglobulin releases T_4, which is converted to triiodothyronine (T_3). T_3 is more potent than T_4 and is responsible for the majority of thyroid hormone effects. Measurement of TSH and free T_4 are useful screening tests for the diagnosis of thyroid disorders (Table 21.4). Pregnancy results in a relative hyperthyroid state due to decreased thyroglobulin. Without

Table 21.4 Hormone abnormalities in thyroid dysfunction		
Disorder	TSH	Free T_4
Hyperthyroidism	↓	↑
Primary hypothyroidism	↑	↓
Secondary hypothyroidism	↓	↓
Pregnancy	Normal	↑

the normal levels of carrier protein, a greater fraction of T_4 is unbound and able to exert its effects.[17]

MOLECULAR PHARMACOLOGY

The thyroid receptor belongs to the steroid hormone superfamily.[18] The mechanism of action of T_3 and T_4 are similar to other members of this family, e.g. the glucocorticosteroid receptor. T_3 and T_4 are transported intracellularly and bind to the thyroid receptor in the cytoplasm. The hormone/receptor complex is transformed into the active state, crosses into the nucleus and binds to DNA recognition sites to regulate gene expression. Upregulation (increased number) of cardiac β-adrenergic receptors results from T_3-mediated gene activation.

HYPERTHYROIDISM

Hyperthyroidism has multiple causes, including diffuse toxic goitre (Grave's disease), pituitary tumours, pregnancy, excess iodine ingestion and excessive thyroid hormone therapy. Grave's disease is the most common cause of hyperthyroidism. It is an autoimmune disorder in which immunoglobulin activation of TSH receptors results in the hyperthyroid state. Thyroid hormone therapy (thyroxine) is an iatrogenic cause of hyperthyroidism, and should be considered when appropriate.

The changes in the cardiac system are the most relevant to anaesthetists.[19] Sinus tachycardia is common, with heart rates above 120 beats per min in severe cases. Atrial fibrillation and premature ventricular contractions are commonly associated arrhythmias. Hyperthyroidism, like anaemia, can result in high output cardiac failure where oxygen delivery is unable to meet tissue metabolic demands. A widened pulse pressure results from an increased systolic and decreased diastolic blood pressure. Patients are susceptible to dehydration from the hypermetabolic state.

The most serious complication of hyperthyroidism is thyroid storm (thyrotoxic crisis). This is an acute exacerbation of hyperthyroidism with marked tachycardia, fever, mental status changes and haemodynamic collapse. Triggers of thyroid storm include surgery, trauma, parturition and critical illness. Thyroid storm is frequently fatal; therefore proper preoperative preparation must proceed all elective operations.

Drugs used in hyperthyroidism

Traditionally young patients have been treated with drugs, surgery being reserved for failure of drug therapy or when there is mechanical compression of the trachea. Drugs can control the disease but do not cure it, since they do not affect the underlying mechanism, which is often autoimmune.

Thioureylenes

These are the most important of the antithyroid drugs. The main compounds are carbimazole, methimazole and propylthiouracil. They all contain a thiocarbamide group $(S=C-N)$ which is essential for their activity. They decrease the production of thyroid hormones by inhibiting the incorporation of iodine and coupling of iodotyrosines. Propylthiouracil also inhibits the removal of an iodine molecule from T_4 to form T_3. Carbimazole is a prodrug which is rapidly converted to the active compound methimazole. All these drugs are given orally. They may take 3–4 weeks to achieve an effect, partly because of the long half-life of thyroxine but also because the thyroid has large stores of preformed hormones, which must first be depleted. The main adverse effect is agranulocytosis, but this is rare (incidence < 1%) and reversible when the drug is stopped. The incidence is greater with propylthiouracil than carbimazole.

Iodine

Iodine alone is no longer used to treat thyrotoxicosis, because of its unreliable effect. It is, however, occasionally used in combination with one of the thioureylenes, particularly because of its fast onset of action, within 1 to 2 days. The exact mechanism of its action is poorly understood, but may include interference with the iodination of thyroglobulin. In high doses it reduces the vascularity of the hyperactive thyroid, and as such it is frequently used in the preparation of patients for thyroidectomy. Radioactive iodine, in the form of the isotope ^{131}I, is used to destroy hyperactive thyroid tissue. It is given orally as a single dose, and is taken up and processed by the thyroid in the same way as dietary iodide. Treatment with ^{131}I often results in hypothyroidism which requires replacement therapy with thyroxine. Tracer doses of ^{131}I are also used as a test of thyroid function.

PREOPERATIVE MANAGEMENT

Hyperthyroid patients should be rendered euthyroid prior to surgery with antithyroid drugs and/or radioactive iodine. A saturated solution of potassium iodide provides negative feedback on thyroid hormone synthesis and reduces vascularity. For patients with iodine allergy, lithium carbonate may be substituted. Radioactive iodine (^{131}I) will ablate the thyroid gland over several weeks. A single dose is often effective, and may reduce the need for thyroidectomy. Furthermore, radioactive thyroid results in decreased goitre size, making airway management easier. Thyroid hormone replacement is required after chemical or surgical thyroid gland ablation. β-Adrenergic receptor antagonists are useful adjuncts to control the cardiovascular effects of hyperthyroidism. Judicious sedation will depress the sympathetic response; however, anticholinergic agents should be avoided.

Intraoperative anaesthetic management
The primary goal is to avoid excess sympathetic stimulation. Drugs which may promote or mimic sympathetic responses are best avoided (i.e. ketamine, pancuronium, ephedrine). Some clinicians consider thiopentone the drug of choice for induction of anaesthesia in hyperthyroid patients since, due to its chemical structure, it may inhibit thyroid hormone release. Hyperthyroidism produces an apparent increase in minimum alveolar concentration (MAC). Although the MAC for inhalational anaesthetics is unchanged by hyperthyroidism, the increased cardiac output will result in greater volatile agent uptake from the lungs. Clinically, it appears as if the MAC has increased. Hyperthyroidism may increase susceptibility to cardiac arrrhythmias. Caution should be exercised if adrenaline is administered (e.g. with local anaesthetics), especially if halothane is used.

If a thyroid storm develops immediate therapy should be directed towards the cardiovascular system and hyperpyrexia. Propylthiouracil, (0.6–1 g) or methimazole (60–100 mg) should be administered orally or by nasogastric tube. Clinical effect should commence in approximately 1 h, at which time saturated potassium iodide solution (30 drops) should be administered. Intravenous sodium iodide (0.5–1 g every 8 h) can be substituted for potassium iodide. Propranolol and dexamethasone also inhibit peripheral conversion of T_4 to the more potent T_3 and should be administered. β-adrenergic receptor antagonists will decrease sinus tachycardia and the risk of additional arrhythmias. Dexamethasone will treat the relative adrenal insufficiency. Aggressive cooling and hydration should be instituted. Aspirin is contraindicated in the treatment of fever in thyroid storm since it displaces thyroid hormone from its protein binding sites.

HYPOTHYROIDISM
Hypothyroidism is a slowly developing condition. Anaesthetists may encounter mild hypothyroidism in patients with inadequate hormone replacement after thyroid ablation (surgical or radiation therapy). Replacement therapy is with oral thyroxine (25–150 μg daily). The most common primary cause is Hashimoto's thyroiditis, an autoimmune disease afflicting mainly women, with resultant fibrosis of the thyroid gland. Cretinism results from untreated congenital hypothyroidism. Iodine deficiency is an important cause in underdeveloped countries. Patients with hypothyroidism have a diminished response to hypercarbia, so that reduced doses of sedating drugs should be given along with vigilant monitoring.

Severe hypothyroidism manifests as nonpitting oedema (myxoedema) producing ascites, pleural and pericardial effusions and thick puffy features. Progression leads to mental status changes (lethargy, somnolence) and eventually myxoedema coma. A large tongue may make airway management difficult. A hoarse voice may indicate vocal cord oedema. Cardiac involvement results in bradycardia and decreased cardiac output. Adrenal cortex suppression exacerbates haemodynamic perturbations.

Recent clinical interest in the potential inotropic properties of T_3 has led to its use following cardiopulmonary bypass. Although T_3 may have a role in hypothyroid or critically ill cardiac surgical patients, routine use is not supported by currently available data.[20]

DIABETES INSIPIDUS

Antidiuretic hormone (ADH; vasopressin) is a posterior pituitary gland hormone which permits resorption of free water in the renal tubules to help maintain intravascular fluid volume. ADH secretion is increased in response to various stimuli (Table 21.5). The renal effects of ADH are mediated through V_2 receptors in the basolateral membrane of the cells of the distal tubules and collecting ducts. It increases the permeability of the membrane to water, allowing water conservation by producing a concentrated, hyperosmolar urine. The actions of ADH on smooth muscle, especially vascular smooth muscle, are mediated via V_1 receptors. These have a much lower affinity for ADH than the V_2 receptors, and effects such as vasoconstriction occur only

Table 21.5 Stimulus for increased ADH secretion

↓ Intravascular volume (↑ osmolarity)
Head trauma
Nausea
Pain
Positive airway pressure
Positive end-expiratory pressure (PEEP)
Surgery

at much higher doses than those producing a renal effect.

Diabetes insipidus is a condition resulting from a relative or absolute deficiency of ADH. Without ADH, the kidneys produce a high volume of dilute urine despite serum hyperosmolarity. Urinary output of 2 to 5 litres daily is common and can lead to hypovolaemia and hypernatraemia. Patients with adequate access to water avoid severe dehydration by marked increases in water intake. Patients to whom access to water is restricted, e.g. after surgery, are at risk of hypovolaemia. Anaesthetic management of patients with diabetes insipidus revolves around close monitoring of fluid status. In ambulatory patients, allowing unrestricted access to water may be sufficient.

Loss of posterior pituitary function can occur from trauma, hypophysectomy, postpartum haemorrhage (Sheehan's syndrome), tumour or sarcoidosis. The absence of pituitary ADH results in central diabetes insipidus. Nephrogenic diabetes insipidus is caused by failure of the renal ADH receptor to respond. Aetiologies of nephrogenic diabetes insipidus include renal disease (obstructive renal failure, chronic renal insufficiency), electrolyte abnormalities (hypokalaemia, hypercalcaemia), drugs (lithium, demeclocycline) and metabolic disorders (sickle cell anaemia, amyloidosis). Differentiation between central and nephrogenic causes is important as central diabetes insipidus may be treated with replacement therapy. Nephrogenic diabetes insipidus is difficult to treat, although thiazide diuretics may produce a paradoxical fall in urine output.

Desmopressin is a synthetic vasopressin analogue selective for the V_2 receptor with 12 times the antidiuretic potency of ADH but only 0.4% of its vasopressor activity. It can be administered subcutaneously, intravenously or intranasally to treat central diabetes insipidus. Administration is guided by urine output; repeat doses are typically required every 6–18 h. An unrelated action of desmopressin is to increase the release of factor VIII (von Willebrand factor) and is used as prophylactic therapy in patients with haemophilia or von Willebrand's disease. It is also used in dialysis-dependent patients to reduce bleeding after cardiac surgery. Chlorpropamide (an antidiabetic drug) and carbamazepine (an antiepileptic drug) potentiate the actions of ADH and are also used in the treatment of diabetes insipidus.

SYNDROME OF INAPPROPRIATE ANTIDIURETIC HORMONE SECRETION (SIADH)

This syndrome occurs when ADH release continues despite hypoosmolality.[21] Hyponatraemia is the main concern with SIADH. Exogenous ADH secretion can occur from malignant tumours, particularly lung small cell (oat) and pancreatic carcinoma. SIADH can develop in response to either a primary lung pathology (pneumonia, tuberculosis) or secondary to positive pressure ventilation. Stroke, head trauma, neurosurgery and infectious disease of the CNS are other causes of SIADH. A number of drugs may also give rise to SIADH (Table 21.6). The diagnosis of SIADH is made by sodium and osmolarity measurements of urine and plasma. Hyponatraemia and decreased plasma osmolarity with paradoxical urine concentration (osmolarity urine > plasma) and urinary sodium excretion (> 20 mmol l^{-1}) confirms the diagnosis.

The mainstay of medical treatment is fluid restriction. This may not be appropriate in the surgical and critical care patient population. Severe (< 120 mmol l^{-1}) or symptomatic hyponatraemia (mental status changes, seizure) requires more aggressive therapy to reduce cerebral oedema. Infusion of hypertonic saline to increase plasma sodium concentrations to 120–125 mmol l^{-1} alleviates symptoms. Slow correction ($\leq$ 2 mmol l^{-1} each hour) is indicated. Rapid correction of hyponatraemia increases the risk of permanent neurological sequelae. Adjunct therapy with demeclocycline (600 mg/daily) may assist management in resistant SIADH. Demeclocycline is a tetracycline antibiotic which inhibits the actions of ADH at the renal tubules.

Table 21.6 **Drugs associated with SIADH**
Carbamazepine
Chlorpropamide
Clofibrate
Opioids
Nicotine
Phenytoin
Thiazide diuretics
Vinca alkaloids (vinblastine, vincristine)

REFERENCES

1. Jorgensen B, Holm H. Anaesthetic implications of long term diabetic complications. *Acta Anaesthesiol Scand* 1995; **39**: 560–562.
2. Atkinson M, Maclaren N. The pathogenesis of insulin-dependent diabetes mellitus. *N Engl J Med* 1994; **331**: 1428–1436.
3. Polonsky K, Sturis J, Bell G. Non-insulin-dependent diabetes mellitus: a genetically programmed failure of the beta cell to compensate for insulin

resistance. *N Engl J Med* 1996; **334**: 777–783.

4. Kuhl C. Etiology and pathogenesis of gestational diabetes. *Diabetes Care* 1998; **21**: B19–B26.

5. White M. The IRS-signalling system: a network of docking proteins that mediate insulin and cytokine action. *Recent Prog Horm Res* 1998; **53**: 119–138.

6. Watkins P. The enigma of autonomic failure in diabetes. *J R Coll Physicians Lond* 1998; **32**: 360–365.

7. Fuloria M, Friedberg MA, DuRant RH, Aschner JL. Effect of flow rate and insulin priming on the recovery of insulin from microbore infusion tubing. *Pediatrics* 1998; **102**: 1401–1406.

8. Bolli GB. Rapid-acting insulin analogues. *Curr Opinion Endocrinology Diabetes* 1997; **4**: 277–281.

9. Stith BJ, Woronoff K, Wiernsperger N. Stimulation of the intracellular portion of the human insulin receptor by the antidiabetic drug metformin. *Biochem Pharmacol* 1998; **55**: 533–536.

10. Bailey CJ. Metformin and its role in the management of type II diabetes. *Curr Opinion Endocrinology Diabetes* 1997; **4**: 40–47.

11. Bailey CJ, Turner RC. Metformin. *N Engl J Med* 1996; **333**: 574–579.

12. Saltiel AR, Olefsky JM. Thiazolidinediones in the treatment of insulin resistance and type II diabetes. *Diabetes* 1996; **45**: 1661–1669.

13. Kelly DE, Killian D. Troglitazone. *Curr Opinion Endocrinology Diabetes* 1998; **5**: 90–96.

14. Sheaves R, Chew S, Grossman A. The dangers of unopposed beta-adrenergic blockade in pheochromocytoma. *Postgrad Med J* 1995; **71**: 58–59.

15. Funder J. Glucocorticoid and mineralocorticoid receptors: biology and clinical relevance. *Annu Rev Med* 1997; **48**: 231–240.

16. Pratt W. The role of heat shock proteins in regulating the function, folding, and trafficking of the glucocorticoid receptor. *J Biol Chem* 1993; **268**: 21455–21458.

17. Edwards R. Thyroid and parathyroid disease. *Int Anesthesiol Clin* 1997; **35**: 63–83.

18. Brent G. The molecular basis of thyroid hormone action. *N Engl J Med* 1994; **331**: 847–853.

19. Woeber K. Thyrotoxicosis and the heart. *N Engl J Med* 1992; **327**: 94–98.

20. Bennett-Guerrero E *et al.* Cardiovascular effects of intravenous triiodothyronine in patients undergoing coronary artery bypass graft surgery: a double-blind, placebo-controlled trial. *JAMA* 1996; **275**: 687–692.

21. Miller M. Inappropriate antidiuretic hormone secretion. *Curr Ther Endocrinol Metab* 1997; **6**: 206–209.

22

RL Harter, FL Christofi

GASTROINTESTINAL PHARMACOLOGY

GASTROINTESTINAL PHYSIOLOGY

The gastrointestinal (GI) tract contains three physiological effector systems, the intestinal mucosa, visceral smooth muscle and the vasculature, each controlled by the enteric and autonomic nervous systems. The enteric nervous system, with as many neurons as the spinal cord, can function as an independent integrative system to control ion transport, motility and mucosal blood without any extrinsic sensory or autonomic input.[1] Neurons of the mysenteric nerve plexus control GI motility and peristalsis, whereas neurons of the submucosal nerve plexus are involved in the regulation of ion transport and mucosal blood flow.

Abnormalities of GI motility are often involved in gastrooesophageal reflux disease (GORD), dysphagia, nonulcer dyspepsia and irritable bowel syndrome. GORD may cause pain by reflux-induced oesophageal spasm, acute acid stimulation of oesophageal chemoreceptors, or oesophageal inflammation from chronic acid exposure. Dyspepsia is a very common and persistent problem with a poorly understood pathophysiology. About 25–50% of patients with nonulcer dyspepsia have delayed gastric emptying. Nonulcer dyspepsia may involve an abnormality in central processing of afferent information from the GI tract involving central 5-hydroxytryptamine (5-HT_{1a}) receptors.[2] Drugs such as digoxin, antibiotics and nonsteroidal antiinflammatory drugs (NSAIDs) may also induce dyspepsia.

REGULATION OF GASTRIC SECRETION

An important group of GI tract diseases are related to abnormalities of gastric secretion. The stomach secretes about 2.5 litres of gastric juice daily, containing pepsinogens produced by the peptic cells and hydrochloric acid and intrinsic factor from the parietal cells. The three major pathways regulating parietal acid secretion are neural stimulation via the vagus nerve, endocrine stimulation via gastrin released from antral G cells, and paracrine stimulation by local release of histamine from enterochromaffin-like cells (Fig. 22.1). Both neurally secreted acetylcholine and circulating gastrin have direct and indirect effects on parietal cells. Acetylcholine acts directly on muscarinic M_3 receptors to stimulate acid production, and indirectly via muscarinic M_1 receptors on histamine-containing paracrine cells to cause release of histamine. The released histamine acts on parietal cell H_2 receptors to stimulate acid production. Similarly, gastrin acts directly on parietal cell gastrin receptors to stimulate acid production and indirectly by stimulating the release of histamine from paracrine cells. Activation of parietal cell muscarinic M_3 receptors, H_2 receptors or gastrin receptors stimulates activation of H^+–K^+-adenosine triphosphatase (ATPase) on parietal cells, leading to the secretion of H^+ at rates between 20 and 40 mmol l^{-1} h^{-1}. The result is an accumulation in the gastric lumen of H^+ to a concentration of about 0.1 mol l^{-1}. The H^+–K^+-ATPase ('proton pump') of the apical membrane of the parietal cell is the ultimate mediator of acid secretion. This pump is unique to gastric parietal cells.

The gastric mucosa also contains cells that secrete mucus and bicarbonate ions, which are trapped in the mucus. The mucus and the bicarbonate form a protective gel-like layer preventing mucosal damage by acid. There is a pH gradient from 1–2 in the lumen of the stomach to 6–7 at the mucosal surface. The secretion of mucus and bicarbonate is stimulated by prostaglandins, explaining the ulcerogenic effects of NSAIDs, which inhibit prostaglandin synthesis. Prostaglandin (PG)E_2 and (PG)I_2 also reduce acid secretion by inhibiting histamine-stimulated adenylyl cyclase activity in the parietal cell (Fig. 22.1). Bile and alcohol can disrupt the mucus–bicarbonate layer.

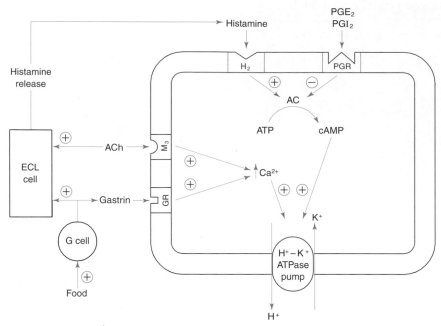

Fig. 22.1 Regulation of acid production by the gastric parietal cell. Gastrin, secreted by G cells in the antrum of the stomach, and acetylcholine (ACh) released from vagus nerve terminals increase intracellular Ca^{2+} concentration, which in turn stimulates H^+–K^+ adenosine triphosphatase (ATPase) (the proton pump) to release hydrochloric acid (HCl). Gastrin and ACh also stimulate enterocromaffin-like (ECL) cells to release histamine, which then acts on histamine H_2 receptors on the parietal cell. Activation of the H_2 receptors stimulates the adenylyl cyclase (AC) system, while the prostaglandins PGE_2 and PGI_2 inhibit AC and thus inhibit acid secretion. M_3, muscarinic M_3 receptor; GR, gastrin receptor; cAMP, cyclic adenosine monophosphate; PGR, prostaglandin receptor.

MANAGEMENT OF DYSPEPSIA

ANTACIDS

The function of antacids is to neutralize the hydrochloric acid secreted by gastric parietal cells and thus raise the pH of the stomach contents. Increasing the gastric pH also reduces the damaging effects of pepsin, which is pH dependent. A straightforward means of raising the gastric pH is the oral administration of alkali antacids such as sodium citrate or aluminium or magnesium salts, which neutralize the acid:

$$Al(OH_3) + 3HCl \rightarrow AlCl_3 + 3H_2O$$

Alkalization of the gastric contents also increases gastric motility through an action on gastrin. Aluminium ions can directly relax stomach smooth muscle and delay gastric emptying while magnesium ions have the opposite effect. Many antacid preparations therefore contain a combination of aluminium and magnesium salts. Aluminium and magnesium also bind and inactivate pepsin. Sodium citrate (15–20 ml), either alone as a 0.3 mol l^{-1} solution or combined with 0.6 mol l^{-1} citric acid, is an effective preoperative antacid, reducing gastric

acidity and thereby the risk of pulmonary injury if the patient should aspirate. Simply raising gastric pH does not necessarily reduce the risk of pulmonary injury, however, if a particulate antacid is used. Various animal studies have shown increased gross and microscopic lung injury when particulate antacids are used, compared with nonparticulate antacids. Because sodium citrate is absorbed, repeated use can result in metabolic alkalosis. The *milk-alkali syndrome* is caused by the ingestion of large quantities of Ca^{2+} and absorbable alkali, such as large doses of antacids with milk. The effects consist of hypercalcaemia, reduced secretion of parathyroid hormone, retention of phosphate, precipitation of Ca^{2+} salts in the kidney and renal insufficiency. Aluminium and magnesium hydroxide are not absorbed but can affect absorption of other drugs. These salts have greater buffering capacity than sodium citrate and are more appropriate for the management of peptic ulcer symptoms.

HISTAMINE H₂-RECEPTOR ANTAGONISTS

Early in the twentieth century, Sir Henry Dale discovered the role of histamine in the production of gastric secretions. Standard antihistamine preparations at

---

Summary box 22.1 Drug therapy for dyspepsia and peptic ulceration

- Alkali antacids (e.g. sodium citrate, aluminium hydroxide and magnesium hydroxide) neutralize hydrochloric acid:

  - aluminium and magnesium salts also inactivate pepsin

  - Al^{3+} delays gastric emptying, Mg^{2+} increases gastrointestinal motility and can cause diarrhoea.

- Histamine H_2 antagonists – cimetidine, ranitidine, famotidine and nizatidine:

  - histamine is an important stimulus for production of hydrochloric acid

  - cimetidine is an inhibitor of the cytochrome P450 enzyme

  - cimetidine has antiandrogenic properties and increases prolactin secretion; high doses can produce gynaecomastia in men or galactorrhoea in women.

- Proton pump inhibitors – omeprazole, lansoprazole and pantoprazole:

  - reduce secretion of H^+ by parietal cell H^+–K^+-ATPase (proton pump).

- Anticholinergic agents (e.g. pirenzepine and telenzepine).

- Cytoprotective agents:

  - prostaglandin analogues (e.g. misoprostol) stimulate secretion of mucus and bicarbonate and inhibit acid secretion

  - sucralfate, an aluminium–sucrose complex which forms a viscous gel at pH < 4, protecting the mucosa from degradation by pepsin.

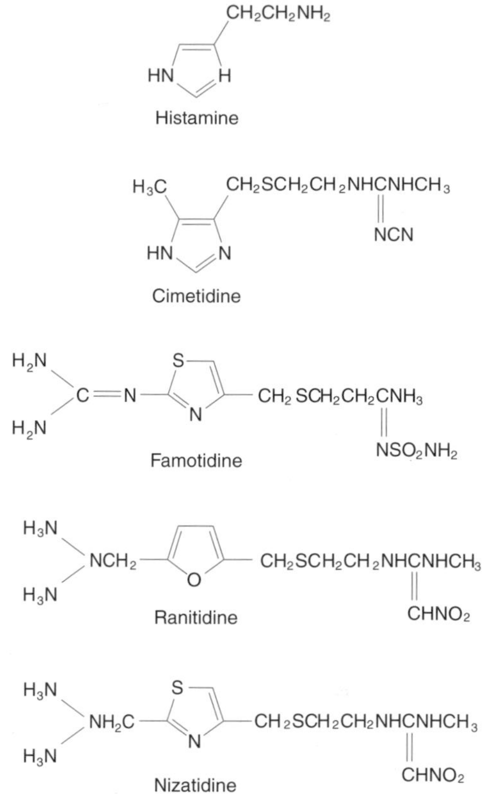

Fig. 22.2 Structure of histamine H_2 antagonists.

Cimetidine

Cimetidine is effective in reducing gastric acid secretion and is readily absorbed from the gut. It is relatively free from significant side-effects. The hepatic first-pass effect is low and bioavailability is 70%. A single 300-mg oral dose significantly reduces gastric acidity and gastric juice volume for up to 8 h. The effect begins 60–90 min after oral administration, and 15–45 min after intravenous administration. Cimetidine and the other H_2 antagonists do not have a significant effect on the rate of gastric emptying, on lower oesophageal sphincter pressure or on pancreatic secretion.

Adverse effects, which occur in less than 2% of patients receiving cimetidine, include headache, dizziness, fatigue, fever, muscle pain, constipation, diarrhoea and skin rashes. Reversible increases in serum transaminase levels and rare cases of hepatic necrosis have been reported. Cimetidine has weak antiandrogenic properties and increases prolactin secretion. Particularly in patients taking very high doses, for example those with the Zollinger–Ellison syndrome, this can produce gynaecomastia in men or galactorrhoea in women. Infrequently, intravenous administration produces cardiac arrhythmias and cardiac arrest. Although cimetidine

that time, which were selective H_1-receptor antagonists, were ineffectual at blocking gastric secretion. It is now known that histamine H_2 receptors are responsible for controlling gastric secretion. Synthesis of the first H_2-receptor antagonist (cimetidine) was achieved by modification of histamine's ethylamine side-chain. In the newer H_2 antagonists, a furan (ranitidine) or a thiazole (famotidine, nizatidine) group replaces the imidazole ring of histamine (Fig. 22.2).

penetrates the blood–brain barrier poorly, central nervous system (CNS) toxicity manifesting as agitation, confusion or coma has been reported, particularly among elderly patients or those with renal insufficiency. Cimetidine inhibits hepatic cytochrome P450 drug metabolism, producing many clinically significant drug interactions (see Chapter 28). It also reduces hepatic flow, which can delay the metabolism of any hepatically cleared drug.

Ranitidine

Ranitidine is five to eight times more potent than cimetidine in antagonizing gastric acid secretion. Like cimetidine, it is rapidly absorbed from the gastrointestinal tract, producing peak plasma concentrations 30–60 min after an oral dose. The bioavailability is 50%. A single 150-mg dose inhibits gastric acid secretion for 8–12 h in healthy adults. About 50% of administered ranitidine is excreted unchanged in the urine.

Side-effects are much less common than with cimetidine. Although ranitidine binds to hepatic cytochrome P450, its affinity is much lower than that of cimetidine, and it does not cause enzyme inhibition. Like cimetidine it reduces hepatic blood flow. Rapid intravenous administration can rarely produce bradycardia and cardiac arrest.[3] Transient reversible increases in serum transaminase levels have been reported. Androgen receptor binding and subsequent gynaecomastia do not occur with rantidine therapy.

Famotidine

Famotidine is nearly four times as potent as ranitidine in inhibiting gastric acid secretion. A single 40-mg oral dose inhibits gastric acid secretion for up to 12 h. As with ranitidine, it has minimal affinity for cytochrome P450. Unlike cimetidine and ranitidine, it has minimal effect on hepatic blood flow and is virtually devoid of significant cardiovascular effects, even with intravenous administration. CNS toxicity has been reported in patients after neurosurgery, associated with raised levels of famotidine in the cerebrospinal fluid.[4] Preoperative administration of famotidine may augment core hypothermia under general anaesthesia, presumably by inhibiting centrally mediated thermoregulatory control.[5]

Nizatidine

Nizatidine's structure is similar to that of famotidine; its potency is comparable to that of ranitidine. Unlike the other H_2 antagonists, first-pass metabolism is negligible and bioavailability is nearly 100%. Renal excretion is the primary route of elimination. Nizatidine is the only H_2 antagonist to have an active metabolite, which has 60% of the activity of the parent drug. It does not bind significantly to cytochrome P450. A single oral dose of 150 mg on the morning of operation reduces preoperative gastric acidity.[6]

PROTON PUMP INHIBITORS

The H^+–K^+-ATPase 'proton pump' of the parietal cell apical membrane is the final common step in gastric acid secretion. The first inhibitors of this enzyme were the substituted benzylimidazoles, of which omeprazole was the first to gain commercial release. They are typically used for patients with hypergastrinaemia, or for those with peptic ulcer disease refractory to other forms of antacid therapy.

Omeprazole

Omeprazole is a weak base (pK 4.0). It is a prodrug that is inactive at neutral pH but in the acidic conditions of the parietal cell it is converted to the active sulphenamide form. This binds the sulphhydryl groups of cysteine residues on the extracellular surface of H^+–K^+-ATPase, irreversibly inhibiting the enzyme's activity. Because omeprazole is degraded in an acidic environment it is formulated in pH-sensitive granules that limit its degradation by gastric acid, permitting intestinal absorption. Bioavailability of initial doses of this formulation is 50%, but this increases to 70% with repeated administration, possibly due to the increase in gastric pH reducing gastric degradation. Peak effect after an oral dose occurs in 2–4 h, and lasts up to 24 h. There is significant individual variation in inhibition of hydrogen chloride secretion, ranging from 30% to 100%.

The side-effects of omeprazole are generally minor and include headache, skin alterations, diarrhoea and nausea. These effects occur in less than 2% of patients. Transient increases in the level of hepatic aminotransferases may occur in less than 3% of patients. Long-term therapy may decrease absorption of vitamin B_{12}. Omeprazole inhibits specific cytochrome P450 isoenzymes and can inhibit the hepatic metabolism of the R isomer of warfarin, phenytoin and diazepam. The metabolism of propranolol and theophylline, however, does not appear to be affected.

Lansoprazole and pantoprazole are second-generation proton pump inhibitors with effects similar to those of omeprazole. Lansoprazole has a significant antibacterial effect and is the most potent of the proton pump inhibitors at inhibiting Helicobacter pylori.[7] This bacterium plays a role in the pathogenesis of both duodenal and gastric ulcers.

ANTICHOLINERGIC DRUGS

Acetylcholine influences gastric physiology via three subtypes of muscarinic cholinergic receptors: M_1, M_2 and M_3. The reduction in gastric acid secretion that is produced by nonspecific muscarinic antagonists such as atropine, glycopyrrolate and hyoscine is accompanied by a significant reduction in gastrointestinal motility and delayed gastric emptying. Lower oesophageal sphincter tone is also decreased, increasing the risk of gastrooesophageal reflux. Intravenous atropine 0.6 mg reduces lower oesophageal sphincter pressure for at least 40 min. Glycopyrrolate 0.2–0.3 mg intravenously produces a similar reduction in lower oesophageal sphincter pressure. Additionally, at doses necessary to produce a significant reduction in gastric acid secretion, the nongastrointestinal effects of the nonspecific antimuscarinics, such as the tachycardia, antisialogogue, mydriatic and cycloplegic effects, will undoubtedly occur. Antimuscarinic drugs selective for the M_1 receptor, such as pirenzepine and telenzepine, reduce gastric acid secretion with much less inhibition of gastrointestinal smooth muscle function.

Pirenzepine
Pirenzepine is the first M_1 receptor antagonist to become available. An oral dose of 50 mg produces a moderate reduction in basal and stimulated acid secretion, but with lower efficacy than that of the H_2-receptor antagonists. Pirenzepine also inhibits salivary gland secretion. Because it is relatively selective for M_1 receptors, it has minimal effect on heart rate, vision or bladder function since these mainly involve M_2 and M_3 receptors. Although pirenzepine causes a mild reduction in gastrointestinal transit time due to smooth muscle relaxation, this is compensated by stimulation of the gastrointestinal intramural neuromuscular plexus.[8]

Telenzepine
Telenzepine is an analogue of pirenzepine that is 10 to 25 times more potent at inhibition of gastric acid secretion. It inhibits salivary production more than pirenzepine, but is less likely to produce blurred vision. Overall gastrointestinal transit time is unaffected by telenzepine, although orocaecal transit time is prolonged.

CYTOPROTECTIVE AGENTS
Prostaglandins synthesized by the gastric mucosa inhibit the secretion of acid and stimulate the secretion of mucus and bicarbonate. Three prostaglandin analogues, misoprostol, rioprostil and enprostil, are used for peptic ulcer therapy. Sucralfate, an aluminium–sucrose complex, has a different mechanism.

Misoprostol
Misoprostol is a synthetic prostaglandin (PG) E_1 analogue that inhibits both basal gastric acid production and that occurring in response to food, histamine or pentagastrin by a direct action on parietal cells. It also increases the secretion of mucus and bicarbonate, and has a protective effect on the gastric and duodenal mucosa. It is rapidly absorbed after an oral dose and is metabolized to the free acid. Misoprostol is as effective as H_2 antagonists in treating gastric and duodenal ulcers. It has also been used to reduce ulceration caused by NSAIDs, although there is little evidence supporting this.[9]

The most common side-effects associated with misoprostol administration are diarrhoea, nausea and vomiting and abdominal pain. These effects seem to be dose related. As with any of the prostaglandin analogues, their use should be avoided in patients with known or suspected pregnancy, due to their abortifacient potential.

Rioprostil
Rioprostil is another PGE_1 analogue with effects similar to those of misoprostol. It may be slightly more efficacious than misoprostol in the treatment of gastric and duodenal ulcers. Its efficacy in peptic ulcer healing is equivalent to that of cimetidine. Diarrhoea occurs in 6–10% of patients, and in about 1% is severe enough to prompt discontinuation of therapy.

Enprostil
Enprostil is a potent PGE_2 analogue. It is much less effective than ranitidine for the long-term treatment of duodenal ulcers. Its side-effect profile is similar to that of the other prostaglandin analogues, with a predominance of gastrointestinal effects.

Sucralfate
Sucralfate is a complex formed from sucrose octasulphate and polyaluminium hydroxide used in the management of peptic ulcers and reflux oesophagitis. It is given orally before meals. Since the preparation is activated by acid, sucralfate should not be administered within 30 min of the administration of antacids. At a pH below 4, sucralfate undergoes extensive polymerization and cross-linking to form a viscous gel, which protects the mucosa from degradation by pepsin. Even though the pH in the duodenum is well above 4, the gel retains its viscid, demulcent properties. Sucralfate also binds bile salts, which are implicated in the pathogenesis of gastric ulcers. A variety of mechanisms have been proposed to account for the cytoprotective and healing effects of sucralfate, including stimulation of PGE_2 synthesis, adsorption of pepsin, and stimulation of local production of epidermal growth factor. Side-effects are few: only constipation due to aluminium (in 2% of patients) and a dry mouth (less than 1%) appear significant. Sucralfate can adsorb and thereby reduce the bioavailability of a number of drugs, including tetracycline and fluoroquinolone antibiotics, ketoconazole, phenytoin, digoxin and amitriptyline. Interactions may be minimized by taking these drugs 2 h before sucralfate.

INFLAMMATORY BOWEL DISEASE

Inflammatory bowel disease is a collective term that refers to Crohn's disease and ulcerative colitis. The aetiology remains unclear, but appears to result from a complex interplay between environmental and genetic factors. An alteration in the mucosal immune system is also thought to play a part. Together, they lead to an inappropriate, exaggerated or prolonged inflammatory response. Common treatment strategies are used to treat these diseases.

Salicylates

Sulphasalazine is a combination of sulphapyridine (a sulphonamide) and 5-aminosalicylic acid. The latter is the active constituent and is released following cleavage of sulphasalazine by colonic flora. Newer compounds are mesalazine (5-aminosalicylic acid itself) and olsalixine, which consists of two molecules of 5-aminosalicylic acid linked by a diazo bond. Bacteria in the colon break down this bond to release the active drug. The mechanism of action of aminosalicylates in inflammatory bowel disease is unknown, but may be by inhibition of leucocyte chemotaxis or of leucotrine and prostaglandin synthesis. They may also act as free radical scavengers. Sulphasalazine is partially absorbed intact from the gut, but most reaches the colon where it undergoes bacterial cleavage. Absorption of sulphapyridine is responsible for many of the side-effects of this drug. Common side-effects include rash, fever, headache and photosensitivity. Less common, but more severe, side-effects include anaemia, agranulocytosis, reversible male infertility, neutropenia, pancreatitis and hepatitis.

Corticosteroids

Prednisolone or hydrocortisone is used to induce remission in patients with active inflammatory bowel disease. Following remission the dose is gradually tapered to minimize side-effects. For severe or extensive disease, the drugs are given intravenously, followed by oral therapy when it is brought under control. Corticosteroids are also effective as retention enemas or rectal foam. These are useful for disease limited to the rectum and descending colon. Newer steroid preparations delivered in enema form, such as tixocortol or beclomethasone dipropionate, may offer adequate efficacy with a lower incidence of systemic side-effects.

Short-chain fatty acids

Short-chain fatty acids, particularly butyrate, are the preferred energy substrates for distal colonic epithelial cells. Decreased faecal concentrations of fatty acids occur in patients with ulcerative colitis, but not in those with Crohn's disease. Short-chain fatty acid therapy is slightly less effective than steroids or salicylates, but the effect is improved when given concurrently with other agents.

Metronidazole

Antibiotic therapy with metronidazole is based on the premise that infectious agents play a role in the aetiology or exacerbation of Crohn's disease or ulcerative colitis. The use of antibiotics in the treatment of inflammatory bowel disease has generally yielded disappointing results. A notable exception is metronidazole, which appears to be useful for treating mild or moderately active Crohn's disease, especially when the disease is limited to the colon.

Immunosuppressive agents

Immunosuppressive agents, such as 6-mercaptopurine and azathioprine, are used for patients with inflammatory bowel disease that is difficult to control with steroids or aminosalicylates. Cyclosporine is very effective in severe ulcerative colitis, allowing avoidance of immediate colectomy for patients that are not candidates for surgery. Long-term, low-dose methotrexate therapy leads to the intracellular accumulation of adenosine, which has potent antiinflammatory effects.

DIARRHOEA

Diarrhoea is a symptom of many bowel diseases as well as a consequence of drug therapy, infection, etc. Most currently available antidiarrhoeal agents work primarily by slowing intestinal transit and increasing the contact time with the absorbing epithelium. If no absorbing surface is available, as in severe secretory diarrhoea, the use of an agent to slow transit may merely serve transiently to reduce stool output by temporarily pooling a larger volume of fluid intraluminally.

OPIOIDS

The three main opioids used to manage diarrhoea are codeine phosphate, diphenoxylate and loperamide. The antisecretory effects of opioids are probably mediated via enteric nerves, mainly by δ opioid receptors, whereas their effects on transit are mediated by μ opioid receptors. The release of noradrenaline and 5-HT from enteric nerves may also play a role. Opioids or other antiperistaltic agents should be used with caution in patients with severe colitis, who may develop toxic megacolon. There is also some concern about their use in acute infectious diarrhoea, when diarrhoea may be the mechanism of clearing a pathogen from the body.

Codeine

Codeine phosphate is an effective and inexpensive treatment for chronic diarrhoea in adults. It decreases gut motility at a lower dose than that which is required to produce analgesia. This effect is maintained even with prolonged use, although addiction concerns arise with chronic use. Oral solutions or tablets are available. The recommended daily adult dose is 15–60 mg. Respiratory depression has been reported with relatively low doses in children.

Diphenoxylate

Diphenoxylate hydrochloride is typically combined with a small dose of atropine, to discourage drug abuse by producing anticholinergic side-effects if taken in excessive doses. This combination may cause respiratory depression in children less than 4 years of age. Anticholinergic side-effects include decreased salivary and bronchial secretions and decreased sweating. Increasing doses will produce mydriasis, urinary retention and reduced gastrointestinal motility. Very high doses can produce opioid effects, including circulatory and respiratory arrest.

Loperamide

Loperamide hydrochloride is a synthetic opioid analogue with essentially no abuse potential. It slows the passage of fluid through the gut, increasing the time available for absorption. Loperamide does not cross the mature blood–brain barrier and thus produces fewer CNS adverse effects than codeine. In combination with oral rehydration, it is generally an effective treatment for acute watery diarrhoea in adults. Adverse effects occur in less than 1% of patients, and include abdominal cramps, headaches, dizziness and skin reactions, including urticaria. Paralytic ileus has also been reported. Loperamide is not recommended in children under 4 years of age, as it can cause shock, enterocolitis, ileus and potentially fatal intestinal obstruction.

Acetorphan

The endogenous opioid peptides, especially enkephalins, have potent antisecretory properties by inhibiting intestinal fluid and electrolyte secretion. Unfortunately their rapid degradation by enkephalinase precludes their therapeutic use. Acetorphan is an orally active inhibitor of enkephalinase in the wall of the gastrointestinal tract, preventing inactivation of endogenous opioid peptides released by submucosal and myenteric neurons. It does not appear to affect gastrointestinal motility. Acetorphan inhibits infectious and chemically induced diarrhoea and is a promising agent with therapeutic potential.[10]

SOMATOSTATIN ANALOGUES

Somatostatin and octreotide are successful in treating diarrhoea due to peptide-secreting tumours (e.g. VIPomas). They act by reducing the tumour size, as well as the secretion of peptides and their effects on the GI tract. Octreotide is more effective in treating chemotherapy-induced diarrhoea than loperamide, and ameliorates the symptoms of dumping syndrome. In this syndrome, uncontrolled gastric emptying causes osmotic movement of fluid into the intestine, producing an exaggerated release of enteric peptides into the circulation, with subsequent hypovolaemia, hypotension, flushing and diarrhoea. Octreotide is administered intravenously or subcutaneously.

ADSORBENTS

Adsorbents such as kaolin, activated charcoal and binding resins are widely used to treat diarrhoea. The binding resin cholestyramine is used in the management of diarrhoea caused by excess bile acids entering the colon, as occurs after vagotomy, terminal ileal resection and cholecystectomy. It reduces the bile salt pool, and is thus potentially lithogenic. Cholestyramine can bind orally administered drugs such as digoxin and warfarin, decreasing their bioavailability. In addition to being unpalatable, it may produce hyperchloraemic acidosis.

BISMUTH

The antibacterial agent bismuth subsalicylate is useful in the prevention and treatment of traveller's diarrhoea and acute diarrhoea in children. Whether it is of benefit in nonbacterial diarrhoea is controversial. When used for short periods, black stools are formed due to the production of bismuth sulphide in the colon.

CONSTIPATION

Constipation is a symptom in about 2% of the general population who seek medical attention, but in as many as 24% of elderly patients, and 45% of hospice patients with advanced cancer. Colonic motility involves mass movements and segmental contractions. Mass movements transport the faeces towards the rectum for evacuation, whereas segmenting contractions are non-propulsive and inhibit the passage of stool. Opioids stimulate segmenting contractions. Constipation is caused by immobility, chronic illness, drugs, prolonged use of laxatives, poor nutrition, obstruction and endocrine disorders. Constipation is usually self-limiting, or it often responds to dietary changes and/or the addition of dietary fibre. Increasing the dietary fibre intake by 25–40% with the addition of bran can eliminate and prevent constipation in up to 60% of patients. When this and other lifestyle management strategies are unsuccessful, laxatives are used to treat chronic constipation. Intermittent use of laxatives is recommended because their prolonged use may cause severe side-effects. Laxative drugs can be classified as:

- Dietary fibre and bulk-forming laxatives.

- Stimulant laxatives.
- Osmotic laxatives.
- Stool softeners or lubricants.
- Prokinetic drugs.

BULKING AGENTS

Bulk-forming agents are nondigestible polysaccharides and semicellulose derivatives such as psyllium, agar, methylcellulose and tragacanth. They stimulate intestinal motility and retention of water. Acidic metabolites formed by bacterial metabolism may further stimulate defaecation. Psyllium is administered with generous amounts of fluids, to prevent impaction in the oesophagus and proximal intestine. Some psyllium products contain as much as 50% dextrose, so diabetics should use psyllium products that are devoid of sugar. The commonly reported side-effects are flatulence and abdominal distension. Large bowel obstruction and perforation occur very rarely. They are contraindicated in patients with intestinal strictures. Pectin and oat bran reduce gut absorption of the serum cholesterol-lowering agent lovastatin. Ispaghula can cause an immunoglobulin E-mediated hypersensitivity reaction resulting in rhinoconjunctivitis, skin rash and urticaria, asthma, GI symptoms and even anaphylaxis.

STIMULANT LAXATIVES

Stimulant or irritant laxatives include the anthraquinones senna, rhubarb, danthron and cascara sagrada. Colonic bacterial action forms active metabolites that exert their effects within 6–24 h. Catharsis is possibly due to a net accumulation of water and sodium in the colon. Diphenylmethane laxatives such as bisacodyl and phenophthalein stimulate the mucosal nerve plexus of the colon, leading to fluid and electrolyte secretion. A common side-effect is abdominal pain. Long-term use of anthraquinone-type laxatives may cause pseudomelanosis coli, associated with brown pigmentation of the colonic mucosa. The effect is completely reversible with discontinuation of therapy. Chronic use of stimulant laxatives can cause permanent damage to nerves or muscles of the gut.

OSMOTIC LAXATIVES

Osmotic agents include magnesium hydroxide, magnesium sulphate, sodium phosphates and sodium sulphates. They may also release cholecystokinin, which contributes to catharsis by inhibiting fluid and electrolyte absorption from the distal small bowel. The hyperosmotic agent lactulose is metabolized to short-chain fatty acids, which contributes to its laxative effect. Common side-effects, occurring in up to 70% of patients, include flatulence, abdominal pain and colic. These symptoms often abate after a few days. Hypertonic salt laxatives can cause significant systemic dehydration un-less adequate oral rehydration is maintained. Osmotic salt laxatives must be used with caution in patients with renal failure or congestive heart failure because of enhanced cation absorption.

STOOL SOFTENERS

Docusate sodium and docusate calcium are stool softeners that act by lowering the surface tension at the oil–water interface of the stool. This permits penetration by water and fat. They are of marginal benefit in the treatment of chronic constipation. Docusate potentiates hepatotoxicity produced by other drugs.

PROKINETIC DRUGS

Cisapride, a serotonin 5-HT$_4$ agonist, is an oral gastrointestinal prokinetic drug chemically related to metoclopramide and domperidone, but unlike these compounds is devoid of CNS depressant or antidopaminergic effects. It reduces intestinal transit time, and may be a viable option for patients with chronic idiopathic constipation that is refractory to conventional therapy. It also lowers lower oesophageal sphincter tone. Treatment for 8–12 weeks may be needed for optimal results. Headache and urinary frequency have been occasionally reported with the use of cisapride. Cisapride has been associated with acquired long QT syndrome and ventricular arrhythmias such as torsades de pointes which produces sudden cardiac death. These cardiotoxic effects can be due to blockade of one or more types of K$^+$ channel currents in the human heart.[11] These side-effects are potentiated by macrolide antibiotics, which inhibit cytochrome P450 enzymes responsible for cisapride metabolism, leading to raised blood concentrations of cisapride.[12]

ANTIEMETICS

PHYSIOLOGY OF EMESIS

Vomiting, the forceful expulsion of GI contents from the mouth, is initiated by the vomiting centre of the brainstem medulla. The vomiting centre receives inputs from many sources and sends efferents to the pharynx, larynx, and upper GI tract, as well as to the nuclei of respiration and the salivatory and vasomotor centres (Fig. 22.3). During a vomiting episode the striated muscles of the thorax, diaphragm and abdomen contract. Just before vomiting, there is inhibition of gastric motility by an unknown inhibitory transmitter, followed by a powerful reverse peristalsis. Vomiting occurs in response to local GI tract activation of afferents of the vagus and sympathetic nerves. Neurons from the chemoreceptor trigger zone (CTZ) in the area postrema synapse with neurons in the nucleus ambiguus and dorsal motor nucleus projecting to the vomiting centre, and with neurons in the nucleus tractus solitarius (NTS).

The area postrema, which lies outside the blood–brain barrier, has neurons extending to the NTS and receives vagal afferent inputs. The NTS also receives strong afferent input from vagal and sympathetic afferent neurons.

Vomiting may be induced by signals from higher centres in the cortex (e.g. induced by pain and unpleasant sights and smells). Afferents in the trigeminal and glossopharyngeal nerves transmit sensory impulses from the fauces to the vomiting centre indirectly through the NTS. The vestibular apparatus in the inner ear sends impulses to the vomiting centre, which can trigger nausea, vomiting and motion sickness. Receptor subtypes for serotonin (5-HT), histamine, acetylcholine and dopamine are present in the GI tract and in the central nuclei involved in vomiting. Most antiemetic drugs act on one or more of these receptors.[12]

Drug-induced vomiting is particularly common with chemotherapeutic agents, opioids, aminoglycoside antibiotics, levodopa and cholinomimetics. The mediators released or produced by radiation therapy activate both peripheral and central sites involved in the vomiting reflex. Premedication with opioids is a major contribution to postoperative vomiting. Their emetic effect is due to an action at the CTZ. Ambulatory patients are more affected than those confined to bed, suggesting a vestibular component in the effect. The emetic action of opioids is complicated by an antiemetic effect exerted at the vomiting centre. Emetic symptoms are more likely when opioids are given intravenously than by intramuscular injection. This may reflect either higher concentrations or more rapid changes in concentration with the intravenous route.

Common causes of chronic vomiting are gastric motility disorders such as gastroparesis, psychogenic factors and structural lesions of the GI tract mucosa such as peptic ulcer disease. Episodic, abrupt, explosive vomiting implies a central disorder with increased intracranial pressure. A viral infection is suggested by symptoms of acute onset of vomiting with diarrhoea and fever. GI tract obstruction may lead to vomiting which is preceded by colicky abdominal pain and abdominal distension. Vomiting of large volume with partly digested food particles suggests gastroparesis. Opioid analgesics, anticholinergics, antidepressants, calcium channel blockers, somatostatin, octreotide or aluminium-containing antacids may induce drug-induced gastroparesis. The incidence of postsurgical gastroparesis is highest with truncal vagotomy and rare with parietal cell vagotomy. About 5% of patients who undergo vagotomy with antral resection develop gastroparesis. Excessive enterogastric reflux after certain types of operation may produce alkaline (or bile) reflux gastritis, which is associated with nausea and bilious vomiting, weight loss, and epigastric pain that is exacerbated by meals.

PHARMACOTHERAPY

Summary box 22.2 Antiemetic drugs

- Act on one or more of 5-HT_3, D_2, H, or muscarinic receptors.

- 5-HT_3 antagonists (e.g. ondansetron), are very effective for the management of emesis due to cytotoxic drugs and radiation therapy, and are also used for postoperative nausea and vomiting.

- Specific H_1 antagonists (e.g. diphenhydramine or cyclizine) are effective in the prevention and treatment of emesis due to middle ear surgery and motion sickness.

- Muscarinic receptor antagonists, especially hyoscine, are particularly effective against motion sickness.

- Metoclopramide:

  - centrally, blocks dopaminergic receptors in the CTZ

  - peripherally, increases lower oesophageal sphincter pressure, increases gastric emptying and small intestinal motility.

- Dopamine D_2 antagonists include the butyrophenones, droperidol and haloperidol.

- Domperidone, structurally related to droperidol, is a dopamine D_2 antagonist which acts centrally at the CTZ and peripherally on the GI tract to increase gastric emptying and gastrointestinal motility.

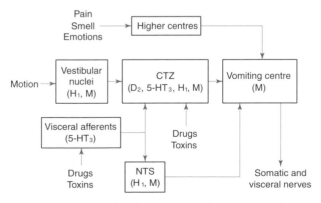

Fig. 22.3 Factors and pathways involved in the control of vomiting. CTZ, chemoreceptor trigger zone of the area postrema; NTS, nucleus tractus solitarius. The location of histamine (H_1), dopamine (D_2), 5-hydroxytryptamine (5-HT_3) and muscarinic (M) receptors are shown in parentheses.

Phenothiazines

The main mechanism for the antiemetic effect of the phenothiazines is antagonism of dopaminergic receptors in the CTZ. However, many also have actions on histamine and muscarinic receptors. Chlorpromazine, promethazine, prochlorperazine and perphenazine have all been used extensively as antiemetics, particularly in conjunction with the administration of opioids. The phenothiazines are moderately effective at treating postoperative nausea and vomiting. However, their use is limited by severe, albeit uncommon, side-effects, especially extrapyramidal effects. These can range from restlessness to oculogyric crisis, and are obviously undesirable in the perioperative period. Furthermore, all phenothiazines produce significant sedation, which makes them less than desirable for day-case surgery.[13] It is unclear whether the phenothiazines are free from teratogenic effects. If a risk is indeed present, it appears to be minimal.[14]

Butyrophenones

The neuroleptic droperidol is the butyrophenone most frequently used as an antiemetic after operation. Haloperidol, which is seldom used following surgery, has similar actions to droperidol but is longer acting. Domperidone, which is structurally related to droperidol, is a dopamine D_2-receptor antagonist. It acts centrally at the CTZ and peripherally on the GI tract to increase gastric emptying and GI motility. The latter effects may be related to blocking of a_1 adrenoceptors in the GI tract. It crosses the blood–brain barrier to a lesser extent than droperidol, so CNS side-effects are less common. Droperidol antagonizes CNS dopamine D_2 receptors and can cause infrequent but disturbing side-effects, including dysphoria, anxiety, restlessness and extrapyramidal reactions. The sedative effects of droperidol can delay discharge after day-case surgery, particularly when doses of $50–75\,\mu g\ kg^{-1}$ are used in paediatric patients, or 2.5–5 mg in adults. Lower doses ($10–20\,\mu g\ kg^{-1}$) are effective in preventing nausea for moderately emetogenic procedures such as laparoscopy, but are generally ineffective for highly emetogenic procedures, such as strabismus surgery.[13] Droperidol is a mild a-adrenoceptor antagonist and can cause hypotension in some patients.

Antihistamines

Histamine H_1 antagonists, such as diphenhydramine, hydroxyzine, dimenhydrinate and cyclizine, are more effective than the phenothiazines in the prevention and treatment of emesis due to middle ear surgery and motion sickness. The piperazine antihistamines, hydroxyzine and cyclizine, produce sedative effects and have been used for preoperative medication, often in conjunction with an opioid. Cyclizine, diphenhydramine and dimenhydrinate have all been used extensively during pregnancy and appear to be relatively safe. Dimenhydrinate appears to be tocolytic early in pregnancy, but is oxytocic in the term uterus, with a potential for uterine hyperstimulation or rupture.[14]

Anticholinergics

Hyoscine (scopolamine) exerts antiemetic effects by acting at specific muscarinic receptors in the cerebral cortex and pons. Hyoscine is an effective treatment for motion sickness where its action on the vestibular apparatus may contribute to its effectiveness. A transdermal preparation is available and, in addition to its use for motion sickness, has been used to decrease the incidence of severe nausea and vomiting after laparoscopy and epidural morphine administration. Therapeutic concentrations for the transdermal route are reached only after 5 h, so the patch should be applied several hours before operation in order to be effective. The use of hyoscine is limited by its side-effects, which predominantly involve the CNS, including dysphoria, confusion and restlessness. These are seen particularly with transdermal administration.[13]

Benzamides

The benzamides that have been used as antiemetics include metoclopramide, trimethobenzamide, cisapride, alizapride, domperidone, clebopride and levosulpride. The most widely used benzamide is metoclopramide.

Metoclopramide

Metoclopramide has both central and peripheral sites of antiemetic action. Centrally, it blocks dopaminergic receptors in the CTZ of the area postrema. Peripherally, it increases lower oesophageal sphincter pressure, increases gastric emptying and small intestinal motility. These actions may be due to actions at the 5-HT_4 receptor. It also has mild peripheral cholinergic actions. High doses of metoclopramide ($1–2\,mg\ kg^{-1}$) are used to manage chemotherapy induced emesis, although significant sedative effects and a relatively high incidence of extrapyramidal reactions can occur with these doses. With high doses actions on 5-HT_3 may predominate over those on dopamine receptors. Doses of $0.1–0.2\,mg\ kg^{-1}$ are typically used for the prophylaxis and treatment of postoperative emesis, with relative freedom from sedative and extrapyramidal effects. The duration of action is, however, short, so repeated doses are often required. Metoclopramide was initially introduced in Europe for the treatment of nausea and vomiting during pregnancy, without evidence of teratogenic or abortifacient effects.

Other Benzamides

Trimethobenzamide is a less potent antiemetic than metoclopramide, but can be administered rectally. Cisapride releases acetylcholine at the myenteric plexus, resulting in increased motility throughout the GI tract, as well as increased lower oesophageal sphincter tone. It has no effect on central dopaminergic receptors, and is therefore devoid of extrapyramidal side-effects. Cisapride is more effective than metoclopramide in treating gastric stasis induced by morphine administration.[13]

Serotonin antagonists

Serotonin (5-HT), acting at the 5-HT_3 receptor, is an important mediator of the emetic response. 5-HT_3 antagonists, ondansetron, granisetron and tropisetron, were introduced for the prophylaxis and treatment of chemotherapy and radiation-induced emesis, but are also used to treat postoperative nausea and vomiting. Chemotherapeutic agents such as cisplatin cause the release of 5-HT from enterochromaffin cells within the intestinal mucosa. The released 5-HT is thought to activate splanchnic and vagal 5-HT_3 receptors in the GI wall, or to activate 5-HT_3 receptors directly in the CTZ. The 5-HT_3 receptors in the area postrema and the NTS lie on the vagal nerve terminals.

Ondansetron, granisetron and tropisetron competitively antagonize the 5-HT_3 receptor with minimum affinity for 5-HT_1 or 5-HT_2 receptors. They have no effect on gastric emptying or on small intestinal transit, but do delay colonic transit. Ondansetron can be given orally or intravenously. An oral dose of ondansetron is readily absorbed and has 60% bioavailability. The elimination half-life after intravenous administration is 3–5 h. Metabolism is extensive, via oxidative hepatic metabolism, with conjugation to glucuronides and sulphate.

Ondansetron, 4 mg, is as effective as an 8-mg dose at preventing postoperative emesis. However, the higher dose may be more effective in patients with a previous history of postoperative nausea and vomiting. Oral ondansetron is also effective as a prophylactic antiemetic. Side-effects are infrequent and generally minor. Headache, constipation and a sensation of warmth or flushing are the most common. Mild sedation, restlessness, dizziness, xerostomia, rash, intestinal obstruction and transient increases in serum alanine aminotransferase levels have been reported in patients undergoing chemotherapy or radiation therapy, in whom higher doses are usually used. Anaphylactic reactions have been reported in these patients.[15] A major advantage of these drugs in the management of postoperative nausea and vomiting is the lack of interaction with other drugs used perioperatively. The absence of sedation means that they do not affect postoperative recovery.

Propofol

There are many reports that patients anaesthetized with propofol have a lower incidence of postoperative nausea and vomiting than those receiving other anaesthetic drugs. Even subanaesthetic doses of propofol are effective in the treatment of postoperative nausea and vomiting.[16] A low-dose infusion of propofol ($1 \text{ mg kg}^{-1} \text{ h}^{-1}$), started 4 h before chemotherapy and continued for up to 24 h, in patients refractory to 5-HT_3 antagonists prevented chemotherapy induced emesis in 90% of patients.[17] No propofol-associated side-effects were observed. At present, the mechanism of propofol's antiemetic action is unknown, but is not via interactions with the dopaminergic system.[18]

REFERENCES

1. Marcello C, Costa M, Brodres SJM. The enteric nervous system. *Am J Gastroenterol* 1994; **89** (Suppl. 129): S129–S137.

2. Talley NJ. Functional dyspepsia should be targeted on disturbed physiology? *Aliment Pharmacol Ther* 1995; **9**: 107–115.

3. Hinrchsen H, Halabi A, Kirch W. Clinical aspects of cardiovascular effects of H₂-receptor antagonists. *J Clin Pharmacol* 1995; **35**: 107–116.

4. Yoshimoto K, Saima S, Echizen H et al. Famotidine-associated central nervous system reactions and plasma and cerebrospinal drug concentrations in neurosurgical patients with renal failure. *Clin Pharmacol Ther* 1994; **55**: 693–700.

5. Hirose M, Hara Y, Matsusaki M. Premedication with famotidine augments core hypothermia during general anesthesia. *Anesthesiology* 1995; **83**: 1179–1183.

6. Mikawa K, Nishina Y, Maekawa N et al. Gastric fluid volume and pH after nizatidine in adults undergoing elective surgery: influence of timing and dose. *Can J Anaesth* 1995; **42**: 730–734.

7. Nakao M, Malfertheiner P. Growth inhibitory and bactericidal activities of lansoprazole compared with those of omeprazole and pantoprazole against *Helicobacter pylori*. *Helicobacter* 1998; **3**: 21–27.

8. Stockbrugger RW. Clinical significance of M₁ receptor antagonists. *Pharmacology* 1988; **37** (Suppl. 1): 54–63.

9. Walt RP. Misoprostol for the treatment of peptic ulcer and antiinflammatory-drug-induced gastroduodenal ulceration. *N Engl J Med* 1992; **327**: 1575–1580.

10. Roge J, Baumer P, Berard H et al. The enkephalinase inhibitor, acetorphan, in acute diarrhoea. A double-blind, controlled clinical trial versus loperamide. *Scand J Gastroenterol* 1993; **28**: 352–354.

11. Drolet B, Khalifa M, Daleau P, Hamelin BA, Turgeon J. Block of the rapid component of the delayed rectifier potassium current by the prokinetic agent cisapride underlies drug-related lengthening of the QT interval. *Circulation* 1998; **97**: 204–210.

12. Mitchelson F. Pharmacological agents affecting emesis. *Drugs* 1992; **43**: 295–315.

13. Watcha MF, White PF. Postoperative nausea and vomiting. Its etiology,

treatment, and prevention. *Anesthesiology* 1992; **77**: 162–184.

14. Leathem AM. Safety and efficacy of antiemetics used to treat nausea and vomiting in pregnancy. *Clin Pharmacol* 1986; **5**: 660–668.

15. Finn AL. Toxicity and side effects of ondansetron. *Semin Oncol* 1992; **19** (Suppl. 10): 53–60.

16. Borgeat A, Wilder-Smith OHG, Suter PM. The nonhypnotic therapeutic applications of propofol. *Anesthesiology* 1994; **80**: 642–656.

17. Borgeat A, Wilder-Smith O, Forni M, Suter PM. Adjuvant propofol enables better control of nausea and emesis secondary to chemotherapy for breast cancer. *Can J Anaesth* 1994; **41**: 1117–1119.

18. Borgeat A. Subhypnotic doses of propofol do not possess antidopaminergic properties. *Anesth Analg* 1997; **84**: 196–198.

23

H Mattie, PJ van den Broek

CHEMOTHERAPY OF INFECTIONS

The course of an infection is determined by three interacting factors: the microorganism, host resistance and treatment. The most important of these is the interaction between the host and the pathogenic microorganism, i.e. the balance between the virulence of the pathogen and the resistance of the host to the pathogen. Cure of an infection can be achieved only if host resistance is intact. The role of antimicrobial agents, although often decisive, is mainly to shift the balance in favour of the host, giving the host time to mobilize its resistance mechanisms. Since antimicrobial agents act on vital mechanisms of the microorganism that generally have no parallel in the host, or are at least much less sensitive, they tend to have a broad therapeutic window.

Rational treatment of infections is based on three important assumptions. The first is that there is indeed an infection, or an infection risk. This statement is less trivial than it seems. The diagnosis of infection is established mainly on clinical grounds. Some clinical signs of infection, such as fever, are not unique. Malignancy or inflammatory disease can often mimic infection, and the clinical diagnosis of infection should be confirmed by bacteriological examination. However, positive cultures alone are not proof of an infection; for example, bronchial secretions in patients who are intubated are always colonized, often with Gram-negative microorganisms, without any clinical evidence of infection. The second assumption is that it is possible to treat the infection with antibiotics. Often antibiotics need to be combined with, for example, surgical treatment. The final assumption is that it is useful to treat the infection with antibiotics. To assess the possible contribution of antibiotic treatment, the natural course of a particular disease needs to be taken into account. The course of the infection is often less influenced by antibiotic treatment and depends more on the type of infection. Never-

theless, the duration of symptoms, such as fever, may often be shortened by antibiotic treatment.

In this chapter the principles of antimicrobial treatment will be discussed in some detail with respect to antibacterial drugs, but these principles are equally applicable to antifungal and antiviral drugs. In accordance with common usage, antibacterial drugs will be called antibiotics.

ANTIBIOTICS

RESISTANCE AND SENSITIVITY

Some bacterial species are naturally resistant to certain classes of antibiotics, either because they lack the necessary receptor or because their cell wall is impenetrable to the drug. Moreover, many strains of originally sensitive microorganisms have acquired mechanisms of resistance as a result of exposure to antibiotics. There are several ways in which bacteria may acquire resistance. One is by mutation, whereby an individual microorganism becomes resistant to a particular antibiotic. Normally this is no advantage, and the mutant disappears. If the population is exposed to an antibiotic when the mutation occurs, then the mutant gives rise to a new, resistant population. This is referred to as 'one-step' resistance. A common example is the resistance that *Mycobacterium tuberculosis* develops to rifampicin.

The most common mechanism of resistance is that the microorganism acquires an enzyme that destroys the antibiotic. Many Gram-positive bacteria produce an enzyme, β-lactamase, which inactivates β-lactam antibiotics by acetylating the β-lactam ring. This problem arose within a few years of the introduction of penicillin and currently over 80% of staphylococci are resistant to penicillin. Streptococci do not produce this enzyme. Nearly all Gram-negative bacteria have a chromosome that codes for a β-lactamase that is more active against cephalosporins than penicillins. A number of β-lactamase-resistant penicillins have been developed (e.g. cloxacillin and flucloxacillin).

An important factor in the spread of resistance is the transfer of genetic material from one microorganism to another, even from a nonpathogen to a pathogen. This can happen when a microorganism picks up free deoxyribonucleic acid (DNA), but more often plasmids (i.e. transmissible, extrachromosomal particles containing DNA) are transferred directly by conjugation of the microorganisms. This is one of the mechanisms of the spread of β-lactam resistance. Resistance-conferring plasmids have been identified in virtually all bacteria. Genetic material may also be transferred by transduction through viruses (bacteriophages). Acquired resistance is currently an enormous problem with particular types of infections and is the overriding reason for rational, very restricted, use of antibiotics. This is especially so in hospitals, where typically about 25% of patients are exposed to antibiotics at any time and this allows resistant strains to emerge more quickly. Hospital staff play a crucial role in spreading resistant strains from patient to patient.

Sensitivity testing

Sensitivity testing for antibiotics is based mainly on quantitative criteria, such as the minimum inhibitory concentration (MIC). The MIC is the minimum concentration that prevents visible growth of a standard inoculum of bacteria after an 18–24-h incubation. For bactericidal antibiotics, the minimum bactericidal concentration (MBC) is defined as the concentration of an antibiotic that kills 99.9% of bacteria. With most bactericidal agents the MBC is only slightly higher than the MIC.

MECHANISMS OF ACTION

Antibiotics can be either bactericidal or bacteriostatic. Bacteriostatic antibiotics inhibit growth and multiplication of bacterial cells, without killing them, but allow host factors to eliminate the pathogen. Bactericidal antibiotics kill and sometimes lyse the cells. For certain infections (e.g. endocarditis, severe sepsis, infections in immune-compromised patients), a bactericidal drug is essential. However, an antibiotic that is primarily bactericidal may not reach sufficient concentrations to cause adequate killing of bacteria if given in an inadequate dose. It is therefore important that the antibiotic is given in a dose that ensures a bactericidal concentration.

Antibiotics can also be classified according to the mechanism by which they interfere with the cellular or biochemical pathways of the pathogen.

INHIBITION OF CELL WALL SYNTHESIS

The cell wall of most bacteria contains peptidoglycan, which is largely responsible for protecting the cell against osmotic damage. The peptidoglycan molecule consists of a glycan (sugar) portion composed of repeating alternating units of two amino sugars crosslinked by short peptide chains. These crosslinks are essential for the structural integrity of the wall. Penicillins prevent the formation of the crosslinks, resulting in cells with defective walls that are susceptible to osmotic damage

---

Summary box 23.1 Classification of antibiotics according to bactericidal or bacteriostatic activity

Bactericidal	Bacteriostatic
• Penicillins	• Tetracyclines
• Cephalosporins	• Chloramphenicol
• Cephamycins	• Clindamycin
• Aminoglycosides	• Sulphonamides
• Glycopeptides	• Trimethoprim
• Polymixins	• Macrolides
• Bacitracin	
• Monobactams	
• Carbapenems	

(Fig. 23.1). The cell wall of Gram-positive bacteria is a relatively simple structure, whereas that of Gram-negative bacteria is much more complex, with an outer membrane. Endotoxin, derived from this outer membrane, is responsible for many of the signs and symptoms of infection and sepsis. This complex wall is difficult for many antibiotics, such as some penicillins and the macrolides, to penetrate, which explains why they are less active against Gram-negative organisms.

β-Lactam antibiotics

The β-lactam antibiotics, which include the penicillins, cephalosporins, monobactams and the carbapenems, are named after the β-lactam ring by which they bind to the target molecule (Fig. 23.2). The β-lactams bind

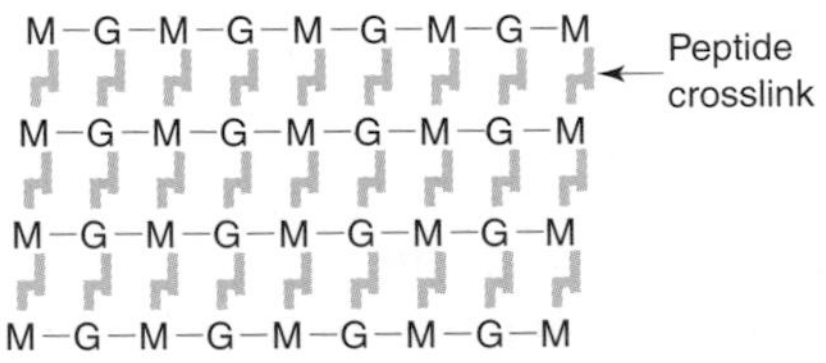

Fig. 23.1 The peptidoglycan molecule, an essential element in the bacterial cell wall, consists of repeating alternating units of the amino sugars N-acetylglucosamine (G) and N-acetylmuramic acid (M), connected by short peptide crosslinks. Penicillins and cephalosporins inhibit the formation of these crosslinks, leading to cell wall disruption.

Summary box 23.2 Classification of antibiotics based on their mechanisms of antibacterial action

Inhibition of cell wall synthesis

- Penicillins
- Cephalosporins
- Cephamycins
- Carbapenems
- Monobactams
- Glycopeptides
- Bacitracin

Inhibition of protein synthesis

- Tetracyclines
- Macrolides
- Aminoglycosides
- Chloramphenicol
- Clindamycin

Inhibition of DNA topoisomerase II

- Fluoroquinolones

Bacterial folate antagonists

- Sulphonamides
- Trimethoprim

penetrate the cell wall. Resistance against β-lactam antibiotics is due mainly to degradation by bacterial β-lactamase.

The pharmacokinetics of many of the β-lactams have much in common.[1] Characteristically the volume of distribution is small, since these substances remain extracellular. Elimination is mostly by the renal route, both by glomerular filtration and active tubular excretion. There are, however, large differences in the extent of tubular excretion, and also in plasma protein binding, leading to marked differences in elimination half-lives (Table 23.1). However, most β-lactams have half-lives shorter than 1–2 h, one notable exception being ceftriaxone, and to a lesser extent cephazolin. In the choroid plexus there is active transport out of the cerebrospinal fluid (CSF), keeping the ratio between CSF and plasma concentrations low. The same holds for the vitreous body of the eye. Probenecid inhibits this transport, and is used to increase the concentration ratio.

Although the mode of action of β-lactams would imply that they are not toxic for humans, they are not altogether harmless. High concentrations of benzylpenicillin and carbenicillin can impair haemostasis, and very high concentrations of penicillins can cause convulsions. Because of the risk of convulsions penicillins, and particularly benzylpenicillin, should not be given intrathecally. β-Lactam antibiotics often give rise to immunological side-effects, due to degradation products forming antigenic complexes with host proteins. In addition to rashes, which are usually innocuous and do not always necessitate discontinuation of the drug, some, in particular flucloxacillin, occasionally cause interstitial nephritis and hepatitis. Much more serious is acute anaphylactic shock in a sensitized patient. Within the group of penicillins there is always cross-allergy, and

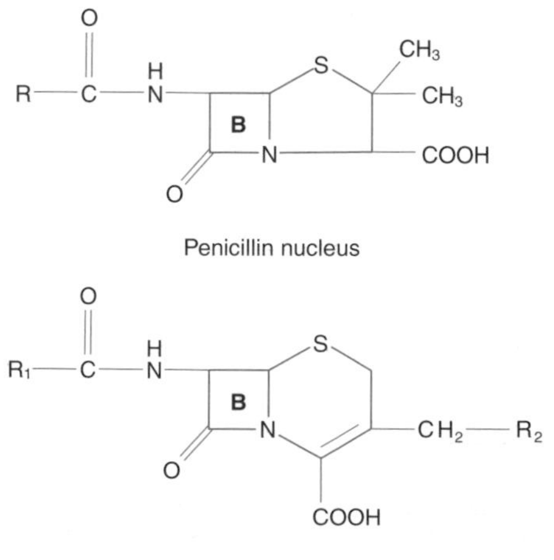

covalently (irreversibly) to penicillin-binding proteins (PBPs), which are involved in transpeptidase reactions responsible for forming crosslinks in the peptidoglycan molecules of bacterial cell walls. Inactivation of PBPs leads to the production of a defective cell wall, cell disruption. These agents are most active against growing bacteria. In situations where the bacteria do not rapidly proliferate (e.g. chronic infections), or if they are combined with antibiotics that inhibit bacterial growth, β-lactam antibiotics are much less active. Although the maximal killing efficacy between the numerous β-lactam antibiotics is similar, there are important differences in their resistance to enzymatic degradation, in intrinsic activity and in their ability to

Fig. 23.2 Molecular structure of β-lactam antibiotics. The common structure (B) is the β-lactam ring.

the same probably holds for cephalosporins. There is no cross-allergy between monobactams, carbapenems and other β-lactams, and little, if any, between penicillins and cephalosporins. Because of possible side-effects the concentration should not be higher than necessary. Since the maximum killing efficacy is obtained at

Table 23.1 Pharmacokinetic parameters of antibiotics (values given are approximate)				
	Half-life (h)	Protein binding (%)	Volume of distribution (l kg^{-1})	Renal elimination (%)
Amoxycillin	1.5	20	0.30	75
Benzylpenicillin	0.5	60	0.30	70
Flucloxacillin	0.8	95	0.30	75
Piperacillin	1.0	20	0.30	80
Cefuroxime	1.5	30	0.17	95
Cefamandole	1.0	70	0.25	80
Ceftazidime	2.0	10	0.20	100
Ceftriaxone	6–9	95	0.15	50
Imipenem	1	25	0.20	70
Meropenem	1	15	0.30	70
Vancomycin	6	50	0.70	95
Teicoplanin	60	90	0.60	95
Erythromycin	1.5	70	0.75	10
Clarithromycin				
Clindamycin	2.5	90	1	10
Gentamicin	2.5	0	0.25	100
Netilmicin	2.5	0	0.25	100
Amikacin	2.5	0	0.25	100
Tobramycin	2.5	0	0.25	100
Doxycycline	18	90	1.6	25
Rifampicin	4	70	1.5	20
Ciprofloxacin	4	30	2.5	60

concentrations only slightly higher than the MIC, higher concentrations are not more effective and are potentially harmful. Continuous administration is more effective than intermittent doses, since most β-lactam antibiotics have short half-lives.[2]

Penicillins

The oldest penicillin is benzylpenicillin, which still is one of the most potent antibiotics against Gram-positive and Gram-negative cocci, and against anaerobes. Its shortcomings are poor penetration in Gram-negative bacteria, but above all its sensitivity to enzymatic degradation. The tubular excretory mechanism is very effective for benzylpenicillin, but is saturable so that at very high concentrations the clearance decreases.

Nafcillin, methicillin, oxacillin, cloxacillin and flu-cloxacillin are mainly active against Gram-positive cocci, less so than benzylpenicillin, but they are resistant to enzymatic breakdown by those organisms. However, resistance of *Staphylococcus aureus* and coagulase-negative staphylococci has emerged, not due to enzymatic breakdown but to an altered target molecule.

Ampicillin was the first penicillin with good activity against Gram-negative bacteria. It has been largely replaced by amoxicillin, which has better oral absorption. Both antibiotics are subject to degradation by β-lactamase, and amoxicillin is often combined with clavulanic acid, in co-amoxiclav. The combination with clavulanic acid increases the otherwise very low risk of hepatitis. Amoxicillin and ampicillin often give rise to a typical rash, which usually appears after about 1 week of treatment. This is seldom due to true penicillin allergy.

Piperacillin is a penicillin with a much broader spectrum than the older ones, active against Gram-positive and Gram-negative aerobic and anaerobic bacteria. It is somewhat resistant to the action of β-lactamases, although it is also combined with tazobactam, another β-lactamase inhibitor.

Cephalosporins and Cephamycins

The development of the cephalosporins began with the observation that cultures of a cephalosporinium fungus obtained from the sea in the vicinity of a sewer outlet in Sardinia inhibited the growth of *S. aureus*. The closely related cephamycins are produced by *Streptomyces* fungi. A large number of semisynthetic broad-spectrum cephalosporins has been produced by alterations to the basic cephalosporin nucleus (Fig. 23.2). The cephalosporins are water soluble and acid resistant. Some are effective if given orally (e.g. cephalexin), but many can be administered only parenterally. Intramuscular injection of some agents can be painful. Like the penicillins, they have varying susceptibility to β-lactamase. However, they are generally more β-lactamase stable than penicillins since the cephalosporin structure is more resistant to this enzyme. Closely related antibiotics are the cephamycins such as latamoxef. The first-generation cephalosporins, such as cephalexin and cephazolin, which are seldom used, and those of a latter generation, cefuroxime and cefamandole, have an extended spectrum against Gram-positive and Gram-negative aerobic bacteria. Newer cephalosporins, like ceftazidime and ceftriaxone, are more potent against Gram-negative bacteria and are also more β-lactamase resistant. Their intrinsic activity against Gram-positive bacteria, however, is much less than that of the penicillins and even the older cephalosporins.

Although they are widely distributed within the body only a few (e.g. cefuroxime, cefotaxime, latamoxef) reach therapeutic concentrations in the CSF,[3] and are used to treat meningitis due to Gram-negative intestinal bacteria. The excretion of the cephalosporins is mainly renal but some, such as ceftriaxone, are also excreted in the bile. Ceftazidime is eliminated only by glomerular filtration and not by tubular excretion, but since it is poorly protein bound its half-life is still relatively short, about 2 h. Ceftriaxone is also excreted only by glomerular filtration but, because it is highly protein bound, its half-life is long, 6–9 h, which gives a more extended concentration profile than for other β-lactams. The toxicity profile of the cephalosporins is broadly similar to that of the penicillins.

Carbapenems and Monobactams

These drugs were developed in response to β-lactamase-producing Gram-negative bacteria that were resistant to broad-spectrum penicillins. Carbapenems such as imipenem and meropenem have high intrinsic activity against most bacteria, both aerobic and anaerobic, and they are very resistant to β-lactamases. Both drugs are eliminated by the kideys. Imipenem, but not meropenem, undergoes hydrolysis by dihydropeptidase in the renal tubule to nephrotoxic products, and therefore it is combined with cilastatin, a specific inhibitor of this enzyme. The combination has some neurotoxic potential, which meropenem lacks. Imipenem is not absorbed orally because of its instability at gastric pH, and is given intravenously.

Aztreonam, the main monobactam, is a simple monocyclic β-lactam resistant to most β-lactamases. Like imipenem, it is not absorbed orally and is given parenterally. Its action is by binding to PBPs in the cell wall. However, it does not bind to the PBPs of Gram-positive or anaerobic bacteria. It thus has a very limited spectrum, being active only against Gram-negative aerobic rods.

β-Lactamase inhibitors

Clavulanic acid, sulbactam and tazobactam are drugs that inhibit β-lactamase by irreversibly inactivating it.

Clavulanic acid is a naturally occurring substance which was isolated from *Streptomyces clavuligerus*. It contains a β-lactam ring but has only minimal antibiotic activity since it binds only poorly to the penicillin-binding protein of most species. It binds irreversibly to serine at the active site of β-lactamase, inactivating the enzyme. β-Lactamases differ in their susceptibility to inhibition by clavulanic acid. Among those readily inhibited are staphylococcal β-lactamase and plasmid-mediated enzymes. However, clavulanic acid does not inhibit chromosomal-mediated β-lactamase produced by *Pseudomonas* or *Enterobacter*. Sulbactam and tazobactam are penicillanic acid derivatives with weak bactericidal activity. Both inhibit the same β-lactamases as clavulanic acid but are two to five times less potent. Combination of these drugs with lactamase-sensitive penicillins such as ampicillin results in reductions in MIC by 10 up to several hundredfold. β-Lactamase inhibitors appear to be free of serious side-effects.

Glycopeptides

Vancomycin and teicoplanin are the main antibiotics in this group. The mechanism of inhibition of cell wall synthesis is different from that of the β-lactams. The glycopeptides block the transport of cell wall molecule precursors over the cell membrane. They are bactericidal to Gram-positive cocci, but much less to Gram-negative cocci since they penetrate the outer membrane of Gram-negative species only with difficulty. Vancomycin is not absorbed from the gastrointestinal tract and is given orally only for treatment of intestinal infections. It is effective mainly against Gram-positive organisms, including methicillin-resistant staphylococci. Vancomycin has a half-life of about 6 h. At the usual dose of 2 g daily, divided in two or four doses, the concentration is continuously well above the MIC for most Gram-positive cocci. This is a relatively high dose compared with the usual dose of β-lactams, and therefore is also sufficient for the treatment of endocarditis. Vancomycin is eliminated by glomerular filtration and the dose has to be adjusted in patients with renal dysfunction, to avoid renal toxicity and ototoxicity. Nephrotoxicity is uncommon when the drug is used alone but the risk may be increased when it is combined with other nephrotoxic drugs. Vancomycin is not removed by haemodialysis or peritoneal dialysis. Rapid intravenous administration can cause histamine release, and therefore vancomycin should be infused over at least 30 min. Intravenous administration can cause phlebitis.

Teicoplanin has somewhat lower intrinsic activity than vancomycin, but is much better tolerated. Like vancomycin, it must be given parenterally. Since it distributes over a large deep compartment, administration is twice daily for the first day and then once daily. At steady state the half-life may exceed 24 h. Also,

because of the extensive plasma protein binding, the total plasma concentration should be considerably higher than that of vancomycin to achieve the same effect. Renal and ototoxicity is less than that of vancomycin.

Bacitracin is a polypeptide bacterial antibiotic which inhibits cell wall synthesis by interfering with the dephosphorylation of the lipid carrier that moves cell wall components through the cell membrane. It has a range of activity similar to that of penicillin, but because of serious renal toxicity is only used topically.

INHIBITION OF PROTEIN SYNTHESIS

Several groups of antibiotics bind to bacterial ribosomes and thereby inhibit protein synthesis. Chloramphenicol, tetracyclines and macrolides do so reversibly, and therefore are essentially bacteriostatic, whereas aminoglycosides bind irreversibly and thus are bactericidal. Although chloramphenicol does not bind to human ribosomes, it does inhibit mitochondrial protein synthesis in humans. This causes a moderate dose-dependent inhibition of haematopoiesis, but in short courses of treatment this is of little clinical consequence. However, in rare instances irreversible aplastic anaemia may occur, which is not dose dependent. For this reason, chloramphenicol is seldom used.

Tetracyclines

Tetracyclines are selectively accumulated in the bacterial cell but less in the human cell. They have a broad antibacterial spectrum and are also effective against other microorganisms such as *Rickettsia*, *Mycoplasma* and *Chlamydia*. Because of this broad spectrum their use may result in disturbance of the intestinal flora and overgrowth by resistant fungi. The most widely used tetracycline, doxycycline, has a long half-life of about 20 h. The untoward effects of tetracyclines are mainly due to their chelating properties with metallic ions, by which they bind to growing bone and teeth. This results in brown-yellow discoloration of the teeth. Binding to bone may lead to depression of skeletal growth, especially in premature infants. They are therefore contraindicated in pregnant women and children. Hepatic toxicity can occur, and is more likely with parenteral administration. Pregnant women are highly susceptible to tetracycline-induced hepatotoxicity.

Macrolides

The term 'macrolide' derives from the structure of these antibiotics: a many-membered lactone ring to which sugar groups are attached. Macrolides, of which erythromycin is the prototype, have their greatest activity against Gram-positive cocci, but also are effective against various other bacteria. The bacteriostatic effect is concentration dependent and reversible. In particu-

lar with Gram-positive cocci, the bacteriostatic effect persists for some time after the antibiotic has been stopped. The half-life of erythromycin is about 4 h; that of other macrolides is often longer.[4,5] Elimination is partly renal, partly hepatic. Gastrointestinal intolerance for erythromycin, due to a direct pharmacological effect on gastrointestinal motility, is its greatest disadvantage. Erythromycin is a potent inhibitor of the hepatic cytochrome P450 enzymes responsible for the metabolism of drugs such as alfentanil, midazolam and theophylline.[6–10] This can result in reduced clearance of these drugs, higher than expected plasma concentrations, and potentially adverse effects. In recommended doses other macrolides have a better gastrointestinal tolerance as well as less inhibition of hepatic drug metabolism.

Clindamycin and lincomycin do not have a macrolide structure, but the mechanism of their antibacterial action is similar. Clindamycin is active against Gram-positive cocci and also against anaerobic bacteria, such as *Bacteroides* and most *Clostridium* species. However, clindamycin is relatively often associated with the emergence of a particular *Clostridium* species (*C. difficile*) in the gut, leading to toxic forms of colitis. It lacks the effect of the macrolides on gastric motility and on drug metabolism.

Aminoglycosides

The main aminoglycosides are gentamicin, streptomycin, amikacin, tobramycin, kanamycin, netilmicin, neomycin and framycetin. They have a complex chemical structure consisting of amino sugars linked through glycosidic bonds to an aminocyclitol ring. They must enter the bacterial cell, where they inhibit protein synthesis by binding to ribosomes to restrict polysome formation and cause misreading of messenger ribonucleic acid (mRNA). Aminoglycosides are strongly bactericidal for a wide range of bacteria, although much more so for Gram-negative than for Gram-positive bacteria. In some instances their efficacy is increased by combination with β-lactam antibiotics, probably because this increases their penetration through the bacterial cell wall. They are highly polar substances and need an active uptake mechanism over the bacterial cell membrane. This oxygen-dependent transport system is absent in anaerobic bacteria and thus the aminoglycosides are not active against anaerobes. They are not absorbed after oral administration. Elimination is solely by glomerular filtration. Their volume of distribution equals the extracellular water space. Because of this and their toxicity, the dose should be adjusted according to renal function, and plasma concentrations should be monitored.

Although their mode of action on the ribosome is highly selective, the toxicity of the aminoglycosides is considerable because of an active uptake mechanism in the proximal tubular cells in the kidney, where they

accumulate. This trapping inside the cell leads to cell death. The toxicity for cochlear and vestibular hair cells is probably due to a similar mechanism. In the kidney the toxicity is reversible because of the formation of new cells, but in the cochlea and the vestibulum it is largely irreversible. The uptake mechanism is saturable, whereas the antibacterial effect is concentration dependent over a large range. Therefore, the therapeutic index is greater at high concentrations than at low concentrations. For this reason infrequent high doses are preferred to frequent low doses. Aminoglycosides may cause a nondepolarizing type of neuromuscular block of skeletal muscle by inhibiting the presynaptic release of acetylcholine and by blocking postjunctional receptor sites. At therapeutic doses this leads to complications only in patients with myasthenia gravis or in combination with nondepolarizing muscle relaxants.

INHIBITION OF BACTERIAL TOPOISOMERASE II

Fluoroquinolones

The fluoroquinolones are synthetic antibiotics that include the broad-spectrum ciprofloxacin, ofloxacin, norfloxacin and pefloxacin and the narrow-spectrum drugs cinoxacin and nalidixic acid used in urinary tract infections. Fluoroquinolones inhibit bacterial DNA topoisomerase II (DNA gyrase), an enzyme that catalyses the supercoiling of bacterial circular DNA, permitting transcription and replication. This enzyme does not occur in humans. Fluoroquinolones are well absorbed after oral administration, although absorption is impeded by metal cations present in aluminium and magnesium antacids. They are broad-spectrum antibiotics, especially active against Gram-negative organisms such as *Pseudomonas aeruginosa*. Apart from gastrointestinal side-effects, their most important toxicity involves the central nervous system (CNS), possibly by competition with γ-aminobutyric acid. The most important of the CNS side-effects, although rare, is seizures. Thus fluoroquinolones are relatively contraindicated in patients with epilepsy.

INTERFERENCE WITH THE SYNTHESIS OF BACTERIAL FOLATE

Folate is essential for the synthesis of precursors of DNA and RNA in both bacteria and mammals, but, whereas mammals obtain folic acid from dietary sources, bacteria must synthesize it. Sulphonamides and trimethoprim inhibit this synthesis, thereby inhibiting bacterial growth. These antibiotics are thus bacteriostatic. Their action can be negated by pus or tissue breakdown products that contain thymidine and purines which the bacteria can use to bypass the need for folic acid.

Sulphonamides, the first antibacterial drugs, compete with the *p*-aminobezoic acid moiety in folic acid for an enzyme involved in the synthesis of purine nucleotides. Most sulphonamides are readily absorbed from the gastrointestinal tract and reach maximum plasma concentrations within 4–6 h. Minor side-effects include nausea and vomiting, and mental depression. Methaemoglobinaemia may occur and present as cyanosis. More serious adverse effects include hepatitis, hypersensitivity reactions and bone marrow depression.

Trimethoprim has a structure that sufficiently resembles the pteridine moiety of folate to confuse bacterial enzymes. It is active against most bacterial pathogens. It is fully absorbed from the gastrointestinal tract and widely distributed within the body. Trimethoprim and sulphonamides block consecutive stages of folate synthesis, act synergistically, and the combination of the two drugs is bactericidal. Co-trimoxazole is a mixture of trimethoprim and sulphamethoxazole.

ANTITUBERCULOSIS DRUGS

Rifampicin
Rifampicin inhibits bacterial DNA-dependent RNA polymerase, thereby blocking protein synthesis and eventually causing cell death. Rifampicin is rapidly bactericidal at very low concentrations for Gram-positive bacteria, *Neisseria meningitidis* and *Haemophilus influenzae*. Moreover, it is the most active cidal drug against *M. tuberculosis*. Because of the rapid development of resistance, due to the emergence of an altered RNA polymerase, rifampicin is practically useless for even short-term treatment of most bacterial infections, but it is very useful for the eradication of *N. meningitidis* in carriers. Its most important use is in the treatment of tuberculosis, always together with a second antituberculous drug, such as isoniazid, to prevent the emergence of resistance. The half-life of rifampicin is variable, from 1 to 6 h. For the treatment of tuberculosis, however, it is given once daily, since *M. tuberculosis* reproduces very slowly. Its absorption is considerably impaired by food. Rifampicin is a potent inducer of hepatic cytochrome P450 activity, thus enhancing the metabolism of other drugs, such as corticosteroids, oral contraceptives and midazolam. The risk of hepatotoxicity of halothane may be enhanced by the same mechanism.

Isoniazid
Isoniazid is limited to the treatment of mycobacterial infections, and is the primary agent for tuberculosis. It is bacteriostatic on resting organisms but can kill multiplying bacteria. The mechanism of its action is unknown. Isoniazid is readily absorbed from the gastrointestinal tract and enters most body compartments and cells. It is thus effective against intracellular bacilli. It is

also actively taken up by tubercle bacilli. In individuals with glucose-6-phosphate deficiency it may cause haemolytic anaemia. It is a cytochrome P450 enzyme inhibitor and decreases the metabolism of a number of drugs, especially antiepileptics such as phenytoin and carbamazepine.

Other drugs used in the treatment of tuberculosis include ethambutol, pyrazinamide, capreomycin, streptomycin and cycloserine. To avoid the emergence of resistant organisms, two or even three antituberculosis drugs are commonly combined.

ANTIFUNGAL DRUGS

In this section only those antifungal agents will be discussed that are used in the treatment of invasive fungal infections. The occurrence of this type of infection has increased steadily over the years since they are typically opportunistic infections in immunocompromised patients. In these patients, therapeutic results are far from favourable. Moreover, in comparison with antibacterial agents, the toxicity of antifungal drugs is much less selective. Therefore, dosage schedules are empiric, and limited by toxic manifestations.

Polyenes
The oldest known antifungal drug belonging to this group is amphotericin B. Nystatin and natamycin are also polyenes, but they are more toxic, and therefore amphotericin B is the only polyene used in the systemic treatment of fungal infections. These drugs are called polyenes because they contain multiple double bonds in a macrolide structure. Due to these double bonds, polyenes bind to ergosterol in the fungal cell membrane. This leads to increased membrane permeability, leakage of potassium and, at high concentrations, cell death. Polyenes are more toxic to fungal cells than to mammalian cells because cholesterol is the main constituent of mammalian cell membranes, and the affinity for cholesterol is less than that for ergosterol. The therapeutic window of amphotericin B is narrow, and clinical toxicity is due mainly to the same mechanism as in fungal cells: renal toxicity, leading to tubular acidosis, potassium loss and decreased glomerular filtration rate. The duration of treatment is therefore limited to less than 6 weeks. Amphotericin B is poorly absorbed when given orally, and for systemic infections it is given intravenously as a colloid suspension since it is insoluble in water. Apart from organ toxicity, infusion of the colloidal suspension causes fever, chills and phlebitis. For this reason hydrocortisone is routinely added to the infusion, and pethidine may be administered to prevent chills in patients who suffer from them. In recent years new administration forms have been developed, such as liposomal preparations, which are better tolerated and less

toxic than the standard colloidal suspension. Amphotericin B is eliminated slowly from the body, if at all, which is an important reason for limiting the duration of treatment. Monitoring of serum concentrations is not useful, since there is no known relation between concentrations and either toxicity or efficacy.

5-Fluorocytosine

5-Fluorocytosine (5-FC) is taken up selectively by fungal cells where it is converted to 5-fluorouracil, an antitumour drug that interferes with RNA synthesis. This is the mechanism of its clinical toxicity, bone marrow depression, although this occurs mainly at higher concentrations, above 100 mg l^{-1}. Serum concentrations should, therefore, be monitored. Fungal cells may become rapidly resistant and therefore 5-FC is used only in combination with other antifungal agents, in particular amphotericin B. In some cases it may improve the efficacy of amphotericin B. Since 5-FC is eliminated exclusively by the kidney, the dose should be adjusted in patients with decreased renal function.

Azole derivatives

Azole derivatives are the imidazoles and the triazoles. For invasive fungal infections, the most widely used drugs are the triazoles, fluconazole and itraconazole. The triazoles contain one or more five-membered rings with three nitrogens. All azoles interfere with the ergosterol synthesis by the fungal cell, leading to increased membrane permeability. In contrast to amphotericin B, however, they are not fungicidal. Nevertheless, in many fungal infections their clinical efficacy is similar to that of amphotericin B, and they are much better tolerated and much less toxic. At high concentrations the azoles also inhibit cholesterol synthesis; because of this, high doses of the imidazole, ketoconazole, are used in the treatment of adrenal tumours. At therapeutic doses fluconazole and, in particular, itraconazole inhibit cytochrome P450 enzymes. The only azole that can be administered intravenously is fluconazole, but all azoles are absorbed well after oral administration. However, for some, in particular ketoconazole and itraconazole, gastric acidity is a condition for good absorption, and antacids can greatly impede absorption.

ANTIVIRAL DRUGS

Antiviral drugs can be grouped in three categories according to their mode of action: DNA polymerase inhibitors, reverse transcriptase inhibitors, and protease inhibitors. The last two types are used in the treatment of human immunodeficiency virus (HIV) infection. DNA polymerase inhibitors are used for the treatment of herpes virus infections.

DNA POLYMERASE INHIBITORS

Aciclovir is the oldest member of this group currently in use. Older drugs such as cytarabine and vidarabine were very toxic and lacked the selectivity that made aciclovir a real breakthrough in antiviral therapy. Selectivity, similar to that of antibacterial drugs, is a hallmark of all the related acyclic guanosine derivatives: ganciclovir, penciclovir, famciclovir and valaciclovir. Aciclovir enters cells infected by herpes virus by diffusion, where it is converted by a viral enzyme, thymidine kinase, to aciclovir monophosphate. It is subsequently converted to aciclovir triphosphate by host cell kinases, which cannot diffuse freely across the cell membrane, so that aciclovir accumulates in infected cells to a far greater extent than in noninfected cells. Aciclovir triphosphate is used by viral DNA polymerase as a false substrate for DNA synthesis, with the consequence that DNA synthesis stops and DNA polymerase is blocked for further use. The selectivity of the drug is thus due to the selective accumulation in infected cells as well as the much higher affinity of the triphosphate for viral than for human DNA polymerase. Foscarnet, a pyrophosphate analogue and DNA polymerase inhibitor, differs from the acyclic guanosine derivatives in that the drug need not be phosphorylated to become active.

Resistance to acyclic guanosine derivatives occurs typically in patients with acquired immune deficiency syndrome receiving prolonged treatment. In most cases resistance is due to mutations in the thymidine kinase, with the effect that the drug is not phosphorylated. Because foscarnet does not need to be phosphorylated, it is active against herpes viruses resistant to aciclovir and related compounds. A less frequent cause of resistance is mutation of viral DNA polymerase.

Aciclovir is indicated for infections by herpes simplex virus and varicella zoster virus. Valaciclovir is a prodrug of aciclovir with better oral absorption than aciclovir. Famciclovir is a prodrug of penciclovir and is used for the same indications. Ganciclovir is specifically used for the treatment of infections by cytomegalovirus. Foscarnet is used as an alternative drug in cases of resistance against acyclic guanosines. It is effective against herpes simplex virus, varicella zoster virus and cytomegalovirus.

Aciclovir is well tolerated and has few side-effects. It should be administered with an ample amount of fluid to prevent impairment of renal function and phlebitis at the site of injection. The most important side-effect of ganciclovir is bone marrow suppression leading to granulocytopenia and thrombocytopenia. Both aciclovir and ganciclovir can cause neurological symptoms such as depressed consciousness, confusion and delirium. The most important side-effects of foscarnet are hypocalcaemia or hypercalcaemia, hypophosphataemia or hyperphosphataemia, headache, epileptic insults, anaemia and neutropenia.

Aciclovir, ganciclovir and foscarnet are excreted mainly by the kidneys. Therefore, the dosage should be adjusted according to renal function. Aciclovir is poorly absorbed after oral administration, but for this purpose the prodrug valaciclovir has been developed, with a bioavailability of about 50%; famciclovir is likewise well absorbed with a bioavailability of about 75%. Ganciclovir is available in an oral formulation but gastrointestinal uptake of the drug is limited.

REVERSE TRANSCRIPTASE INHIBITORS

To this group belong the nucleoside derivatives zidovudine, lamivudine, didanosine, zalcitabine, stavudine and the non-nucleoside compound nevirapine. Their common mode of action is the inhibition of the viral enzyme reverse transcriptase. This enzyme is essential for the synthesis of DNA from the viral RNA as it enters the cell. Like aciclovir and related drugs, the nucleoside derivatives have to be phosphorylated intracellularly. Important side-effects are bone marrow depression (zidovudine, didanosine), peripheral neuropathy (lamivudine, zalcitabine, didanosine, stavudine), pancreatitis (lamivudine, zalcitabine, didanosine), myopathy (zidovudine) and hepatitis (nevirapine). A problem with antiviral therapy of HIV infections is that the virus readily becomes resistant to the drugs. This has led to combination therapy, typically two nucleoside derivatives (e.g. zidovudine and stavudine) and a protease inhibitor, for example indinavir.

PROTEASE INHIBITORS

HIV proteins are synthesized as one long chain of amino acids, which is split into single proteins by a viral proteinase, which is the target for the proteinase inhibitors. Several proteinase inhibitors are now available – saquinavir, ritonavir and indinavir – and others are under development. The proteinase inhibitors are very effective drugs, but HIV becomes readily resistant, so that they are preferably used in combination with other anti-HIV drugs. Ritonavir is a drug with many side-effects (hypertriglyceridaemia, paraesthesia, diarrhoea) and interactions with many other drugs. The most important side-effects of indinavir are nephrolithiasis and hyperbilirubinaemia. The presently available formulation of saquinavir is not optimal because of a low bioavailability.

TREATMENT AND PROPHYLAXIS OF INFECTION

The management of upper respiratory tract infections such as otitis media in children and chronic bronchitis illustrate the principles mentioned in the introduction to this chapter. Otitis is a very painful condition that can be alleviated immediately by paracentesis, but this probably does not influence the final course of the disease or the risk of complications. Antibiotic treatment instead of paracentesis is much debated, but in the end it is probably as good as paracentesis, with the exception of alleviating pain. In chronic bronchitis the bronchial mucosa is permanently damaged and bronchial secretions cannot be eliminated sufficiently. Intercurrent viral infections can lead to bacterial invasion, often with *H. influenzae*. Except in a relatively small group of seriously ill patients, it has not been proven that treatment with antibiotics alters the course of the disease.

Soft tissue infections and infections of bones and joints may be treated by a combination of surgery and antibiotics. Sometimes surgery is sufficient, for example in superficial abscesses, but a complete cure of osteomyelitis often requires the combination of surgery and antibiotics. However, acute osteomyelitis in children can be cured by antibiotics alone, if they are given for sufficiently long periods and at sufficiently high doses. Bacterial endocarditis also requires prolonged antibiotic therapy, for up to 6 weeks, although for some causative microorganisms the use of specific antibiotic combinations may be shortened to 4 weeks, or sometimes even 2 weeks. Treatment of right-sided endocarditis does not need as long a treatment as left-sided endocarditis.

Because of the serious consequences of infections of the CNS, they invariably need to be treated with antimicrobial drugs. This holds not only for bacterial infections, but also for fungal and some viral infections. For the treatment of these infections, important pharmacokinetic aspects have to be considered. Many antibacterial drugs, in particular β-lactam antibiotics and aminoglycosides, are not lipophilic enough to pass easily across the blood–brain barrier into brain tissue and CSF. On the other hand, the majority of β-lactam antibiotics are actively transported out of the CSF. In cases of acute bacterial meningitis, the inflamed meninges are much more permeable and adequate concentrations at the site of infection can easily be obtained, provided sufficiently high doses are given. Low-grade meningitis poses much more difficulty in this respect (e.g. secondary meningitis after neurosurgery). In these cases it is sometimes advisable to block the transport mechanism for β-lactams with probenecid. A viral infection of the CNS that can be treated successfully is herpes simplex encephalitis. This is a serious and often fatal disease, the prognosis of which has improved considerably by treatment with aciclovir.

CHOICE OF ANTIBIOTIC BASED ON PATHOGENS

The correct choice of an antibiotic is based not only on the type of infection but also on the causative micro-organism. In choosing an antibiotic the pharmaco-dynamic and pharmacokinetic characteristics of the drug should be taken into account. Ideally it should be the most active antibiotic against the pathogen and the least toxic for the patient. For this reason the first choice is often a β-lactam antibiotic. In the recommended dose those antibiotics generally exert their maximum effect as long as the unbound plasma concentration is higher than the MIC. However, there is not much difference in the maximum effect between the various β-lactam antibiotics. Sensitivity will thus depend to a large extent on bacterial resistance mechanisms, in particular β-lactamase production.

In several countries S. aureus may be methicillin resistant, which implies that it is not only resistant to benzylpenicillin and amoxicillin by β-lactamase pro-duction, but also to nafcillin and flucloxacillin, due to insensitivity of the receptor. Infections with this type of staphylococcus should be treated with vancomycin or teicoplanin. The same holds for infections with coagulase-negative staphylococci (e.g. S. epidermidis), of which a substantial proportion is methicillin resistant. For the empirical treatment of life-threatening infec-tions with S. aureus, the choice between a penicillin and a glycopeptide therefore depends on the a priori risk of methicillin resistance. Infections with coagulase-negative staphylococci are nearly always foreign-body related, and seldom immediately life threatening. Re-moval of the foreign body is the most efficient treatment, without the need for antibiotics. If this is not feasible, for instance in the case of cardiac valve pros-thesis, long-term treatment with antibiotics is inevit-able, but often not successful.

COMBINATION OF ANTIBIOTICS

The most obvious reason to combine antibiotics is to broaden the spectrum in empirical treatment. This reason is no longer valid when the results of bac-teriological tests become available, and therefore it is good practice to revert to a single drug if possible. However, in some situations combination of antibi-otics does increase the potency. A good example is co-trimoxazole, which is much more potent against Gram-negative microorganisms than its single constitu-ents, sulphamethoxazole and trimethoprim. Also the combination of benzylpenicillin and an aminoglycoside has a greater bactericidal effect against enterococci than either antibiotic alone.

ANTIBIOTIC PROPHYLAXIS

For antibiotic prophylaxis the same principles hold as for treatment. Prophylaxis is intended to prevent in-fections, so there should be a realistic probability that infections will occur in the absence of antibiotic admini-stration. For instance, it has become evident that some types of abdominal surgery carry a considerable risk for wound infections, and it has been shown that antibiotic prophylaxis reduces this risk. Probably the most impor-tant consideration, however, should be whether preven-tion of infection in a number of cases is better than early treatment of infection if it occurs. A good example is prophylaxis for implantation of prosthetic joints or heart valves, where the risk for infection may be low but treat-ment of infection is extremely difficult and often neces-sitates removal of the prosthesis. However, unnecessary prophylaxis is a significant contributor to the emer-gence of antibiotic resistance. It is, therefore, essential that hospitals develop antibiotic policies that give strict indications for prophylaxis.

To prevent wound infections after surgery in con-taminated areas (e.g. abdominal surgery), it is manda-tory that the tissue concentration is maximal at the time of surgery; therefore the antibiotics should be given within 30 min before operation. If this is carried out properly, continuation of administration probably does not decrease the proportion of wound infection further. A second dose is usually indicated only for long procedures. The choice of antibiotics is determined by the microorganism that causes wound infections (i.e. staphylococci and streptococci), and in abdominal surgery also aerobic Gram-negative and anaerobic microorganisms. For neurosurgical operations the risk of infection is primarily from skin bacteria, and flu-cloxacillin is effective. The same holds for prosthetic valve implantation and prosthetic joints, for which staphylococcal infections are the most prominent.

Prophylaxis against bacterial endocarditis is given if surgical or dental procedures can give rise to bac-teraemia with microorganisms that are prone to cause endocarditis. For natural heart valves these are mainly Streptococcus viridans, but for artificial valves other microorganisms may be potentially harmful. Antibiotic administration has to be prolonged, since there should be sustained antibacterial concentrations in the blood to enable the body to clear the circulating bacteria. For the β-lactam antibiotics this goal is obtained either by re-peating administration 6 h after the procedure or by giv-ing a depot preparation or a single very high dose.

For patients being treated with cytotoxic drugs a different approach is often taken. Since the source of infection is often endogenous microflora, selective gastrointestinal decontamination may be used with oral, preferably nonabsorbable, antibiotics with activity against aerobic Gram-negative microorganisms (e.g. an aminoglycoside such as neomycin). This leaves the anaerobic microorganisms undisturbed, guaranteeing a barrier against secondary colonization by exogenous aerobic microorganisms. To this is added a non-absorbable antifungal agent, such as amphotericin B, to prevent secondary outgrowth of fungi. Only if this procedure fails should the patients be treated prophy-lactically with systemic antibiotics directed against invasive aerobic microorganisms. Since this type of patient nevertheless often has to be treated for manifest infections, unnecessary prophylactic treatment may be harmful because of the risk of developing resistant strains.

REFERENCES

1. Bergan T. Pharmacokinetics of beta-lactam antibiotics. *Scand J Infect Dis Suppl* 1984; **42**: 83–98.

2. LeBel M, Spino M. Pulse dosing versus continuous infusion of antibiotics. Pharmacokinetic–pharmacodynamic considerations. *Clin Pharmacokinet* 1988; **14**: 71–95.

3. Bergan T. Pharmacokinetic properties of the cephalosporins. *Drugs* 1987; **34** (Suppl. 2): 89–104.

4. Periti P, Mazzei T, Mini E, Novelli A. Clinical pharmacokinetic properties of the macrolide antibiotics. Effects of age and various pathophysiological states (Part I). *Clin Pharmacokinet* 1989; **16**: 193–214.

5. Periti P, Mazzei T, Mini E, Novelli A. Clinical pharmacokinetic properties of the macrolide antibiotics. Effects of age and various pathophysiological states (Part II). *Clin Pharmacokinet* 1989; **16**: 261–282.

6. Bartkowski RR, Goldber ME, Larijani GE. Inhibition of alfentanil metabolism by erythromycin. *Clin Pharmacol Ther* 1989; **46**: 99–102.

7. Bartkowski RR, McDonnell TE. Prolonged alfentanil effect following erythromycin administration. *Anesthesiology* 1990; **73**: 566–568.

8. Olkkola KT, Aranko K, Luurila H *et al.* A potentially hazardous interaction between erythromycin and midazolam. *Clin Pharmacol Ther* 1993; **53**: 298–305.

9. Periti P, Mazzei T, Mini E, Novelli A. Pharmacokinetic drug interactions of macrolides. *Clin Pharmacokinet* 1992; **23**: 106–131.

10. Gascon M, Dayer P. In vitro forecasting of drugs which may interfere with the biotransformation of midazolam. *Eur J Clin Pharmacol* 1991; **41**: 573–578.

24 DP Desiderio

CHEMOTHERAPEUTIC (ANTINEOPLASTIC) AGENTS

Summary box 24.1 Classification of chemotherapeutic agents

- Alkylating agents:
    - nitrogen mustards
    - nitrosoureas
    - busulphan.
- Platinum analogues.
- Antimetabolites:
    - folate antagonists
    - purine analogues
    - pyrimidine analogues.
- Plant derivatives:
    - *Vinca* alkaloids
    - taxanes.
- Cytotoxic antibiotics.
- Immunotherapy agents.
- Growth factors.

Chemotherapeutic or cytotoxic agents are drugs that inhibit cell division and thus are potentially useful in cancer chemotherapy. A wide range of chemically diverse substances is used for chemotherapy.

Chemotherapeutic agents are an important part of the treatment regimen for patients with cancer. They are used for both primary treatment and, perhaps more importantly, as adjuvant therapy to surgery and/or radiation therapy. Therefore, many patients with cancer who require elective or emergency operation will be undergoing or will have undergone chemotherapy. The clinical benefits of chemotherapeutic agents are often limited by their toxic effects on vital organ systems. Accordingly it is important for the anaesthetist to have a clear understanding of their actions, interactions and toxic effects. A comprehensive preoperative evaluation of these patients is essential, including a detailed history of the exact type and dose of the antineoplastic drugs used and a thorough examination of the organ systems most likely to be affected (Table 24.1).

MECHANISMS OF ACTION

Most antineoplastic agents interfere with the process of deoxyribonucleic acid (DNA) synthesis, replication or transcription within the cancer cell (Fig. 24.1). The cell cycle of dividing cells is divided into several phases, and chemotherapeutic agents can act at different steps in this cycle (Fig. 24.2). Cancer cells are most sensitive to attack when undergoing the process of division. Therefore rapidly growing tumours, where the majority of the cells are undergoing division, will respond more favourably to chemotherapy than those that are slow growing, such as carcinoma of the colon. Cells in the

Table 24.1 Toxicity associated with chemotherapy	
Agent	**Major toxicity**
Cyclophosphamide	Myelosuppression, haemorrhagic cystitis, water retention, pulmonary fibrosis, plasma cholinesterase inhibition
Nitrogen mustard	Myelosuppression, local tissue damage
Vincristine	Neurotoxicity, dilutional hyponatraemia
Vinblastine	Myelosuppression
Methotrexate	Renal tubular injury
5-Fluorouracil and cytarabine	Haemorrhagic enteritis, diarrhoea, myelosuppression
Doxorubicin	Cardiac toxicity
Bleomycin	Pulmonary toxicity
Mitomycin C	Pulmonary toxicity
Cisplatin	Renal toxicity, neurotoxicity
Nitrosoureas	Myelosuppression, renal and pulmonary toxicity
Taxanes	Hypersensitivity reactions, myelosuppression, cardiac and peripheral neuropathy
Interferon and interleukin-2	Immune deficiency syndrome
Growth factors	Pulmonary oedema, pericardial and pleural effusions

resting, G_o, phase are generally resistant to these drugs. Some, however, such as the alkylating agents and cisplatin, can act during the resting phase, although their effects become apparent only later when the cell attempts to undergo division.

ADVERSE EFFECTS

Chemotherapeutic agents are among the most toxic substances used therapeutically, and generally the toxic dose is very close to the therapeutic dose. Because they act on cells that are actively dividing, it is not surprising that toxicity is often manifested in normal tissues that have a rapid cellular turnover, such as gastrointestinal epithelium, bone marrow, hair follicle cells and the reproductive system. Toxicity in these systems is often the dose-limiting factor with these drugs. Partial or complete alopecia may occur, but is usually only temporary.

Gastrointestinal toxicity is common, with nausea and vomiting, anorexia, mucosal ulceration and diarrhoea. Nausea and vomiting, especially common with the alkylating agents and cisplatin, can be extremely severe and prolonged. It starts 1–5 h after initiation of treatment and lasts from 6 to 48 h, depending on the drug. However, because it is predictable, preventive measures can be taken. The most effective drugs are the 5-hydroxytryptamine $(5\text{-}HT)_3$- receptor antagonists, such as ondansetron, in combination with a dopamine D_2-receptor antagonist such as metoclopramide.

Bone marrow suppression is the single most important dose-limiting factor with most chemotherapeutic agents. It results in severe leucopenia, thrombocytopenia and anaemia. As a consequence patients undergoing chemotherapy have a high risk of infection, especially by opportunistic Gram-negative bacteria from the patient's own flora. Action on gonadal cells can result in sterility. Since many cytotoxic drugs are poten-

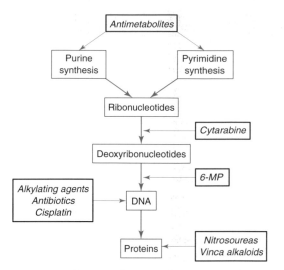

Fig. 24.1 Sites of action of antineoplastic agents that act on dividing cells. 6-MP, 6-mercaptopurine.

tration and acidification are maximal, can lead to a uric acid nephropathy and renal failure. To prevent this complication, it is essential to maintain good hydration during therapy, if necessary with intravenous fluids, along with urine alkalization and the administration of allopurinol.

Many cytotoxic drugs are carcinogenic, and some patients, cured of a primary cancer, develop a second treatment-induced cancer 5–20 years later. The risk seems to be greatest with the alkylating agents and some antimetabolites (mercaptopurine) and antibiotics (doxorubicin). Common secondary cancers include leukaemia, lymphoma and squamous cell carcinoma.

SPECIFIC CHEMOTHERAPEUTIC AGENTS

ALKYLATING AGENTS AND RELATED COMPOUNDS

These were the first drugs to be introduced for the treatment of cancer in the 1940s and they are still being used effectively today. Drugs in this class contain alkyl groups that form strong covalent bonds with cellular molecules, in particular the nucleic acid bases of DNA, especially guanine and cytosine. The alkylated bases can interfere with DNA replication either by being misread or by crosslinking to another base. Most have two alkylating groups, i.e. they are bifunctional, allowing them to interact simultaneously with two DNA nucleic acids to form intrachain and interchain crosslinking

tially teratogenic, pregnant women, whether as patients or medical or nursing staff, should not be exposed to them.

The rapid destruction of tumour mass following chemotherapy can cause an increase in purine and pyrimidine breakdown products of cellular destruction, with a sudden, temporary, rise in uric acid production. Uric acid is sparingly soluble in water and urine, and its solubility decreases at lower pH. Precipitation of uric acid crystals in the distal renal tubules, where concen-

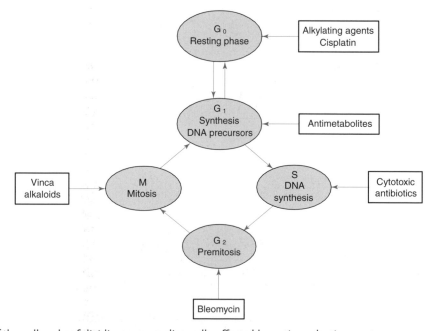

Fig. 24.2 Phases of the cell cycle of dividing mammalian cells affected by antineoplastic agents.

- Most have two alkylating groups that form covalent bonds with cell constituents.

- Form crosslinks with guanine in DNA:

  - interferes with DNA replication

  - causes misreading of message during transcription

  - main effect during DNA synthesis.

- Main side-effects are:

  - myelosuppression

  - sterility

  - risk of carcinogenesis, especially nonlymphatic leukaemia

  - pulmonary toxicity

  - cyclophosphamide inhibits plasma cholinesterase synthesis, prolonging the action of succinylcholine.

- Cisplatin has similar actions, by forming interstrand links in DNA. Main side-effects are:

  - severe nausea and vomiting

  - nephrotoxicity

  - ototoxicity

  - neurotoxicity

  - low incidence of myelosuppression.

(Fig. 24.3). This interferes with DNA transcription and the replication of DNA strands, inhibiting mitosis, although these agents also have actions throughout the cell cycle. To this group of drugs belong the nitrogen mustards, nitrosoureas and busulphan. They have a broad spectrum of antitumour activity and are used in the treatment of lymphoma, breast and ovarian carcinoma, melanoma and multiple myeloma.

NITROGEN MUSTARDS

Examples: Cyclophosphamide, nitrogen mustard, busulphan, melphalan, chlorambucil and ifosfamide.

These drugs were developed from the sulphur-containing 'mustard gas' used during the First World

War. Severe bone marrow suppression resulting in anaemia, agranulocytosis and thrombocytopenia is a dose-limiting factor. This usually occurs during therapy and resolves within a few months after completion. The nitrogen mustards have also been associated with pulmonary toxicity, with fibrosis developing in extreme cases. The exact mechanism is unknown, but a direct effect on the pulmonary epithelium leading to alveolar fibrosis is involved. The symptoms start gradually with a nonproductive cough, dyspnoea and cyanosis. If therapy is not stopped promptly, this can lead to fibrosis and death. The fibrosis, which is not reversible, can be detected by pulmonary function studies, which should be included in the preoperative evaluation.

Cyclophosphamide, one of the most commonly used chemotherapeutic agents, is also used as an immunosuppressive (see Chapter 25). It can be administered orally and intravenously. Nausea, vomiting and alopecia are associated with intravenous use. It is a prodrug that is inactive until metabolized by hepatic cytochrome P450 enzymes to 4-hydroxyphosphamide, which undergoes further nonenzymatic biotransformation to the active cytotoxic compound, phosphoramide mustard, and acrolein. Acrolein, which has much less

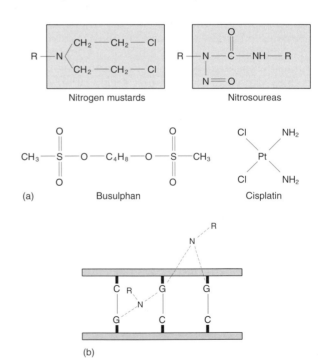

Fig. 24.3 (a) Structure of the alkylating agents and related compounds. The portions of the molecules contained within the shaded boxes are the nitrogen mustard or nitrosourea groups. (b) Two of the mechanisms whereby alkylating agents and related compounds interact with the nucleic acid bases of DNA to form intra- and interstrand crosslinks. This interferes with DNA replication and transcription.

cytotoxic activity than phosphoramide mustard, is responsible for most the adverse side-effects of cyclophosphamide. The excretion of acrolein in the urine causes haemorrhagic cystitis (which also occurs with the related drug, ifosfamide), which may require surgical coagulation. This side-effect can be prevented by increasing fluid intake and the use of sulphydryl donors such as N-acetylcysteine or MESNA (mercaptoethane sulphonate), which interact with acrolein to form nontoxic compounds. Cyclophosphamide can also cause inappropriate water retention due to a direct effect on the renal tubules. Hyponatraemia should be monitored to prevent seizures and coma. Of importance to anaesthetists is inhibition by cyclophosphamide of plasma cholinesterase synthesis, which can lead to a prolongation of the response to succinylcholine.[1,2] Neuromuscular monitoring and documented return of the train-of-four before the administration of a nondepolarizing muscle relaxant are recommended.

Nitrogen mustard (mustine, mechlorethamine) was one of the first agents used for the treatment of lymphoma. Today, however, its use is limited to isolated limb perfusion for metastatic malignant melanoma.[3] This involves the perfusion of the drug directly into the arterial circulation of the affected limb, usually a leg. The arterial inflow tract and the venous outflow tract are cannulated and, via extracorporeal circulation, the perfusion of this agent, as well as that of melphalan and tumour necrosis factor, can be controlled for an exact period of time. The advantage is that the drug is concentrated in the diseased limb, so that exposure to the general circulation is limited. However, there is always a leak, dependent on the surgical ability to isolate the limb. It is important to stabilize pump flow before starting the chemotherapy infusion to avoid an overdose. Online radioisotope labelling can be used to determine leak of the perfusate into the general circulation. Because isolated limb perfusion is intensely painful, lasts about 3–4 h, and nausea and vomiting are common, it is usually carried out under general anaesthesia. Central venous monitoring is helpful to monitor the fluid status during and after the procedure, as there can be considerable leak of the perfusate into the general circulation, as well as blood loss to the pump.

NITROSOUREAS

Examples: Lomustine (CCNU), carmustine (BCNU), semustine (methyl CCNU) and streptozotocin.

This is the other main group of alkylating agents. Nitrosoureas are effective against a wide range of tumours. They are lipophilic and are able to cross the blood–brain barrier; they are therefore effective against brain tumours. Their toxic effects are similar to those of other alkylating agents, but they cause a severe cumu-

lative bone marrow depression that starts within 1–2 months of treatment. Pulmonary toxicity has been reported when doses of lomustine and carmustine exceed 1000 mg m^{-2}. These drugs cause a direct injury to the pulmonary epithelium and lead to alveolar fibrosis. Renal toxicity has also been reported at doses exceeding 1200 mg m^{-2}. Streptozotocin is a monofunctional alkylating agent isolated from *Streptomyces* which has little bone marrow toxicity, but destroys the pancreatic β cells, causing diabetes mellitus.

BUSULPHAN

Busulphan is an alkylsulphonate with selective activity on the bone marrow, suppressing granulocyte and platelet formation; it is used primarily in granulocytic leukaemia. Like the nitrogen mustards, it can cause pulmonary fibrosis.

PLATINUM ANALOGUES

Examples: Cisplatin, carboplatin.

Cisplatin and carboplatin are platinum-containing compounds used in the treatment of testicular, ovarian and bladder carcinomas as well as head and neck tumours. They interact with DNA in a manner similar to the alkylating agents. Cisplatin is a water-soluble compound with a central platinum atom surrounded by two chloride and two ammonia groups. Within the cell, the chloride ions dissociate, leaving a reactive diamine–platinum complex which forms covalent crosslinks between guanine or adenine in the DNA strands, changing its configuration and inhibiting its synthesis. Cisplatin therapy is associated with a high incidence of severe nausea and vomiting. Myelotoxicity is low. The primary dose-limiting toxicities with these agents are nephrotoxicity, ototoxicity and neurotoxicity, which are cumulative and only partially reversible with discontinuation of therapy. There is a high (31%) incidence of severe renal dysfunction. Hydration is a key determinant of the development of renal toxicity, and acute renal failure may occur within 24 h of drug administration in underhydrated patients. Cisplatin is administered by slow intravenous infusion, usually 4–6 h after intravenous hydration and 50 g mannitol. Patients receiving systemic antibiotics such as aminoglycosides have an increased incidence of renal toxicity. The primary pathology in humans is coagulation necrosis of the distal renal tubules and collecting ducts. This causes a reduction of renal blood flow and glomerular filtration rate with concomitant magnesium and potassium wasting. The magnesium loss can lead to symptomatic tetany. Perioperative management of these patients should focus on optimizing renal perfusion, fluid and electrolyte balance. Blood urea nitrogen and creatinine levels are good indicators of renal damage and should be monitored routinely. Appropriate haemodynamic monitoring is essential, and a pulmonary artery catheter may be required for optimal management. Mannitol is the drug of choice for maintaining adequate urine output once intravascular volume status has been assessed and corrected. Anaesthetic agents that might be nephrotoxic as a result of free fluoride release should be avoided.

ANTIMETABOLITES

Antimetabolites are structural analogues of normal cellular constituents, folic acid, purine and pyrimidine. They are accepted by the cell as a substrate and interfere with the synthesis of purine and pyrimidine, which are essential for DNA synthesis and cell division. These agents are used in the treatment of gastrointestinal and pulmonary carcinomas as well as sarcomas and some leukaemias. Antimetabolite drugs can be administered intrathecally for control of central nervous system metastasis. A rise in cerebrospinal fluid pressure may result during and immediately after treatment, and needs to be taken into consideration in anaesthetic planning. The major toxic effects are bone marrow suppression, mucositis, severe diarrhoea, and nausea and vomiting. They have been associated with acute and chronic hepatotoxicity.[4] Liver enzymes rise acutely during high-dose therapy but usually return to normal levels within 1 week after stopping the drug.

FOLATE ANTAGONISTS

The main folate antagonist is methotrexate, an analogue of folic acid. Folic acid is essential for the synthesis of purine and pyrimidine by the enzyme dihydrofolate reductase, and this enzyme is competitively inhibited by methotrexate. Methotrexate is actively transported across the cell membrane into the cytoplasm, where it binds

---

Summary box 24.3 Antimetabolites

- Analogues of folic acid, purine or pyrimidine.

- Interfere with purine and pyrimidine synthesis.

- Block DNA synthesis.

- Main adverse effects are:

  - myelosuppression, especially with cytarabine

  - gastrointestinal epithelial damage

  - renal damage with methotrexate.

---

and inactivates dihydrofolate. Decreased transport is one of the mechanisms that leads to methotrexate resistance. Trimetrexate, a methotrexate analogue, enters the cell by simple diffusion and is therefore useful in treating methotrexate-resistant tumours. It is also used to treat *Pneumocystis carinii* infection. Methotrexate is usually given orally, but may also be given intravenously or intrathecally. In addition to its use in cancer therapy, it is used in the treatment of psoriasis. Methotrexate is associated with serious renal tubular toxicity in 10% of treated patients. This is characterized by rising blood urea nitrogen and serum creatinine levels, with decreasing production of urine. Hydration and urine alkalization are routine with initiation of high-dose methotrexate therapy. Methotrexate can also cause obstructive nephropathy owing to its precipitation in the renal calyx.

PURINE AND PYRIMIDINE ANALOGUES

Examples: 6-Mercaptopurine (6-MP), thioguanine, pentostatin, 5-fluorouracil (5-FU) and cytarabine (cytosine arabinoside).

6-MP and thioguanine, the main purine analogues, are 6-thiol analogues of the purine bases, hypoxanthine and guanine respectively. Both are given orally, although absorption is poor and bioavailability variable. The low bioavailability of 6-MP (5–37%) results from metabolism by xanthine oxidase in the intestinal wall and the liver. Xanthine oxidase is inhibited by allopurine, and its concomitant administration can increase 6-MP bioavailability fivefold. If the dose of mercaptopurine is not appropriately adjusted, this can result in excessive toxicity. Thioguanine is not a substrate for xanthine oxidase and so is not affected by allopurine.

5-FU and cytarabine act primarily by inhibiting pyrimidine synthesis. Pentostatin is a purine analogue that acts by inhibition of adenosine deaminase, the enzyme that converts adenosine to inosine. Inhibition of this critical pathway in the metabolism of purine interferes with cell proliferation. 5-FU is converted by the liver into the 'fraudulent' nucleotide, fluorodeoxyuridine monophosphate which interacts with thymidylate synthetase by covalent coupling to the enzyme, preventing the synthesis of thymidylate. This results in inhibition of DNA, but not ribonucleic acid (RNA) or protein, synthesis. 5-FU may be given orally or intravenously. It readily crosses the blood–brain barrier. 5-FU and its derivative deoxyuridine are also increasingly being administered by intrahepatic arterial infusion in patients with metastases confined to the liver. The high hepatic clearance of these drugs (> 50% for 5-FU and > 95% for deoxyuridine) allows little drug to escape into the systemic circulation. 5-FU and cytarabine can cause a wide variety of pathological changes in the gastrointestinal tract, ranging from superficial ulceration to haemorrhagic enteritis and perforation.

PLANT DERIVATIVES

VINCA ALKALOIDS

This class of agents includes vincristine, vinblastine, vinorelbine and vindesine, all derived from the peri-winkle plant *Vinca rosea*. They bind to and inactivate tubulin, preventing microtubule assembly, and arrest the cell in the metaphase of mitosis. Etoposide, derived from the root of the mandrake plant, has a similar mechanism of action but may also have an effect on topoisomerase II similar to that seen with doxorubicin. The *Vinca* alkaloids are used primarily in the treatment of testicular carcinoma, sarcomas, Hodgkin's and non-Hodgkin's lymphoma and some leukaemias. The major toxic effect of vinblastine, and to a lesser extent that of vindesine and vinorelbine, is on the bone marrow, with some isolated cases of neurotoxicity. Vincristine is not myelosuppressive but is associated with major neurotoxicity. This is manifested as a progressive and disabling sensory and motor peripheral neuropathy, with signs of decreasing deep tendon reflexes, peripheral paraesthesias, ataxia and foot drop. These defects can be permanent. Although muscle damage is uncommon, there can be considerable muscle wasting in severely incapacitated patients. Autonomic neuropathy after a single high dose, and hepatic failure, have been reported. Because of the risk of hyperkalaemia, succinylcholine should be avoided in patients with severe

neurotoxicity. Vincristine has also been associated with stimulation of antidiuretic hormone secretion and dilutional hyponatraemia. The *Vinca* alkaloids are administered intravenously, and great care is needed to avoid drug extravasation, which may cause severe soft tissue injury.

TAXANES

The taxanes, paclitaxel and docetaxel, derived from the bark of the yew tree, are an important new class of chemotherapeutic agents used primarily in the treatment of breast, lung and ovarian carcinomas, and are being tested in combination with other agents. Taxanes enhance tubulin polymerization, a mechanism that is opposite to that of the *Vinca* alkaloids. These microtubules are very stable so that the dynamic reorganization of the microtubule network during mitosis is inhibited. The tubules accumulate in the cell and disrupt cellular division, leading to cell death. Paclitaxel is highly insoluble in water and is emulsified in cremaphor. The risk of anaphylactic reactions to the cremophor necessitates premedication with dexamethasone, diphenhydramine and cimetidine to prevent severe type 1 hypersensitivity reactions. These reactions usually occur with the first or second dose. Docetaxel is more water soluble, and is a more potent antitubule agent. For both drugs, neutropenia is the major dose-limiting side-effect, with counts reaching a minimum in 10 days and returning to normal by 21 days. Surgical procedures should, if possible, be scheduled after recovery of the neutropenia.

Neurotoxicity caused by aggregation of the microtubules in the neurons, axons or Schwann cells also occurs. This results in a painful peripheral sensory neuropathy. Neurotoxicity is not only dose dependent but also seems to be peak concentration dependent. Clinically the symptoms appear 2–3 days after administration and present with numbness, paraesthesia of the toes and then fingertips. Muscle, joint and bone pain may be accompanying features. When administered with other neurotoxic agents (e.g. cisplatin, vincristine and vinblastine), toxicity is accentuated. Cardiac toxicity has been observed, causing bradydysrhythmias and second- and third-degree heart block, as well as ventricular tachycardias.[5] Asymptomatic bradycardia occurs in up to 30% of patients during infusion of taxanes and is clinically insignificant.

CYTOTOXIC ANTIBIOTICS

The anthracycline antibiotics, which include doxorubicin, daunorubicin, bleomycin and mitomycin C, form stable complexes with DNA, thereby inhibiting DNA and RNA synthesis. Doxorubicin, the main anticancer anthracycline antibiotics, also has actions mediated

---

Summary box 24.4 Plant derivatives

- Interact with tubulin, interfering with microtubules to inhibit mitosis:

  - *Vinca* alkaloids and etoposide prevent microtubule assembly

  - taxanes stabilize microtubules

  - etoposide also interacts with topoisomerase II.

- Main adverse effects are:

  - myelosuppression, except vincristine

  - peripheral neurotoxicity – vindesine, vinorelbine and the taxanes

  - hypersecretion of antidiuretic hormone – vincristine

  - cardiac arrhythmias – taxanes.

Summary box 24.5 Cytotoxic antibiotics

- Inhibit DNA and RNA synthesis, or disrupt transcription.

- Doxorubicin's actions on DNA are principally via interference with topoisomerase II.

- Main adverse effects are:

  - cardiotoxicity with anthracyclines

  - pulmonary toxicity with bleomycin and mitomycin. NB: Restrict oxygen concentration to less than 28%

  - renal toxicity and myelosuppression with mitomycin.

Table 24.2 Risk factors associated with doxorubicin and cardiotoxicity

- Total cumulative dose over 550 mg m^{-2}.
- Concomitant cyclophosphamide therapy.
- Previous history of heart disease.
- Age over 65 years.

through an effect on topoisomerase II (a DNA gyrase), the activity of which is markedly increased in proliferating cells. This latter action may be the main anticancer action of this drug. Structurally related to doxorubicin are epirubicin and mitozantrone. The cytotoxic antibiotics are used to treat leukaemias and lymphomas and also for many solid tumours such as those in the breast, lung, thyroid and ovary.

Cardiotoxicity is the major dose-limiting factor. This occurs in two phases, acute and chronic. The acute phase is unrelated to dose and can occur hours to days after the start of treatment. It usually presents as a mild and transient electrocardiographic (ECG) disturbance or, in extreme cases, as overt pump failure related to reduced myocardial contractility. Sudden death has been reported. Benign, nonspecific ECG changes occur in 10% of patients, with an increase in supraventricular tachydysrhythmias, heart block and ventricular dsyrhythmias, which usually resolve 1–2 months after therapy. The incidence is increased in patients with preexisting heart disease. Some patients may develop acute congestive heart failure 24–48 h after starting anthracycline therapy. The chronic phase of cardiotoxicity is a dose-dependent cardiomyopathy that leads to congestive heart failure in 2–10% of patients, and it may be irreversible in up to 59% of patients. The risk factors associated with this cardiotoxicity are listed in Table 24.2.

Anthracycline-induced myocardial injury appears to be the result of oxygen free radical formation. Cardiac tissue is low in catalase, an enzyme that detoxifies free radicals. It is thought that dilatation of the sarcoplasmic reticulum and a build-up of calcium deposits in cardiac myocytes are a result of free radical injury, and this ultimately leads to cardiac failure. Patients receiving these drugs should be followed routinely by serial ECGs and radionucleotide-gated pool studies performed at rest and with exercise. Serial ejection fractions are the most sensitive indicators of myocardial damage.[6] Children are particularly sensitive to these cardiotoxic reactions and may require a heart transplant in their later years.

For the anaesthetist, a thorough preoperative evaluation is essential to determine the degree of cardiac compromise. The clinical signs of congestive heart failure such as dyspnoea, inspiratory râles, peripheral oedema, pleural effusion and an S3 gallop may or may not be present. Patients with overt anthracycline-induced congestive heart failure may require administration of digoxin, diuretics and other inotrophic support; it is essential to optimize their cardiovascular status before surgery. Intraoperative management for those with overt cardiac compromise should include monitoring with a pulmonary artery catheter and, if available, transoesophageal echocardiography. Intraoperative cardiac function is better preserved with an anaesthetic technique that lowers systemic vascular resistance, similar to the recommendations for patients with idiopathic cardiomyopathy.[7]

Bleomycins are a group of metal-chelating glycopeptide antibiotics that degrade preformed DNA. This action is thought to involve chelation of ferrous iron and interaction with oxygen. Bleomycin is used in the treatment of testicular carcinoma, sarcomas, and carcinomas of the oesophagus and lung. It is primarily dose-limited by its pulmonary toxicity, occurring in 5–10% of patients. The antitumour and toxic effects are the result of binding to cellular DNA, causing single- and double-stranded breaks. When bleomycin binds to DNA, a ferrous ion on the bleomycin undergoes oxidation to the ferric state, liberating electrons. The electrons are accepted by oxygen and form superoxide and oxygen free radicals. The lung is a prime target for bleomycin toxicity because of the high oxygen concentration and its low level of the enzyme, bleomycin hydrolase, a metabolic inactivator of the drug.

Experimental models show that the injury occurs in two phases. The first is an exudative phase, occurring 1 week after treatment and characterized by interstitial pulmonary oedema, sloughing of the alveolar lining cells and hyaline membrane formation. The second phase is characterized by interstitial infiltration by inflammatory cells and hyperplasia of type II pneumocytes that eventually leads to pulmonary fibrosis.[8] The clinical signs of bleomycin toxicity include a nonproductive cough, dyspnoea and fever. Symptoms can be delayed for up to 4–10 weeks following therapy. Pulmonary function studies are used to monitor these patients. A restrictive pattern develops and a decrease in the carbon monoxide diffusion capacity denotes pulmonary compromise.[9] Chest radiography shows a progressive bibasilar infiltrate. Risk factors associated with the development of pulmonary toxicity in patients taking bleomycin are noted in Table 24.3. Once the toxicity is recognized, treatment is supportive in nature, with the administration of high-dose corticosteroids in an attempt to prevent progression of the pulmonary fibrosis.

Of concern to the anaesthetist is not only the amount of lung damage that has occurred before operation but also the risk of inducing lung damage by high intraoperative concentrations of oxygen. Numerous animal studies have shown that exposure to increased oxygen concentrations increases the incidence of pulmonary toxicity and death after bleomycin therapy. A fraction of inspired oxygen greater than 0.28 may enhance the risk of developing pulmonary toxicity in the postoperative period,[10] and it is recommended that oxygen concentration be limited to less than 28% in the perioperative period while still mantaining satisfactory arterial oxygenation. This requires vigilant monitoring with pulse oximetry and frequent blood gas determinations. Perioperative fluids should be restricted to prevent the development of pulmonary oedema.

Mitomycin C was first introduced in the 1970s. It has activity against gastrointestinal, lung and breast cancers. Originally its major dose-limiting factor was thought to be myelosuppression. However, mitomycin becomes active by undergoing enzymatic reduction; once activated, it inhibits DNA function and causes cell death. During this activation process, mitomycin forms oxygen free radicals, and there have been several case reports of severe interstitial pneumonitis, similar to that associated with bleomycin.[11] The lung is the likely target for this toxicity because of its high level of nicotinamide adenine dinucleotide phosphate (NADP)

cytochrome P450 reductase, the enzyme responsible for mitomycin activation and the ultimate formation of oxygen free radicals. Unlike the case with bleomycin, pulmonary toxicity is thought not to be dose related. Once pulmonary toxicity develops, there is a very high mortality rate. The use of high-dose corticosteroid at the onset of symptoms may be of benefit. As in the case of bleomycin, there is a triad of symptoms, dyspnoea, cough and fever, often hard to distinguish from other aetiologies. The role of increased oxygen concentration and the development of mitomycin-induced pulmonary toxicity has been raised but never proven in humans. The author's experience has been that patients treated with mitomycin who develop postoperative pulmonary complications are those with impaired diffusion capacities. It is important to compare diffusion capacities before and after chemotherapy in these patients and, if there has been a significant decrease, the use of oxygen concentrations less than 28% while still maintaining adequate oxygenation is recommended.

IMMUNOTHERAPY AGENTS

Interferon and interleukin-2 (IL-2) are used in the treatment of malignant melanoma, renal cell carcinoma, Karposi sarcoma and various leukaemias and lymphomas. Interferon is synthesized in normal cells as a response to a viral infection. The theory underlying its use is that malignancies induced by a virally mediated change in DNA may respond to this agent. IL-2 is used to activate naturally occurring killer T cells and tumour-infiltrating lymphocytes. Patients undergoing treatment with these agents require intensive care management due to the development of severe immune deficiency syndromes, hypotension, hyperthermia and sepsis during treatment. These complications usually resolve after discontinuation of therapy.

GROWTH FACTORS

Although growth factors are not chemotherapeutic agents, they are being used with increasing frequency with all of the chemotherapy protocols. Severe haematopoietic toxicity is the dose-limiting factor for many chemotherapeutic agents. The incorporation of G-CSF granulocyte colony-stimulating factor (G-CSF) and granulocyte–macrophage colony-stimulating factor (GM-CSF) decreases the period of neutropenia, thereby lessening the risk of infection and allowing higher doses of the chemotherapeutic agent to be continued for longer periods. Growth factors work by regulating the development of stem cells into erythrocytes, granulocyte and megakaryocytes. They also have associated toxicity, in particular a generalized leaky capillary syndrome, leading to pleural and pericardial effusions.[12]

Table 24.3 Risk factors associated with bleomycin pulmonary toxicity

- Total cumulative dose over 200 mg.
- Concomitant thoracic radiation therapy.
- Age over 65 years.
- Possibly increased oxygen concentrations.

CONCLUSION

The proper anaesthetic management of the patient with cancer requires a thorough knowledge of the specific anticancer regimen the patient has been undergoing before operation and anaesthesia. This includes a detailed history of the chemotherapeutic agents, their doses and last administration. All the agents have some associated toxic side-effects and a thorough preoperative evaluation is essential. Specific emphasis should be placed on the organ systems most likely affected by the chemotherapeutic regimen utilized for specific cancers. Intraoperative management will depend on these data as well as the general clinical condition of the patient.

REFERENCES

1. Gruman GM. Prolonged apnea after succinylcholine in a case treated with cytostatics for cancer. *Anesth Analg* 1972; **51**: 761–763.
2. Zsigmond EK, Robins G. The effects of a series of anticancer drugs on plasma cholinesterase activity. *Can J Anaesth* 1972; **19**: 75–82.
3. Coit DG. Hyperthermic isolation limb perfusion for malignant melanoma: a review. *Cancer Invest* 1992; **10**: 277–284.
4. Desiderio DP. Anesthetic–antineoplastic drug interactions. *Semin Anesth* 1992; **12**: 68–75.
5. Rowkinsky EK, McGuire WP, Guarieri T *et al*. Cardiac distrubances during the administration of taxol. *J Clin Oncol* 1991; **9**: 1704–1712.
6. Bacon DR, Nuzzo RJ. Anthracycline antineoplastic chemotherapy agents: anesthetic implications. *Semin Anesth* 1993; **XII**: 74–78.
7. Thorne AC, Orazem JP, Shah NK *et al*. Isoflurane versus fentanyl: hemodynamic effects in cancer patients treated with anthracyclines. *J Cardiothorac Vasc Anesth* 1993; **7**: 307–310.
8. Goldiner PL, Shamsi A. Bleomycin–oxygen interaction. *Semin Anesth* 1993; **XII**: 79–82.
9. Sorensen PG, Rossing N, Rorth M. Carbon monoxide diffusing capacity: a reliable indicator of bleomycin-induced pulmonary toxicity. *Eur J Respir Dis* 1985; **66**: 333–340.
10. Goldiner PL, Carlon GC, Cvitkovic E *et al*. Factors influencing postoperative morbidity and mortality in patients treated with bleomycin. *BMJ* 1978; **1**: 1664–1667.
11. Budzar AU, Legha SS, Luna MA. Pulmonary toxicity of mitomycin. *Cancer* 1980; **45**: 236–244.
12. Tobias JD, Furman WL. Anesthetic considerations in patients receiving colony-stimulating factors (G-CSF and GM-CSF). *Anesthesiology* 1991; **75**: 536–538.

25

RJM ten Berge, S Surachno, JM Wilmink, PThA Schellekens

IMMUNOSUPPRESSIVE DRUGS

The immune system defends the body against invading organisms, foreign antigens and abnormal host cells (e.g. tumour cells). In addition it is actively involved in the rejection of transplanted organs and tissues, and in a variety of autoimmune diseases. As knowledge of the function of the immune system is a prerequisite for the proper understanding of the effects of immunosuppressive drugs, some principles relating to the physiology of the immune system will be discussed briefly first.

PHYSIOLOGY OF THE IMMUNE SYSTEM

In every individual, resistance against infection depends on nonspecific and specific mechanisms. The nonspecific mechanisms include mechanical barriers, such as skin and mucous membranes, bactericidal substances in the body fluids such as lysozyme, and phagocytosis of bacteria by specialized cells. Higher species, moreover, are equipped with a second line of defence which responds specifically against microbes or foreign antigens and serves to enhance the efficiency of the nonspecific immune systems by, for example, facilitating adherence of microorganisms to phagocytic cells by coating them with antibody and complement. The specific immune response is one component of an integrated host defence system involving numerous cells and molecules. The specific immune system 'remembers' past encounters with each microbe or foreign antigen, so that subsequent encounters stimulate increasingly effective defence mechanisms. This system also serves to amplify the protective responses of the nonspecific natural immunity.

TYPES OF LYMPHOCYTE

Lymphocytes play a central role in the functioning of the immune system. They are responsible for the specificity of immune responses as they are the only cells in the body capable of specifically recognizing and distinguishing different antigenic material. They originate in the bone marrow from stem cells; as the stem cells mature they differentiate into three distinct subtypes of lymphocyte: B and T lymphocytes and natural killer (NK) cells (Fig. 25.1). B lymphocytes are the only cells capable of producing antibodies. Mature B lymphocytes migrate from the bone marrow to peripheral lymphoid tissues where they can interact with foreign antigens and become activated to produce specific antibodies. Antibody-producing B cells often differentiate into specialized forms called plasma cells. B lymphocytes are found in lymphoid organs and at sites of immune responses, and comprise about 5–15% of the lymphocytes present in peripheral blood. The second major class of lymphocytes consists of cells that migrate from the marrow to the thymus (hence 'T'), where they mature. They then migrate to the peripheral lymphoid organs, for example to the paracortical zones of the lymph nodes, and to the spleen. T lymphocytes have

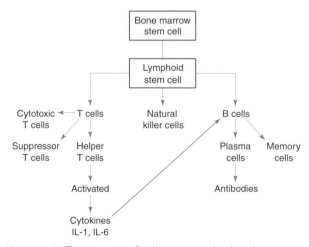

Fig. 25.1 Differentiation of cell types involved in the immune response. Cytokines generated by activated T cells stimulate B-cell proliferation and differentiation. IL, interleukin.

antigen receptors, but recognize only peptide antigens that are presented in the context of proteins belonging to the major histocompatibility complex (MHC) expressed on the surface of accessory cells. When activated they produce cytokines. NK cells are large lymphocytes capable of lysing a variety of tumour and virus-infected cells without overt antigenic stimulation.

SPECIFIC IMMUNE RESPONSES

Specific immune responses take two forms, which usually develop in parallel: humoral and cellular immunity. *Humoral immunity* is characterized by the appearance of globulins known as immunoglobulins or antibodies. These combine with the inducing substance (antigen) that stimulated their production. There are five classes of antibodies: immunoglobulin (Ig) M, IgG, IgA, IgE and IgD. The protection mediated by these antibodies can be transferred from one individual to another by noncellular means (e.g. by serum or colostrum). With the first exposure to an antigen, antibodies can be detected after about 1 week, reaching a maximum at about 2 weeks. These antibodies are mainly of the IgM class. This process is called the primary antibody response. When a second exposure to the antigen occurs, a marked increase in the level of antibody can be detected after only 2 days, and the peak level, which is considerably higher than that associated with the primary response, is reached after about 1 week. A characteristic of secondary antibody responses is the production of IgG, IgA or IgE class antibodies. Thus a primary response conveys both *specificity* and *memory* to the individual for that particular antigen. Humoral immunity can readily be transferred from one individual to another by means of serum containing the antibodies.

Optimum antibody production requires cooperation between T and B lymphocytes. T cells responsible for cooperation with B cells are called helper T cells. They are involved in the switch in antibody production from the IgM class to IgG and IgA classes. IgM antibody production is largely independent of T-helper cell activity. The different lymphocyte populations and subpopulations can be recognized by appropriate monoclonal antibodies directed to characteristic membrane markers referred to by the initials CD (cluster of differentiation), followed by a unique identifying number. For instance, CD3 proteins are expressed by all mature T lymphocytes.

In contrast to humoral immunity, *cellular immunity* cannot be transferred by serum but only by appropriately sensitized T lymphocytes. A few T lymphocytes are specifically activated by antigen and react via their T-cell antigen receptor (TCR) with the antigenic peptide, presented by an antigen-presenting cell (APC). An important feature of antigen presentation is that it occurs in conjunction with one of the MHC antigens. The initial activation signal is provided by binding of the TCR to the antigenic peptide–MHC on the APC surface, and is transmitted through a set of molecules called the CD3 complex, although other costimulatory signals are also involved. After activation and clonal proliferation, T cells produce soluble factors (cytokines) which play an important role in the immune process by facilitating the actions of B cells or other T cells. T cells can mature into delayed-type hypersensitivity (DTH) effector cells. Monocytes and macrophages are recruited and make up most of the infiltrating cells at a site of DTH reaction (e.g. DTH skin tests). The proliferating capacity of these T-DTH lymphocytes can be measured in vitro after stimulation by soluble microbial antigens. In cytotoxic reactions, such as occur in the defence against virus-infected cells, a further subset of T lymphocytes is activated, the cytotoxic T lymphocytes. Cellular immunity is also characterized by specificity and memory. Resistance to intracellular multiplying organisms occurring in some bacterial infections, and a major part of the resistance against viral and fungal infections, depends on cellular immune mechanisms. On the other hand, humoral immunity is mainly responsible for resistance to bacterial infections.

The distinction between humoral and cellular immunity can be traced in the structure, physiology and pathology of the immune system. The tissues primarily engaged in immune responses are the lymph nodes, spleen and bone marrow. Within the lymph node, humoral reactions occur predominantly in the cortex and medulla. After antigenic stimulation, follicles (local accumulations of lymphocytes) in the cortex enlarge to form germinal centres. In the germinal centre, antibody-producing plasma cells are formed from B lymphocytes and migrate to the medulla. Cellular immune reactions are localized in the paracortical zone, between the cortex and the medulla. Lymphocytes within the lymph nodes migrate with the lymph to the blood and reenter the lymph nodes via adhesion molecules on the postcapillary venules. There is thus a recirculation of small lymphocytes between blood and lymphoid tissues, and each lymphocyte may be exchanged between these compartments many times during its lifetime. In this way sensitized lymphocytes originating from a local lymph node become widely distributed throughout the body.

TESTING THE IMMUNE RESPONSE

The integrity of the lymphoid system can be tested both in vivo (Table 25.1) and in vitro. Humoral immunity is tested in vivo by analysing the capacity to produce antibodies of the different immunoglobulin classes after either primary or secondary immunization. Cellular immunity is assessed by skin tests performed in an individual already sensitized (secondary skin tests with recall antigens) or *de novo* sensitized (primary response) with 2,4-dinitrochlorobenzene or keyhole limpet haemo-

Table 25.1 Immune responses in vivo	
	Antigen
Humoral Primary Secondary	KLH Diphtheria toxoid, tetanus toxoid, polio vaccine
Cellular Primary Secondary	DNCB or KLH PPD, varidase, mumps, *Trichophyton, Candida*
KLH, keyhole limpet haemocyanin; DNCB, 2,4-dinitrochlorobenzene; PPD, purified protein derivative from *Mycobacterium tuberculosis*.	

cyanin. After a low dose of antigen has been injected intracutaneously or applied to the skin, a localized inflammatory response occurs which reaches a maximum in 24–48 h, provided the individual has been sensitized at least 2 weeks previously. The diameter of the induration can be readily measured. In vitro, mononuclear cells can be cultured after isolation from the peripheral blood and stimulated to differentiate and divide by various substances, such as phytohaemagglutinin, or more specifically by antigen(s). In general, these reactions are dependent on the proper functioning of T lymphocytes. Proliferative capacity is measured by culturing the cells in the presence of radiolabelled precursors of nucleic acids (e.g. [³H]thymidine).

IMMUNE REACTIVITY
Normally, tissue antigens present in the body do not provoke an immune response. However, under certain conditions an immune response will develop against the body's own tissues. This results in an autoimmune disease. Another example of unwanted immune reactivity is that which develops against antigens present on a transplanted organ, leading to allograft rejection. Immunosuppressive drugs have been developed to suppress these reactions. These drugs exert their influence at different levels of the immune response.

In general, the ultimate goal of an immune response is the elimination of the offending antigen. Fig. 25.2 depicts the different stages by which this goal is reached. The afferent part consists of recognition of the antigen, followed by the central phase in which generation and proliferation of effector T cells and proliferation of B cells that mature into antibody-producing plasma cells occurs. In the effector phase, interaction of effector T cells or antibodies with their respective antigens takes place and an inflammatory response ensues, generally leading to elimination of that antigen. The term 'antiinflammatory action' refers to nonspecific

events that occur as part of the effector phase of an immune response and which may be the target of an immunosuppressive drug. For example, diminished skin reactivity to chemical or microbial antigens may be due not only to a defect somewhere in the specific immune response elicited by the antigen, but also to a defect in subsequent nonspecific events. The latter play a role in the effector phase of the immune response and determine its outcome. Thus, immunosuppressive drugs may inhibit cellular immune responses, humoral immune responses and/or the inflammatory reaction in the effector phase of an immune response.

IMMUNOSUPPRESSIVE DRUGS

CORTICOSTEROIDS
The effects of glucocorticosteroids on the immune system vary among animal species: mouse, rat, hamster and rabbit are 'corticosteroid sensitive', whereas ferret, monkey, guinea-pig and humans are 'corticosteroid resistant'. In all corticosteroid-resistant species, including humans, the major effect of these drugs seems to be to influence lymphocyte traffic. There is a transient decrease in the number of mononuclear cells in peripheral blood following each administration of corticosteroids. However, the precise mechanism for the redistribution of mononuclear cells has not been

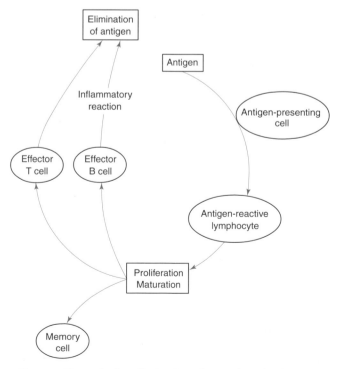

Fig. 25.2 Stages in the elimination of an antigen by the immune system.

Summary box 25.1 Mechanisms of action of immunosuppressive drugs

- Glucocorticosteroids have an inhibitory effect on many cells of the immune system; they suppress the proliferative responses of T cells and the early stages of activation and proliferation of B cells; they inhibit expression of the MHC, IL-1 and IL-2.

- Cytotoxic agents (azathioprine, cyclophosphamide, methotrexate) inhibit the proliferative responses of B and T cells by interfering with DNA.

- Cyclosporin and tacrolimus (FK506) inhibit IL-2 proliferation of T cells.

- Monoclonal antibody anti-CD3 (OKT3) specifically binds to the CD3 molecule on T cells, resulting in their depletion.

defined. In patients receiving long-term glucocorticosteroid therapy, no effect on secondary antibody response has been demonstrated. Current evidence suggests that the main immunosuppressive effect of steroids is not due to inhibition of antigen recognition or of the proliferative phase of the immune response but to some other mechanism, probably an antiinflammatory effect. This may be related to the ability of corticosteroids to block activation of the interleukin (IL)-1 and IL-6 genes in a variety of cells.[1] However, in kidney transplant recipients treated with azathioprine combined with high doses of prednisolone, in addition to the effects mentioned above, the levels of serum immunoglobulins, except IgM, decrease while primary and secondary antibody responses are normal. In contrast, the proliferative response of lymphocytes in vitro after stimulation with the same antigens is low or even absent.[2] This indicates that, although antigen-reactive cells are apparently depleted from the peripheral blood, they may still be present in other lymphoid compartments to provide help for production of antibodies. It appears that lymphocytes are redistributed under the influence of therapy with prednisolone and azathioprine, and that this regimen has only a small effect on the immunocompetence of lymphocytes in vivo.

THIOPURINES

Azathioprine and its biologically active metabolite, 6-mercaptopurine (6-MP), appear to be equally effective for use in organ transplantation and in the treatment of autoimmune diseases. These drugs will therefore be discussed as equivalents. 6-MP undergoes further metabolism to the active antitumour and immunosuppressive thioinosinic acid. This inhibits hypoxanthine–guanine phosphoribosyl transferase, which mediates the conversion of purines to the corresponding phosphoribosyl-5′-phosphates and hypoxanthine to inosinic acid. This leads to inhibition of cell proliferation, and is the mechanism of immunosuppression by azathioprine and 6-MP.

Humans are more sensitive to the toxic effects of 6-MP and azathioprine than other species, in particular as far as the haemopoietic system is concerned. The major limiting toxicity of azathioprine is bone marrow suppression, with leucopenia and thrombocytopenia. These changes are reversible when the drug is stopped. Liver toxicity is another common toxic effect. Since allopurinol inhibits the metabolism of azathioprine, their concurrent use is contraindicated. Azathioprine and 6-MP do not have a distinct effect on secondary humoral or cellular immune responses, but do exert some influence on the primary humoral immune response. However, from a clinical point of view, a drug that can suppress secondary responses is wanted. Azathioprine does influence nonspecific functions that may play a role in the effector phase of the immune response, decreasing the activity of killer and NK cells. These cells may have a nonspecific effector function in the defence against (microbial) antigens, whether antibody-coated or not. The diminished function of these cells may explain the moderate antiinflammatory and thus the corticosteroid-sparing effects of azathioprine.

CYCLOPHOSPHAMIDE

Cyclophosphamide belongs to the family of nitrogen mustard alkylating agents also used for their antineoplastic actions (see Chapter 24). Alkylation refers to the covalent attachment of alkyl groups to other molecules, such as the nucleic acids of deoxyribonucleic acid (DNA). In the body cyclophosphamide undergoes a combination of enzymatic and chemical activation to form the active phosphoramide mustard. Cyclophosphamide is used for the treatment of autoimmune diseases and to prevent graft rejection. Therapy with cyclophosphamide affects both primary and secondary humoral immune responses; in addition it suppresses primary cellular immune reactivity.[3] The effects of treatment with cyclophosphamide on the outcome of the primary humoral immune response in humans seem to be highly dependent on the dose of the drug, as well as on the time interval between administration of the drug and antigenic challenge.

Cyclophosphamide may induce a profound lymphocytopenia involving both T and B cells. Serum levels of immunoglobulins as well as primary and secondary antibody responses are depressed. Proliferative responses of lymphocytes in vitro and secondary cellular immune responses in vivo remain intact, but the primary cellular immune response in vivo is depressed.

Because of the life-threatening toxicity that may occur with cyclophosphamide, particularly myelosuppression, haemorrhagic cystitis and cardiomyopathy, extreme care should be taken to ensure that the minimal effective dose is administered. Use of this drug has significantly decreased with the advent of cyclosporin.

Cyclophosphamide reduces the activity of plasma cholinesterase by 50% and may be associated with prolonged apnoea following succinylcholine.[4] However, the safe use of succinylcholine in a patient who was treated with cyclophosphamide and had a plasma cholinesterase activity of about one-third normal has been reported.[5] Thus, although succinylcholine may be safe in these patients, it should be used cautiously and monitored with a nerve stimulator.

CYCLOSPORIN

Cyclosporin (cyclosporin A) is a cyclic peptide derived from a fungus. The introduction of cyclosporin revolutionized immunosuppressive therapy by virtue of its highly selective inhibition of T cells, and was one of the major influences in the improvement of early graft survival in the 1980s. Cyclosporin strongly suppresses primary humoral and cellular immune responses, whereas most humoral immune responses not requiring T cells are spared.[6] Unlike cytotoxic immunosuppressive drugs such as cyclophosphamide or azathioprine it does not cause myelosuppression in therapeutic doses – a major advantage of cyclosporin.

The major toxic effect of cyclosporin is renal, with reduced glomerular filtration and damage to the proximal tubules. Nephrotoxicity is a common and dose-limiting side-effect of this drug. The other major side-effect is hepatotoxicity with cholestasis and hyperbilirubinaemia. Neurotoxicity is observed in about 20% of patients, and about 50% develop moderate hypertension. Some patients develop hypersensitivity to the drug vehicle. Cyclosporin is metabolized by the hepatic cytochrome P450 enzyme system, and enzyme induction by phenobarbitone, phenytoin, carbamazepine or rifampicin will drastically increase the clearance of cyclosporin.[7–9] Concurrent administration of these drugs, for seizures or tuberculosis, has caused rejection of transplanted organs. Conversely, the use of enzyme inhibitors such as erythromycin or the azole antifungal agents (e.g. ketoconazole) increases the blood concentrations of cyclosporin leading to an increased risk of toxic side-effects.

TACROLIMUS (FK506)

Tacrolimus is a lactone–lactam antibiotic with immunosuppressive properties. Although chemically different, tacrolimus has many similarities to cyclosporin. Like cyclosporin it inhibits the IL-2-dependent proliferation of T cells. It is a very active immunosuppressive drug in both the prevention and treatment of liver and renal allograft rejection in humans. It has been regarded as the immunosuppressive of choice for small bowel transplantation.[10] On a gram for gram basis, tacrolimus is many times more potent than cyclosporin, but the side-effects are remarkably similar. It has a major potential for nephrotoxicity, as well as being neurotoxic and diabetogenic.[11] The drug seems superior to cyclosporin with regard to efficacy. To the authors' knowledge, no studies on the influence of tacrolimus on primary and secondary immune responses in vivo in humans have yet been performed.

MYCOPHENOLATE MOFETIL

Mycophenolate mofetil is a noncompetitive reversible inhibitor of eukaryotic but not prokaryotic inosine monophosphate dehydrogenase with a selective effect on immunocompetent cells. Clinical trials have indicated that the drug is capable of lowering the incidence of acute allograft rejection and reversing acute rejection crises.[12] Side-effects appear to be mild and consist mainly of a dose-dependent gastrointestinal toxicity. Other new antimetabolite agents are mizoribine and brequinar sodium.

POLYCLONAL ANTIBODIES, ANTITHYMOCYTE GLOBULINS

Polyclonal antibodies or antithymocyte globulins (ATGs) are obtained by injecting animals (horse or rabbit) with human thymocytes and then separating the resulting immune sera to obtain purified γ-globulin fractions. These preparations have been used for organ transplantation since the 1970s and have proved to be more effective than corticosteroids for reversing acute allograft rejection. Each polyclonal immunoglobulin preparation varies in its constituent antibodies. As a consequence, treatment is associated with variable efficacy as well as with adverse reactions. Batch standardization and assessment of immunosuppressive potency are difficult. Unwanted antibodies can cause thrombocytopenia and granulocytopenia. Owing to the development of host antibodies to the animal polyclonal immunoglobulin, serum sickness commonly occurs during treatment.

There are several possible mechanisms by which ATG may exert its immunosuppressive effect. These include classic complement-mediated lympholysis, clearance of lymphocytes in the mononuclear phagocytic system, and masking of T-cell antigens resulting in inhibition of lymphocyte function.

MONOCLONAL ANTIBODY ANTI-CD3, OKT3

OKT3 is a murine monoclonal antibody of the IgG_{2a} class, directed against the CD3 molecule which is present on the surface of human thymocytes and mature T cells. The CD3 molecule is closely associated with the TCR in the so-called CD3–TCR complex. In vivo administration of OKT3 initially results in coating of all circulating T cells. Within minutes, these OKT3-coated cells disappear almost completely from the circulation. After 2–5 days of treatment, CD3-negative T cells reappear in the circulation, but are functionally inactive. It is generally assumed that the disappearance of the CD3 molecule from the surface of the T lymphocyte (a process called 'antigenic modulation') contributes to the immunosuppressive effect of anti-CD3 moabs monoclonal antibodies.[13] The detection of large numbers of OKT3-coated cells in the circulation during OKT3 treatment suggests that masking of the CD3 molecule may also play a role. However, it is not certain which of these mechanisms – blocking and/or modulation of the CD3–TCR complex or disappearance of T cells from the circulation – is most responsible for the immunosuppressive effect of OKT3.

OKT3 is a very powerful immunosuppressive agent in renal transplantation. It is superior to high-dose steroids as the first-line treatment of acute renal allograft rejection. Furthermore, it is comparable to ATG in treating steroid-resistant rejection, and is also effective as rescue treatment in ATG- and antilymphocyte globulin-resistant rejection.[14] A prophylactic course of OKT3 may be beneficial in immunologically high-risk patients and in patients with delayed graft function.

The initial use of OKT3 is accompanied by side-effects which are usually transient and seldom life threatening, provided overhydration has been corrected and steroids have been given before the first administration. The side-effects are attributed partly to the release of cytokines as a result of mononuclear cell activation or lysis.[15] In addition, complement activation and subsequent activation of neutrophils, and activation of the coagulation and fibrinolytic system, may play a role in the pathogenesis of side-effects.[16,17] There is an increased incidence of infections and posttransplant lymphoproliferative disease and lymphomas associated with OKT3.[18,19] However, it is not yet clear whether this is due to OKT3 as such, or whether it merely reflects the total burden of immunosuppression. Xenosensitization (i.e. development of human antimouse antibodies) represents an important limitation to OKT3 treatment, although a second or third course can still be effective in patients with low antibody titres. Because of concerns about the risk of infection and malignancy, OKT3 is not used for the treatment of autoimmune diseases.

SIDE-EFFECTS

Table 25.2 provides a summary of the major side-effects of immunosuppressive drugs. Because in recent years there has been a tendency to reduce the dosage of these drugs, especially of prednisolone, some of the complications (e.g. infections) are seen less often than in the past. However, immunosuppressive drug therapy remains a two-sided sword, which may preserve life but which may also create serious illness.

USE OF IMMUNOSUPPRESSIVE DRUGS IN NONTRANSPLANT-RELATED DISEASES

RENAL DISEASE

Therapy with corticosteroids induces a prompt and complete response of minimal change nephrotic disease in children. Adults tend to respond somewhat less often and more slowly: about 80% of adult patients have complete remission of proteinuria. Cyclophosphamide or chlorambucil for 8–12 weeks may induce remission in steroid-resistant patients or increase its duration in frequent relapsers.[20] Cyclosporin often sustains remission in such cases, but relapse may occur when the drug is stopped. Because of the danger of irreversible nephrotoxicity, its use is still experimental and should be reserved for therapy-resistant cases. Although focal and segmental glomerulosclerosis has, in the past, been considered to have a uniformly poor prognosis, about 25% of patients experience partial or complete remission upon treatment with corticosteroids. In cases of relapsing proteinuria, a short course of cyclophosphamide may lead to prolonged remission. Preliminary evidence suggests that cyclosporin will induce remission in about 30% of steroid-resistant adults with focal sclerosis.[21] The overall benefit of corticosteroids and cytotoxic drugs in patients with membranous nephropathy seems to be limited to short-term alterations in the course of this disease. Only patients at high risk and those who are obviously losing renal function rapidly seem to benefit from treatment with prednisolone and chlorambucil. The outcome of treatment of antiglom-

---

Summary box 25.2 Clinical uses of immunosuppressive drugs

- Suppression of organ and tissue rejection after transplant surgery.

- Treatment of diseases with an autoimmune component:

  - renal diseases (e.g. glomerulonephritis, some nephrotic syndromes)

  - connective tissue diseases – systemic lupus erythematosus, rheumatoid arthritis

  - systemic vasculitis.

- Therapy is often limited by the high incidence of side-effects (see Table 25.2).

erular basement membrane nephritis depends on the severity of renal failure. Nonoliguric patients with anti-glomerular basement membrane nephritis whose serum creatinine concentration is less than $600\,\mu$mol l^{-1} have a high response rate to treatment with plasma-pheresis combined with corticosteroids and cyclophos-phamide, whereas in patients with oliguria or creatinine levels above $600\,\mu$mol l^{-1} recovery of renal function is unusual.

SYSTEMIC VASCULITIS

Treatment of patients with rapidly progressive glom-erulonephritis and/or systemic vasculitis (polyarteritis nodosa, microscopic polyarteritis, Wegener's granulo-matosis, Churg–Strauss disease) with corticosteroids in combination with oral cyclophosphamide will generally result in acute control of these diseases. In an attempt to minimize the considerable toxicity of cyclophos-phamide, azathioprine may be substituted once the acute phase of the disease has been controlled.

CONNECTIVE TISSUE DISEASES

The beneficial effects of corticosteroids on extrarenal manifestations of systemic lupus erythematosus (SLE) have long been recognized, but prolonged use of high doses of corticosteroids is associated with a high inci-dence of adverse effects. Treatment with intravenous pulses of methylprednisolone followed immediately by a low oral maintenance dose of corticosteroids appears to be as effective as the conventional oral scheme in inducing remission of severe acute renal disease. Cyto-toxic drugs are usually reserved for the patient with lupus who cannot tolerate corticosteroids or who suffers from intolerable steroid side-effects, whose extrarenal disease is not controlled with corticosteroids, or whose renal function is deteriorating and/or whose renal his-tology reveals proliferative glomerulonephritis.

The position of systemic corticosteroids in the therapy of rheumatoid arthritis remains controversial: controlled trials demonstrating its efficacy are not avail-able. It is recognized that under treatment with corti-costeroids the disease may progress with development of new articular erosions and other joint damage, while otherwise being adequately suppressed clinically. Gen-erally, low-dose corticosteroids are recommended only for severe disabling disease, certain forms of extraartic-ular disease and acute systemic rheumatoid vasculitis, or while awaiting the onset of action of second-line agents. In recent years, methotrexate (discussed in Chapter 24) has been shown to be beneficial in short-term double-blind controlled studies, but its efficacy in long-term treatment is less impressive. The effect of methotrexate on the ultimate course of rheumatoid arthritis is unknown. Azathioprine is currently pres-cribed only for patients who are intolerant to or have failed on methotrexate.

CONCLUDING REMARKS

Optimal immunosuppression can be defined as sup-

Side-effect	Examples of cause
Table 25.2 Side-effects of immunosuppressive drugs	
Caused by immunosuppression	
Infection	Viral, bacterial, fungal
Malignancy[*]	
Caused by side-effects of each individual drug	
Bone marrow suppression	Azathioprine, cyclophosphamide
Diabetes mellitus	Prednisolone, tacrolimus
Aseptic necrosis of the bone	Prednisolone
Gingival hypertrophy	Cyclosporin
Hirsutism	Cyclosporin
Nephrotoxicity	Cyclosporin, tacrolimus
Haemorrhagic cystitis	Cyclophosphamide
Infertility	Cyclophosphamide
Teratogenicity	Cyclophosphamide
Liver toxicity	Azathioprine
Venoocclusive disease of the liver	Azathioprine
Gastrointestinal toxicity	Mycophenolate mofetil
Drug-induced pneumonitis	Cyclophosphamide, azathioprine (rare)

[*] Particularly malignant lymphomas and skin cancers.

Table 25.3 Effects of immunosuppressive drugs: immune responses in vivo				
	Humoral		Cellular	
	Primary	Secondary	Primary	Secondary
Corticosteroids	=	=	↓↓	↓
Azathioprine	=	=	?	?
Cyclophosphamide	↓	(↓)	↓	=
Cyclosporin	↓↓	=	↓↓	=
CD3 monoclonal antibody	↓	(↓)	↓↓	↓↓

pression of humoral or cellular immune responses induced by particular antigens without affecting immune responses against all other antigens. Until now, this goal is far from being achieved.

Table 25.3 summarizes the point of attack of several immunosuppressive drugs in the immune system. In contrast to azathioprine and glucocorticosteroids, cyclophosphamide, cyclosporin, tacrolimus and mycopheno-

late mofetil seem to affect more the immune system itself and to have less influence on nonspecific reactions in the effector phase of the immune response. Monoclonal antibodies anti-CD3 suppress cellular immunity specifically. However, they are nonselective with regard to the antigens that induce cellular immunity. Much additional research is necessary to develop drugs with increased specificity and lower toxicity.

REFERENCES

1. Knudsen PJ, Dinarello CA, Strom TB. Glucocorticoids inhibit transcription and post-transcriptional expression of interleukin-1. *J Immunol* 1987; **139**: 4129–4134.
2. ten Berge RJM, Schellekens PTA, Surachno S, The TH, ten Veen JH, Wilmink JM. A longitudinal study on the effects of azathioprine and high doses of prednisone on the immune system of kidney-transplant recipients. *Clin Immunol Immunopathol* 1982; **24**: 33–46.
3. ten Berge RJM, van Walbeek HK, Schellekens PTA. Evaluation of the immunosuppressive effects of cyclophosphamide in patients with multiple sclerosis. *Clin Exp Immunol* 1982; **50**: 495–502.
4. Davis L, Britten JJ, Morgan M. Cholinesterase. Its significance in anaesthetic practice. *Anaesthesia* 1997; **52**: 244–260.
5. Dillman JB. Safe use of succinylcholine during repeated anesthetics in a patient treated with cyclophosphamide. *Anesth Analg* 1987; **66**: 351–353.
6. van der Heyden AAPAM, Bloemena E, Out TA, Wilmink JM, Schellekens PThA, van Oers MHJ. The influence of immunosuppressive treatment on immune responsiveness in vivo in kidney transplant recipients. *Transplantation* 1989; **48**: 44–47.
7. Freeman DJ, Laupacis A, Keown PA, Stiller CR, Carruthers SG. Evaluation of cyclosporin–phenytoin interaction with observations of cyclosporin metabolites. *Br J Clin Pharmacol* 1984; **18**: 887–893.
8. Gillum JG, Israel DS, Polk RE. Pharmacokinetic drug interactions with antimicrobial agents. *Clin Pharmacokinet* 1993; **25**: 450–482.
9. Charles BG, Ravenscroft PJ, Rigby RJ. The ketoconazole–cyclosporin interaction in an elderly renal transplant patient. *Aust N Z J Med* 1989; **19**: 292–293.
10. Parrott NR. Transplantation; where are we now? *Int J Intensive Care* 1996; **3**: 126–133.
11. Hooks MA. Tacrolimus, a new immunosuppressant – a review of the literature. *Ann Pharmacother* 1994; **28**: 501–511.
12. Danovitch GM. Mycophenolate mofetil in renal transplantation: results from the US randomized trials. *Kidney Int* 1995; **48** (Suppl. 52): S93–S96.
13. Bowen A, Edwards LC, Gailiunas P, Helderman JH. Lymphocyte function in patients treated with monoclonal anti-T3 antibody for acute cadaveric renal allograft rejection. *Transplantation* 1984; **38**: 489–493.
14. Norman DJ, Barry JM, Bennett WM et al. The use of OKT3 in cadaveric renal transplantation for rejection that is unresponsive to conventional anti-rejection therapy. *Am J Kidney Dis* 1988; **11**: 90–93.
15. Chatenoud L, Ferran C, Reuter A et al. Systemic reaction to the anti-T-cell monoclonal antibody OKT3 in relation to serum levels of tumor necrosis factor and interferon-gamma. *N Engl J Med* 1989; **320**: 1420–1421.
16. Raasveld MHM, Bemelman FJ, Schellekens PTA et al. Complement activation during OKT3 treatment: a possible explanation for respiratory side effects. *Kidney Int* 1993; **43**: 1140–1149.
17. Raasveld MHM, CE Hack, ten Berge RJM. Activation of coagulation and fibrinolysis following OKT3 administration to renal transplant recipients: association with distinct mediators. *Thromb Haemost* 1992; **68**: 264–267.
18. Oh CS, Stratta RJ, Fox BC, Sollinger HW, Belzer FO, Maki DG. Increased infections associated with the use of OKT3 for treatment of steroid-resistant rejection in renal transplantation. *Transplantation* 1988; **45**: 68–73.
19. Penn I. The changing pattern of posttransplant malignancies. *Transplant Proc* 1991; **23**: 1101–1103.
20. Meyrier A, Simon P. Treatment of corticoresistant idiopathic nephrotic syndrome in the adult: minimal-change disease and focal-segmental glomerulosclerosis. *Adv Nephrol* 1988; **17**: 127–150.
21. Ponticelli C, Rizzoni G, Edefonti A et al. A randomized trial of cyclosporin in steroid resistant idiopathic nephrotic syndrome. *Kidney Int* 1993; **43**: 1377–1384.

26 D Royston

DRUGS ACTING ON THE HAEMOSTATIC SYSTEM

HEPARINS

Heparin is a naturally occurring negatively charged sulphated polysaccharide with a complex structure. It is a glycosaminoglycan formed from alternating residues of D-glucosamine and L-iduronic acid. The uronic acid residues bind two sulphate groups to produce one of the strongest acids found in nature. Heparin is mostly located in lungs, intestine and liver in mammals, with the skin, lymph nodes and thymus being less plentiful sources. The finding of heparin in tissues rich in mast cells suggests that these are the prime source of the compound. Heparin was originally isolated from liver during investigations to ascertain whether the phospholipid component of cephalin would cause clotting. Since heparin's discovery in 1916 by McLean,[1] numerous physiological actions have been proposed for this agent.

As a linear anionic compound, heparin demonstrates a wide spectrum of activity with enzymes, hormones, biogenic amines and plasma proteins. Heparin has a direct antiinflammatory action in humans. The finding of heparin-rich mast cells in tissues where the inside and outside of the body are in close proximity suggests a primary antiinflammatory or immunological role for this agent. This concept is strengthened when we consider (1) that heparin alone has no effects on coagulation and (2) it is found in lower orders of the animal kingdom, such as molluscs, which lack a coagulation system. None the less, about one-third of the molecules of heparin contain a pentasaccharide sequence which binds to antithrombin III (ATIII). ATIII, also called the heparin cofactor, is a naturally occurring, slow-acting inhibitor of coagulation. Binding with heparin dramatically increases this inhibitory effect. The heparin–AT III complex was thought initially to inactivate thrombin alone. It is now known to have a wider effect as the complex will bind to a number of serine proteases including coagulation factors XIIa, XIa, Xa, IXa, plasmin and kallikrein. Other functions of heparin are related to a role in angiogenesis and, as it is a precursor of lipoprotein lipase, a role in lipid metabolism.

Standard preparations of heparin are unfractionated, derived from either porcine intestine or bovine lung and prepared as calcium or sodium salts. The number and sequence of the saccharides is variable, producing a heterogeneous collection of polysaccharides. Molecular weights range from 3000 to 30 000 Da, with a mean of 15 000 Da representing 40 to 50 saccharides in length. There is no apparent difference between any of the available forms of unfractionated heparin (UFH) with respect to their pharmacology or anticoagulant profile.[2]

PHARMACOKINETICS AND PHARMACODYNAMICS OF UNFRACTIONATED HEPARIN

The pharmacokinetics of heparin are complex. Heparins are poorly absorbed from the gastrointestinal tract and can cause haematomas after intramuscular injection. They are therefore usually administered by subcutaneous or intravenous injection. Intravenous injection is the preferred route when a rapid anticoagulant effect is needed. Even so, similar levels of anticoagulation can easily be achieved by the subcutaneous route if sufficient doses are used and onset is only delayed by 1–2 h,[2] which can be overcome by using an intravenous loading dose. Studies suggest the safety of the two routes is comparable.

The heterogeneity of heparin molecules produces great variability in the plasma concentration of the agent in relation to the dose administered. A three-compartment model best describes heparin kinetics in humans. After intravenous injection, plasma levels initially decline rapidly due to redistribution and possible uptake by endothelial cells. More than 50% of heparin circulates bound to a number of plasma proteins including platelet factor 4, histidine-rich glycoprotein, vitronectin, fibronectin and von Willebrand factor. The first three of these also neutralize heparin's activity and reduce its bioavailability. Raised levels of these proteins may account for the heparin resistance sometimes seen in malignancy and inflammatory disorders.[1]

Elimination occurs by two separate processes; a rapid mechanism which is readily saturated in the therapeutic ranges used clinically, and a slower process involving first-order kinetics. Heparin clearance is therefore nonlinear: as the dose of heparin is increased, the elimination half-life appears to lengthen and the anticoagulant response is exaggerated. The rapid saturable phase of heparin clearance is thought to be due to cellular degradation. In particular macrophages internalize the heparin, then depolymerize and desulphate it. Saturation occurs when all the receptors have been utilized, and further clearance depends on new receptor synthesis. This process explains the poor bioavailability after low-dose subcutaneous injection, as the slow rate of absorption barely exceeds the capacity of cellular degradation. Significant plasma levels can only be achieved once these receptors have been saturated following a loading dose. The slower phase of heparin elimination is due to renal excretion. Surprisingly, no consistent report of the effects of renal or hepatic dysfunction on the pharmacokinetics of heparin has been made.[1,2]

PHARMACOKINETICS AND PHARMACODYNAMICS OF LOW MOLECULAR WEIGHT HEPARIN

Low molecular weight heparins (LMWHs) are produced from UFH by depolymerization. This depolymerization produces marked changes in the properties of LMWHs and leads to their clinical advantages over UFH.[3,4] LMWHs have mean molecular weights of 4000–6500 Da, although the range is 2000–10 000 Da. There are significant variations between the different commercial preparations according to the method used in their production.

The LMWHs differ also in the distribution of their fragment molecular weights, their in vitro potency (anti-Xa, antithrombin and anticoagulant activities) and, consequently, in their biodynamic patterns, recommended dose regimen, and efficacy : safety ratio.[5] Since they are mainly administered subcutaneously, compared with UFH they are almost completely absorbed and, in contrast to UFH, exhibit linear pharmacokinetics with proportionality between anti-Xa (and anti-IIa in some cases) plasma concentration and dose, and stationary distribution volume and clearance processes when the dosage is increased. Unlike UFH their distribution volume is close to the blood volume. Similar to UFH they

are partially metabolized by desulphation and depolymerization. Urinary excretion of anti-Xa activity for enoxaparin, dalteparin and nadroparin, all given at doses for prevention of venous thrombosis, is between 3% and 10% of the injected dose. However, these LMWHs differ in the extent of their nonrenal clearance, resulting in different apparent elimination half-life values and relative apparent bioavailability. When given at doses recommended for prevention of venous thromboembolism, the LMWHs do not significantly cross the placenta and their excretion profiles are only slightly altered in severe renal disease. Because of the differences among LMWHs, the clinical profile of a given LMWH cannot be extrapolated to another or generalized to the whole LMWH family.

The affinity of plasma proteins for LMWHs is much less than that for UFH so that only 10% is protein bound. This increased bioavailability ensures a more predictable anticoagulant action. LMWHs have nearly complete bioavailability at all doses when given by subcutaneous injection, compared with 40% for low-dose subcutaneous UFH. Similarly LMWHs do not bind to endothelial cells or macrophages, and so are not subject to the rapid degradation that UFH suffers. Although the clearance of LMWH is dependent on renal excretion, producing a half-life two to four times as long as that of UFH, this is not clinically apparent until low creatinine clearance values (< 15 ml min^{-1}) are achieved.

MECHANISM OF ACTION OF UNFRACTIONATED HEPARIN

The anticoagulant activity of heparin requires the presence of a plasma cofactor, ATIII. ATIII has an intrinsic low level of anticoagulant activity, mediated by an arginine centre that binds to and inactivates the activated serine proteases of the coagulation cascade. A critical pentasaccharide sequence of heparin binds to and induces a conformational change in ATIII, greatly enhancing its activity. The binding of heparin to ATIII is highly specific, reversible, and does not inactivate the heparin molecule. Approximately one-third of heparin molecules contain the pentasaccharide and are capable of binding to ATIII; these heparin molecules are responsible for the main anticoagulant effect.

The coagulation factors affected by the heparin–ATIII complex are the activated forms of thrombin (factor II) and factors IX, X and XII. The most avid reaction is with thrombin, the inhibition of which requires that heparin binds not only ATIII but also to thrombin itself, to form a ternary complex. Only heparin moieties with more than 18 saccharides are able to do this. In contrast, the inhibition of factors IXa, Xa and XIIa requires only that the heparin should bind ATIII to form the heparin–ATIII complex.[2] The inhibition of thrombin activation also prevents the feedback by thrombin on factors V and VII, which normally amplifies the clotting cascade.

Heparin has actions in addition to the anticoagulant effects mediated via ATIII. At high blood levels ($>$ 4 units ml^{-1}), heparin is capable of binding heparin cofactor II, potentiating its inactivation of bound activated thrombin.[6] This action does not require the specific ATIII binding site but does require heparins greater than 7200 Da or 24 units in length. At present the clinical importance of this antithrombotic action is unclear. Heparin also stimulates the release of tissue factor plasma inhibitor (TFPI), which binds and neutralizes the tissue factor–VIIa complex, reducing prothrombinase production via the extrinsic pathway. Plasma concentrations of TFPI rise two- to sixfold following heparin injection. This rise occurs with UFH and LMWH.[7]

Although bound thrombin can be inactivated by the heparin–ATIII complex, much higher concentrations are required than to inactivate free thrombin.[8] In addition, platelets secrete platelet factor 4, which neutralizes heparin. Clinically this is seen as a requirement for much higher levels of heparin to prevent the extension of venous thrombosis compared with those required to prevent initiation of thrombosis.[1,2]

In contrast to this requirement to inhibit clot formation, heparin will also impair platelet aggregation mediated by von Willebrand factor and by collagen, and inhibits platelet function by direct binding to platelets. It is the higher molecular weight heparin molecules with the lower affinity for ATIII that interfere most with platelet function.[9] These actions may be responsible for heparin-induced haemorrhage by a mechanism that is separate to its anticoagulant actions.

Heparin also inhibits vascular smooth muscle proliferation and is involved in regulating angiogenesis.

MECHANISM OF ACTION OF LOW MOLECULAR WEIGHT HEPARINS

The molecular weight profiles of LMWHs vary significantly, so their anticoagulant properties are not necessarily identical.[10] The exact mechanism underlying the anticoagulant effects of LMWH remains uncertain. The proportion of LMWH containing the critical pentasaccharide responsible for binding ATIII is less than in the parent UFH.[3,4] The smaller size of the molecules in LMWH results in less in vitro inhibition of thrombin via ATIII, while the ability to inhibit Xa remains intact. When in vivo measurements are performed, the anti-IIa action is much greater, and the anti-Xa is less than would be predicted. Although the LMWHs have weak anti-IIa action, their high bioavailability and long half-life mean that both the anti-Xa and the anti-IIa action are four times greater than for UFH. The potency of LMWHs is further increased by their resistance to inac-

tivation by platelet factor 4 and by lack of protein binding. Like UFH, the main action of LMWHs is to prevent the formation of prothrombinase and amplification of the coagulation cascade. LMWHs are as effective as UFH in stimulating endothelial release of TFPI,[11] and directly inhibit the activation of VII. This further reduces the production of prothrombinase.

MONITORING HEPARIN

There is marked variation in response between individuals to the anticoagulant effect of a fixed dose of UFH. The response to increasing doses of UFH is nonlinear due to saturation of the cellular degradation process described above. Furthermore, as there is good evidence that maintaining the anticoagulant effect of UFH above the lower limit of the therapeutic range minimizes the risk of recurrent thromboembolism,[12,13] monitoring is routinely performed during therapy with UFH.

Direct measurement of heparin concentration is not possible, although protamine titration can be used to ascertain blood levels. The commonly used laboratory test of heparin function is the activated partial thromboplastin time (APTT), which measures the effect of heparin on thrombin and factors IXa and Xa. The therapeutic range most commonly quoted is an APTT between 1.5 and 2.5 times the control value. However, the commercially available kits for measurement of APTT differ in their sensitivity to heparins. This suggests that the protamine titration method of monitoring may be more robust.

The higher bioavailability of LMWHs and their longer half-life produce a more predictable anticoagulant response. These properties allow once-daily subcutaneous administration for prophylaxis of deep venous thrombosis without laboratory monitoring.[4,12]

CLINICAL USE OF HEPARIN

For thromboembolic prophylaxis, UFH is administered as either 'low dose' (5000 units subcutaneously every 8 or 12 h) or 'adjusted dose' heparin (3500 units every 8–12 h, which is then adjusted to maintain the APTT at 1–3 s above the control level). For treatment of established thromboembolic disease, full therapeutic doses of heparin are used either by intravenous infusion or by subcutaneous injection following an intravenous loading dose. Long-term heparin therapy is only used during pregnancy (because, unlike warfarin, neither UFH nor LMWH is able to cross the placenta) and in patients who have suffered recurrent thromboembolic complications while taking adequate doses of warfarin.

Low-dose UFH is a safe and effective prophylactic treatment for surgical patients at risk of venous thromboembolism. Overviews of clinical trials have shown that low-dose subcutaneous UFH produces a marked and statistically significant reduction in the incidence of venous thrombosis, and in fatal and nonfatal pulmonary embolism. Although these papers demonstrated an increased incidence of wound haematomas, there was no increase in major or fatal haemorrhage. LMWHs have been shown to be as safe and effective as UFH in placebo-controlled and in numerous comparative trials. Meta-analysis of these trials suggests low-dose LMWHs are slightly superior to low-dose UFH,[14] particularly in reducing the incidence of pulmonary embolism. As yet there is little evidence of the predicted decreased risk of haemorrhage with LMWHs compared with UFH.

Patients undergoing major orthopaedic procedures represent a group with a particularly high risk of thromboembolism. Without prophylaxis, patients undergoing total hip replacement have an incidence of deep vein thrombosis of 50%, and a pulmonary embolus-related mortality rate of 3–6%. Low-dose subcutaneous UFH reduces the risk by only 30–40%, compared with the 70% reduction produced in other groups of surgical patients. In contrast low-dose LMWHs are able to reduce the risks by 70–80% without any increase in haemorrhage compared with low-dose UFH, which has been confirmed by meta-analysis.[14]

While relatively low doses of heparin are sufficient to provide thromboprophylaxis, much higher concentrations are needed to prevent thrombus propagation. Recommended regimens for the treatment of deep vein thrombosis with UFH include an intravenous loading dose of 5000–10 000 units, then a continuous infusion of 1300 units h^{-1}, adjusted to maintain the APTT at 1.5–2.5 times the control value. This should be continued until warfarin therapy has prolonged the prothrombin time into the therapeutic range for at least 24 h.[13] Studies have shown that this regimen reduces the recurrence of venous thrombosis and death from pulmonary embolism.[1,2] The most common reason for failure of treatment is inadequate anticoagulation, particularly within the first 24 h, a problem that is overcome by the large intravenous loading dose.[13] These treatment protocols have been compared with twice-daily subcutaneous LMWHs without laboratory assessment. In an analysis of the randomized trials, Green et al.[15] concluded that LMWHs were safer and more effective, with significant and important reductions in recurrence of thrombosis and major haemorrhage. It is likely that LMWHs will replace UFH in the treatment of established thromboembolic disease, allowing patients to be treated outside hospital.

SIDE-EFFECTS OF HEPARIN

Although haemorrhage is rare in patients on prophylactic doses of either UFH or LMWHs, it is a frequent complication of therapeutic heparin therapy. The greater the dose of heparin, and therefore the greater its anticoagulant effect, the greater the risk of haemorrhage. When comparable doses are used, the risks are similar using either the continuous intravenous or subcutaneous route of administration.[1,2] Many patient factors are known to increase the risk of haemorrhage, including the length of treatment, presence of cardiac, hepatic or renal dysfunction, aspirin or other nonsteroidal therapy, and recent surgery, trauma or invasive procedures. Approximately 30% of patients who suffer anticoagulant-related haemorrhage are found to have previously undiagnosed predisposing lesions, particularly of the gastrointestinal and genitourinary tracts. The incidence of major bleeding in anticoagulated patients has been estimated as approximately 5%. A recent review estimated the daily frequencies of fatal, major and all types of haemorrhage in patients receiving therapeutic anticoagulation as 0.05%, 0.8% and 2.0% respectively, approximately twice the level expected in the absence of anticoagulation.[16]

Studies of LMWHs given for prophylaxis suggest they cause an increase in wound haematomas but no change in the incidence of haemorrhage. In contrast, a significant reduction in major haemorrhage is seen when LMWHs are used to treat established thrombosis.[4,13]

Heparin-induced thrombocytopenia (HIT) is a relatively common complication. The incidence is 1.1% and 2.3% in patients receiving therapeutic doses of intravenous porcine and bovine heparin respectively. Affected patients are generally receiving high doses of UFH, but rare cases have been reported in patients on low-dose subcutaneous heparin prophylaxis and have even been attributed to flushing lines with heparin. The risk of HIT is less with LMWH than with UFH, perhaps due to the lesser interaction with platelets. Two distinct clinical syndromes have been described.[17] Type I involves a mild thrombocytopenia with a platelet count that rarely falls below $100 \times 10^9 \, l^{-1}$ which occurs during the first few days of treatment and usually recovers rapidly even if heparin is continued. The patient is normally asymptomatic and no specific treatment is required. The underlying mechanism probably involves the action of heparin as a mild platelet aggregator.[17] The importance of type I HIT is in its distinction from the less benign type II HIT.

Type II HIT is characterized by a delayed onset of a severe, progressive thrombocytopenia with platelet counts below $100 \times 10^9 \, l^{-1}$ and often below $50 \times 10^9 \, l^{-1}$. The platelet count does recover unless heparin therapy is stopped, and recurs promptly if heparin is restarted. Recovery usually occurs within 1 week but may occasionally be prolonged. An immune mechanism has been suggested, in which heparin binds to platelet factor 4 to form a molecule that stimulates the production of an immunoglobulin (Ig)G antibody. This antibody binds the heparin–platelet factor 4 molecule to produce an immune complex, all three parts of which are capable of binding to platelets. These complexes have two separate effects. First, they coat platelets and increase their removal from the circulation by the reticuloendothelial system. Second, they cause activation of platelets and the coagulation cascade, leading to a hypercoagulable state.[17] Haemorrhage is uncommon and resistance to anticoagulation may occur due to heparin-induced release of platelet factor 4.

A high index of suspicion is necessary, since only immediate withdrawal of heparin will reduce mortality and morbidity rates. The condition is underdiagnosed and should be considered in all patients receiving heparin who develop a new thrombosis or heparin resistance.[17] Confirmation requires a platelet count to show thrombocytopenia, a blood film to demonstrate clumping, exclusion of other causes for thrombocytopenia and the presence of a heparin-dependent antiplatelet antibody.[17] A rapid platelet aggregation test can be used to detect the antibody and confirm the diagnosis.

The most serious complication associated with type II HIT is new thromboembolic events, due to platelet-rich thrombi, which continue to form until the heparin is withdrawn. Platelet counts should be monitored closely as precipitous falls may herald the onset of thrombosis even without absolute thrombocytopenia. Arterial and venous thrombosis may occur either alone or together, and multiple sites are often involved. Of patients receiving therapeutic doses of porcine heparin, 0.4% exhibited manifestations of thrombosis, most commonly lower-limb thrombosis, thrombotic cerebrovascular accident or acute myocardial infarction.[18] In one series of surgical patients the incidence was reported as 0.3%, but 80% (eight of the ten patients) suffered major thromboembolic morbidity, five of these eight requiring limb amputation. Warfarin should be started as early as possible but the 3–5 days it takes to reach a therapeutic level will need to be covered with an alternative antithrombotic agent. LMWHs have a high incidence of cross-reaction with the heparin-dependent antibody, which can be ascertained by means of the platelet aggregation test. If no cross-reaction occurs, successful anticoagulation can be safely undertaken.[17] Organan, a low molecular weight heparinoid which contains no heparin, has a low cross-reaction rate and appears to produce a good outcome. Ancrod, a defibrinogenating agent, has been used for short-term treatment, although antibodies to the drug are produced and reduce its effectiveness. Both organan and ancrod have been used to enable patients with HIT to undergo cardiopulmonary bypass (CPB).[17]

REVERSAL OF ACTION: ANTIDOTES TO HEPARINS

The effects of UFH wear off so rapidly that an antagonist is rarely required, except after the high doses administered to facilitate CPB. If it is necessary to reverse the action of UFH, equimolar amounts of protamine sulphate can be used to neutralize the anticoagulant and antithrombotic effects. Protamine is a basic protein which combines with heparin to form a stable, inactive complex; 1 mg protamine will reverse the actions of 100 units (1 mg) UFH. Careful titration of protamine dosage is required, since in excess it may exert an anticoagulant effect of its own. With LMWHs, protamine is able to neutralize the anti-IIa action but not the anti-Xa, due to inability to bind the smaller molecules.

Recombinant platelet factor 4 (rPF4) has been proposed as an alternative to protamine. The effective heparin neutralization dose of rPF4, compared with the standard agent protamine, in human blood activated through exposure to the CPB suggested a 2:1 (weight:weight) reversal ratio for rPF4 and protamine. The safety and efficacy of rPF4 have been shown in a randomized placebo-controlled study.[19]

PROTAMINE

SOURCE AND PREPARATION

Most vertebrate species synthesize a protamine that is found in sperm. Human protamine closely resembles that of other species. Fish, especially salmon, milt provides the source of protamine used clinically. Protamine is produced following a salt and alcohol extraction, together with filtration, of these fish parts. The final product, a dried powder, is commonly reconstituted as a 10 mg ml^{-1} solution. Like insulin and some other protein products, it is stable without refrigeration for several weeks. Protamine is available as sulphate and chloride salts. Protamine chloride may have a more rapid onset compared with protamine sulphate. Nevertheless, clinical studies reveal no superiority of one preparation over the other.

USES AND ACTIONS

Neutralization of heparin-induced anticoagulation remains the primary use of protamine. Formation of complexes with the sulphate groups of heparin forms the basis for this effect. Protamine neutralizes the antithrombin effect of heparin far better than its anti-Xa effect. This distinction may arise from the need for thrombin, but not factor Xa, to remain complexed to heparin in order that ATIII can exert its inhibitory effect. Since porcine mucosal heparin has more potent anti-Xa activity than bovine lung heparin, the latter source of heparin may prove a better choice when depending upon protamine neutralization.

Protamine as a cause of bleeding

Protamine exhibits antihaemostatic properties by affecting platelets and by releasing tissue plasminogen activator (tPA) from endothelial cells. Thrombocytopenia follows protamine administration. Heparin–protamine complexes inhibit thrombin-induced platelet aggregation.[20] In addition, protamine appears to bind to thrombin, inhibiting its ability to convert fibrinogen to fibrin. Attempts to document an in vivo antihaemostatic effect of protamine have proved unsuccessful.[20] Rapid degradation of protamine by circulating proteases may account for this discrepancy.

PHARMACOKINETICS AND DYNAMICS

Neutralization of heparin occurs following intravenous injection of protamine. Subcutaneous administration is limited to prolongation of insulin absorption. In the presence of circulating heparin, protamine forms large complexes with heparin. Excess protamine creates larger complexes. The time course of protamine disappearance from plasma in patients remains poorly investigated. Protamine degradation in vivo proceeds by the action of circulating proteases, among them carboxypeptidase N, an enzyme that also clears anaphylatoxins and kinin pathway products.

The recommended dose of protamine to neutralize heparin varies widely. Reports of the optimal ratio of milligrams of protamine to units of heparin cite values as low as zero (i.e. do not neutralize heparin) to as much as 4 mg per 100 units. This variability arises from differences in timing, temperature and other environmental factors, choices for coagulation tests together with personal prejudice based on unproved assumptions.

Protamine titration tests at the conclusion of CPB can determine the amount of heparin remaining in the circulating blood pool. Semiautomatic systems of heparin management utilizing protamine titration have been compared with empirical dosing methods. Of interest is that utilization of such systems produced increased heparin and reduced protamine dose.

Gross protamine overdose may anticoagulate patients. Dogs given excess protamine exhibited a dose-dependent prolongation of the Activated Clotting Time (ACT), with the ACT nearly doubling following a protamine dose four times that needed to neutralize heparin. At a tenfold dose, the APPT was prolonged and thrombocytopenia developed. Without previous administration of heparin, the coagulation test abnormalities occurred at lower protamine doses.

ADVERSE REACTIONS

Adverse reactions to protamine include rash, urticaria, bronchospasm, raised pulmonary artery pressure and hypotension, which leads at times to cardiovascular collapse and death.[21,22]

Cardiovascular dysfunction following protamine administration

Not all adverse responses to protamine are allergic reactions. Rapid protamine injection decreases blood pressure. Indeed, protamine infusion is one of the most common causes of hypotension following cardiac surgery. The hypotension can be related to:

1. *Rapid administration.* Systemic hypotension follows rapid infusion of protamine. This hypotension is not associated with changes in pulmonary artery pressures but is associated with decreases in systemic vascular resistance, without changes in cardiac output. This hypotension is unaffected by the site of administration.
2. *Anaphylactoid (and anaphylactic) reactions.* Despite profound systemic hypotension with IgE-mediated anaphylactic reaction, there is usually little change in the pulmonary artery pressure.
3. *Raised pulmonary arterial resistance.*

Available evidence strongly indicates that this different response to protamine is probably caused by IgG antibodies. As with the other causes, systemic hypotension occurs 2–3 min after protamine, but in this case it will be accompanied by pulmonary hypertension with an associated increase in thromboxane A_2. When IgG interacts with protamine, the complement cascade is activated, and thromboxane A_2 has been shown to be the mediator of the pulmonary vasoconstrictor response.

Previous protamine exposure, fish (usually shellfish) allergy or previous vasectomy remain theoretical risk factors for a true protamine allergy. Insulin-dependent diabetics are a group of patients at risk for protamine reaction. Neutral protamine Hagedorn (NPH) insulin contains 0.35–0.4 mg protamine per 100 units. Continued administration of NPH insulin may potentially sensitize patients to protamine.[21]

USE OF LOCAL ANAESTHESIA IN THE PATIENT RECEIVING HEPARIN

Therapeutic anticoagulation is a contraindication to central nerve blockade unless the coagulation profile is corrected to normal. The risks associated with epidural or spinal anaesthesia in patients receiving heparin prophylaxis has been a controversial subject.[23] The best estimate of the frequency of clinically significant spinal haematomas, in patients not taking anticoagulants, following spinal or epidural anaesthesia is less than 1 in 100 000 blocks.[24] The rarity of this complication and the fact that it may occur spontaneously in patients receiving anticoagulant therapy (including LMWH) have hampered attempts to estimate the increased risk attached to performing central blockade in patients on heparin therapy.

PHARMACOLOGICAL INTERVENTIONS TO REDUCE BLEEDING

A number of pharmacological interventions are now available to inhibit bleeding after surgery and trauma. None of the commonly available agents is new; most have been used for over 30 years. What is new is their use to prevent bleeding.

The agents with proven benefit to reduce bleeding include desmopressin, the lysine analogue antifibrinolytics and the serine protease inhibitors. The major part of this section will compare and contrast the effects of the lysine analogues and aprotinin.

DESMOPRESSIN

The actions of desmopressin are dose related. The recommended dose is $0.3 \mu g$ kg^{-1} given over a 20–30-min period. The principal action of desmopressin is to induce the release of the larger multimers of von Willebrand factor. This action increases the adhesion of platelets to the endothelium. Once the platelet has adhered to the endothelium it will undergo a shape change and express receptors which will allow the process of coagulation to be initiated and amplified. There are no data to suggest that desmopressin specifically affects any of the clotting factors directly. Administration of desmopressin will also produce a release of tPA and prostacyclin. Rapid administration of desmopressin is associated with a significant fall in blood pressure and a decrease in systemic vascular resistance. Whether this vasodilatation is related to the known action of desmopressin to induce prostacyclin release or by stimulation of the vasopressin V_2 receptors is currently unknown.

The prostacyclin release induced by desmopressin will inhibit platelet function. None the less, the majority of conditions where desmopressin has been shown to have a major benefit are in situations where platelet function is abnormal before the bleeding episode. This is especially true for patients with uraemia or those taking aspirin therapy in whom administration of desmopressin has been shown to shorten prolonged bleeding time and to reduce bleeding and the need for blood and blood products.

LYSINE ANALOGUES

Human plasminogen contains lysine binding sites which are important to allow binding to a_2-antiplasmin and fibrin. The binding of plasminogen to fibrin and the heavy chain of plasmin to fibrin monomer is mediated through these binding sites. This interaction is almost completely blocked by the synthetic antifibrinolytic amino acids. The potency of the aminocarboxylic acids depends on the presence of free amino and carboxylic groups, and on the distance between the carboxylic group and the carbon atoms to which the amino group is attached.

Native human plasminogen contains one high-affinity and four or five low-affinity lysine binding sites. The high-affinity site of plasminogen is involved primarily in its binding to fibrin. Saturation of this binding site with a lysine analogue displaces plasminogen from the fibrin surface. This results in retardation of fibrinolysis because, no matter how rapidly plasmin is formed, it cannot bind to fibrinogen or fibrin monomers. Conversely, when the lysine binding sites of plasmin are blocked by tranexamic acid, inactivation by a_2-antiplasmin is virtually impossible.

ε-Aminocaproic acid

ε-Aminocaproic acid or 6-aminohexanoic acid (molecular weight 131 Da) was the first synthetic representative of the antifibrinolytic agents. The clinical pharmacology of ε-aminocaproic acid has been known since the early 1960s. Oral doses (100 mg per kg body weight) are rapidly and nearly completely absorbed, giving peak plasma concentrations of 30 mg l^{-1} after about 2 h. The elimination half-life is between 1 and 2 h. The drug is distributed throughout the extravascular space; it readily crosses the erythrocyte membrane and diffuses into various tissues. Oral ε-aminocaproic acid is concentrated and excreted in the urine in a chemically unchanged active form, 80% being excreted within 12 h; only a small amount of the absorbed dose is believed to be metabolized. The rapid excretion means that parenteral administration for a systemic effect should be by continuous infusion.

Intravenous administration of 100 mg kg^{-1} ε-aminocaproic acid produces an initial serum concentration of about 1500 mg l^{-1}, which falls to 35 mg l^{-1} within 3–4 h. About 90% of the administered dose is found in the urine within 4–6 h. Thus, ε-aminocaproic acid is concentrated many times during excretion, urinary levels being 50–100 times those found in plasma. Because of its short half-life, therapy requires relatively large doses to reach and sustain an effective plasma concentration. An intravenous loading dose of 10 g followed by 1 g h^{-1} gives the desired blood level.

There is a vast literature on the clinical use of ε-aminocaproic acid, but its effectiveness has been documented by controlled clinical trials in only a limited number of circumstances. As tranexamic acid is seven to ten times more potent than ε-aminocaproic acid and has the same low toxicity, the latter drug is now little used clinically and has no licence for use in many countries such as the UK. In countries such as the USA, licence still exists for prophylactic use only in dental surgery and for the treatment of bleeding only where excess fibrinolysis has been documented from laboratory tests.

Tranexamic acid

Tranexamic acid is the trans-stereoisomer of 4-aminomethylcyclohexane carboxylic acid, with a molecular weight of 157 Da. Initial investigations with the drug were performed using a preparation containing a mixture of isomers, but it was subsequently found that only the *trans* stereoisomer has antifibrinolytic activity.

At therapeutic concentrations (5–10 mg l^{-1}), tranexamic acid is very weakly protein bound. The 3% protein binding is almost all accounted for by binding to plasminogen. The elimination half-life has been reported to be 80 min. Following intravenous administration of tranexamic acid 10 mg kg^{-1}, plasma concentrations at 1, 3 and 5 h after injection were 18, 10 and 5 mg l^{-1} respectively. About 30% of the administered dose is recovered in the urine during the first hour after intravenous administration of 10 mg kg^{-1}, a total of about 45% during the first 3 h, and about 90% after 24 h. Tranexamic acid produces substantial inhibition of urinary fibrinolytic activity for at least 24 h after a single dose.

Tranexamic acid displays a considerably higher and more sustained antifibrinolytic activity in tissues than ε-aminocaproic acid, and is able to cross the blood–brain barrier. Owing to subtle chemical differences, tranexamic acid is, on a molar basis, more potent than ε-aminocaproic acid but has the same acute and chronic toxicity profile. As tranexamic acid also displays a considerably higher and more sustained antifibrinolytic activity in tissues than ε-aminocaproic acid, and has a longer half-life, tranexamic acid would appear to be the most logical choice of lysine analogue.

The main indications for the use of tranexamic acid are the prevention of excessive bleeding after tonsillectomy, in prostatic surgery, after cervical conisation, and in primary or intrauterine device-induced menorrhagia. It is possible that gastric and intestinal bleeding can also be reduced, as well as recurrent epistaxis. Tranexamic acid could prove useful after ocular trauma. The value of fibrinolysis inhibitors in the prevention of bleeding after tooth extraction in patients with haemophilia is well documented, as is the treatment of hereditary angioneurotic oedema.

Tranexamic acid is licensed for use in Europe as a prophylactic agent to prevent bleeding following dental surgery in patients with haemophilia and as a treatment for menorrhagia. Tranexamic acid currently has no licence for use in North America for other indications.

APROTININ

Aprotinin is a naturally occurring inhibitor of proteolytic enzymes. It was discovered independently by Kraut *et al.* in 1930 and by Kunitz and Northrop in 1936 as the trypsin–kallikrein inhibitor from bovine tissue. This serine protease inhibitor is a single-chain polypeptide of 6512 Da and consists of 58 amino acid residues in a single polypeptide chain crosslinked by three disulphide bridges; the reactive site bond of this strongly basic protein being Lys-15–Ala-16.[25] The concentration and activity of commercial preparations of aprotinin are usually given in KIU (kallikrein inactivator units). Some 100 000 KIU are equivalent to 14 mg of the pure polypeptide or 2.15 μmol l^{-1} aprotinin respectively.

Aprotinin acts as an inhibitor of human trypsin, plasmin, plasma kallikrein and tissue kallikreins by forming reversible stoichiometric enzyme–inhibitor complexes. This is achieved by the formation of aprotinin–proteinase complexes at the active serine site of the enzyme.

The combination with various proteases shows, however, certain differences between dissociation constants. The binding with trypsin is most stable. The binding with human plasmin is not so tight and is reversible. The complex of aprotinin with human plasma kallikrein is relatively loose but still within the therapeutic range of aprotinin achieved with the high-dose regimen.

Aprotinin not only binds to isolated enzymes but also to enzymes already complexed by a third binding partner, provided there is still free access to the active site of the enzyme. Thus, aprotinin will efficiently inhibit free plasmin and also the plasmin–streptokinase complex.

Aprotinin is inactive when given orally and needs to be administered by the intravenous route. The half-life in plasma is biphasic, with an initial elimination half-life of about 1 h. It follows that the compound has to be given by continuous infusion if the plasma concentration is to be maintained.

Aprotinin is highly resistant to proteolysis and processes associated with moderate chemical degradation. One of the noteworthy aspects of the pharmacokinetics of aprotinin is the affinity of the drug for renal tissue, especially the brush border and proximal convoluted tubule. This may in part be due to the neuraminic acid content of the brush border in the kidney, together with the basic nature of the drug.

Aprotinin prevents the bleeding associated with a number of different types of surgery. The largest number of studies have been in patients having extracorporeal circulation and open heart surgery. There are also studies showing efficacy in orthopaedic and trauma surgery, neurosurgical, vascular, genitourinary and gynaecological surgery, and various transplant procedures.[25]

Other serine protease inhibitors such as nefamostat (FUT-175) should have similar efficacy. The one published controlled trial showed a reduction in drain loss of 34% and a reduction in red cell transfusion of 82%.

For the lysine analogues the only studies to show consistent efficacy apart from open heart surgery are reports of the use of tranexamic acid in patients having knee replacements.

MECHANISM OF ACTION

There is a considerable difference between the mechanism of action of these two groups of agents in relation to their ability to effect haemostasis and clot lysis. The body's naturally occurring plasmin inhibitor is a_2-antiplasmin, or a_2-plasmin inhibitor (a_2-PI), which has a number of properties related to site-specific activation. If free plasmin is found in the circulation then a_2-PI will react and neutralize this plasmin with a time constant of approximately 0.01 s. Free plasmin is a digestive enzyme and will degrade a number of intravascular proteins including the clotting factors. In contrast to the rapid inhibition of free enzyme, if plasmin is generated on the fibrin strand then a_2-PI will only slightly inhibit this process. It is therefore apparent that a_2-PI is a powerful inhibitor of free plasmin (associated with 'pathological' fibrinolysis) but does not act as an antifibrinolytic agent for 'appropriate' or 'physiological' fibrinolysis (Fig. 26.1).[8] a_2-PI does, however, have an interesting effect on the haemostatic process. Administration of tPA produces an increase in bleeding from cut wounds. The administration of a_2-PI inhibits this process and returns the duration and quantity of skin bleeding towards normal values (Fig. 26.1).[8] This site specificity of a_2-PI ensures that haemostasis will be maintained and physiological or appropriate clot lysis will not be prevented.

Aprotinin and the serine protease inhibitors act in the same way as a_2-PI rapidly to inactivate free plasmin but have little effect on bound plasmin. Separate studies have shown that lysis of clot, induced by tPA, is not inhibited significantly in the presence of high doses of aprotinin (Fig. 26.2).[26] None the less, and as found with a_2-PI, the haemostatic defect induced by tPA, prolonged and increased bleeding from cutaneous wounds, is inhibited in the presence of high doses of aprotinin (Fig. 26.2).[27]

The mode of action of the lysine analogue antifibrinolytics is in complete contrast to the actions of the plasmin inhibitors. The lysine analogues are designed to prevent excessive plasmin formation by mimicking lysine, fitting into plasminogen's lysine binding site, and thus preventing the binding of plasminogen to fibrin.

It is thus not surprising that results from similar studies to those described above contrast with results achieved with plasmin inhibitors (a_2-PI or aprotinin). The lysine analogues have no effect on the tPA-associated bleeding (Fig. 26.3)[27] but significantly impede normal clot lysis.[26]

COMPARATIVE EFFICACY

The efficacy of any pharmacological agent will exhibit a dose–response effect. It is assumed that with increasing dosage there will be an increasing benefit of administering more drug until a plateau is reached. With the majority of chemical entities, the higher the dose the more likely will be a toxic effect, and this will define

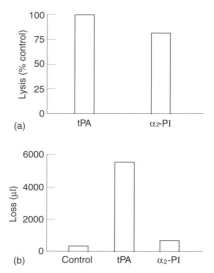

Fig. 26.1 Effect of a_2-plasmin inhibitor (a_2-PI) on tissue plasminogen activator (tPA) clot lysis (a) and induced bleeding (b). From Weitz et al.[8]

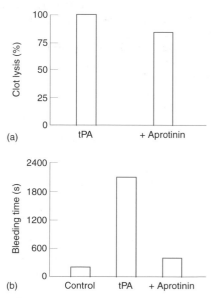

Fig. 26.2 Effect of aprotinin on tissue plasminogen activator (tPA) clot lysis (a) and induced bleeding (b). Data for clot lysis are from Fears et al.[26] and those for bleeding times are from de-Bono et al.[27]

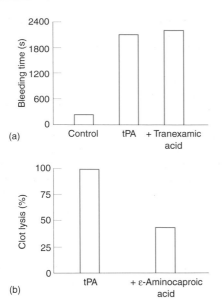

(a)

(b)

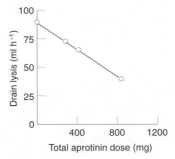

Fig. 26.4 Relationship between total aprotinin dose and postoperative drain loss for patients enrolled in randomized double-blind placebo-controlled studies of the use of aprotinin in reoperation surgery conducted in North America. Doses of aprotinin were 0 mg (placebo patients, n = 156), 280 mg ('pump prime' dose, n = 68), 420 mg ('half Hammersmith' dose, n = 113) and 840 mg ('full Hammersmith' dose, n = 143). Line derived by regression analysis. Data from Bayer Corporation.

Fig. 26.3 Effect of the lysine analogues, tranexamic acid or ε-aminocaproic acid, on tissue plasminogen activator (tPA)-induced bleeding (a) and clot lysis (b). Data for bleeding times are from de-Bono et al.[27] and clot lysis data are from Fears et al.[26]

the upper dosage limit. There should also be a 'no-effect' dose.

Dose–response for efficacy can be demonstrated for aprotinin by analysis of the data provided in the manufacturer's package insert for Trasylol and obtained in controlled randomized double-blind studies conducted in patients in North America.[28] Efficacy to reduce perioperative blood loss (Fig. 26.4) and the need for blood product transfusions (Fig. 26.5) against the total administered dose of aprotinin follows a tight relationship. However, this relationship was defined from multicentre studies and thus may not be predictive for any one centre or specific surgeon. The data for drain losses showed that the pump prime-only regimen was not of significant benefit in the reduction of total drain loss.[29] This dose can thus be considered the 'no-effect' dose. The so-called half-dose had statistically significant benefits compared with control losses and transfusion requirements, which were further increased with the increased dosage. In addition, these data suggest that the plateau for efficacy has not been achieved with the doses studied thus far.

Analysis of dose–response for the lysine analogue agents is confounded by a lack of placebo-controlled randomized double-blind studies. Horrow and colleagues[30] demonstrated that administration of tranexamic acid above a total dose of about 3 g failed to bring about any further benefit to reduce drain losses. This dose will reduce losses by between 20% and 35%. In

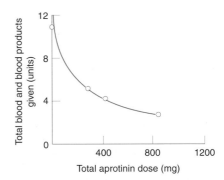

Fig. 26.5 Relationship between total aprotinin dose and the total blood product transfusion for patients enrolled in randomized double-blind, placebo-controlled studies of the use of aprotinin in reoperation surgery conducted in North America. Doses of aprotinin are 0 mg (placebo patients, n = 156), 280 mg ('pump prime' dose, n = 68), 420 mg ('half Hammersmith' dose, n = 113), and 840 mg ('full Hammersmith' dose, n = 143). Line derived by regression analysis. Data from Bayer Corporation.

addition these studies failed to show any benefit of the reduction in drain losses in relation to the transfusion requirements of patients, which were not altered by this therapy.

A recent meta-analysis of the data for the various agents confirmed there was a reduction in drain losses of about 20–40% in patients receiving the lysine analogues.[31] However, a more recent meta-analysis which used transfusion requirements was not as positive.[32] In particular, the analysis failed to show a significant benefit of the use of ε-aminocaproic acid. More interesting were the data to suggest that any blood-sparing effects of tranexamic acid were not observed in patients at higher risk of bleeding, such as those taking aspirin before operation or having reoperation. In these patients the proportion not receiving blood fell by 3–5% with tranexamic acid compared with a 26–32% reduction in those receiving aprotinin therapy (Fig. 26.6).

This difference in efficacy to inhibit bleeding was also demonstrated by the lack of difference in patients requiring re-exploration for bleeding when given tranexamic acid compared with the fourfold reduction in those given aprotinin.

EFFECTS OF PHARMACOLOGICAL INTERVENTIONS ON ORGAN AND TISSUE FUNCTION

Organ systems and tissues may have altered functions during surgery, especially cardiac surgery. Three organ systems are principally affected:

1. The brain and nervous system.
2. The heart and myocardium.
3. The kidney.

The next section will discuss briefly some aspects of the actions of pharmacological interventions to prevent bleeding on these systems.

CEREBRAL CIRCULATION

The use of lysine analogue antifibrinolytic agents in patients with subarachnoid haemorrhage is associated with an increase in mortality and morbidity rates due to the development of cerebral vasospasm and ischaemia. This is in contrast to the vasodilating effects of aprotinin and other serine protease inhibitors, which have been advocated as a therapy to improve outcome after subarachnoid haemorrhage.

The concept for the potential for aprotinin to reduce

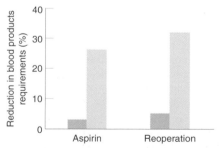

Fig. 26.6 Reduction in the proportion of patients requiring blood products when receiving tranexamic acid (■) or aprotinin (■) therapy. Data show lack of efficacy of tranexamic acid with higher-risk patients. These include those receiving preoperative aspirin and patients having reoperation. Significant reductions in patients exposed to blood are achieved with aprotinin therapy in these cases. From Laupacis and Fergusson.[32]

the incidence of stroke following cardiac surgery was investigated in a meta-analysis of data from studies performed within North America in order to achieve regulatory approval for the drug. These pooled data showed that, of the patients allocated to the randomized studies investigating high-dose aprotinin (1721 patients in total), 2.4% of those in the placebo group were reported as suffering stroke. This was reduced to 0.7% of patients with the use of aprotinin therapy. This reduction achieved statistical significance ($P = 0.027$).[33]

The lack of large-scale randomized prospective studies investigating the use of lysine analogues in similar groups of cardiac patients prevents a comparative analysis of the incidence of stroke between the two different pharmacological therapies.

HEART AND MYOCARDIUM

A number of studies have investigated the role of the use of serine protease inhibitors to protect the myocardium.[34]

In humans, morbidity and mortality rates following myocardial infarction are reduced with aprotinin therapy. This was largely as a result of a decrease in the incidence and severity of infarction, shown by a significant reduction in enzyme release, and arrhythmia. With surgical patients the use of aprotinin in cardioplegic solutions is reported to produce a better preservation of myocardial function at the end of surgery.

Data from earlier studies of the use of aprotinin therapy during primary myocardial revasularization show that perioperative myocardial infarction occurred in 8.0% of patients in the control group and in 6.3% of patients receiving high-dose aprotinin therapy. In studies from a single German centre, the mortality rate in 882 treated patients was 2.7% and in 907 nontreated patients was 3.5%.[28] These data have been mirrored recently in the results of a large multicentre study, where myocardial infarction (definite and probable) occurred in 8.6% of patients receiving aprotinin and in 9.1% of those having placebo. The mortality rate was 1.4% and 1.6% respectively.[35]

There are no controlled data for the effects of lysine analogues on myocardial recovery after ischaemia.

PULMONARY CIRCULATION

For the pulmonary vascular bed there are studies to show that pulmonary hypertension and raised transpulmonary pressure gradients are reduced with aprotinin therapy, both in paediatric surgery associated with single-ventricle palliation such as bidirectional Glenn shunt or Fontan procedures, or following heart transplantation in adults (Fig. 26.7). A study of implantation of left ventricular assist devices showed a significant reduction in the need to establish a right ventricular assist device at the same time, which may be related to the action of aprotinin in reducing abnormally high pulmonary vascular tone.[28,34]

KIDNEY AND RENAL FUNCTION
Early toxicology studies suggested that the administration of high doses of aprotinin over prolonged periods (about 6 weeks) was associated with the development of hyaline casts in the renal tubule. The reason for this is that the kidney recognizes that aprotinin is a small polypeptide and actively transports the compound into the proximal tubule. It may also be related to the high neuramidase concentration in the renal brush border. This led to some original concerns about renal function in patients given high doses of aprotinin.

Renal function has been specifically investigated in a number of studies.[34] The first, in patients having first-time revascularization surgery, showed an increase in urine volume and free water and sodium clearance during the operative and early postoperative period in those given aprotinin therapy. In the second study, in patients having reoperation coronary artery bypass grafting, there was an increase in average creatinine clearance from 110 ml min^{-1} in the control nontreated patients to 132 ml min^{-1} in patients given high-dose aprotinin therapy. However, this change was not statistically significant.

Despite this apparent benefit, there is also a body of evidence suggesting a biochemical abnormality, implying altered renal function some 3–5 days after the

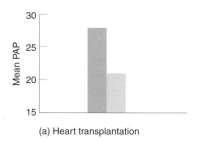

(a) Heart transplantation

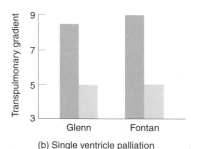

(b) Single ventricle palliation

Fig. 26.7 Action of aprotinin to reduce mean pulmonary artery pressure (PAP mmHg) and improve pulmonary and right heart function, in patients during the posttransplantation period (a) and during surgery for single ventricle palliation with the Glenn shunt or Fontan procedure (b). ■, Control; ■, aprotinin. From Royston.[28]

procedure with an increase in plasma creatinine, but not blood urea nitrogen, levels at that time. Typically plasma creatinine values are within the normal range but are about 0.5 mg higher in aprotinin-treated than in placebo-treated patients. This rise in creatinine concentration is not associated with, or dependent on, the baseline creatinine concentration nor is it associated with any deleterious event or need for renal support with dialysis.[28]

None the less, data have been reported following insertion of a left ventricular assist device with the use of aprotinin therapy and in patients who had valve replacement who were also insulin-dependent diabetics. These reports show a significant rise in creatinine concentration to above the normal range, without any concomitant change in the blood urea nitrogen levels, or an increase in morbidity or early mortality rates in these patients. Early evidence that aprotinin therapy may have an effect in increasing the chance of renal failure has not been confirmed in studies describing this in larger groups of patients.

The effect of lysine analogues on renal function in association with cardiac surgery has been less well categorized. There have been reports of acute renal failure and severe proteinuria associated with the use of ε-aminocaproic acid. There are similar articles cautioning against the use of such agents because of the potential renal toxicity profile. Indeed, tranexamic acid is excreted predominantly via the kidney, and the package insert and product information approved by the Food and Drug Administration in the USA highlights this caution and recommends that the dose of tranexamic acid administered should be reduced if preoperative renal dysfunction exists.

SPECIFIC AREAS OF CONCERN WITH USE OF LYSINE ANALOGUES AND APROTININ

HYPERSENSITIVITY RESPONSES
The published evidence concerning hypersensitivity and anaphylactic reactions to the lysine analogue antifibrinolytics is sparse. In contrast, there have been a number of reports of cardiovascular effects when high-dose aprotinin has been administered. Hypersensitivity reactions are rarely reported in patients with no previous exposure to aprotinin. The recent literature suggests that the incidence of hypersensitivity reactions on first-time exposure will vary from minor skin rashes and minor changes in blood pressure, to true anaphylactic reactions in between 0.3% and 0.6%. These values approximate those anticipated with use of muscle relaxants or synthetic volume replacement during cardiac surgery.

The overall incidence of anaphylactic reactions to aprotinin in patients who have had a definite previous exposure is estimated to be 2.5%. In patients who received aprotinin within 3–6 months of their first exposure, the incidence was 5.0%. This fell to 0.9% of patients re-exposed more than 6 months after the primary exposure.[28]

THROMBOTIC EPISODES

It is not surprising that the majority of reports of thrombotic complications have been anecdotal case reports. Reports of thrombotic episodes in patients receiving lysine analogue antifibrinolytics cover a wide range of vascular beds, although the cerebral circulation predominates. Notwithstanding this, there is an increasing literature to show that abnormal clot formation can occur in any organ or tissue and in association with indwelling vascular catheters. In contrast to this broad spectrum, the current literature shows that with aprotinin therapy reported problems are confined to native and grafted myocardial blood vessels and indwelling catheters.[28]

Thus far, the focused studies on the effects of apro-

tinin on graft patency after myocardial revascularization have not shown any consistent detrimental effect for the use of aprotinin. A recent report of angiographic graft patency (about 11 days postsurgery) showed that graft patency was impaired in patients receiving aprotinin at only one of 13 centres involved in this multicentre study.[35] A number of suggestions can be made to explain these observations. The most commonly discussed aspect is the control of anticoagulation in these patients. If the celite-activated ACT is maintained at approximately 400 s, it is almost certainly true that the patient is not adequately heparinized. The suggestion at present is to maintain the celite-activated ACT at > 750 s or the kaolin-activated ACT at > 500 s. Other suggested strategies include fixed-dose heparin regimens or monitoring heparin by protamine titration.

The most intriguing observation from this study was that myocardial infarction was not universally related to the presence of an occluded graft. Similarly, despite more graft occlusions at this one centre, mortality and morbidity were not affected.

REFERENCES

1. Hirsh J. Heparin. *N Engl J Med* 1991; **324**: 1565–1574.
2. Hirsh J, Dalen JE, Deykin D, Poller L. Heparin: mechanism of action, pharmacokinetics, dosing considerations, monitoring, efficacy, and safety. *Chest* 1992; **102**: 337s–351s.
3. Hirsh J, Levine MN. Low molecular weight heparin. *Blood* 1992; **79**: 1–17.
4. Hirsh J, Levine MN. Low molecular weight heparin: laboratory properties and clinical evaluation. A review. *Eur J Surg Suppl* 1994; **571**: 9–22.
5. Frydman A. Low-molecular-weight heparins: an overview of their pharmacodynamics, pharmacokinetics and metabolism in humans. *Haemostasis* 1996; **26** (Suppl.2): 24–38.
6. Tollefsen DM, Majerus DW, Blank MK. Heparin cofactor II. Purification and properties of a heparin-dependent inhibitor of thrombin in human plasma. *J Biol Chem* 1982; **257**: 2162–2169.
7. Bregengaard C, Nordfang O, Ostergaard P *et al*. Pharmacokinetics of full length and two-domain tissue factor pathway inhibitor in combination with heparin in rabbits. *Thromb Haemost* 1993; **70**: 454–457.
8. Weitz JI, Hudoba M, Massel D, Maraganore J, Hirsh J. Clot-bound thrombin is protected from inhibition by heparin–antithrombin III but is susceptible to inactivation by antithrombin III-independent inhibitors. *J Clin Invest* 1990; **86**: 385–391.
9. Salzman EW, Rosenberg RD, Smith MH, Lindon JN, Favreau L. Effect of heparin and heparin fractions on platelet aggregation. *J Clin Invest* 1980; **65**: 64–73.
10. Fareed J, Walenga JM, Hoppensteadt D, Huan X, Racanelli A. Comparative study on the in vitro and in vivo activities of seven low-molecular-weight heparins. *Haemostasis* 1988; **18** (Suppl. 3): 3–15 [published erratum appears in *Haemostasis* 1988; **18** (4–6): following 389].
11. Abildgaard U. Heparin/low molecular weight heparin and tissue factor pathway inhibitor. *Haemostasis* 1993; **1**: 103–106.
12. Hull RD, Pineo GF. Low molecular weight heparin treatment of venous thromboembolism. *Prog Cardiovasc Dis* 1994; **37**: 71–78.
13. Litin SC, Gastineau DA. Current concepts in anticoagulant therapy. *Mayo Clin Proc* 1995; **70**: 266–272.
14. Nurmohamed MT, Rosendaal FR, Buller HR *et al*. Low-molecular-weight heparin versus standard heparin in general and orthopaedic surgery: a meta-analysis. *Lancet* 1992; **340**: 152–156.
15. Green D, Hirsh J, Heit J, Prins M, Davidson B, Lensing AW. Low molecular weight heparin: a critical analysis of clinical trials. *Pharmacol Rev* 1994; **46**: 89–109.
16. Landefeld CS, Beyth RJ. Anticoagulant-related bleeding: clinical epidemiology, prediction, and prevention. *Am J Med* 1993; **95**: 315–328.
17. Chong BH. Heparin-induced thrombocytopenia. *Br J Haematol* 1995; **89**: 431–439.
18. Warkentin TE, Kelton JG. Heparin-induced thrombocytopenia. *Annu Rev Med* 1989; **40**: 31–44.
19. Dehmer GJ, Lange RA, Tate DA *et al*. Randomized trial of recombinant platelet factor 4 versus protamine for the reversal of heparin anticoagulation in humans. *Circulation* 1996; **94**: Ii347–352.
20. Ellison N, Edmunds LH Jr, Colman RW. Platelet aggregation following heparin and protamine administration. *Anesthesiology* 1978; **48**: 65–68.
21. Levy JH, Schwieger IM, Zaidan JR, Faraj BA, Weintraub WS. Evaluation of patients at risk for protamine reactions. *J Thorac Cardiovasc Surg* 1989; **98**: 200–204.
22. Lowenstein E, Johnston WE, Lappas DG *et al*. Catastrophic pulmonary vasoconstriction associated with protamine reversal of heparin. *Anesthesiology* 1983; **59**: 470–473.
23. Liu S, Carpenter R, Neal J. Epidural anesthesia and analgesia: their role in postoperative outcome. *Anesthesiology* 1995; **82**: 1474–1506.
24. Bullingham A, Strunin L. Prevention of postoperative venous thromboembolism. *Br J Anaesth* 1995; **75**: 622–630.
25. Royston D. High-dose aprotinin therapy: a review of the first five years' experience. *J Cardiothorac Vasc Anesth* 1992; **6**: 76–100.
26. Fears R, Greenwood J, Hearn J, Howard BS, Morrow G, Standring R. Inhibition of the fibrinolytic and fibrinogenolytic activity of plasminogen activators in vitro by the antidotes ε-aminocaproic acid, tranexamic acid and aprotinin. *Fibrinolysis* 1992; **6**: 79–86.
27. de-Bono DP, Pringle S, Underwood I. Differential effects of aprotinin and

tranexamic acid on cerebral bleeding and cutaneous bleeding time during rt-PA infusion. *Thromb Res* 1991; **61**: 159–163.

28. Royston D. Aprotinin versus lysine analogues: the debate continues. *Ann Thorac Surg* 1998; **65**: S9–19.

29. Levy J, Pifarre R, Schaff H *et al*. A multicenter double-blind, placebo-controlled trial of aprotinin for reducing blood loss and the requirement for donor-blood transfusion in patients having repeat coronary artery bypass grafting. *Circulation* 1995; **92**: 2236–2244.

30. Horrow JC, Van Riper DF, Strong MD, Grunewald KE, Parmet JL. The dose–response relationship of tranexamic acid. *Anesthesiology* 1995; **82**: 383–392.

31. Fremes SE, Wong BI, Lee E *et al*. Metaanalysis of prophylactic drug treatment in the prevention of postoperative bleeding. *Ann Thorac Surg* 1994; **58**: 1580–1588.

32. Laupacis A, Fergusson D. Drugs to minimize perioperative blood loss in cardiac surgery: meta-analyses using perioperative blood transfusion as the outcome. The International Study of Peri-operative Transfusion (ISPOT) Investigators. *Anesth Analg* 1997; **85**: 1258–1267.

33. Smith PK, Muhlbaier LH. Aprotinin: safe and effective only with the full-dose regimen. *Ann Thorac Surg* 1996; **62**: 1575–1577.

34. Royston D. Preventing the inflammatory response to open-heart surgery: the role of aprotinin and other protease inhibitors. *Int J Cardiol* 1996; **53** (Suppl): S11–37.

35. Alderman EL, Levy JH, Rich JB *et al*. Analyses of coronary artery graft patency after aprotinin use: results from the International Multicenter Aprotinin Graft Patency Experience (IMAGE) trial. *Ann Thorac Surg* 1998; **116**: 716–730.

27

NC Bhaskaran, JE Peacock

ANAPHYLAXIS AND OTHER ADVERSE REACTIONS DURING ANAESTHESIA

Summary box 27.1 Adverse reactions to drugs

- Extension of the pharmacological effects of the drug (drug interaction or overdose).

- Immunological.

- Idiosyncratic.

- Physicochemical.

During the conduct of anaesthesia and surgery it is necessary to administer a large number of drugs of different chemical composition, and it is not surprising that there is a significant incidence of adverse reactions. There has been an apparent increase in these reactions in recent years and this is probably secondary to an increased awareness of reactions as well as improved vigilance and monitoring during anaesthesia.[1] In addition, the availability of sophisticated diagnostic tests has contributed to a better understanding of the problem, since the mechanisms of such adverse actions are diverse.

An adverse reaction may be defined as any unwanted response following the administration of a drug; the causes of such reactions are extremely varied. Adverse reactions may be the result of immunological, idiosyncratic or physicochemical interactions, and may be either predictable (chemical interaction between drugs or drug additives) or unpredictable (idiosyncratic reactions). Adverse reactions may also be an extension of the desired response of the drug, perhaps the result of an absolute or relative overdose, or they may follow pharmacokinetic or pharmacodynamic interactions (see Chapter 28). The present chapter focuses primarily on reactions that are mediated via immunological mechanisms. To understand the pharmacology of anaphylaxis, we first have to understand the immunological principles involved.

IMMUNOLOGICAL REACTIONS

Immunological reactions such as increased plasma histamine levels or minor clinical observations can occur in over 1% of anaesthetic administrations.[2] The incidence of more serious immunological reactions is uncertain, with estimates ranging from 1 in 600 to 1 in 20 000 anaesthetics. Similarly the estimated mortality rate varies widely between 1% and 9% of severe reactions.[3] Such reactions may be allergic, anaphylactic, anaphylactoid or hypersensitivity reactions. Each of the above terms has a specific meaning, although they are frequently interchanged in the clinical setting. To avoid the use of specific terms when the mechanism is not known, the term 'anaphylactoid' will be used here, although 'histaminoid' has also been recommended.[3]

DEFINITIONS

An *allergic* reaction refers to a hypersensitive state acquired through previous exposure to a specific antigen, with rexposure usually resulting in a severe immunological reaction caused by preformed antibodies. *Anaphylaxis* refers to such a reaction when it is the result of the release of immunoglobulin (Ig) E-mediated vasoactive substances. A clinical presentation similar to anaphylaxis but caused by other immune mechanisms is called an *anaphylactoid* reaction, and this is also the preferred term when the precise mechanism awaits immunological confirmation. *Hypersensitivity* is a state of heightened reactivity in which the body mounts an exaggerated immune response to an agent, whether or not there has been previous exposure to it.

MECHANISM OF IMMUNOLOGICAL ADVERSE REACTION

Immunological reactions are characterized by specific antigen–antibody and/or effector cell responses, and these are reproducible when the patient is challenged with the specific antigen. Any molecule that has the capacity to initiate immunospecific antibody production or lymphocyte activation is called an antigen. The size of the molecule and the degree to which it is recognized as foreign are critical determinants of the immunogenicity of an antigen. Only a small number of drugs have a molecular size large enough to initiate an immunological response by themselves (e.g. streptokinase, protamine and insulin). Other drugs with a smaller molecular size bind first to a host antibody or protein, and the complex thus formed initiates immune stimulation. Such antigens are called incomplete antigens or 'haptens', and the host proteins or antibodies are known as 'carrier molecules'.

Antibodies are protein macromolecules with the ability to combine specifically with the antigen that initiated their production. Following an antigenic stimulus, B lymphocytes transform to plasma cells in a complex but well regulated process which results in the synthesis of the antibodies. Antibodies have a Y-shaped structure, with the base conferring the ability to attach to effector cells and activate complement, while the antigen-binding sites are located on the two wings. There are five different types of antibodies (IgG, IgA, IgM, IgD and IgE), each playing a physiologically different and specific role. The antigen also stimulates lymphocytes in lymph nodes, Peyer's patches of the intestine and other reticuloendothelial organs involving T lymphocytes which are primarily involved in cell-mediated immunity and help in the process of antigen recognition.

TYPES OF IMMUNOLOGICAL REACTION

Based on the immunological mechanism involved in hypersensitivity, reactions can be classified into four types, I–IV.

Summary box 27.2 Immunological (hypersensitivity) reactions

- Type I (allergic release): mediated by IgE antibodies. Often (but not always) manifests as rapidly occurring anaphylactic reaction. Frequently exhibits two phases: immediate (5–30 min) and delayed (2–8 h).

- Type II (cytotoxic release): delayed response produced by protein complexes. Mediated by IgG or IgM antibodies. Examples include ABO blood transfusion reactions and some reactions to protamine.

- Type III (complement-mediated release): insoluble antibody–antigen complexes deposited in organs such as kidneys, joints or skin, producing serum sickness.

- Type IV (cell-mediated or delayed release): involves combination of antigen with T cells. Reactions delayed for 18–24 h. Examples include tuberculin testing and graft rejection.

Type I: immediate hypersensitivity reactions

This is a rapidly occurring reaction which follows the combination of an antigen with an antibody that has previously bound to the surface of mast cells or basophils, resulting in crosslinking of the antibodies (Fig. 27.1). It is mediated exclusively by IgE antibody.

Crosslinking results in the release of preformed chemical mediators that manifest the clinical changes. However, not all type I reactions manifest clinically as full-blown anaphylaxis. Other examples of type I reactions are extrinsic asthma, allergic rhinitis, bee-sting reactions and penicillin allergy. It is recognized that many type I reactions have two well-defined phases. The initial response is characterized by vascular changes and smooth muscle spasm, which usually becomes evident within 5–30 min after exposure to an antigen and tends to subside within 60 min. In many individuals a second 'late phase' reaction commences 2–8 h afterwards without an additional antigenic challenge, and may last for several days. The synthetic mediators play a predominant role in sustaining the altered physiological state.

Type II: cytotoxic reactions

Type II hypersensitivity reactions involve the IgG or IgM types of antibodies. The antigens are usually an integral component of cell membranes (e.g. blood group antigens) or haptens adhered to the cell membranes (e.g. penicillin). Antigen–antibody interaction activates either the complement system, which in turn lyses the cells

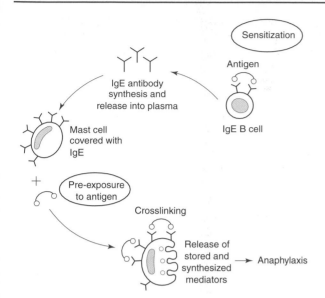

Fig. 27.1 Type I: immediate hypersensitivity reactions – rapidly occurring, following the combination of an antigen with an antibody that had previously bound to the surface of mast cells or basophils, resulting in crosslinking of the antibodies.

(e.g. ABO-incompatible transfusion reactions, Rh disease of the newborn, drug-induced or autoimmune haemolytic anaemia, and Goodpasture syndrome), or the target cell is lysed by killer cells (Fig. 27.2).

Type III: immune complex reactions

Antibodies and circulating soluble antigens may form insoluble complexes that are too small to be removed effectively by liver and spleen macrophages. Deposition of immune complexes in various organs can initiate local activation of the complement system and chemotactic accumulation of neutrophils, which are important components of this type of immunological injury. Drug-induced systemic lupus erythematosus and penicillin-induced vasculitis are examples of this type of reaction.

Type IV: cell-mediated immune or delayed hypersensitivity reactions

These reactions are important in dealing with intracellular antigens and pathogens such as viruses and fungi. Thymus-derived lymphocytes (T cells) when activated by cellular antigens and circulatory proteins can directly kill the foreign cells or produce lymphokines, which mediate an immune response. These reactions are slow, taking 18–24 h to develop and reaching a maximum in 48 h. Tuberculin testing and graft rejection are examples of this type of reaction, and they are uncommon mechanisms in the immediacy of anaesthetic situations. However, one of the subpopulations of T cells (cytotoxic suppressor cells), when altered by

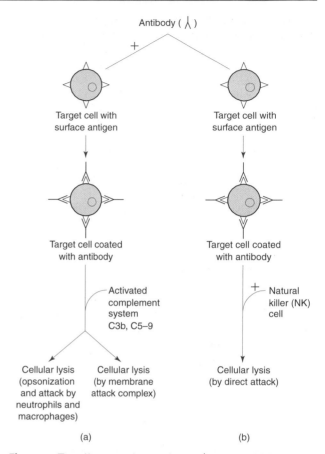

Fig. 27.2 Type II: cytotoxic reactions – hypersensitivity reactions involve the IgG or IgM types of antibodies. The antigens are usually an integral component of cell membranes or haptens adhered to the cell membranes. Antigen–antibody interaction activates either the complement system, which in turn lyses the cells, or the target cell is lysed by killer cells.

infection with human immunodeficiency virus, predisposes to opportunist infections such as *Pneumocystis carinii* and lymphoproliferative syndromes such as Kaposi sarcoma.

COMPLEMENT SYSTEM

Complement is a series of at least 20 distinct plasma and cell membrane proteins that can be activated by one of two mechanisms: classical (antigen–antibody complex mediated) and alternative pathways (Fig. 27.3). Once activated, the series of actions follows a sequential pattern similar to the clotting cascade. The net effect of activated complement is the production of biological effector proteins that lyse susceptible targets, promote phagocytosis by coating targets with protein fragments, or generate peptides that activate other humoral amplification systems such as coagulation, fibrinolysis and release of kinins. Plasmin and heparin–protamine complex activate the classical pathway, whereas radiocontrast media, endotoxin, exotoxin, protamine and other drugs activate the alternate pathway of the complement system.

MEDIATORS OF IMMUNE REACTION

The life-threatening responses during anaphylactic reaction are the result of end-organ responses to preformed mast cell and basophil granular contents (primary or stored mediators) and newly synthesized mediators such as arachidonic acid metabolites (secondary or synthesized mediators) (Table 27.1).

Histamine is the most important of the stored mediators, and also the best studied. Human lung, intestine and skin contain high concentrations of stored histamine. Within 3 min of mast cell stimulation, degranulation occurs and released histamine causes intense vasodilatation of arterial and venous capacitance vessels, and increased capillary permeability. Histamine also stimulates the airway smooth muscles to contract, causing bronchospasm. H_1 receptors are involved in the mediation of coronary, peripheral and pulmonary vasodilatation, increases in vascular permeability, and stimulation of pulmonary histamine receptors. Although H_2 receptors are also involved in coronary and peripheral vasodilatation, they mediate bronchodilatation, pulmonary vasoconstriction and the positive inotropic and chronotropic effects on the heart. The individual clinical picture may depend on the relative preponderance of H_1 or H_2 receptors involved. Tryptase, chemotryptase and glycoaminoglycans such as heparin are other mediators stored in granules and released together with histamine.

The degranulation of stored mediators also triggers the synthesis of lipid- and protein-derived mediators. Arachidonic acid is liberated from membrane lipids by the action of phospholipase A_2, and is processed into cyclooxygenase products, such as prostaglandins, thromboxanes and prostacyclins, and 5-lipooxygenase products such as leukotrienes. Prostaglandins mainly affect

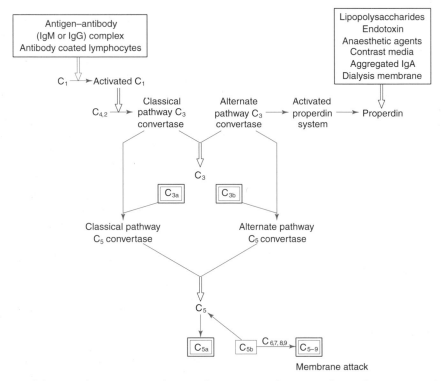

Fig. 27.3 Activation of the complement system by two alternative mechanisms: classical (antigen-antibody complex mediated) and alternative pathways.

Table 27.1 Mediators of anaphylactic reaction	
Mediator	**Biological effects**
Preformed mediators released by mast cell degranulation	
Histamine	Vasodilatation, increased capillary permeability, bronchoconstriction, ?direct cardiac effects
Heparin	Anticoagulant
Tryptase	Activation of C_3
Platelet-activating factor	Shock, further mediator release
ECF and NCF	Eosinophil and neutrophil chemotaxis
Newly synthesized mediators; synthesis triggered by mast cell degranulation	
Cyclooxygenase pathway Prostaglandins and thromboxanes	Vasodilatation, platelet aggregation and effect on bronchial smooth muscle
Lipooxygenase pathway Leukotrienes C_4 and D_4 (SRS-A)	Vasoactive, bronchoconstriction and chemotaxis

ECF, eosinophilic chemotactic factor; NCF, neutrophilic chemotactic factor; SRS-A, slow releasing substance of anaphylaxis.

the bronchial smooth muscle, while the leukotrienes are responsible for a reduction in organ perfusion affecting mainly the kidneys and myocardium. Platelet-activating factor (PAF), another lipid derivative, has negative inotropic effects and is a potent vasodilator; it is the single most potent initiator of shock. Of the protein derivatives of synthesized mediators, prekallikrein and bradykinin have been identified in anaphylaxis within various species.

DRUGS COMMONLY IMPLICATED IN ANAPHYLACTOID REACTIONS

A drug reaction involving hypotension and/or bronchospasm may be the result of a classical type I hypersensitivity reaction involving IgE antibody, classical complement activation involving IgG or IgM antibody, alternative complement activation where no antibody is involved, or it may be the direct pharmacological effect of the drug. In anaesthetic practice, any of the classes of drugs commonly used may be involved, although certain agents are more likely to predispose to a reaction than others.

INDUCTION AGENTS
Of the intravenous anaesthetic agents, thiopentone is the most commonly implicated agent. Although previous exposure to thiopentone has no predictive value, it seems to predispose patients to anaphylaxis. IgE, IgG and direct histamine release have been implicated

in thiopentone allergy, which occurs in 1 in 23 000–36 000 administrations.[4] The secondary pentyl and ethyl groups attached at position 5 of the pyramidine ring nucleus are the antigenic determinants.[5] Reactions to thiopentone are more common in women, and delayed reactions are not uncommon. It is also possible that precipitants formed by direct mixing of thiopentone and suxamethonium or atracurium given in the intravenous tubing may be responsible for a few reported adverse reactions. Etomidate, and propofol formulated in soya bean oil and purified egg phosphatide, have only rarely been implicated in anaphylaxis. A significant, although small, rise in plasma concentrations of histamine may occur following benzodiazepine administration; however, no severe reactions to midazolam have been reported. Ketamine also seems to be free of adverse reactions. Althesin, propanidid and the original formulation of propofol were cremophor-based drugs that have been withdrawn from the market because of an unacceptably high incidence of reactions.

NEUROMUSCULAR BLOCKING DRUGS
Over 80% of reported reactions during anaesthesia involve neuromuscular blocking drugs, with suxamethonium accounting for about one-half of these. IgE antibodies from most patients cross-react with other muscle relaxants and unrelated compounds containing quaternary nitrogen ions. These occur most commonly between suxamethonium and gallamine, alcuronium and d-tubocurarine, and pancuronium and vecuron-

ium. Cisatracurium and atracurium are antigenically identical and there appears a high incidence of cross-sensitivity between rocuronium and vecuronium but, surprisingly, not pancuronium.[6] It is important to recognize that many drugs, including neostigmine, trimetaphan and morphine, as well as normal cell membrane constituents contain quaternary nitrogen ions. In addition certain foods, cosmetics and industrial materials may provide an opportunity for sensitization. Flexible molecules with simple carbon chains (e.g. suxamethonium) can stimulate and sensitize cells more strongly than rigid molecules (e.g. pancuronium).

ANALGESIC DRUGS

Although IgE antibodies to pethidine and morphine have been detected, most of the reactions seen with these opioids are related to histamine release. In most instances, combined H_1- and H_2-receptor blocking drugs given prophylactically will reduce the severity of reactions. The *N*-methyl group and the cyclohexanyl ring with a hydroxyl at C-6 have been identified as the antigenic determinants, which result in immune stimulation and the rare instances of anaphylaxis seen with this group of drugs. Fewer than 20 cases have been reported in the literature. Cross-reactivity has been recognized among morphine, codeine and papaveretum.[7] Buprenorphine is unique among opioids in that it is the only drug that is known to stimulate the synthesis of vasoactive eicosanoids (prostaglandins and leukotrienes). Other synthetic opioids such as fentanyl, alfentanil, sufentanil and remifentanil do not cause significant histamine release.

The increased use of nonsteroidal antiinflammatory drugs (NSAIDs) in the perioperative period may have been responsible for an apparent rise in reported adverse reactions to this group of drugs. Approximately 8–20% of asthmatics develop bronchospasm with NSAIDs[8] and this incidence doubles if there is an additional history of nasal polyps or allergic rhinitis. A history of aspirin-induced or NSAID-induced reactions is most valuable as a predictor of such reactions, and in nearly 60–85% of these patients adverse respiratory reactions are seen.

LOCAL ANAESTHETIC AGENTS

Anaphylactic reactions to local anaesthetics are extremely rare. Some of the reactions may be related to the additives in local anaesthetics.[9] Methylparaben and sodium bisulphate, used in the past as preservatives with most local anaesthetic agents, have been implicated as causing adverse reactions. Methylparaben is a contact sensitizer, and has a structural similarity to the ester moiety in procaine and similar ester-type local anaesthetics. Whilst reactions to these two preservatives may have accounted for a number of initially reported

reactions, the picture is far from clear because of incomplete investigation of suspected cases, and the rarity with which these are seen. Available data suggest that contact sensitivity and contact dermatitis do not predict that immediate hypersensitivity reactions will occur when the drug exposure is by other routes.

INTRAVENOUS FLUIDS AND BLOOD PRODUCTS

Almost all intravenously infused fluids have been reported to be responsible for anaphylactoid reactions (Table 27.2). With crystalloids reactions are more likely to be the result of high molecular weight, chemical contaminants or preservatives such as benzyl alcohol or sulphites. Heat treatment of plasma proteins may result in the formation of protein aggregates, which are the main suspects for reactions seen with plasma protein solutions such as human serum albumin, plasma factors and immunoglobulins. Gelatins cause nonspecific histamine release, while dextran-related reactions are mainly complement mediated. Hydroxyethyl starch, stroma-free haemoglobin solutions and synthetic perfluorochemicals have all been shown to cause immunological reactions in various animal and experimental studies.

ALLERGIC REACTIONS TO BLOOD PRODUCTS

Febrile reaction is the most commonly observed side-effect of blood transfusion in patients who are awake. There is at least a $1\,°C$ rise in temperature, and this is sometimes associated with headache and backache. After multiple transfusions or pregnancies, antibodies may appear in response to transfused white blood cells, and febrile reactions occur frequently. In such individuals further transfusions should consist of red

---

Table 27.2 Nonanaesthetic agents associated with hypersensitivity reactions during anaesthesia

Intravenous fluids
  Blood derivatives
    Whole blood
    Factor VIII concentrates
  Other intravenous fluids
    Gelatin, haemaccel, hetastarch

Other drugs
  Radiocontrast media
  Antibiotics
  Protamine
  Formaldehyde
  Ethylene oxide
  Chymopapain

Latex

blood cells that have been washed or specially filtered to remove white blood cells.

Hypersensitivity reactions to an unknown component in donor blood are common, and usually due to allergens in donor plasma, or less often from an allergic donor. Immunized IgA-deficient patients may develop anaphylactoid reactions to IgA in donor plasma. In a patient with a history of allergies or an allergic transfusion reaction, prophylactic administration of histamine H_1 and H_2 antagonists may be useful. If symptoms of allergy occur, the transfusion should be stopped; the more serious cases may occasionally need treatment with adrenaline and steroids.

LATEX

Since it was first described in 1979, latex allergy has become one of the clinically most important allergic reactions, and may account for as many as 15% of reactions in the perioperative period. Most patients with latex sensitivity are females. The reaction may be local or generalized and may manifest as angioedema, rhinitis, bronchospasm or even anaphylactoid shock. Immediate allergic reactions are IgE dependent. Typically, sensitization occurs through direct contact between skin or mucosa and latex during surgical or dental procedures, vaginal examination, application of adhesive bandages or from infant pacifiers. Inhalation of latex allergens attached to the cornstarch powder in surgical gloves may also be an important means of exposure. Latex allergy is more common in those who have atopy. Children with spina bifida or congenital urological abnormalities have a 20–65% chance of having a latex allergy, which may arise from repeated surgical exposure and a need for multiple catheterization. Cross-reactivity between latex and foods such as kiwi fruit, banana, avocado and chestnut have been found, all antigenically similar to latex.[10]

PROTAMINE

Protamine sulphate is a polycationic, strongly basic polypeptide used to reverse heparin anticoagulation. It is also used to retard absorption of certain types of insulins, namely neutral protamine Hagedorn (NHP) and protamine zinc insulin (PZI). Protamine may be an incomplete or monovalent antigen which must first combine with a tissue macromolecule or possibly heparin to become a complete antigen capable of immune stimulation. In diabetics treated with protamine insulins there is a 10–30-fold increased risk of life-threatening reactions when protamine is given intravenously as after cardiac surgery to reverse heparin anticoagulation. Two different types of reaction may occur: a classical anaphylactic reaction and a syndrome producing pulmonary hypertension and right heart failure.[11]

HALOTHANE

Halothane hepatitis is discussed more fully elsewhere (see Chapter 4), but many patients with halothane hepatitis have IgE antibodies in response to the oxidative metabolite trifluoroacetyl halide. This hapten appears to be responsible for the antigenicity associated with this disease.

CLINICAL PRESENTATION

A high index of suspicion is vital in making the diagnosis of anaphylaxis, as the multiple clinical signs that occur may also be caused by other conditions which must be considered in the differential diagnosis (see below). In general a sudden onset of hypotension with or without bronchospasm that occurs in temporal relation to the administration of a drug in any clinical setting can be due to anaphylaxis.

The frequency of anaphylactic or anaphylactoid reactions to intravenous anaesthetics varies between 1 in 5000 to 1 in 7000 in different studies. Further evaluation would suggest that 90% of these are due to type I (IgE mediated) reactions, and occur within the first 10 min after injection of the substance. Non-immunological histamine release and activation of complement may account for the rest. Allergic reactions due to latex typically occur 30 min to 2 h after the exposure.

Females are three times more prone to react to neuromuscular blocking agents, and four times more likely to react to thiopentone. Teenagers and young adults are also more likely to develop such reactions. Although genetic factors have been suspected of playing a role, the evidence for this is mainly from animal studies using a variety of haptens and low molecular weight polymers. It is not clear how relevant genetic factors are in humans, except that the degree of antigenic challenge necessary to mount a similar immune response varies between different groups. The presence of atopy has been suggested as a risk factor, but the evidence for this is inconclusive. Similarly, a history of bronchial asthma may by itself not increase the global risk of drug-related reactions, but the consequences of intense bronchospasm-related hypoxia can be very severe when such reactions occur. Clearly aspirin-related aggravation of bronchospasm is an important predictor for reactions to NSAIDs.

Cardiovascular collapse and mucocutaneous signs are the predominant features of anaphylactoid reactions. Itching, burning, tingling and a bright red erythematous rash in areas richest in mast cells (neck, the upper chest and face) may often be the first clues to an impending cardiovascular collapse. Mucocutaneous oedema is a late feature and may affect the eyelids, lips, tongue and respiratory tract. These cutaneous signs of histamine release may be absent in sudden, severe, cardiovascular collapse as a result of significant compromise of the cutaneous circulation. Hypotension and tachycardia are the rule and, although the degree of hypotension is variable, a 20% reduction in blood pressure is common. Rhythm and conduction disorders occur within the first 30 s after the onset of anaphylaxis and may be life threatening. In patients treated with β-adrenoceptor antagonists bradycardia may occur, and the degree of cardiovascular collapse is usually severe. Cardiac arrest is usually secondary to severe hypoxaemia from intractable bronchospasm or severe hypotension.

In one-third of cases, respiratory signs are present. Initially the reaction may present with a dry cough, tachypnoea or even frank bronchospasm with difficulty in ventilating the patient's lungs. If the patient is not already intubated, it is impossible to ventilate the lungs with a mask and airway. Bronchoconstriction is partly due to the action of histamine on H_1 bronchial receptors, but other mediators such as leukotrienes released with histamine are more important (see Chapter 19). In the presence of severe cardiovascular collapse, pulmonary oedema can occur, probably mediated by PAF. Profuse diarrhoea may be a further manifestation of generalized smooth muscle contraction.

Cerebral hypoxia resulting in cerebral oedema may present with convulsions, sphincteral incontinence or even motor deficits. Often a delayed awakening, not related to the amount of administered anaesthetic agents, is noted. In less severe reactions, disorientation, agitation and fear of dying (as with other causes of hypotension) are not uncommon.

The differences in clinical manifestation of anaphylactoid reactions may be related to differential sensitivity of mast cells in anatomically different locations, and whether preformed or secondary mediator release is triggered. In some special subgroups, such as pregnant women, the clinical picture is especially serious. In IgE-mediated reactions, the placenta serves to filter this antibody and the fetus suffers only the haemodynamic consequences of the mother. However in IgG-mediated reactions, such as occurs with dextrans, the antibody crosses the placental barrier and the fetus is at increased risk. Even with only a moderate degree of maternal hypotension, the outcome can be fatal for the fetus.

Complications of anaphylactoid reactions are related to the degree and duration of cardiovascular collapse. Cardiogenic shock, renal failure, adult respiratory distress syndrome, disseminated intravascular coagulation, a sudden rise in intracranial pressure and altered hepatic function are well recognized complications.

DIFFERENTIAL DIAGNOSIS

In the awake patient the onset of sudden collapse following injection of a drug may be due to a vasovagal attack. Cutaneous histamine reactions are distinctly absent, and bronchospasm is not a feature of this condition. In the perioperative period, dysrhythmias, myocardial infarction, pulmonary embolism, bronchial asthma, disconnection of vasoactive drug infusions and drug overdose are important conditions to consider whilst initiating immediate treatment of sudden onset, severe hypotension.

MANAGEMENT OF ANAPHYLACTOID REACTIONS

Retrospective studies of anaphylactic shock indicate a mortality rate as high as 9%. Where possible, prophylactic measures to prevent anaphylactoid responses should be taken to avoid or minimize the complications of an anaphylactoid reaction. Similarly the mortality and morbidity rates of anaphylactoid reactions are directly related to the speed with which therapy is instituted. With early diagnosis and treatment, the prognosis of anaphylactoid reactions is in general good if there are no other risk factors present. The earlier treatment is instituted, the better is the outcome.[12] Because of the urgency of the situation, much can be said for the presence of an action plan well in advance of any possible occurrence, such as that produced by the Association of Anaesthetists of Great Britain and Ireland.

The important goal of initial therapy is to maintain oxygenation and tissue circulation. To this end immediate cessation of anaesthetic agents likely to have contributed to the reaction, maintenance of a good airway, administration of 100% oxygen, acute expansion of intravascular volume and administration of adrenaline are the mainstays of immediate therapy.

A treatment protocol emphasizing the relevant steps, such as in Table 27.3, must be instituted without delay once the diagnosis has been made. With less severe forms of reactions, where cardiac and respiratory functions are relatively stable, it may be possible to proceed with emergency surgery under an appropriate anaesthetic, taking care to avoid all unnecessary medications. Elective surgery should probably be suspended until a complete investigation has been completed, and must be rearranged in a planned manner with all resuscitation measures readily to hand.

In mild forms where the condition is not life threatening, secondary therapy such as antihistamines and corticosteroids may be all that is necessary. In more severe forms, adrenaline is the preferred first-line treatment (0.5 ml of a 1 in 1000 (1 mg ml^{-1}) solution intramuscularly or 3–5 ml of a 1 in 10 000 (100 μg ml^{-1}) solution intravenously). This can be repeated every 5 min, or an infusion may be started if required. When carefully titrated, the risk of intravenous adrenaline is small. The importance of simultaneous intravascular volume expansion, initially with 1–2 litres of colloid solution, cannot be overstated. This may reduce the need for further adrenaline and its associated arrhythmogenic side-effects, which may be severe in the presence of hypoxia and respiratory and metabolic acidosis, and in patients with preexisting cardiac disease.

Adrenaline is also effective in treating bronchospasm. Other bronchodilators such as nebulized or intravenous β-adrenoceptor agonists (e.g. salbutamol), or intravenous aminophylline may need to be considered and most patients will respond to this treatment. When continuing histamine release may be a problem, antihistamines such as chlorpheniramine may be given intravenously, but the value of this is questionable. Severe bronchospasm that is resistant to the above mea-

---

Table 27.3 Management protocol for anaphylactoid reactions

Immediate therapy

1. Stop all suspected anaesthetic drugs.

2. Summon more help.

3. Intubate if not already done so, and ventilate with 100% oxygen.

4. Lay flat and elevate both legs to 45° to increase venous return.

5. Titrate 50–100 μg aliquots of adrenaline intravenously for hypotension.

6. Start intravascular volume expansion.

7. Repeated assessments of cardiovascular and respiratory systems.

Secondary mangement

1. Investigations:
   • full blood count, urea and electrolytes, coagulation screen (baseline), tryptase levels, immunoglobulin and complement assay as appropriate.

2. Treatment of resistant cardiovascular shock:
   • adrenaline, isoprenaline or noradrenaline infusion
   • corticosteroids
   • bicarbonate (for metabolic acidosis compromising myocardial function).

3. Treatment of resistant bronchospasm:
   • aminophylline infusion
   • β₂ agonists infusion
   • reassessment of airway oedema, before extubation.

4. Antihistamines.

5. Intensive monitoring and observation in an intensive care area.

6. Postdischarge investigation measures and drawing up future anaesthetic plan.

---

sures may necessitate the patient to be ventilated under isoflurane or ketamine sedation. Intravenous corticosteroids commenced early will reduce the inflammatory component of the process, and large doses of steroids (e.g. 1 g methylprednisolone) have been particularly effective when complement-mediated reactions are suspected (e.g. following protamine administration or transfusion reactions).

When hypotension does not respond to fluids, severe acidosis should be suspected. Sodium bicarbonate can justifiably be used only when circulatory collapse is complicated by acidosis and a vicious cycle has been set up with an increasing degree of acidosis causing further depression of myocardial function.

The progression of anaphylaxis varies, and in 5% of patients it recurs after an initial recovery without any additional challenge. This clinical relapse may occur between 1 and 72 h after the acute event. Anaphylactic reactions may also be protracted and, as stated above, the incidence of serious life-threatening complications will depend on the duration and severity of the cardiovascular collapse. The onset of complications such as disseminated intravascular coagulation, renal and liver dysfunction in the following 24 h must be borne in mind. Further invasive haemodynamic monitoring with a direct arterial line, as well as central venous pressure and pulmonary artery occlusion pressure measurements, may be necessary in severe cases. These patients should be managed on the intensive care unit, be observed for at least 24 h and have a proper airway assessment before an elective extubation.

INVESTIGATION OF A PATIENT WITH SUSPECTED ALLERGIC REACTION

Despite appropriate treatment, about 6–9% of the patients who have suffered a severe anaphylactic reaction die. It is therefore of utmost importance to develop a rational approach to try to minimize the risk for future anaesthetics by identifying possible risk factors and, again, there should be guidelines directing the investigation. However, any investigation should follow immediate treatment of an emergency, and the diagnosis of anaphylaxis will be made primarily on clinical grounds.

The majority of the 'precipitous manifestations' of anaphylactoid reactions are due to chemical mediators released from mast cell degranulation, most notably histamine. Histamine has a very short half-life (2 min), and it is clearly impractical to assay plasma levels of histamine for confirmation of diagnosis. Tryptase is another enzyme released at the time of mast cell degranulation and is a good marker of severe reactions, although not minor ones. After a severe reaction, plasma tryptase levels reach a peak concentration in about 1 h, and remain raised for at least 3 h. It is important to take blood samples at 4-h intervals for the first day, and the plasma should be frozen at −20°C for further analysis.

Basic tests require the quantification of immunoglobulins, IgG, IgA, IgM and IgE, complement components C3, C4, C-1 inhibitor and albumin by conventional immunochemical methods. The plasma albumin and IgM ratios provide a useful measure to assess both haemoconcentration and haemodilution as a result of management with fluids.

The specific identification of the causative agent is not easy in view of cross-sensitivity among drugs with similar antigenic determinants. However, it is an important part of the investigation as it helps to identify drugs that may be used safely in a future anaesthetic. Intradermal tests should be performed at least 4 weeks after the suspected episode. Drugs such as antihistamines, sympathomimetics, xanthine derivatives, steroids and cromoglycates must be stopped for at least 48 h before testing because of their effect on mast cells. However, skin tests may be of little value in predominantly complement-mediated reactions such as those due to radiocontrast media and colloids.

The investigation of transfusion reactions should be conducted by or with the advice of a regional transfusion centre. The value of IgE assays, measurement of antibodies using radioallergosorbent test (RAST) and enzyme-linked immunosorbent assay (ELISA) in routine clinical practice remains to be established, probably because of the prohibitive costs of such tests. No single test can accurately predict the safety or otherwise of a drug, and diagnosis usually rests with accurate history-taking and other collaborative evidence supplemented with appropriate intradermal testing.

MANAGEMENT OF A FUTURE ANAESTHETIC

A detailed history of the clinical manifestations and temporal sequence of the reaction, with a review of anaesthetic records, is essential before a future anaesthetic is planned. Where the history is consistent with an allergic reaction, all suspected drugs must be strictly avoided, although cross-sensitivity is a particular feature of muscle relaxants. Where a reaction to relaxants is suspected, an immunological evaluation is of considerable help in trying to identify safe muscle relaxants. The use of NSAIDs should probably be avoided after an anaphylactoid reaction in patients who have known aspirin- or exercise-induced asthma, rhinosinusitis, nasal polyps or a history of atopy. As anxiety is recognized to contribute to adverse reactions, effective premedication with benzodiazepines may help, although there is no scientific evidence to support this practice.

Even after complete investigation of a reaction, surgical procedures should be done under local or regional anaesthesia where possible. Where a general anaes-

thetic is warranted, pretreatment with antihistamines (H_1- and H_2-receptor antagonists), steroids and sympathomimetics (e.g. ephedrine) have been used. There has been a reduction in the incidence and severity of reactions due to radiocontrast media following such prophylaxis. However, the role of such pretreatments in well established IgE-mediated reactions is less clear.

In other 'at-risk' patients, in addition to specific measures aimed at predisposing factors, one may consider giving H_1- and H_2-receptor antagonists for 16–24 h before anaesthesia to alter the physiological dose–response curve to histamine. However, antihistamines do not prevent secondary mediator release after mast cell or basophil activation. Corticosteroids may be given in large divided doses for at least 24 h before surgery, but again their value remains unquantified.

IDIOSYNCRATIC REACTIONS

This is an imprecise term to describe the unusual responses occasionally seen in some patients. The mechanism of these reactions is diverse but idiosyncrasy can be defined as a genetically determined abnormal reactivity to a chemical where the underlying mechanism is predominantly genetic. The term should not be confused with drug allergy, for which an external means of exposure and sensitization is required. Idiosyncratic reactions occur in a small proportion of patients, and the unusual response observed has no relation to the dose of the drug administered. For example, about 10% of males of African extraction have a deficiency of glucose-6-phosphate dehydrogenase enzyme activity in their red blood cells and develop serious haemolytic anaemia when exposed to primaquine. Similarly, a genetically determined alteration in the receptor for warfarin results in resistance to warfarin anticoagulation.

In anaesthetic practice malignant hyperthermia, succinylcholine apnoea and porphyria are examples of genetically linked responses. Carcinoid syndrome is also associated with an idiosyncratic response but this is related to the release of humoral mediators from a tumour into the systemic circulation.

MALIGNANT HYPERTHERMIA

Malignant hyperthermia is a subclinical myopathy where, in the presence of triggering agents, there is acute loss of intracellular control of calcium. The sudden increase in free ionized and unbound calcium results in intractable contraction of skeletal muscles and, with it, an uncontrolled and rapid rise in body temperature. The presence of high intracellular calcium concentrations stimulates further intracellular mobilization of calcium, and without timely intervention the mortality rate is as high as 80%.

Malignant hyperthermia is a pharmacogenetic disease with autosomal dominant inheritance with impaired penetrance. The responsible gene has been located on the long arm of chromosome 19. The reported incidence is about 1 in 64 000 anaesthetic administrations, with four times as many suspected cases. Succinylcholine and volatile agents are responsible for most cases reported under anaesthesia. Succinylcholine affects the cell membrane, resulting in calcium release from the T tubules, whereas the volatile agents trigger the condition by altering the intracellular calcium dynamics.

A sudden rise in the metabolic rate to approximately five times normal results initially in muscle rigidity, increased carbon dioxide production and an increase in heart rate. This is rapidly followed by hyperkalaemia, hypoxia, hypercarbia and acidosis, and the body temperature rises at a rate of 2°C per h. Once considered, all suspected agents should be discontinued, and the patient ventilated with 100% oxygen through a 'clean' (vapour free) machine. Dantrolene is the mainstay of treatment of this condition and its administration should not be delayed. Other supportive measures to correct hyperthermia, acidosis, hypercarbia and hyperkalaemia should be instituted as appropriate. Even when treated with the above, the mortality rate may be around 5%.

After initial therapy, the patient and the family should be referred to a centre with facilities to investigate the disorder further. This is important for safe conduct of future anaesthesia in these patients and their families.

PORPHYRIA

The porphyrias are a group of disorders of porphyrin metabolism caused by a genetically determined absence of specific enzymes involved in the pathway for haem synthesis. This results in an overproduction and accumulation of intermediates known as porphyrins. Certain toxic agents such as hexachlorobenzene may also cause one type of porphyria (porphyria cutanea tarda).

The type of porphyria that concerns the anaesthetist most is acute intermittent porphyria.[13] It is a dominantly transmitted disorder that can exist in a latent form indefinitely. Acute attacks are precipitated by various environmental (e.g. exposure to drugs and infection) and endogenous (e.g. starvation and crash dieting) factors. The basic enzyme defect in this disorder is a 50% decrease of uroporphyrinogen I synthetase. The manifest disease is more common in women, and occurs in all races.

Drugs that have been implicated in precipitating acute attacks of the disease include barbiturates, etomidate, benzodiazepines except midazolam, alcuronium, pentazocine, phenytoin, sulphonamides, imipramine,

ergot alkaloids, methyldopa, chloramphenicol, griseofulvin, meprobamate and glutethimide. Enflurane is not recommended, and use of halothane and isoflurane remains contentious. Propofol, suxamethonium, curare, vecuronium, morphine, pethidine, fentanyl, codeine, paracetamol, hyoscine, nitrous oxide, aspirin, prochlorperazine, promethazine, diphenhydramine, atropine, neostigmine, steroids and most antibiotics are probably safe to use in the suspected individuals. Ketamine, atracurium, pancuronium, alfentanil and sufentanil are probably best avoided as the evidence for their safety is questionable.

Symptoms of the acute attack result from nervous system damage. Any part of the nervous system may be affected and, as such, the clinical findings can vary through a wide spectrum. The outcome varies from complete recovery to death, and some patients may be left with a permanent neurological deficit. Autonomic neuropathy is common and causes abdominal pain, vomiting, labile hypertension, sinus tachycardia, sweating and postural hypotension. Sensory or motor neuropathy, seizures, cerebellar and basal ganglion manifestations are also well recognized. Respiratory paralysis may require assisted ventilation and carries a high mortality rate. Profound hyponatraemia is thought to be secondary to gastrointestinal and renal loss of sodium, and inappropriate release of antidiuretic hormone. Depression may be a presenting symptom of this disorder.

Patients who are known to have acute intermittent porphyria are at risk from an acute attack following prolonged preoperative starvation, the stress of surgery, dehydration, pain and exposure to medications that are not safe. These patients should receive regional anaesthesia where practical, and meticulous attention should be paid to correcting the above factors in the conduct of anaesthesia.

CARCINOID SYNDROME

Carcinoid syndrome is a collection of symptoms resulting from release of vasoactive peptides into the systemic circulation. Release of mediators may occur from hepatic metastases or from a primary tumour with its venous drainage outside of the portal circulation. Although 5-hydroxytryptamine (5-HT) is the mediator used for diagnostic purposes, the mediators that cause symptoms are varied and also include histamine, bradykinin, prostaglandins and kallikreins. Symptoms include abdominal pain, flushing, diarrhoea and asthma, and cardiac involvement may involve tricuspid or pulmonary valve disease and may progress to right heart failure. Anaesthesia may be problematic because severe hypotension or hypertension may occur during induction or maintenance following direct release of mediators by anaesthetic agents or surgical manipulation.

Early attempts at preoperative control by the use of histamine antagonists, 5-HT antagonists and corticosteroids were not always successful, especially at controlling severe hypotension. More recently octreotide (a somatostatin analogue) has been used as preoperative prophylaxis and for symptomatic control of hypotension, with good effect. Avoidance of anaesthetic techniques or agents that release catecholamines or histamine is also of benefit. The use of ketanserin as a 5-HT antagonist to control the hypertension has also been effective.[14]

PHYSICOCHEMICAL REACTIONS

Bacterial contamination, instability of drugs in solution and direct chemical combination resulting in precipitation may cause adverse effects on occasions.

Aseptic precautions in preparing and handling of drugs are important. Propofol is made up in egg phosphatide emulsion, and contains no antimicrobial preservatives. Bacterial contamination has resulted in clinical disease and this is preventable by using the drug within the recommended time interval after opening the vial. Likewise it is important to observe careful aseptic practice when handling all drugs.

Some drugs are unstable when made up in solution. Amoxycillin, ampicillin, benzylpenicillin, tetracycline, flucloxacillin and cephradine lose their activity in solution, either in saline or dextrose, within 6–12 h. Sodium nitroprusside, amphotericin, frusemide and certain phenothiazines are unstable in the presence of light. Similarly, when lipophilic drugs formulated in solubilizing agents are diluted, the solution may become unstable. Thiopentone and etomidate have a high pH in solution and they may precipitate when mixed with acidic drugs or solutions.

Drug incompatibility may be due to direct chemical interaction. Total parenteral nutritional solutions are delicately balanced solutions, and the addition of drugs or electrolytes to fat-containing solutions may result in aggregation or precipitation of the mixture. When penicillin derivatives are added to infusions containing amino acids, drug–protein complexes can be formed. The resulting complexes may induce the formation of antibodies with the risk of a future anaphylactoid reaction. Mixing thiopentone and *d*-tubocurarine in the same syringe, or even administering these drugs into the same intravenous cannula, results in a precipitation reaction. Alcuronium, pancuronium, vecuronium and atracurium may form precipitates with thiopentone. Suxamethonium and thiopentone precipitates have been implicated in anaphylactoid reactions.

CONCLUSION

Hypersensitivity reactions occur in clinical practice with varying incidence and severity. With greater understanding of pathophysiology of these reactions, and speedy institution of treatment, mortality and morbidity rates can be reduced. The importance of investigating a suspected or frank anaphylactoid reaction in the planning of a future anaesthetic in the affected patient cannot be overemphasized.

REFERENCES

1. Fisher MM. Epidemiology of anaesthetic anaphylactic reactions in Australasia. *Anaesth Intensive Care* 1981; **9**: 226–234.
2. Thornton JA, Lorenz W. Histamines and antihistamines in anaesthesia and surgery. Report of a symposium. *Anaesthesia* 1983; **38**: 373–379.
3. McKinnon RP, Wildsmith JAW. Histaminoid reactions in anaesthesia. *Br J Anaesth* 1995; **74**: 217–228.
4. Beamish D, Brown DT. Adverse response to intravenous anaesthetics. *Br J Anaesth* 1981; **53**: 55–58.
5. Harle DG, Baldo BA, Fisher MM. The molecular basis of IgE antibody binding to thiopentone. Binding of IgE from thiopentone-allergic and non-allergic subjects. *Mol Immunol* 1990; **27**: 853–858.
6. Whittington T, Fisher MM. Anaphylactic and anaphylactoid reactions. *Baillieres Clin Anaesthesiol* 1998; **12**: 301–323.
7. Harle DG, Baldo BA, Coroneos NJ, Fisher MM. Anaphylaxis following administration of papaveretum. Case report: implication of IgE antibodies that react with morphine and codeine, and identification of an allergenic determinant. *Anesthesiology* 1989; **71**: 489–494.
8. Szczeklik A. Adverse reactions to aspirin and non-steroidal anti-inflammatory agents. *Ann Allergy* 1987; **59**: 113–118.
9. Kajimoto Y, Rosenberg ME, Kytta J *et al.* Anaphylactoid skin reactions after intravenous regional anaesthesia using 0.5% prilocaine with or without preservative – a double-blind study. *Acta Anaesthesiol Scand* 1995; **39**: 782–784.
10. Kam PCA, Lee MSM, Thompson JF. Latex allergy: an emerging clinical and occupational health problem. *Anaesthesia* 1997; **52**: 570–575.
11. Horrow JC. Protamine: a review of its toxicity. *Anesth Analg* 1985; **64**: 348–361.
12. Fisher M. Treatment of acute anaphylaxis. *BMJ* 1995; **311**: 731–733.
13. Harrison GG, Meissner PN, Hift RJ. Anaesthesia for the porphyric patient. *Anaesthesia* 1993; **48**: 417–421.
14. Veall GRQ, Peacock JE, Bax NDS, Reilly CS. Review of the anaesthetic management of 21 patients undergoing laparotomy for carcinoid syndrome. *Br J Anaesth* 1994; **72**: 335–341.

28 J Vuyk

DRUG INTERACTIONS IN ANAESTHESIA

Drug interactions occur when the actions of one drug are altered by the concurrent administration of another. When combinations of drugs are used, such as during anaesthesia, there is always the possibility of drug–drug interactions. Also, many patients will be taking drugs related to their surgical or medical condition that may interact with drugs given during anaesthesia. In the first half of this chapter therapeutic (beneficial) drug interactions will be discussed, followed by interactions that have the potential to cause adverse effects.

TERMINOLOGY

The relationship between the blood or plasma concentration of a drug and its effect can be described by four modalities, potency, efficacy, slope and variability. Potency reflects the sensitivity to the drug, and is defined by the location of the concentration–effect relationship curve on the x-axis. It is often described in terms of the EC_{50} or minimum alveolar concentration (MAC), the median effective concentration for intravenous drugs and inhalational anaesthetics. These parameters allow definition of the effectiveness of different drugs with respect to a specific effect, and of the effectiveness with which a single drug exerts different effects. For intravenous and inhalational drugs, different clinical endpoints can be used to define EC_{50} or MAC. Efficacy, or maximum efficacy, is the (maximum) effect that a drug can produce, and allows agonists and partial agonists to be differentiated. The slope of the concentration–effect curve is related to the mechanism of action of the drug, for example receptor binding. The steepness of the curve describes the concentration range between almost no effect and maximum effect. Most anaesthetic drugs have steep concentration–effect curves. Finally, the interindividual variability in concentration–effect relationships is reflected by the standard deviation or standard error of the EC_{50} or MAC.

Berenbaum[1] defined three classes of drug interaction: zero interactions, and supra- and infra-additive interactions. A zero interaction, more commonly referred to as an additive interaction, is one where the effect of the combination of two drugs is exactly the sum of the effects of the drugs given separately. When the effect of the combination is greater than that expected from the concentration–effect relationships of the individual drugs, the interaction is supra-additive. Synergism and potentiation are often used as synonyms for supra-additivity. In this case, relatively less of the combination is needed to obtain a given effect than when the drugs are given separately. An interaction is infra-additive (sometimes erroneously referred to as antagonistic) when the effect of the combination is less than the sum of the effects of the individual drugs. Relatively more of each drug is then needed to obtain the effect produced by either drug given alone. Pharmacological antagonism occurs when the effect of a combination is less than that of one of its constituents; for example, the combined effect of alfentanil and naloxone is less than that of alfentanil alone.

The 'isobolographic method' is commonly used to analyse drug interactions. An isobole is a line connecting equipotent dose or concentration combinations of two (or more) drugs that exert a similar effect. To illustrate this method, consider two drugs, A and B, which when given separately in doses (or concentrations) D_a

---

Summary box 28.1 Drug interactions: terminology

- Additivity – the effect of the combination of two drugs is the sum of the effects of the drugs given separately.

- Supra-additivity (synergism or potentiation) – less of the combination is needed to obtain a given effect than when the drugs are given separately.

- Infra-additivity – relatively more of each drug is needed to obtain the effect produced by either drug given alone.

and D_b each produce effect E. If combinations of A and B in doses (or concentrations) d_a and d_b also produce effect E, then the interaction between A and B can be represented by eqn [1]:

$$\frac{d_a}{D_a} + \frac{d_b}{D_b} = x \qquad [1]$$

where x is called the interaction index. When $x = 1$, the interaction is additive and points representing different combinations producing effect E lie on a straight line (Fig. 28.1). Such a line is an isobole (isoeffect line). For example, the interaction between nitrous oxide and the volatile anaesthetics is additive so that 0.6 MAC nitrous oxide plus 0.4 MAC isoflurane is equipotent to 1 MAC isoflurane. When $x < 1$, the isobole represented by eqn [1] is concave-up and the interaction is supra-additive or synergistic. For example, only one-eighth of the dose of drug A required for effect E may need to be combined with five-eighths of the dose of drug B to achieve effect E. Points representing isoeffective combinations lie below and to the left of the line of additivity. Conversely, when $x > 1$, points representing isoeffective combinations lie above and to the right of the line of additivity; the isobole joining these points is concave-down and the interaction is infra-additive. In this situation one-eighth of the dose of drug A may need to be combined with eleven-eighths of drug B to produce effect E. For a combination of three drugs, the isobole is a surface in three dimensions and, for example, the zero-interaction isobole is a flat plane.

Isoboles may be inconsistent, in that they may cross the line of zero interaction (Fig. 28.2).[2] This occurs when drug combinations exert synergistic and infra-additive effects when mixed in different ratios. Finally, the character of the interaction may be different for different clinical endpoints. Two drugs may act synergistically with respect to one effect and infra-additively with respect to another. It has also been

argued that combinations of two drugs with dissimilar dose–response curves can generate curved isoboles even if there is no interaction.

MECHANISMS OF DRUG INTERACTIONS

The mechanisms involved in drug interactions may be one of three types: pharmaceutical, pharmacokinetic or pharmacodynamic. Pharmaceutical interactions refer to

---

Summary box 28.2 Drug interactions: classification

- Pharmaceutical – direct chemical interactions between drugs or their absorption into the material of their containers.

- Pharmacokinetic – when one drug changes the pharmacokinetic disposition of another by altering its:

  - absorption

  - distribution (e.g. by alteration in protein binding)

  - clearance (e.g. enzyme induction or inhibition, changes in renal or hepatic blood flow). The cytochrome P450 enzyme system is one most commonly involved in anaesthesia-related drug interactions.

- Pharmacodynamic – cooperation or competition for receptor sites.

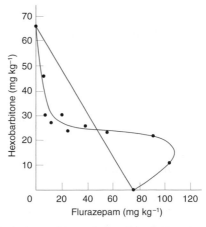

Fig. 28.2 Isobolographic analysis of the interaction between flurazepam and hexobarbitone for producing electroencephalographic burst suppression of more than 1 s in rats. The isobole is markedly inconsistent, with different regions showing supra-additive, infra-additive interactions and antagonism. From Norberg and Wahlström.[2]

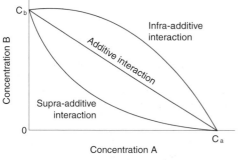

Fig. 28.1 Interaction diagram with, on the x- and y-axis, concentrations of the compounds studied and the line of additivity; the areas represent infra-additive and supra-additive interactions.

direct chemical combinations between drugs, or their absorption into the material of their containers. A pharmacokinetic interaction occurs when a drug alters the distribution, redistribution, metabolic clearance and/or the excretion of another drug. This may be the result of an alteration in protein binding, induction or inhibition of the enzymes responsible for drug metabolism, or a change in renal or hepatic clearance. A pharmacodynamic interaction occurs when one drug influences the actions of another drug at the effect site, which for general anaesthetic agents is generally the central nervous system but could also be, for example, the cardiovascular or respiratory system. Underlying mechanisms for pharmacodynamic interactions include cooperation or competition at similar receptor sites.

THERAPEUTIC DRUG INTERACTIONS

PHARMACEUTICAL INTERACTIONS

An example of a therapeutic pharmaceutical interaction is the reversal of the anticoagulant effects of heparin by protamine by the formation of an inactive chemical complex between the two substances. In general, however, pharmaceutical interactions are more likely to give rise to adverse effects.

PHARMACOKINETIC INTERACTIONS

Therapeutic pharmacokinetic interactions are uncommon in anaesthesia. One example is the second gas effect, where the concomitant administration of one volatile agent increases the rate of uptake and, after termination of administration, the rate of decrease of the end-tidal concentration of a second agent.

PHARMACODYNAMIC INTERACTIONS

Interpatient variability in the pharmacodynamics of anaesthetic drugs is in the order of 300–400%, compared with the interindividual variability in pharmacokinetics of approximately 60–80%. Pharmacodynamic interactions between anaesthetic agents can influence this variability, and are thus of greater clinical importance than pharmacokinetic interactions. The pharmacodynamic interactions of importance to anaesthesia can be divided into those between inhalational agents, between inhalational and intravenous drugs, and between the various intravenous drugs.

Interactions between inhalational agents

Inhalational agents shift the concentration–response relationships of other inhalational agents to the left. It is generally accepted that inhalational agents interact in an additive manner (Fig. 28.3). This means that, when combined, the potencies of the individual drugs may be added to determine the potency of the mixture.

Halothane 0.5 MAC (0.38%) combined with nitrous oxide 0.5 MAC (55%) results in a combination with a potency of 1 MAC. However, in rats there is an infra-additive interaction between cyclopropane and nitrous oxide or ethylene, and between nitrous oxide and enflurane. There is also evidence that the interaction between nitrous oxide and halothane, enflurane or isoflurane in rats is nonlinear for nitrous oxide concentrations exceeding 30%.[3]

Interactions between inhalational and intravenous agents

Interactions between Inhalational Agents and Opioids

Morphine, fentanyl, sufentanil and alfentanil all reduce the MAC of inhalational agents in animals and in humans. However, there is a ceiling to this effect, with the maximum MAC reduction being about 65%, providing evidence that opioids alone cannot produce complete anaesthesia (Fig. 28.4).[4,5] The maximum MAC reduction possible with partial opioid agonists such as butorphanol and nalbuphine is much less than that of the full agonists, about 8–11%. The nature of the interaction between opioids and inhalational agents differs depending on the endpoint studied. Morphine and halothane interact additively with respect to the suppression of purposeful movement in response to noxious stimuli, but infra-additively with respect to the increase in heart rate due to noxious stimuli.

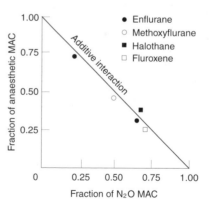

Fig. 28.3 Interaction between inhalational anaesthetic agents. The vertical axis represents the fraction of minimum alveolar concentrations (MAC) in patients for four anaesthetics. The value 1.0 represents 1 MAC, or 1.68% enflurane, 0.76% halothane, 0.16% methoxyflurane or 3.4% fluroxene. The horizontal axis represents the MAC fraction of nitrous oxide; in this case 1 MAC represents 101% nitrous oxide. The straight line connecting the 1.0-MAC points represents the line of simple addition. From Torri G, Domia G, Fabian ML. Effect of nitrous oxide on the anaesthetic requirement of enflurane. *Br J Anaesth* 1974; **46**: 468–472, with permission.

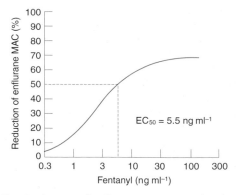

Fig. 28.4 Reduction of enflurane minimum alveolar concentration (MAC) versus plasma concentration of fentanyl on a log scale. A ceiling effect is evident. From Schweiger *et al.*,[5] with permission.

Interactions between Inhalational Agents and Induction Drugs
Benzodiazepines decrease the MAC of inhalational anaesthetic agents and exhibit a ceiling effect similar to that seen with opioids. The ceiling effect in the reduction of MAC by benzodiazepines suggests that they, like the opioids, are not complete anaesthetics. This is in contrast to, for example, propofol and α_2-adrenoreceptor agonists, which at sufficient concentrations can produce a 100% reduction in MAC.

Interactions between Intravenous Anaesthetic Drugs
With the introduction of short-acting intravenous drugs, characterization of the interaction between different intravenous anaesthetics has gained clinical importance and has been studied extensively. Interactions are possible between intravenous anaesthetic drugs acting via the same receptor as well as between drugs producing the same clinical endpoint via different receptors.

Interactions between Induction Agents
Although seldom combined during the induction of anaesthesia, the interaction between intravenous induction agents has been studied extensively. In general, most induction agents interact in a synergistic manner. The steroid anaesthetic alphahexatone and midazolam interact synergistically with barbiturates with respect to the loss of righting reflex in rats. The synergistic interaction may be the result of an interaction between these agents at the benzodiazepine and the barbiturate effector site on the γ-aminobutyric acid (GABA)$_A$ receptor, where these drugs facilitate GABA-mediated inhibition of neurotransmission. Similar synergism exists between midazolam and both thiopentone and methohexitone in humans with respect to loss of consciousness. Propofol, which also acts at the GABA$_A$ receptor, inter-

acts in a synergistic manner with respect to loss of consciousness when combined with midazolam or thiopentone.

Interactions between Intravenous Anaesthetics and Opioids
Opioids are commonly used with intravenous anaesthetics during induction of anaesthesia and are increasingly combined during operation with drugs such as propofol and midazolam for total intravenous anaesthesia. Most interactions between intravenous anaesthetics and opioids are synergistic, although the degree of synergism may vary depending on the chosen endpoint. Both morphine and fentanyl act infra-additively in combination with thiopentone for the suppression of purposeful movements to tail clamping, but interact synergistically for the loss of righting reflex in rats. With increasing stimulus intensity (increasing pressure applied during tail clamping), the ability of morphine to reduce the ED_{50} of pentobarbitone for the suppression of arousal to a noxious stimulus decreases markedly.[6] The interaction between opioids and intravenous induction agents is also characterized by a ceiling effect.

The interaction between fentanyl and midazolam also appears to be concentration dependent. In dogs, the interaction with respect to the suppression of a response to tail clamping is additive with fentanyl infusion rates from 0.05 to 0.2 μg kg^{-1} min^{-1}, whereas at higher infusion rates the interaction becomes infra-additive.[5] It is possible that the development of acute tolerance to fentanyl may have contributed to this observation. In contrast, in patients midazolam and alfentanil interact in a supra-additive manner with respect to loss of consciousness. Even subanalgesic doses of alfentanil (3 μg kg^{-1}) significantly reduce the concentration of midazolam needed to induce loss of consciousness, suggesting that the magnitude of this interaction may be based on a functional relationship between the GABA$_A$ and opioid receptors in producing hypnosis. Intrathecal morphine and midazolam interact synergistically to suppress thermally evoked pain, an interaction that is antagonized by naloxone.[7] Both fentanyl and alfentanil reduce the dose requirements of thiopentone and midazolam for induction of anaesthesia, and midazolam and propofol interact synergistically with alfentanil with respect to loss of consciousness in patients. The triple combination of propofol, midazolam and alfentanil is strongly synergistic with respect to loss of consciousness in adult patients.

Opioids decrease propofol requirements during induction of anaesthesia. Fentanyl reduces the induction dose of propofol but aggravates the haemodynamic depressant effects of propofol after induction of anaesthesia but before intubation. Fentanyl concentrations of 0.6 ng ml^{-1} reduce the propofol EC_{50} for purposeful movement to skin incision by 50%. Alfentanil decreases the blood propofol concentration required for the loss of the eyelash reflex and loss of consciousness. However, this positive effect is not reflected in greater haemodynamic stability since alfentanil, like fentanyl, potentiates the haemodynamic depressant effects of propofol.[8]

The synergistic interaction between opioids and induction agents is even more pronounced for the suppression of intraoperative responses. In patients undergoing cardiac surgery anaesthetized with target-controlled infusions of alfentanil and propofol, increasing the target propofol concentration from 2 to 6 μg ml^{-1} reduced the EC$_{50}$ of alfentanil for intubation from 232 to 51 ng ml^{-1}, for skin incision from 126 to 2 ng ml^{-1} and for sternotomy from 103 to 16 ng ml^{-1}.[9] Comparable strongly synergistic interactions between propofol and alfentanil occur for stimuli during abdominal surgery (Fig. 28.5).[10]

By using data from interaction studies such as those discussed above together with pharmacokinetic–dynamic modelling techniques, it is possible to obtain estimates of the optimum concentrations of opioid and intravenous anaesthetic that will ensure both adequate intraoperative anaesthesia and rapid recovery at the end of surgery. This technique has been applied to the combination of alfentanil and propofol.[10,11] The predicted optimum concentrations were propofol 3.5 μg ml^{-1} and alfentanil 85 ng ml^{-1}. After 3 h of anaesthesia, 50% of patients are likely to recover within 10 min with this combination of concentrations. Higher intraoperative blood propofol concentrations delay recovery, whereas with lower propofol levels the higher alfentanil requirements also lead to prolonged recovery.

Duration of infusion and the choice of opioid influence the optimum propofol concentration that ensures both adequate anaesthesia and rapid recovery. For the combination with fentanyl and sufentanil, the optimum propofol concentration is approximately similar to that with alfentanil. In contrast, when propofol and remifentanil are combined, the decay in remifentanil concentration after termination of the infusion is very much more rapid than that of propofol, so that it is advisable from the point of view of recovery to maintain anaesthesia with a lower blood propofol concentration (2.5 μg ml^{-1}) combined with a relatively higher remifentanil concentration.

Finally, the length of infusion affects the optimal propofol concentration differently for the various opioids. The steeper the decay in the opioid concentration relative to the decay in the propofol concentration after termination of an infusion, the more the propofol–opioid concentration combination shifts to a lower propofol and a higher opioid concentration. As a consequence, with increasing duration of infusion, the optimum blood propofol concentration increases when combined with alfentanil, sufentanil and fentanyl, but decreases when combined with remifentanil. Length of infusion increases the time to awakening after termination of the infusion more for the combination of propofol with alfentanil, sufentanil and fentanyl than for the combination of propofol with remifentanil.[12]

ADVERSE DRUG INTERACTIONS

As with therapeutic drug interactions, it is useful to classify adverse interactions according to their mechanisms as pharmaceutical, pharmacokinetic or pharmacodynamic.

PHARMACEUTICAL INTERACTIONS

A common example of a direct chemical interaction is the precipitation that occurs when a solution of thiopentone (highly alkaline) is mixed with acidic solutions such as suxamethonium or adrenaline. When thiopentone and vecuronium are administered consecutively, a white precipitate of thiopentone acid forms, which is insoluble in plasma and which may occlude intravenous tubing. Aminoglycosides and penicillin should never be mixed in the same container since the penicillin inactivates the aminoglycoside to a significant degree. Glyceryl trinitrate is inactivated by binding to polyvinyl chloride, and insulin can adhere to the surface of glass or plastic syringes. The net result is that the patient receives a lower than expected dose of the drug, with a reduction in clinical effect. In general, however, pharmaceutical interactions are seldom a problem in anaesthesia if sensible precautions are taken. Problems are more likely to arise in the intensive care unit.

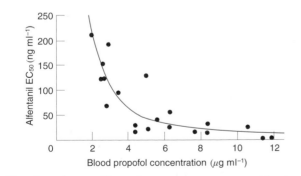

Fig. 28.5 Plasma alfentanil concentrations versus blood propofol concentrations associated with a 50% probability of no response to intraabdominal surgical stimulation. Symbols represent the EC$_{50}$ of alfentanil at corresponding mean blood propofol concentrations for suppression of responses. The curve describing the interaction was fitted to the data by nonlinear logistic regression. From Vuyk *et al.*,[10] with permission.

PHARMACOKINETIC INTERACTIONS

Absorption

The absorption of a drug from the gastrointestinal tract may be influenced by gastric and intestinal pH, speed of gastric emptying, the pK_a of the drug, its lipid solubility and its pharmaceutical formulation. Premedication with opioids and anticholinergics delays gastric emptying and drug absorption, whereas metoclopramide, which increases the rate of gastric emptying, increases the rate of absorption of benzodiazepines. Interactions between drugs within the gut can affect absorption. Tetracycline antibiotics chelate with calcium, aluminium and bismuth present in dairy products and antacids to form complexes that are poorly absorbed and have reduced antibacterial effect.

Distribution

Alfentanil can increase blood propofol concentrations by 20% when the two drugs are given in combination at concentrations associated with a moderate degree of sedation (Fig. 28.6). The mechanism of this interaction is unknown. One factor may be a reduction in the first-pass pulmonary uptake of propofol, which has been described with fentanyl.[13] This would increase the initial blood propofol concentration after a bolus dose administration. The plasma concentration of alfentanil is also increased in the presence of propofol. Inhibition of the oxidative metabolism of alfentanil by the cytochrome P450 isoenzyme, CYP3A, may explain the increased plasma alfentanil concentrations in the presence of propofol.[14] Propofol also inhibits the metabolism of sufentanil and possibly also of fentanyl.[14] Since the metabolism of midazolam is also catalysed by CYP3A isoenzymes, propofol also interferes with the metabolism of midazolam. For propofol, midazolam and the opioids, the relationship between dose and blood concentration changes by approximately 10–20% as a result of these pharmacokinetic interactions. Because the interindividual pharmacokinetic variability of single drugs is about 60–80%, the rather small additional variability due to pharmacokinetic interactions is unlikely to give rise to significant problems in clinical practice.

Metabolism and elimination

The most important elimination process for many drugs is phase I hepatic biotransformation catalysed by one of the more than 60 cytochrome P450 enzymes. There are three P450 families, CYP1, CYP2 and CYP3, based on the similarity of their amino acid sequences. These are further divided into subfamilies, denoted by a capital letter, and specific enzymes denoted by an Arabic numeral. CYP3A4, the isoform with highest expression in human liver, and also present in high concentrations

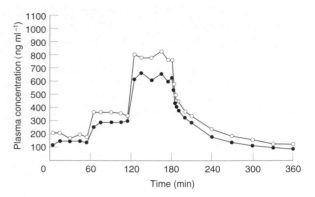

Fig. 28.6 Mean plasma propofol concentrations during infusion (0–180 min) and washout (180–360 min) in the same volunteers receiving the same infusion scheme of propofol in the presence and absence of a target-controlled infusion of alfentanil at a target concentration of 40 ng ml^{-1}. ●, Propofol alone; ○, propofol and alfentanil.

in the intestine, catalyses the metabolism of a large number of drugs, including midazolam and alfentanil. Many drugs interact with the cytochrome P450 system, either increasing (induction) or inhibiting enzyme activity (Table 28.1), both of which can cause adverse drug interactions. Phase II reactions, involving conjugation with glucuronide or sulphate, are less commonly involved in drug interactions.

Enzyme induction

The major enzyme responsible for the metabolism of the fluorinated volatile anaesthetics is CYP2E1, leading to the formation of products that can cause renal or hepatic toxicity. Enzyme induction by the antituberculous drug, rifampicin, a potent inducer of P450 enzymes, was implicated in a near-fatal case of hepatoxicity in a patient given this drug immediately after anaesthesia with halothane.[15] Halothane undergoes oxidative metabolism to form trifluoroacetyl halide (TFA), a pathway metabolized mainly by CYP2E1. Most TFA is excreted by the kidneys but a small proportion binds covalently to lipoproteins and proteins, including P450 enzymes, to form a TFA–hapten which in susceptible individuals may be responsible for halothane hepatitis. This pathway is enhanced by induction of P450, and it is therefore advisable to avoid using halothane in patients taking potent enzyme inducers. The metabolism of methadone is increased by up to 30% in patients treated with rifampicin, and it is likely that the metabolism of other opioids is similarly increased, so that higher than normal doses would be required.

Midazolam undergoes extensive hepatic metabolism by CYP3A enzymes, and its oral bioavailability, elimination half-life and clinical effects are significantly

Table 28.1 Drugs that inhibit or induce cytochrome P450 enzymes	
Inhibitors	**Inducers**

Antibiotics
    Macrolides
        Troleandomycin
        Erythromycin
    Fluoroquinolones
    Isoniazid
 	
Azole antifungal agents
    Ketoconazole
    Itraconazole
 	
Calcium entry blockers
    Diltiazem
    Verapamil
 	
Omeprazole
 	
Cimetidine
 	
Propofol
 	
Grapefruit juice
	Barbiturates
	
	Antiepileptics
	    Carbamazepine
	        Phenytoin
	        Primidone
	
	Rifampicin
	
	Dichloralphenazone
	
	Ethanol
	
	Tobacco smoke

reduced by inducers of these enzymes, such as rifampicin (Fig. 28.7).[16] The changes caused by enzyme induction are less marked when midazolam is given intravenously, but might become important with prolonged infusions, when the increased hepatic clearance will result in lower than expected steady-state concentrations.

Phenobarbitone was one of the earliest drugs to be recognized as an enzyme inducer. Other antiepileptic drugs, especially carbamazepine and phenytoin, also are potent P450 enzyme inducers, in particular the CYP3A isoforms, although carbamazepine also induces other isoforms as well as glucuronyl transferases. The oxidation of cyclosporin A, which is catalysed by CYP3A enzymes, is increased by phenytoin and carbamazepine, resulting in lowered plasma concentrations and an increased risk of transplant rejection. Carbamazepine and other antiepileptic drugs accelerate the metabolism of warfarin and dicoumarol, reducing the anticoagulant effect.

Carbamazepine and phenytoin also enhance the biotransformation of benzodiazepines. In the case of diazepam, this causes an increased production of the pharmacologically active metabolite, nordiazepam, which can minimize the decrease in therapeutic efficacy. Although midazolam does have an active metabolites, enzyme induction decreases pharmacological effect. In patients taking either carbamazepine or phenytoin, a single dose of oral midazolam (15 mg) produced no sedative effects, whereas there was a clear sedative effect lasting 2–4 h in control subjects.[17] The AUC (area under the curve) of midazolam in patients was only 5.7%, the peak midazolam concentration 7.4% and the elimination half-life 42% of the values in control subjects. Carbamazepine, phenytoin and barbiturates also enhance the hepatic metabolism of opioids. These pharmacokinetic and pharmacodynamic changes need to be taken into account when administering drugs metabolized by P450 enzymes to patients on chronic antiepileptic therapy.

Inhibition of Drug Metabolism

Although the number of compounds that inhibit enzyme activity is fewer than that producing enzyme induction, their potential for causing serious adverse reactions is probably much greater.

Antibiotics. The macrolide antibiotics and azole antifungal drugs are potent enzyme inhibitors and can cause significant adverse drug interactions. Macrolides produce a dose-dependent inhibition of CYP3A4 by forming a stable inactive complex with the enzyme. Coadministration of erythromycin with midazolam or alfentanil results in delayed excretion (Fig. 28.8)[18,19] and, in the case of alfentanil, prolonged respiratory depression.[20] Erythromycin does not appear to inhibit the metabolism of sufentanil. It increases the oral bioavailability and decreases clearance of midazolam, with excessively long-lasting hypnotic and amnesic effects. Exceptionally high midazolam concentrations and deep unconsciousness were reported in a child being treated with intravenous erythromycin who was given oral midazolam as premedication.[21] These effects are much less when midazolam is given intravenously.

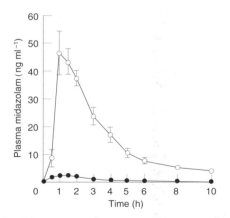

Fig. 28.7 Mean ± SEM plasma concentrations of midazolam after a 15-mg oral dose following pretreatment with placebo or 600 mg rifampicin once daily for 5 days in 10 healthy subjects. ○, After placebo; ●, after rifampicin. From Backman *et al.*,[16] with permission.

Antifungal agents. The common mechanism of action of the azole antifungal drugs is inhibition of a fungal cytochrome P450, but they also inhibit human enzymes from all three P450 enzyme families. Ketoconazole is 10 times more potent as an enzyme inhibitor than itraconazole and 500 times more potent than fluconazole. Ketoconazole inhibition of cyclosporin has even led to the suggestion that it could be used to reduce the dose, and thus the cost, of cyclosporin treatment. Ketoconazole and itraconazole are potent inhibitors of benzodiazepine metabolism, increasing oral bioavailability up to 27-fold and the elimination half-life six- to sevenfold.[22]

Calcium channel blockers. Diltiazem, and probably also verapamil, are metabolized by CYP34A, and both are potent inhibitors of this enzyme. They significantly increase the oral bioavailability of midazolam and triazolam, and prolong the elimination half-life. These

changes may be associated with profound and prolonged sedative effects. They also interact with a variety of other drugs including propranolol, carbamazepine and cyclosporin.

Grapefruit juice. Grapefruit juice is not a substance usually associated with anaesthesia. However, it increases the bioavailability of a number of drugs, especially the dihydropyridine calcium channel blockers, cyclosporin and the antihistamine terfenadine. All of these compounds are metabolized by CYP3A4, and the inhibitory effect of grapefruit juice is due to inhibition of this enzyme. This effect is found only with grapefruit juice and not with other citrus fruits, and is thought to be caused by flavinoids and other ingredients of the grapefruit. Of more direct relevance to anaesthetic practice are the changes produced by drinking this juice on the pharmacokinetics of oral benzodiazepines. Pretreatment with grapefruit juice resulted in a 56% increase in peak plasma midazolam concentrations, and an increase in bioavailability from 24% (control) to 35% (grapefruit juice).[23] Oral midazolam is commonly used for premedication of children and the concomitant drinking of grapefruit juice could cause a more profound sedative effect than anticipated.

Propofol. Propofol undergoes oxidative metabolism in the liver by cytochrome P450 enzymes. As such, it has the potential to interact with other drugs metabolized by this enzyme system. Propofol impairs the intrinsic clearance of propranolol, a P450 substrate, and inhibits the enzymatic degradation of alfentanil and sufentanil.[14] The mechanism for this latter interaction is unclear. Whereas alfentanil and sufentanil are metabolized by cytochrome P450 CYP3A enzymes, current evidence suggests that the P450 isoforms responsible for the biotransformation of propofol are primarily CYP2A1 and CYP2B1.

Proton pump inhibitors. The proton pump inhibitors, omeprazole, lansoprazole and pantoprazole, are used for the treatment of peptic ulcers and other hypersecretory conditions. They undergo extensive hepatic metabolism mediated by CYP2C19. Other substrates for CYP2C19 include *S*-mephenytoin, propranolol, diazepam and a number of tricyclic antidepressants. About 2–6% of caucasians are poor metabolizers of *S*-mephenytoin, the prototype substrate for CYP2C19, whereas in Asian populations the proportion of poor metabolizers is higher (12–20%). In poor metabolizers of *S*-mephenytoin, diazepam is more slowly metabolized than in subjects who are extensive metabolizers. Omeprazole has no effect on the pharmacokinetics of diazepam in poor metabolizers since these individuals are deficient in CYP2C19 and the conditions for an

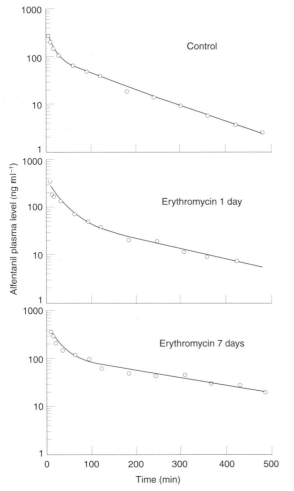

Fig. 28.8 Plasma alfentanil concentrations in a subject who had taken no drugs (control) and after erythromycin 500 mg for 1 or 7 days. From Bartkowski *et al.*,[19] with permission.

interaction therefore do not exist. However, omeprazole significantly decreases the mean clearance and increases the half-life in extensive metabolizers. Whether this interaction between omeprazole and diazepam has clinical relevance remains to be established. However, in view of the wide therapeutic safety index of diazepam, the changes produced are unlikely to cause serious adverse effects. Pantoprazole and lansoprazole do not seem to have a major effect on diazepam metabolism.

H₂-receptor antagonists. The H₂-receptor antagonist, cimetidine, is a potent inhibitor of the hepatic cytochrome P450 enzymes responsible for the phase I metabolism of many drugs, including opioids, benzodiazepines, lignocaine and warfarin. This inhibition leads to a higher than expected plasma drug concentration and a more pronounced clinical effect, which also may be prolonged. The inhibition of P450 by cimetidine results from a direct interaction with the P450 haem iron through one of the nitrogen atoms of the imidazole nucleus. Ranitidine, which contains a furan ring in place of imidazole, does not inhibit P450, although it does form a complex with hepatic cytochrome P450, but more weakly than cimetidine. As far as is known, neither famotidine nor nizatidine inhibits P450 enzymes.

Monoamine oxidase inhibitors. Monoamine oxidase (MAO) catalyses the oxidative deamination of over 15 monoamines, including adrenaline, noradrenaline, dopamine and serotonin (5-hydroxytryptamine; 5-HT). There are two subtypes of MAO, MAO-A and MAO-B, which differ in substrate preference, inhibitor specificity and tissue distribution. MAO-A preferentially deaminates 5-HT, noradrenaline and adrenaline, whereas MAO-B preferentially deaminates nonpolar aromatic amines. Tyramine and dopamine are substrates for both. The monoamine oxidase inhibitors (MAOIs) developed in the 1950s as the first effective antidepressant agents bind irreversibly with MAO-A and MAO-B. Because the formation of fresh MAO is a slow process, the potential for drug interactions with these drugs persists for up to 2 weeks after stopping the drug. The newer generation of MAOIs, in contrast, are competitive (reversible) inhibitors of MAO-A (RIMAs). Specific MAO-B inhibitors such as selegiline (*l*-deprenyl) have been developed, but are less efficient than MAO-A inhibitors as antidepressants. Selegiline is used for the treatment of Parkinson's disease. Because of the widespread inhibition of MAO, and other enzyme systems, by MAOIs there is considerable potential for adverse interactions with other drugs as well as certain foods such as cheese and yeast extracts that contain tyramine. Of most concern to anaesthetists are interactions with sympathomimetic agents and opioids.

Indirectly acting sympathomimetic drugs such as amphetamine, ephedrine and metaraminol act partly by stimulating the release of endogenous noradrenaline from sympathetic nerve terminals. Following reuptake of noradrenaline into the nerve terminal it is metabolized by MAO and catechol-*O*-methyltransferase (COMT) (Fig. 28.9). During treatment with MAOIs, large amounts of noradrenaline accumulate in the brain and in the sympathetic terminals, and administration of an indirectly acting sympathomimetic will cause an exaggerated release of noradrenaline and a potentially fatal hypertensive response. Indirectly acting sympathomimetic agents should therefore be avoided in patients treated with MAOIs. Directly acting agents (adrenaline, isoprenaline, methoxamine or phenylephrine) are safe to use in these patients.

Pethidine (meperidine) is the opioid most commonly associated with an adverse reaction with MAOIs. Although only a small proportion of patients taking MAOIs will react adversely to pethidine, there is no sure way of predicting those in whom the combination could produce severe, life-threatening reactions. These can present in two distinct forms. The excitatory form is characterized by sudden agitation, delirium, headache, hypotension or hypertension, rigidity, hyperpyrexia, convulsions and coma. It is possibly caused by an increase in cerebral 5-HT concentrations due to inhibition of MAO. This is potentiated by pethidine, which

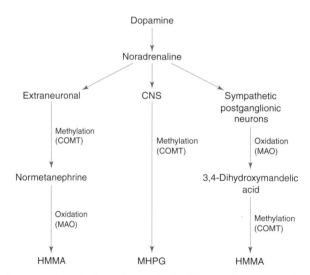

Fig. 28.9 Metabolic pathways in the biotransformation of noradrenaline involve the enzyme monoamine oxidase (MAO). Inhibition of MAO by the class of antidepressant drugs known as MAO inhibitors can lead to important and potentially life-threatening adverse drug interactions. CNS, central nervous system; COMT, catechol-*O*-methyltransferase; HMMA, 4-hydroxy 3-methoxy mandelic acid; MHPG, methyoxy-hydroxy phenyl-ethelene glycol.

blocks neuronal uptake of 5-HT. The depressive form, which is frequently severe and fatal, presents as respiratory and cardiovascular depression and coma. It is the result of a reduced breakdown of pethidine due to the inhibition of hepatic N-demethylase by MAOIs, leading to accumulation of pethidine. The risk of adverse reactions to pethidine may be less likely with the newer, specific MAO-A inhibitors. Interactions with other opioids such as morphine and pentazocine have been reported, but are less common. Other opioids appear to be safe in combination with MAOIs, with the possible exception of phenoperidine, which is metabolized to pethidine, norpethidine and pethidinic acid.

Prolongation of the action of suxamethonium has been reported with phenelzine. This seems to be a specific interaction with phenelzine, which decreases pseudocholinesterase concentration. The use of non-depolarizing muscle relaxants is not contraindicated in the presence of MAOIs, although pancuronium should be used with care because of its ability to release noradrenaline.

PHARMACODYNAMIC INTERACTIONS

Adverse drug interactions can occur when two drugs acting at the same or a related receptor are given concomitantly. For example, β-adrenoceptor antagonists diminish the effectiveness of β agonists such as salbutamol or terbutaline. On other occasions, interactions involve drugs with quite different mechanisms; for example, the inhibition of prostaglandin production by nonsteroidal antiinflammatory drugs (NSAIDs) can sometimes cause marked loss of antihypertensive control in patients receiving treatment with β-adrenoceptor antagonists, diuretics or angiotensin-converting enzyme inhibitors.

Antidepressants

The tricyclic and tetracyclic antidepressants act by specifically blocking the reuptake of endogenous catecholamines and serotonin into nerve terminals, by competing for the active transport mechanism. In patients receiving these drugs the circulatory effects of adrenaline are potentiated two to three times, and that of noradrenaline by up to ninefold. A marked increase in hypertensive effect also occurs with other directly acting sympathomimetics. Pancuronium and ketamine also inhibit the neuronal reuptake of catecholamines and should be used with caution in patients taking these drugs. Conversely, the release of noradrenaline by indirectly acting vasoconstrictors such as ephedrine is partially or completely prevented in the presence of tricyclic and tetracyclic antidepressants, resulting in a diminished effect.

Electrolyte disturbances

Electrolyte disturbances caused by diuretics, for example, can result in important pharmacodynamic interactions. The incidence of toxic effects of the cardiac glycosides is increased by potassium depletion brought about by potassium-depleting diuretics. Hypokalaemia caused by diuretics may potentiate the activity of non-depolarizing muscle relaxants leading to prolonged paralysis. The elimination of lithium occurs almost entirely by the kidney, and lithium clearance is reduced by thiazide diuretics so that plasma lithium concentrations can rise to toxic levels. Diuretic-induced sodium depletion may also result in lithium toxicity due to compensatory increases in proximal tubular reabsorption of lithium. Clinically important increases in lithium levels have been reported in patients taking angiotensin-converting enzyme inhibitors. The mechanism is unclear but may involve altered sodium reabsorption. Lithium toxicity has also been associated with calcium entry blockers, NSAIDs, tricyclic antidepressants and a wide variety of antipsychotic drugs such as haloperidol, phenothiazines and clozapine. Interactions with antipsychotics usually involve some form of neurotoxic reaction ranging from extrapyramidal symptoms to the neuroleptic malignant syndrome.

Protein binding and pharmacodynamics

Changes in protein binding are generally clinically important only for highly bound drugs. A reduction in binding from 95% to 90% represents a 100% increase in unbound (free) fraction of drug, whereas a reduction from 35% to 30% corresponds to only a 7.7% increase in the free fraction that is responsible for the pharmacological effect. The effects of altered protein binding are complex and often involve changes in clearance and volume of distribution that may mitigate the expected increase in free drug concentration. Concomitantly administered drugs can compete with one another for binding sites on plasma proteins, resulting in displacement interactions that may lead to increased pharmacological effect and the possibility of toxicity. Drugs likely to be involved in displacement interactions are those that are highly protein bound, have a small volume of distribution, a high clearance and a narrow therapeutic range of concentrations. One of the best documented examples is the displacement of warfarin and other anticoagulants that are highly bound to albumin, by acidic drugs such as chloral hydrate, phenylbutazone, mefenamic acid and sulphinpyrazone. However, although such displacement can result in increased anticoagulation, the effect is usually transient. Other mechanisms are probably of equal importance, in particular inhibition of metabolism.

The pharmacodynamics of the coumarin anticoagulants is also increased by some antibiotics such as the aminoglycosides and cephalosporins. The mechanism is not well understood, but one possibility is that the reduction in bacteria in the gut responsible for producing vitamin K reduces production of the vitamin. However, this is normally not an essential source of vitamin K and a more likely explanation is that vitamin K absorption is reduced by the antibiotics as part of a general antibiotic-induced malabsorption syndrome.

Interactions with muscle relaxants

Several classes of antibiotics possess neuromuscular blocking actions, including the aminoglycosides, tetracyclines, polymixins and linocosamides. Most of the aminoglycosides are comparatively potent in their ability to potentiate muscle relaxants. Potentiation of neuromuscular block by the aminoglycosides can occur with relatively small doses of the drugs, and sufficient drug can be absorbed from irrigation of the intrapleural space, peritoneal cavity or even a wound to give rise to clinical problems. The only aminoglycoside that has not

been implicated in this type of interaction is netilmicin, which does not seem to have any neuromuscular action. Aminoglycosides inhibit neuromuscular transmission by preventing the presynaptic release of acetylcholine, tetracyclines by chelating extraneuronal calcium. These drugs can prolong the recovery from nondepolarizing muscle relaxants, with the possible exception of atracurium. Aminoglycoside-induced block may be overcome by calcium salts and 4-aminopyridine, but the block caused by the other groups cannot be reversed reliably by pharmacological means.

Chronic therapy with antiepileptic drugs, phenytoin, carbamazepine or sodium valproate, has been associated with resistance to the nondepolarizing muscle relaxants. There is an increase in the dose of muscle relaxant required to achieve a given degree of block and a reduction in the duration of action. The mechanisms of these effects may be a decrease in the sensitivity of the postjunctional membrane to acetylcholine.

REFERENCES

1. Berenbaum MC. What is synergy? *Pharmacol Rev* 1989; **41**: 93–141.
2. Norberg L, Wahlström G. Anaesthetic effects of flurazepam alone and in combination with thiopental or hexobarbital evaluated with an EEG-threshold method in male rats. *Arch Int Pharmacodyn Ther* 1988; **292**: 45–57.
3. Cole DJ, Kalichman MW, Shapiro HM, Drummond JC. The nonlinear potency of sub-MAC concentrations of nitrous oxide in decreasing the anesthetic requirement of enflurane, halothane, and isoflurane in rats. *Anesthesiology* 1990; **73**: 93–99.
4. Murphy MR, Hug CC. The anesthetic potency of fentanyl in terms of its reduction of enflurane MAC. *Anesthesiology* 1982; **57**: 485–488.
5. Schwieger IM, Hall RI, Hug CC Jr. Less than additive antinociceptive interaction between midazolam and fentanyl in enflurane-anesthetized dogs. *Anesthesiology* 1991; **74**: 1060–1066.
6. Kissin I, Stanski DR, Brown PT, Bradley EL Jr. Pentobarbital–morphine anesthetic interactions in terms of intensity of noxious stimulation required for arousal. *Anesthesiology* 1993; **78**: 744–749.
7. Yanez A, Sabbe MB, Stevens CW, Yaksh TL. Interaction of midazolam and morphine in the spinal cord of the rat. *Neuropharmacology* 1990; **29**: 359–364.
8. Vuyk J, Engbers FHM, Griever GER, Burm AGL, Vletter AA, Bovill JG. Interaction between propofol and alfentanil when given for induction of anesthesia. *Anesthesiology* 1996; **84**: 288–299.
9. Mora CT, Henson M, Bailey J, Szlam F, Hug CC. Propofol plasma concentration affects alfentanil requirements for cardiac surgery. *Anesthesiology* 1992; **77**: A408.
10. Vuyk J, Lim T, Engbers FHM, Burm AGL, Vletter AA, Bovill JG. The pharmacodynamic interaction of propofol and alfentanil during lower abdominal surgery in female patients. *Anesthesiology* 1995; **83**: 8–22.
11. Stanski DR, Shafer SL. Quantifying anesthetic drug interaction. *Anesthesiology* 1995; **83**: 1–5.
12. Vuyk J, Mertens MJ, Olofsen E, Burm AGL, Bovill JG. Propofol anesthesia and rational opioid selection. Determination of optimal EC_{50}–EC_{95}

propofol–opioid concentrations that assure adequate anesthesia and a rapid return of consciousness. *Anesthesiology* 1997; **87**: 1549–1562.
13. Matot I, Neely CF, Katz RY, Neufeld GR. Pulmonary uptake of propofol in cats. Effect of fentanyl and halothane. *Anesthesiology* 1993; **78**: 1157–1165.
14. Janicki PK, James FHM, Erskine WAR. Propofol inhibits enzymatic degradation of alfentanil and sufentanil by isolated liver microsomes in vitro. *Br J Anaesth* 1992; **68**: 311–312.
15. Most JA, Markle BG. A nearly fatal hepatoxic reaction of rifampicin after halothane anaesthesia. *Am J Surg* 1974; **127**: 593–595.
16. Backman JT, Olkkola KT, Neuvonen PJ. Rifampin drastically reduces plasma concentrations and effects of oral midazolam. *Clin Pharmacol Ther* 1996; **59**: 7–13.
17. Backman JT, Olkkola KT, Ojala M, Laaksovirta H, Neuvonen PJ. Concentrations and effects of oral midazolam are greatly reduced in patients treated with carbamazepine or phenytoin. *Epilepsia* 1996; **37**: 253–257.
18. Olkkola KT, Aranko K, Luurila H *et al.* A potentially hazardous interaction between erythromycin and midazolam. *Clin Pharmacol Ther* 1993; **53**: 298–305.
19. Bartkowski RR, Goldber ME, Larijani GE. Inhibition of alfentanil metabolism by erythromycin. *Clin Pharmacol Ther* 1989; **46**: 99–102.
20. Bartkowski RR, McDonnell TE. Prolonged alfentanil effect following erythromycin administration. *Anesthesiology* 1990; **73**: 566–568.
21. Hiller A, Olkkola KT, Isohanni P, Saarnivaara L. Unconsciousness associated with midazolam and erythromycin. *Br J Anaesth* 1990; **65**: 826–828.
22. Olkkola KT, Backman JT, Neuvonen PJ. Midazolam should be avoided in patients receiving the systemic antimycotics ketoconazole or itraconazole. *Clin Pharmacol Ther* 1994; **55**: 481–485.
23. Kupferschmidt HHT, Ha HR, Ziegler WH, Meier PJ, Krähenbühl S. Interaction between grapefruit juice and midazolam in humans. *Clin Pharmacol Ther* 1995; **58**: 20–28.

29

BJ Swanton, WP Blunnie

DRUGS IN SPECIAL PATIENT POPULATIONS

THE ELDERLY

The rational use of drugs by the elderly is challenging to patient and physician. Decline in physiological functions as part of the normal ageing process can lead to altered drug pharmacokinetics and pharmacodynamics. Chronic illness and multiple diseases contribute to increased drug use and thus more adverse reactions in the elderly. Decisions about drug selection and dosage in the elderly are based largely on trial and error, anecdotal data and clinical impression. Reliable information on drug disposition and tissue or cellular responses to drugs in the elderly has been obtained only recently.

PHYSIOLOGICAL CHANGES AND AGEING

Several physiological functions decline linearly, beginning between 30 and 45 years of age, with important influences on pharmacokinetic processes. An important caveat, however, is that the rates of decline with ageing are highly individualized and some elderly people show little change compared with population means. Cardiac output decreases by about 1% per year beginning at 30 years of age. In the elderly, this is associated with redistribution of blood flow favouring brain, heart and kidney, and a reduction in hepatic blood flow. The proportion of lean body mass declines with age, such that body fat increases from 18% to 35% in men and from 33% to 48% in women between 18 and 55 years of age. Total body water decreases by 10–15% between 20 and 80 years of age. Plasma albumin concentrations are lower in the elderly, particularly in the chronically ill or poorly nourished. The concentrations of a_1-acid glycoprotein (AAG) increase, but they do so more sharply in response to acute illness than simply to ageing. Glomerular filtration rate (GFR) and effective renal plasma flow decline steadily with advancing age. Note that serum creatinine concentration does not increase as a function of ageing in spite of a smaller lean body mass. Tubular secretory capacity declines in parallel with GFR.

PHARMACOKINETIC CHANGES ASSOCIATED WITH AGEING

DRUG ABSORPTION

Several physiological alterations in gastrointestinal function occur with ageing: (1) decreased gastric parietal cell function with (2) a corresponding rise in gastric pH, (3) a slower rate of gastric emptying, and decreased active transport of glucose, vitamin B_{12} and other nutrients. The rate and extent of absorption of most drugs are determined by passive diffusion in the proximal small bowel. This probably accounts for the general lack of clinically significant alterations in drug absorption in the elderly. One exception is a threefold increase in the bioavailability of levodopa due to reduced activity of dopa decarboxylase activity in the stomach wall.

DRUG DISTRIBUTION

Reduced lean body mass, reduced total body water, increased fat and decreased plasma albumin levels in the elderly can contribute to alterations in drug distribution. The effect of body composition on drug distribution depends largely on the physiochemical properties of individual drugs. Lipid-soluble drugs such as diazepam and lignocaine have a larger volume of distribution in the elderly; water-soluble drugs such as paracetamol and ethanol have a smaller volume of distribution.[1] Digoxin has a lower volume of distribution in the elderly, and therefore doses must be reduced. There is a slight trend to lower plasma albumin concentrations in the healthy elderly patient, whereas the hospitalized or poorly nourished elderly may have 10–20% decreased plasma albumin concentrations. This can result in increased unbound or free concentration of drug, the consequences of which can be complex. There are no guidelines available based on objective data for dosage modification to compensate for decreased protein binding.

DRUG METABOLISM

The decline in the ability of the elderly to metabolize most drugs is relatively small and difficult to predict. In general, hydroxylation and N-dealkylation reactions catalysed by hepatic microsomal mixed-function oxidase enzymes decrease slightly with ageing. Total hepatic content of cytochrome P450 enzymes decreases by about 30% after 70 years of age, although there is considerable variation between the different P450 isoenzymes.[2] As a result there is reduced metabolism of some drugs (e.g. paracetamol, barbiturates, benzodiazepines and nifedipine), with no age-related change for others (e.g. warfarin, β-adrenoceptor antagonists and tricyclic antidepressants).[3] Conjugation reactions such as glucuronidation are not greatly affected by ageing.[4] Effects of cigarette smoking, diet or alcohol consumption may be more important than physiological hepatic changes. Decreased dietary protein intake or reduction in cigarette consumption may lead to decreased liver microsomal enzyme activity. Studies in ageing animals are not predictive in humans because of pronounced sex and species differences.

In the elderly, first-pass metabolism may be of clinical importance, requiring decreased dosages. Total liver blood flow declines by 40–45% with ageing, partly as a result of reduced cardiac output. Diseases such as congestive heart failure may further compromise hepatic blood flow. As hepatic blood flow declines, clearance of flow-dependent drugs will usually decrease and blood concentrations will rise. In general, the ability of hepatic mixed-function oxidases to respond to enzyme inducers is retained. For example, cigarette smoking and phenytoin induce hepatic theophylline metabolism to a similar degree in young and old. Also, the ability of cimetidine to inhibit microsomal drug metabolism is the same in young and old.

DRUG ELIMINATION

Drug clearance is often directly proportional to creatinine clearance whether elimination is by tubular secretion or glomerular filtration. Interpretation of serum creatinine concentration in the elderly requires caution. Because creatinine is a product of muscle metabolism, less is produced as lean body mass declines. Thus an 80-year-old man with a serum creatinine concentration of 1 mg dl^{-1} may have a creatinine clearance of 60 ml min^{-1}, only 50% that of a 40-year-old man with the same serum creatinine level.

There are no absolute guidelines, but two general principles apply. First, most elderly patients do not have 'normal' renal function when serum creatinine concentration appears 'normal'. Second, most elderly patients require dose adjustments for drugs that are eliminated primarily by the kidneys. These include the aminoglycosides, lithium carbonate, chlorpropamide and digoxin. Because of reduced clearance, the half-lives of many drugs are prolonged in the elderly (Fig. 29.1).

DRUG RESPONSE CHANGES ASSOCIATED WITH AGEING

Drug responses often change with ageing. In general, an enhanced response can be expected. For example, the extent of sensory block after spinal or epidural local anaesthetics is greater in the elderly compared with

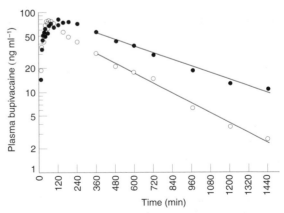

Fig. 29.1 Plasma concentration profiles after intrathecal administration of 0.5% bupivacaine in a patient aged 64 years (●; $t_{1/2}$ 449 min; (Cl) 219 ml min^{-1}) and one of 35 years (○; total plasma clearance $t_{1/2}$ 286 min, Cl 423 ml min^{-1}). From Veering BT, Burm AGL, Spierdijk J. Spinal anaesthesia with hyperbaric bupivacaine. Effects of age on neural blockade and pharmacokinetics. *Br J Anaesth* 1988; **60**: 187–194, with permission.

younger patients (Fig. 29.2). However, reduced responses to some drugs do occur, and a revised dosage schedule is recommended to prevent serious side-effects. Factors that affect the sensitivity or intensity of drug responses are discussed below.

AGE-RELATED CHANGES IN RECEPTORS AND POSTRECEPTOR MECHANISMS

In general, there is little evidence for specific alterations causing altered sensitivity or intensity in responses. The sensitivity of the β-adrenergic system of the heart is decreased in elderly subjects, and the increase in heart rate caused by isoprenaline is less in the elderly than in younger subjects. This is not caused by alterations in β-adrenoceptors but to changes in the cyclic adenosine monophosphate second-messenger system or in other postreceptor events proximal to calcium–troponin interaction.

The magnitude of the increased responses to benzodiazepines in the elderly cannot be explained totally by pharmacokinetic differences. The occurrence of flurazepam-induced adverse effects increases dramatically with ageing.

IMPAIRED HOMEOSTATIC MECHANISMS

With advancing age, several critical physiological control mechanisms become increasingly inefficient. These include decreased activity of aortic and carotid body chemoreceptors, reduced baroreceptor reflexes, impaired thermoregulation, inappropriate response of blood glucose and insulin to an orally administered glucose load, and altered neurological control of bowel and bladder. Decreased baroreflexor sensitivity may lead to increased risk of orthostatic (postural) hypotension. In the elderly, this is a common problem with some

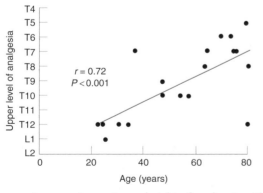

Fig. 29.2 Increase in maximum height of analgesia with age following intrathecal administration of 0.5% bupivacaine. From Veering BT, Burm AGL, Viletter AA, van den Hoeven RA, Spierdijk J. The effect of age on systemic absorption and systemic disposition of bupivacaine after subarachnoid administration. *Anesthesiology* 1991; **74**: 250–257, with permission.

phenothiazines and antidepressants (those with significant adrenergic antagonist properties), nitrates and antihypertensives such as prazosin and α-methyldopa. The normal homeostatic response of the aortic and carotid body chemoreceptors to opioid-induced respiratory depression is to increase respiratory stimulation. Impaired chemoreceptor activity may lead to greater than expected respiratory depressant effects of opioids. Chlorpromazine and many other psychoactive drug may cause hypothermia.

DISEASE-INDUCED CHANGES

Multiple chronic diseases are common in the elderly. One-third have three or more chronic diseases such as diabetes, glaucoma, hypertension, coronary artery disease and arthritis. This leads to polypharmacy, an increased frequency of drug interactions, and adverse drug reactions. Moreover, disease may increase the risk of adverse drug reaction or preclude the use of the otherwise most effective or safest drug for another problem. For example, anticholinergic drugs may cause urinary retention in men with enlarged prostate glands or precipitate glaucoma, and drug-induced hypotension may cause ischaemic events in persons with vascular disease.

Age-related morphological changes, electrolyte disturbances, comorbidity and polypharmacy each make elderly patients more susceptible to the cardiac toxicity of antiarrhythmic drugs.[5] Therefore, treatment with these drugs is discouraged in patients with nonlife-threatening arrhythmias.

DRUG INTERACTIONS

Multiple drug therapies may lead to confusion, medication errors and further drug interactions. An often overlooked factor is the common use among the elderly of over-the-counter antacids, laxatives, analgesics, antihistamines, sleeping pills and vitamins. Inadequate dietary potassium increases the likelihood of diuretic-induced hypokalaemia, whereas excessive sodium chloride ingestion may attenuate the effects of antihypertensive drugs. Most drug–nutrient problems, however, are pharmacokinetic in nature.

EXAMPLES OF DRUG PROBLEMS AND PRESCRIBING IN THE ELDERLY

ANTICHOLINERGIC DRUG TOXICITY

Anticholinergic drug toxicity illustrates some of the inherent problems of drug treatment in the elderly. A large number of drugs possess atropine-like activity, for example tricyclic antidepressants (e.g. amitryptiline), antiarrhythmics (e.g. disopyramide) and antihistamines (e.g. diphenhydramine). For some drugs, the anticholinergic response is the desired pharmacological effect, but for others this may be an unwanted side-effect. It is common for elderly patients to receive several of these atropine-like drugs concurrently. This can result in additive effects and toxicity, such as the anticholinergic syndrome.[6] Some elderly patients will be more susceptible than others to anticholinergic toxicity because of impaired autonomic bowel or bladder innervation, glaucoma, benign prostatic hypertrophy or impaired cognitive capacity. Some are especially sensitive to cognitive disruption caused by anticholinergic drugs. Thus, in the elderly, great care must be taken to avoid excessive antimuscarinic effects and to be observant for potential toxicity.

BENZODIAZEPINE-BASED CENTRAL NERVOUS SYSTEM DEPRESSION

Benzodiazepines are more likely to cause greater central nervous system (CNS) depression in elderly than in younger patients, due to altered pharmacokinetics and increased sensitivity. Benzodiazepines that undergo oxidative hepatic metabolism, such as diazepam, have reduced metabolic clearance, a disproportionately longer plasma half-life and an increase in volume of distribution. This is attributed to the relative increase in body fat and a small decline in plasma albumin concentration with ageing. Oxazepam, lorazepam and temazepam, which are all metabolized by conjugation, exhibit little alteration in metabolism and clearance with ageing, but still are associated with an increased sensitivity in

response.[7] The molecular basis for the altered sensitivity remains unknown, but in the elderly lower doses should be employed and drugs with extremely long half-lives avoided if possible.

PREGNANCY

Understanding the use of drugs during pregnancy has lagged far behind the development of knowledge in other areas of therapeutics. This is partly because the thalidomide tragedy has slowed research that entails giving a drug to a pregnant woman.

About 35% of women in the UK take drugs (excluding iron and vitamin supplements) at least once during pregnancy, although only 6% take a drug during the first trimester.[8] The most commonly used drugs are nonopioid analgesics (13%), antibiotics (10%) and antacids (7%). In the puerperium the use of drugs increases substantially.

MATERNAL–PLACENTAL–FETAL UNIT

MATERNAL PHARMACOKINETIC VARIABLES

The physiological changes that occur during pregnancy alter maternal pharmacokinetics of drugs administered during pregnancy. Generally two principal factors deter-

---

Summary box 29.1 Guidelines for drug prescribing in the elderly

Drug prescribing in the elderly can be safe and effective by adherence to the following principles:

- Know all the patient's medical problems.

- Ascertain all drugs being taken, including over-the-counter preparations.

- Know the pharmacology of the drugs.

- Start with small doses and titrate the drug based on response.

- Keep dosage regimens simple.

- Be sure that visual, motor or cognitive impairments will not result in errors or noncompliance.

- Review treatment plan and response frequently.

- Regularly consider that new symptoms or problems may be drug induced.

Summary box 29.2 Factors affecting pharmacokinetics and pharmacodynamics of drugs in the mother and fetus

- Altered maternal absorption.

- Increased maternal unbound (free) fraction.

- Increased maternal volume of distribution.

- Altered hepatic drug clearance in mother.

- Increased maternal renal blood flow and glomerular filtration rate.

- Placental transfer.

- Possible placental metabolism.

- Placental blood flow.

- Maternal and fetal pH.

- Immature fetal blood–brain barrier.

- Immature fetal enzyme activity.

- Increased fetal unbound fraction.

mine the changes in drug kinetics during pregnancy: maternal physiological changes and the effect of the placental–fetal compartment (Fig. 29.3).[9] Maternal pharmacokinetics ultimately determine fetal therapeutic and toxic responses to drugs, drug metabolites or toxic compounds that cross the placenta.

Maternal drug absorption may be enhanced or decreased by a combination of delayed gastric emptying and decreased motility. Absorption from sites other than the gastrointestinal tract also may be affected. For example, increased pulmonary absorption may result from greater minute ventilation and increased cutaneous absorption as a result of greater blood flow.

The apparent volume of distribution of many drugs increases during pregnancy as maternal plasma volume expands 30–50% during the first trimester. For example, the apparent volume of distribution of ampicillin increases by 70% at term. Changes of similar magnitude occur in cardiac output and GFR. The greater apparent volume of distribution, together with an increase in renal clearance, leads to lower plasma concentrations than in nonpregnant women receiving the same dose. Hepatic blood flow remains constant, and so the percentage of total cardiac output distributed to the liver tends to decrease. This may diminish the metabolism of drugs that undergo 'first-pass' hepatic clearance and result in unanticipated increases in plasma drug concentrations. Cholestasis frequently develops during pregnancy and may result in decreased hepatic clearance of drugs that undergo biliary excretion.

THE PLACENTA

The functions of the placenta during gestation are protection of the fetus, maintenance of pregnancy, possible prevention of maternal rejection of the pregnancy as foreign tissue, transportation of nutrients and wastes, metabolism of endogenous and drug substances, and endocrine activity. However, any substance that gains access to the maternal bloodstream should be considered capable of crossing the placenta and reaching the fetus unless demonstrated otherwise. As the placenta develops during pregnancy its structure and function alters, and this can result in varying fetal drug exposure during pregnancy. For example, the maternal to fetal transfer of gentamicin, when infused continuously to the mother, increases from the first half of gestation to term (Fig. 29.4).[10]

PLACENTAL PROCESSES

For the transfer of many substances, the placenta can be viewed as a lipid membrane, which drugs cross by passive diffusion.[11,12] The Fick equation describes the transfer of substances by simple diffusion as:

$$\text{Rate of diffusion} = D \times \Delta c \times A/d$$

where D is the diffusion constant of the drug, Δc is the concentration gradient across the placenta (maternal − fetal plasma drug concentration), A is the area across which transfer occurs, and d is the membrane thickness. In general, lipophilic, un-ionized, low molecular weight drugs in their free nonprotein-bound state will cross the placenta easily. Some, such as barbiturates, opioids and local anaesthetics, are 'flow limited' in their placental transfer because a decrease in maternal blood flow to the placenta may reduce their placental passage.[13] Given time, however, most drugs will achieve roughly equal concentrations on each side of the placenta. Thus the practical view to take when prescribing drugs during pregnancy is that transfer of drugs to the fetus is inevitable. There are exceptions to this rule, such as heparin, insulin and nondepolarizing muscle relaxants.

Normal uterine contractions during labour, oxytocic drugs, exogenously administered sympathomimetics

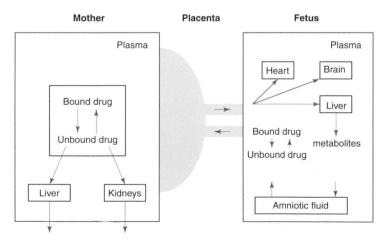

Fig. 29.3 Drug disposition in the maternal–placental–fetal system. Modified from Loebstein *et al*, with permission.[9]

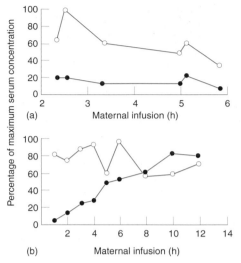

(a) Maternal infusion (h)

(b) Maternal infusion (h)

Percentage of maximum serum concentration

Fig. 29.4 Developmental differences in maternal (○) to fetal (●) transfer of gentamicin in humans during maternal administration of a loading dose followed by a continuous infusion. (a) At 18 weeks' gestation; (b) at term. From Pacifici and Nottoli, with permission.[10]

and β-adrenoceptor antagonists all affect maternal and fetal haemodynamics, and therefore may modify maternal drug distribution and placental transfer. As mentioned above, for some drugs maternal–fetal transfer may change during gestation.

The human placenta contains multiple enzyme systems, including those responsible for drug oxidation, reduction, hydrolysis and conjugation. These systems are involved primarily with endogenous steroid metabolism; however, the activities of these enzymes are usually minor compared with those of maternal or fetal organs (including liver, kidney and adrenal gland). Thus the presence of drug metabolizing systems in the placenta does not contribute greatly to overall drug clearance from the maternal–placental–fetal unit. The transfer of many substances across the placenta requires energy or special carriers.

FETAL DRUG DISPOSITION

Fetal biotransforming enzyme systems begin to develop at 5–8 weeks of gestation, and their activity increases until 12–14 weeks, when it reaches up to 30% of adult activity. It is not until approximately 1 year after birth that liver enzymatic activity is comparable to that of the adult. The first system expressed is the cytochrome P450 group of enzymes, which develops at around 40–60 days' gestation. It is most active in the adrenal gland and less active in the fetal liver. The fetal kidney and gut systems also have detectable P450 activity. Human fetuses generally have well developed conjugating enzyme activities, except for glucuronidation, which

remains low until shortly before term. For endogenous compounds, conjugation may enhance activity. For example, certain steroid glucuronides and sulphates have greater potencies than the parent compound.

Considering the limited protection afforded by the placenta, the ability of the fetus to metabolize drugs may appear fortuitous. However, it can sometimes be detrimental, by generating potentially toxic metabolites. Further, induction of metabolism *in utero* may alter postnatal drug metabolism, which may enhance metabolism of the same or unrelated agents. For example, the ability of the newborn infant to metabolize bilirubin by conjugation may be induced by prenatal maternal phenobarbitone therapy.

TERATOLOGY

To be considered a teratogen, an agent must have little effect on the mother, since the presence of maternal toxicity precludes ascribing effects on the fetus directly to the agent. The substance must cause transient or permanent, physical or functional disorders in the fetus in the absence of toxic effects in the mother. Not all adverse effects on prenatal development result in malformations. Death and growth retardation are not considered as teratogenic events *per se*. The term developmental toxicity is proposed as a broader categorization of outcomes. Developmental toxicity comprises four possible manifestations of abnormal development: altered growth (growth retardation), death, malformations and functional deficits or impairments.

The concept of a behavioural teratogen is an agent that disrupts normal behavioural development after prenatal exposure. Because some agents clearly produce mental but not physical disturbances, it is a useful subdivision of the concept of teratogens. Mutagens are substances that cause permanent change in germ cell lines secondary to changes in deoxyribonucleic acid. All mutagens are teratogens, but not all teratogens are mutagens.

There are several factors in the development of teratogenesis:

1. The fetus has varying susceptibility depending on the stage of gestation.
2. Pharmacokinetic characteristics of absorption, distribution, metabolism and elimination effect fetal drug exposure.
3. The higher the dose, the more likely is a teratogenic effect. There may be a threshold dose for some teratogens.
4. Poorly understood fetal genetic characteristics can greatly influence teratogenic potential.
5. The same defect can be produced by different agents acting by varying mechanisms.

Vitamin A is an example of how these principles can be applied to specific agents, as well as their shortcomings in characterizing all teratogens. Dietary vitamin A (as β-carotene) is not associated with developmental toxicity in animals or humans. However, high-potency vitamin A prepared as retinol or retinyl esters is an animal teratogen. At daily doses of 15–75 mg kg^{-1} and higher, it produces cranial, brain, cardiovascular, limb or genitourinary malformations. Human malformations are associated with daily doses of 25 000 international units of vitamin A or more, but no epidemiological studies are available to quantify the risk to humans. Isotretinoin, an isomer of retinoic acid used for the treatment of cystic acne, may produce craniofacial, cardiac, thymic and CNS abnormalities in humans. Etretinate, a vitamin A congener used in the treatment of psoriasis, is also a documented animal teratogen with similar potential in humans.

Direct teratogenic effects depend on the achievement of drug or active metabolite concentrations in the fetus at a critical time period, especially during gestation weeks 3–12 (period of organogenesis). Thus the changes in maternal pharmacokinetic parameters and dosing requirements during pregnancy may be expected to influence the risk of malformations. Because few agents appear to demonstrate a minimum teratogenic concentration for production of defects, it is a difficult task to determine the concentration at which a specific drug is safe in humans. It should also be noted that animal models are frequently used to assess the teratogenic potential of drugs and chemicals, and drug-induced animal malformations sometimes do not correlate with malformations in humans (e.g. thalidomide).

ADVERSE EFFECTS OF DRUGS ON THE FETUS AND NEONATE

To have a teratogenic effect, a drug must present during the critical time when organogenesis occurs, between 18 and 55 days after conception. Some commonly used drugs that are teratogens are given in Table 29.1. Several commonly used drugs can also influence the growth and physiological function of the fetus during the period of growth and development from the end of organogenesis up to delivery.

Angiotensin-converting enzyme inhibitors interfere with fetal renal function, producing oligohydramnios and neonatal anuria by mechanisms that are not understood. They should not used during pregnancy. Warfarin and heparin can both cause problems, one to the baby and the other to the mother. Warfarin has been associated with fetal intracranial haemorrhage, even though the maternal international normalized ratio (INR) is in the therapeutic range. This presumably reflects differing sensitivity to warfarin between fetal and maternal tissues. Heparin can lead to osteoporosis in the mother.

Table 29.1 Some commonly used drugs that are teratogenic in humans		
Drug	**Defects most commonly reported**	**Incidence**
Phenytoin	Craniofacial, limb	2–26%
Carbamazepine	CNS, limb, cardiac	0.6–36%
Valproate	Neural tube, other?	1–2%
Warfarin	Chondrodysplasia punctata	10–25%
Retinoids	Multiple	High
Lithium	Cardiac	< 5%
Danazol	Masculinization	Not known

This has been associated particularly with daily doses above 15 000 units for more than 6 months. There is about a 25% risk of intrauterine growth retardation when β-adrenoceptor antagonists are taken in early pregnancy; they do not impair growth when given in the third trimester. The mechanism of this effect is unknown.

Tetracyclines, which concentrate in fetal tissues, will cause tooth discoloration, but this does not become a problem until the teeth begin to calcify at 5–6 months' gestation. There is no evidence that tetracyclines are teratogenic. However, they may cause fatty necrosis of the liver and pancreatitis in pregnant women, and should be avoided during pregnancy.[14] Aspirin in analgesic doses can cause minor neonatal haemorrhage when taken within 5 days before delivery. Indomethacin has been used in pregnancy both as an antiinflammatory drug and in the treatment of preterm labour. Preterm infants exposed to indomethacin have a high incidence of adverse effects, including necrotizing enterocolitis and intracranial haemorrhage. When used at the end of pregnancy, indomethacin may cause premature closure of the ductus arteriosus.

FETAL DRUG THERAPY

Fetal responses to some drugs have been exploited to provide pharmacological therapy to the fetus.[10] Potent glucocorticoid stereoisomers, betamethasone and dexamethasone, have been intentionally administered to the mother to induce fetal enzymes needed for production and release of surfactant to prevent hyaline membrane disease after birth. Certain types of fetal arrhythmias and heart failure have been treated with drugs such as digoxin and procainamide, which reach the fetus across the placenta after administration to the mother or by direct fetal injection intramuscularly or intravenously. Adrenal enzyme defects may cause the fetus to overproduce androgens that alter the development of external female genitalia. These may require extensive surgical correction after birth. Female fetuses, identified by family history and enzyme analysis, may be exposed to sufficient glucocorticoids transplacentally to suppress the fetal adrenal gland and prevent masculinization. Directed pharmacological treatment of the fetus may become more important in the future with improved prenatal diagnosis of fetal disease.

EFFECT OF PREGNANCY ON DRUG DISPOSITION

Total body water increases by as much as 8 litres during pregnancy, and this provides a substantially increased volume within which drugs can be distributed. Serum proteins relevant to drug binding undergo considerable changes in concentration. Albumin, which binds acidic drugs such as phenytoin, decreases in concentration by up to 10 g l^{-1}. The main implication of this change is in the interpretation of drug concentrations, which is discussed below.

Some liver metabolic pathways are induced during pregnancy, but blood flow in the liver is unchanged. The blood concentration of drugs with a low hepatic extraction, whose elimination depends on liver enzyme activity, can be decreased markedly during pregnancy, probably as a result of increased metabolic clearance. The clearance of phenytoin, for example, doubles during pregnancy.[15] In contrast, drugs whose elimination is dependent mainly on liver blood flow, such as propranolol, show no change in clearance during pregnancy.[16]

Renal plasma flow has almost doubled by the last trimester of pregnancy, and drugs that are eliminated unchanged by the kidney are usually eliminated more rapidly. For example, the clearance of both lithium and ampicillin doubles during pregnancy.

THERAPEUTIC DRUG MONITORING DURING PREGNANCY

Two points that should be considered when interpreting drug concentrations during pregnancy are protein binding and therapeutic range.

Protein binding
The reduction in albumin concentration during pregnancy leads to a decrease in the mean plasma concentrations of drugs that are highly bound, such as phenytoin. The amount of unbound drug will, however, be increased and this is available for both distribution out of blood and elimination from the body. The net result is that the total level falls but the free concentration is virtually unchanged. Similar arguments apply for basic drugs that bind to AAG, which decreases during pregnancy. For this reason free drug concentrations should be requested; if these are not available, the concentrations in saliva are a good approximation.

Therapeutic range
It is not clear whether pregnancy alters the effects of drugs. Established therapeutic ranges might be inappropriate during pregnancy because of changes in the relation between drug concentration and effect.

BREASTFEEDING

Virtually all drugs cross into breast milk. However, dilution in the mother's body, coupled with the volume of milk consumed, usually means that the amount taken by the baby is clinically unimportant. There are three main categories of drugs to be considered:

1. Drugs that will not harm the baby if given to a nursing mother, such as warfarin and aminoglycosides, which are not absorbed from the gastrointestinal tract of normal infants, since negligible concentrations are reached in the infant.
2. Drugs that reach the baby but in an insignificant amount include most drugs used in everyday practice: nonsteroidal antiinflammatory drugs, penicillin and cephalosporin antibiotics, antihypertensive drugs, inhaled bronchodilator and anticonvulsants (with the exception of barbiturates).
3. Drugs that reach the baby in sufficient amounts to be harmful.

CONCLUSION

The use of drugs during pregnancy and in the puerperium requires that a fine balance should be maintained. No harm should be allowed to befall the baby because of the drug, but equally no harm must come to the mother or baby because a disease is being treated inadequately.

NEONATES AND INFANTS

THERAPEUTIC OVERVIEW

Limited understanding of the clinical pharmacology of specific drugs in paediatric patients, particularly infants, predisposes this population to problems with rational drug treatment. Pharmacological data derived primarily from adults is seldom appropriate for dosage guidelines in children. The problem of establishing efficacy and

Summary box 29.3 Drugs that should be avoided by women who are breast feeding

- Amiodarone:
  - iodine content may cause neonatal hypothyroidism.
- Aspirin:
  - risk of Reye's syndrome.
- Barbiturates:
  - drowsiness.
- Benzodiazepines:
  - lethargy.
- Carbimazole:
  - use lowest effective dose to avoid hypothyroidism.
- Contraceptives (combined oral):
  - may diminish milk supply and reduce nitrogen and protein content.
- Cytotoxic drugs:
  - potential problems include immune suppression and neutropenia.
- Ephedrine:
  - irritability.
- Tetracyclines:
  - tooth discoloration.

Summary box 29.4 Factors affecting drug responses in neonates

- Total plasma protein concentration is low at birth and does not reach adult values until 1 year of age.
- The concentration of plasma a_1-acid glycoprotein (AAG) is one-third that in maternal plasma:
  - less drug will be needed to achieve the desired effect
  - basic drugs such as local anaesthetics, propranolol and most opioids bind to AAG.
- Hepatic clearance is decreased in the neonate, due to either a diminution of uptake or immaturity of the intrinsic metabolic pathways.
- Enzymes involved in glucuronide conjugations are not fully developed at birth:
  - compounds eliminated mainly by glucuronidation have greatly prolonged half-lives or are conjugated by different pathways compared to those in children and adults.
- Renal function is reduced at birth and adult levels are not reached until 6 months of age.
- Many receptors involved in drug activity are not fully developed in the neonate, especially in premature infants.

dosing guidelines for use in infants is further complicated, since the pharmacokinetics of many drugs change appreciably as the child ages from birth (sometimes prematurely) to several months after birth. The dose–response relationships of some drugs may change markedly during the first few weeks after birth. Prematurely born neonates are now surviving at gestations as short as 24 weeks. This is a stage of fetal development when both structure and function are quite immature, with important implications for drug therapy.

NEONATAL PHARMACOLOGY

The same basic pharmacological principles that apply to adults also apply to neonates and children. However, some processes of absorption, distribution, metabolism and elimination differ in the fetus and neonate.

DRUG ABSORPTION

At birth, gastric pH is usually between 6 and 8 but falls rapidly to 1.5–3.0 within several hours; however, this fall is variable and appears to be independent of birthweight and gestational age. In the premature infant, hydrochloric acid level is decreased before 32 weeks of gestational age, and the time of acid production may be related to the initiation of enteral feedings.

The rate of gastric emptying is an important determinant of the overall rate and extent of drug absorption. The rate of gastric emptying is variable during the neonatal period and is affected by gestational maturity, prenatal age and type of feeding. In addition, the presence of pyloric stenosis, gastrooesophageal reflux, respiratory distress syndrome and congenital heart disease delay gastric emptying and reduce drug absorption.

Drugs and chemical agents applied to the skin of a premature infant may result in inadvertent poisoning. For example, steroid creams may result in extensive absorption through the thin skin of a neonate and result in adrenal suppression. Extreme caution should be exercised in using topical therapy on newborn infants.

DRUG ADMINISTRATION

Intravenous drug administration is recommended for the treatment of sick neonates to ensure effective circulating drug concentrations and to avoid the unpredictability of gastrointestinal drug absorption. The small size of extremely premature neonates presents unique problems during parenteral drug delivery. Fluid infusion rates are as low as $2\,\mathrm{ml\,h}^{-1}$, sometimes divided between two infusion sites. Even though a drug is infused via intravenous tubing, it may not reach the patient in the desired length of time. In small neonates, accurate infusion pumps must be used to deliver the drug as close to the circulation as possible.

Intramuscular drug administration may be used occasionally in larger infants, but is generally not recommended. As with adults, the rate of absorption of drug from the intramuscular site is directly related to blood flow. Newborn infants are often hypothermic and exhibit vascular constriction, which limits circulation to muscles. With a small muscle mass, intramuscular therapy may lead to sterile abscesses, which may later require surgical intervention.

DRUG DISTRIBUTION

There are important differences in drug–protein binding between newborns and adults. In general, there is a reduction in binding of drugs to plasma proteins during the neonatal period. The affinity of albumin for acidic drugs and total plasma protein concentration increase from birth into early infancy, but do not reach normal adult values until 10–12 months of age. In addition, although plasma albumin concentrations may reach adult values shortly after birth, the concentration of albumin in blood is directly proportional to gestational age. Basic drugs such as local anaesthetics, propranolol and most opioids bind to plasma AAG. The concentration of AAG in healthy term neonates is about one-third that in maternal plasma so that the level of the active (unbound) form will be greater and thus less drug will be needed to achieve the desired effect. Bilirubin binds noncovalently to albumin, and this association is reversible. The bilirubin-binding affinity of albumin at birth is independent of gestational age and is less for the newborn than the adult. The binding affinity of albumin for bilirubin increases with age and reaches adult values by approximately 5 months of age. The lower bilirubin-binding affinity of albumin in neonates is believed to be a contributing factor in their susceptibility to kernicterus. Other factors, such as the effect of hypothermia, acidosis, hypoglycaemia, hypoxia, sepsis, birth asphyxia and hypercapnia on the permeability of the blood–brain barrier and on bilirubin–albumin binding, must also be considered.

DRUG METABOLISM

Drugs are taken up into hepatocytes by diffusion or by one of several carrier-mediated transport mechanisms. Decreased hepatic clearance of a drug in the neonate may reflect either a diminution of uptake or immaturity of the intrinsic metabolic pathways. In contrast, metals such as copper, iron and zinc may accumulate in the liver of neonates and reach higher concentrations than in adults. During fetal life, some drug-metabolizing enzymes are present at about 30% of adult activity in vitro. After correction for differences in liver weight, the specific activity in vitro for many drug-metabolizing enzymes approaches adult activities. Postnatally, the hepatic cytochrome P450 monooxygenase system appears to mature rapidly. For example, phenytoin and its metabolites appear in the urine of newborns and adults in similar proportions. Furthermore, the decline in plasma drug concentration parallels the rate of urinary metabolite excretion, an indication that the rate of excretion reflects the rate of hepatic metabolism of phenytoin.

The enzymes uridine diphosphate (UDP)–glucose dehydrogenase and UDP–glucuronyl transferase required for glucuronide conjugations are poorly developed at birth, so that compounds that rely on glucuronidation for elimination have greatly prolonged half-lives or are conjugated by different pathways than in children and adults. For example, the clearance of morphine, which is metabolized principally by glucuronidation, is dependent on the age of the patient (Fig. 29.5) and is significantly lower, and the half-life longer, in neonates than in children or young adults.[17] There is a very large interindividual variability in the pharmacokinetics of morphine, particularly in premature infants and during the first week of life, probably due to the changes in enzyme activity that occur in this period.

RENAL DRUG ELIMINATION

Renal function is reduced at birth compared to that in the adult. Renal blood flow increases with age as a result of increased cardiac output and reduced peripheral vascular resistance. Within the first 12 h after birth, the kidneys receive only 4–6% of cardiac output, increasing to 8–10% during the first week. In adults the kidneys receive 25% of cardiac output. The distribution of intrarenal blood flow away from the cortex and to the medulla immediately after birth further reduces glomerular filtration. Adult levels of renal function are usually reached by 6 months of age. These developmental changes in renal tubular and glomerular function contribute to rapid changes in the elimination

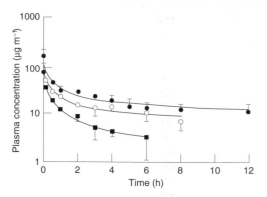

Fig. 29.5 Relationship between age and morphine plasma disposition following a single dose of morphine 0.1 mg kg^{-1} intravenously. The mean half-life was 8.1 h in neonates younger than 1 week (●), 5.4 h in infants aged from 1 week to 2 months (○), and 2.6 h in infants aged from 2 to 6 months (■). From Pokela ML, Olkkoa KT, Seppala T, Koivisto M. Age-related morphine kinetics in infants. *Dev Pharmacol Ther* 1993; **20**: 26–34, with permission.

kinetics of drugs cleared by the kidneys. At birth, the GFR is directly proportional to gestational age over 34 weeks. Before 34 weeks of gestation, GFR remains relatively constant at low rates. In the first 2–3 days of postnatal life, there is a rapid two- to threefold increase in GFR of full-term babies, compared to increases in neonates of less than 34 weeks of gestation of one- to twofold. Adult values for GFR are reached by 2.5–5 months. An example of the clinical implications of the maturation of GFR is the decreasing half-life for gentamicin with increasing gestational age in infants aged less than 7 days. Gentamicin is eliminated almost entirely by glomerular filtration.

Proximal convoluted tubules in the normal kidney of a full-term infant are small in relation to their corresponding glomeruli. This glomerulotubular imbalance is reflected by functional differences in the secretory capacity of the proximal tubular cells. A tenfold increase in para-aminohippuric acid secretion occurs in the first year of life, with adult values (based on body surface area) attained by 30 weeks of age. Therefore, tubular drug secretion matures at a slower rate than glomerular drug filtration function.

PHARMACODYNAMICS

The ability of the developing fetus, newborn and child to respond to a particular concentration of drug may involve a complex sequence of events. Inadequate response to an effective concentration of a drug may result from an absence or immaturity of receptors, inadequate drug–receptor binding, inadequate transduction of the receptor–drug interaction to an intracellular message, or the ability of the organ or tissue to respond to that intracellular message. Each of these events progresses during development at different rates.

RECEPTOR MATURATION

The cardiovascular system exemplifies some of the developmental steps in receptor maturation. When fully matured, many cardiovascular tissues exhibit a balance between sympathetic and parasympathetic nervous system control. During development, however, these two systems mature at different rates among different tissues. This may produce imbalances in the responsiveness of postjunctional organs or tissues innervated by parasympathetic or sympathetic mediators such as acetylcholine and noradrenaline. Thus, failure of the fetal or newborn heart to respond to β-adrenergic stimulation may reflect incomplete innervation, lack of β-adrenoceptors or neurotransmitter. Once receptors are present, interactions between the agonist and receptor may differ significantly between newborn and the adult. In ventricular muscle, the binding affinity for the β-adrenoceptor is greater in the adult, where there are more receptors. There are also important differences between neonates and older children or adults in the coupling between the receptor and the adenylate cyclase system. The newborn heart exhibits a greater increase in adenylate cyclase activity for a smaller number of β-adrenergic receptor interactions than does an infant. Dose–response studies using β-adrenergic agonists comparing fetal and maternal sheep have revealed similar responses, but much higher doses are required to achieve comparable responses in fetal tissues. Differences have been noted between contractile responses and chronotropic responses to β-adrenoceptor stimulation.

CLINICAL PROBLEMS

Certain drugs pose unusual therapeutic challenges when used in the perinatal period because of the unique character of their distribution or elimination in these patients or because of the unusual side-effects they may cause. These drugs include the antibiotics, digoxin, methylxanthines and indomethacin.

Bacterial sepsis, pneumonia, necrotizing enterocolitis and meningitis, as primary or secondary diseases of infants and newborns, are effectively treated with β-lactam, aminoglycoside or glycopeptide antibiotics. Because these drugs are primarily eliminated from the body unchanged through the kidneys, the renal function of the patient is an important variable in establishing doses and dosage intervals. In neonates, cephalosporins have potential renal and bone marrow toxicity, and high-dose penicillins may cause reversible bone marrow suppression. Routine monitoring of serum creatinine concentration and white cell counts is advisable when these drugs are administered in the neonatal period.[14] High plasma concentrations of amino-glycosides may contribute to orotoxicity.

Another type of antibiotic, chloramphenicol, is associated with cardiovascular collapse and the 'grey baby' syndrome, a direct result of excessively high and prolonged plasma concentrations (usually above 50–75 mg l^{-1}). The 'grey baby' syndrome results from accumulation of the drug due to immaturity of neonatal liver glucuronyl transferase enzymes and reduced glomerular filtration. For these reasons chloramphenicol is no longer indicated in the newborn. Care is also warranted with sulphonamides in the newborn because of the risk of raised bilirubin levels due to displacement from albumin.

Digoxin is a commonly used cardiac glycoside in the treatment of myocardial disturbances in neonates, infants and children. Extensive clinical experience shows that available data describing digoxin biodisposition in neonates and infants require cautious interpretation. The neonatal heart is also less sensitive to the cardiac glycosides than is the adult heart.

The methylxanthine, theophylline, is used as a bronchodilating drug and in the treatment of apnoea of prematurity. However, the efficacy of theophylline in this latter syndrome may be related to the additive or synergistic action of caffeine, a metabolite of theophylline, which accumulates in the plasma of infants. The N-methylation of theophylline to caffeine appears to be unique to preterm and newborn infants, and is clinically important because of its prolonged elimination half-life. Caffeine is rarely detectable in the plasma of older infants, children or adults receiving theophylline alone. The pharmacokinetics of theophylline in neonates are considerably different from those for older infants, children and adults. These differences are probably attributable to different body-water compartmentalization and/or decreased plasma protein binding in neonates (average 36% in neonates and 56% in adults). Although neonates can metabolize theophylline, it is excreted largely unchanged in newborn urine, compared with only approximately 10% as unchanged drug in older children and adults.

The use of indomethacin in neonates to stimulate ductus arteriosus closure is associated with potentially serious drug-induced complications and thus is not without risk.

REFERENCES

1. Frontera WR, Hughes VA, Lutz KJ et al. A cross-sectional study of muscle strength and mass in 45 to 78-yr-old men and women. *J Appl Physiol* 1991; **71**: 644–650.
2. Sotaniemi EA, Arranto AJ, Pelkonen O, Pasanen M. Age and cytochrome P450-linked drug metabolism in humans: an analysis of 226 subjects with equal histopathologic conditions. *Clin Pharmacol Ther* 1997; **61**: 331–339.
3. Kinirons MT, Crome P. Clinical pharmacokinetic considerations in the elderly: an update. *Clin Pharmacokinet* 1997; **33**: 302–312.
4. Schmucker DL. Aging and drug disposition: an update. *Pharmacol Rev* 1985; **37**: 133–148.
5. Van Gelder IC, Brügemann J, Crijns HJGM. Pharmacological management of arrhythmias in the elderly. *Drugs Ageing* 1997; **11**: 96–110.
6. Peters NL. Snipping the thread of life. Antimuscarinic side effects of medications in the elderly. *Arch Intern Med* 1989; **149**: 2414–2420.
7. Swift CG, Ewan JM, Clarke P et al. Responsiveness to oral diazepam in the elderly; relationship to total and free plasma concentrations. *Br J Clin Pharmacol* 1985; **20**: 111–118.
8. Bonati M, Bortolus R, Marchetti F, Romero M, Tognoni G. Drug use in pregnancy: an overview of epidemiological (drug utilization) studies. *Eur J Clin Pharmacol* 1990; **38**: 321–328.
9. Loebstein R, Lalkin A, Koren G. Pharmacokinetic changes during pregnancy and their clinical relevance. *Clin Pharmacokinet* 1997, **33**: 328–343.
10. Pacifici GM, Nottoli R. Placental transfer of drugs administered to the mother. *Clin Pharmacokinet* 1995; **28**: 235–269.
11. Bourget P, Roulot C, Fernandez H. Models for placental transfer studies of drugs. *Clin Pharmacokinet* 1995; **28**: 161–180.
12. Simone C, Derewlany LO, Koren G. Drug transfer across the placenta. Considerations in treatment and research. *Clin Perinatol* 1994; **21**: 463–481.
13. Edwards MS. Antibacterial therapy in pregnancy and neonates. *Clin Perinatol* 1997; **24**: 251–266.
14. Ward RM. Pharmacological treatment of the fetus. Clinical pharmacokinetic considerations. *Clin Pharmacokinet* 1995; **28**: 343–350.
15. Lander CM, Smith MT, Challc JB et al. Bioavailability in pharmacokinetics of phenytoin during pregnancy. *Eur J Clin Pharmacol* 1984; **27**: 105–110.
16. O'Hare MF, Kinney CD, Murnaghan JA, McDevitt DG. Pharmacokinetics of propranolol during pregnancy. *Eur J Clin Pharmacol* 1984; **27**: 583–587.
17. Jacqz-Aigrain E, Burtin P. Clinical pharmacokinetics of sedatives in neonates. *Clin Pharmacokinet* 1996; **31**: 423–443.

INDEX